Textbook of
PHARMACOVIGILANCE
Ensuring the Safe Use of Medicines

Textbook of
PHARMACOVIGILANCE
Ensuring the Safe Use of Medicines

SECOND EDITION

Chief Editor

SK Gupta PhD DSc FIPS FIACS
Distinguished Professor
Delhi Pharmaceutical Sciences and Research University
New Delhi, India

Formerly
Professor and Head
Department of Pharmacology
All India Institute of Medical Sciences
New Delhi, India
&
Dean and Director General
Institute of Clinical Research (India)
New Delhi, India

Co-Editor

Sushma Srivastava PhD PDCR
Senior Consultant
Indian Pharmacopoeia Commission
Ministry of Health and Family Welfare, Government of India
Ghaziabad, Uttar Pradesh, India

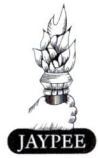

JAYPEE BROTHERS MEDICAL PUBLISHERS
The Health Sciences Publisher
New Delhi | London | Panama

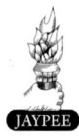 **Jaypee Brothers Medical Publishers (P) Ltd**

Headquarters
Jaypee Brothers Medical Publishers (P) Ltd
4838/24, Ansari Road, Daryaganj
New Delhi 110 002, India
Phone: +91-11-43574357
Fax: +91-11-43574314
Email: jaypee@jaypeebrothers.com

Overseas Offices
J.P. Medical Ltd
83 Victoria Street, London
SW1H 0HW (UK)
Phone: +44 20 3170 8910
Fax: +44 (0)20 3008 6180
Email: info@jpmedpub.com

Jaypee-Highlights Medical Publishers Inc
City of Knowledge, Bld. 235, 2nd Floor
Clayton, Panama City, Panama
Phone: +1 507-301-0496
Fax: +1 507-301-0499
Email: cservice@jphmedical.com

Jaypee Brothers Medical Publishers (P) Ltd
Bhotahity, Kathmandu, Nepal
Phone: +977-9741283608
Email: kathmandu@jaypeebrothers.com

Website: www.jaypeebrothers.com
Website: www.jaypeedigital.com

© 2019, Jaypee Brothers Medical Publishers

The views and opinions expressed in this book are solely those of the original contributor(s)/author(s) and do not necessarily represent those of editor(s) of the book.

All rights reserved. No part of this publication may be reproduced, stored or transmitted in any form or by any means, electronic, mechanical, photocopying, recording or otherwise, without the prior permission in writing of the publishers.

All brand names and product names used in this book are trade names, service marks, trademarks or registered trademarks of their respective owners. The publisher is not associated with any product or vendor mentioned in this book.

Medical knowledge and practice change constantly. This book is designed to provide accurate, authoritative information about the subject matter in question. However, readers are advised to check the most current information available on procedures included and check information from the manufacturer of each product to be administered, to verify the recommended dose, formula, method and duration of administration, adverse effects and contraindications. It is the responsibility of the practitioner to take all appropriate safety precautions. Neither the publisher nor the author(s)/editor(s) assume any liability for any injury and/or damage to persons or property arising from or related to use of material in this book.

This book is sold on the understanding that the publisher is not engaged in providing professional medical services. If such advice or services are required, the services of a competent medical professional should be sought.

Every effort has been made where necessary to contact holders of copyright to obtain permission to reproduce copyright material. If any have been inadvertently overlooked, the publisher will be pleased to make the necessary arrangements at the first opportunity. The **CD/DVD-ROM** (if any) provided in the sealed envelope with this book is complimentary and free of cost. **Not meant for sale.**

Inquiries for bulk sales may be solicited at: jaypee@jaypeebrothers.com

Textbook of Pharmacovigilance

First Edition: 2011
Second Edition: 2019
Reprint: **2024**

ISBN 978-93-5270-703-4

Printed at: Sterling Graphics Pvt. Ltd.

Contributors

Arani Chatterjee MBBS MPhil MD
Senior Vice President
Department of Clinical Research
Aurobindo Pharma Ltd
Hyderabad, Telangana, India

Arun Gupta MD
Head
Department of Medical Affairs and Clinical Research
Dabur India Ltd
Ghaziabad, Uttar Pradesh, India

Kamal Akhtar MSc
Assistant Professor
Institute of Clinical Research (India)
New Delhi, India

Manoj Sharma PhD
Senior Manager
Panacea Biotec Ltd
Department of Global Pharmacovigilance
Win-Medicare Private Ltd
New Delhi, India

Mohit Hans
Research Scholar
Delhi Pharmaceutical Sciences and
Research (DPSR) University
New Delhi, India

Mugdha Chopra
Associate Vice President
APCER Life Sciences
New Delhi, India

Puneet Agarwal MD
Ophthalmologist
Department of Ophthalmology
International Medical University
Bukit Jalil, Kuala Lumpur, Malaysia

Rajani Mathur PhD
Assistant Professor
Delhi Institute of Pharmaceutical Sciences and
Research (DIPSAR)
New Delhi, India

Renu Agarwal PhD
Professor
Faculty of Medicine
Universiti Teknologi Mara
Selangor, Darul Ehsan, Malaysia

Sanjeev Miglani MD
Vice President
APCER Life Sciences
New Delhi, India

SK Gupta PhD DSc FIPS FIACS
Distinguished Professor
Delhi Pharmaceutical Sciences and
Research (DPSR) University
New Delhi, India

Sushma Srivastava PhD PDCR
Senior Consultant
Indian Pharmacopoeia Commission
Ministry of Health and Family Welfare
Government of India
Ghaziabad, Uttar Pradesh, India

Preface to the Second Edition

Pharmacovigilance has evolved and growing at a faster pace in India meeting the expectations of the people and the demands of modern public health. It has been deemed necessary to have a reliable system of pharmacovigilance in our country for public health and for the rational, safe and cost-effective use of medicines. India is striving hard to achieve the goals through its pharmacovigilance programme.

The bustling pharmacovigilance activities all over the country have also led to the increase in career opportunities. Besides healthcare professionals, the pharmaceutical companies are also sensitized towards pharmacovigilance programme. Now the pharma companies are establishing their own pharmacovigilance cells. Pharmacovigilance is also being included in the curriculum by academic institutions or is in the process of inclusion, thereby increasing the demand for the books on pharmacovigilance as ready reference. In consideration of this, we put our best efforts to update the first edition and now with immense pleasure we brought out the updated second edition of the *Textbook of Pharmacovigilance: Ensuring the Safe Use of Medicines*.

Adverse drug reactions (ADRs) have become a global problem and a major concern of patient safety and clinical practice. Today, most of the patients are treated with multiple drugs or in simple terms. The concept of polypharmacy has led to an increase in the number of ADRs that are inevitable. Understanding the healthcare burden of ADRs as well as the relevant types and drugs involved represents an important gap in our knowledge. Keeping in view several regulatory and organizational changes that occurred within a span of few years, the chapters have been updated and new chapters like Pharmacoepidemiology and Pharmacovigilance, Hospitalization due to Adverse Drug Reactions and its Economic Burden, and Vigilance Systems for Medical Devices have been added.

This book will be useful for the healthcare professionals, postgraduate students, industry professionals and those engaged in clinical research at academia and the pharmaceutical industry.

Bringing out the book has not been possible without cooperation and assistance of a large number of individuals. As editors, we express our heartfelt gratitude to the contributors of the chapters. We express our deep grateful thanks to Shri Jitendar P Vij (Group Chairman), Mr Ankit Vij (Managing Director), Mr MS Mani (Group President), and dedicated team of M/s Jaypee Brothers Medical Publishers (P) Ltd, New Delhi, India, who all joined to convert this dream project into reality.

SK Gupta
Sushma Srivastava

Preface to the First Edition

Modern medicines have changed the way in which diseases are managed and controlled. However, despite their benefits, adverse drug reactions (ADRs) to medicines are common. Pharmacovigilance—an umbrella term used to describe the processes for monitoring and evaluating ADRs—is a key component to effective drug regulation systems, clinical practice and public health programs. The principal concern of pharmacovigilance is the detection of ADRs in real world clinical trial that are novel by virtue of their clinical nature, severity and/or frequency as soon as possible with minimum patient exposure.

The scope of pharmacovigilance needs to be extended beyond the strict confines of detecting new signals of safety concerns. Globalization, consumerism and the resulting explosion in free trade and communication across borders, and increasing use of the Internet have all changed the way medicinal products and information about them is accessed. These changing patterns in drug use require a shift in the approach to pharmacovigilance. The system and the key players in the field have to be geared up to be more closely linked, and more responsive towards the management of the ADRs.

Although many drugs have been extensively used and studied, their safety profile cannot necessarily be generalized. Special thrust needs to be laid on measures to improve drug safety monitoring. Effective links have been forged between Ministry of Health (CDSCO) and other stakeholders. The Indian government through its National Pharmacovigilance Program is encouraging collaboration between academic investigators, drug companies, and regulatory agencies to undertake clinical studies in order to develop and compile database on common ADRs. This will need an extensive infrastructure and trained healthcare providers.

I had the opportunity to be at the helm of the affairs and saw the dawn of pharmacovigilance in India as Chief Coordinator, National Pharmacovigilance Center at AIIMS, New Delhi, associated with WHO International Drug Monitoring Center, Uppsala. For the past decade, I have been closely associated with the various aspects of pharmacovigilance including, Education, Reporting, Data Mining, Signal Detection, Regulations, etc. This book *Textbook of Pharmacovigilance* has been the concentrated effort to compile all the theoretical and practical aspects of pharmacovigilance, for easy accessibility to any new entrant in the field and serve as a ready reference for those actively involved in the area. The book introduces basic definitions, classifications, objectives and elaborates the practical aspects including setting up of pharmacovigilance center, regulations in various countries, data mining, risk-benefit assessment, etc. It also provides latest updates on key issues like pharmacogenetics and herbal drug monitoring.

SK Gupta

Contents

1. **Key Definitions in Pharmacovigilance** — 1
   Renu Agarwal, SK Gupta
   - Sources 7

2. **Pharmacovigilance: Historical Perspective** — 9
   Renu Agarwal, SK Gupta
   - Pharmacovigilance before 18th Century 9
   - Pharmacovigilance in 18th Century 9
   - Pharmacovigilance in 19th Century 11
   - Pharmacovigilance in 20th Century: Prethalidomide Era 11
   - Pharmacovigilance in 20th Century: Thalidomide Disaster and Post-thalidomide Era 13
   - McBride's Famous Letter to the Lancet Thalidomide Infant 13
   - Pharmacovigilance: The Current Status 14
   - Pharmacovigilance: The Current System in India 14

3. **Pharmacovigilance: Need and Objectives** — 17
   Renu Agarwal
   - Need for Pharmacovigilance and Widening Horizons 17
   - Purpose of Pharmacovigilance 19
   - Specific Aims of Pharmacovigilance in View of Widening Horizons 19
   - Priority Areas of Pharmacovigilance 19
   - Outcome and Impact of Current System 21

4. **Current Methods of Pharmacovigilance** — 25
   Arani Chatterjee, Manoj Sharma, SK Gupta
   - Methods for Vaccine Safety 33

5. **Adverse Drug Reactions: Classification, Mechanism and Interaction** — 40
   SK Gupta, Manoj Sharma, Arani Chatterjee
   - Adverse Event (or Adverse Experience) 40
   - Adverse Drug Reaction (ADR) 40
   - Adverse Drug Reactions: Importance 41
   - Risk Factors for Adverse Drug Reactions 42
   - Pharmacological Classification 44
   - Causality Classification (WHO-UMC Classification) 45
   - Severity Classification 47
   - Seriousness Classification 47
   - Frequency Classification 48
   - Mechanism Classification 48
   - Statistical Classification 49

- Mechanism of Adverse Drug Reactions 49
- Adverse Drug Interactions 56

6. Signal Detection in Pharmacovigilance 63
Renu Agarwal, Puneet Agarwal
- Sources and Methods of Signal Detection 65
- Automated Quantitative Signal Detection 69
- Application of Quantitative Methods for Signal Detection 71
- Vigi Methods and Tools 72
- The UMC Signaling Process 73
- WHO and UMC Leadership in Signal Detection 74

7. Postmarketing Surveillance 77
Manoj Sharma, SK Gupta
- Need of Postmarketing Surveillance: Why 78
- Postmarketing Surveillance Methodologies 80

8. Setting up of a Pharmacovigilance Centre 100
Sushma Srivastava
- Initiation of Drug Monitoring Centres 101
- Practicalities in the Organization of a Pharmacovigilance Centre 102
- Pharmacovigilance Centres in India 108
- Pharmacovigilance Programme of India (PvPI) 109

9. Benefit-Risk Assessment in Pharmacovigilance 111
Renu Agarwal, SK Gupta
- Adverse Health Effect 111
- Actual Versus Perceived Benefits and Risks 112
- Benefit-Risk Assessment: A Dynamic Process 112
- Factors Affecting Benefit-Risk Balance 114
- Stepwise Approach to Benefit-Risk Assessment 115
- Benefit-Risk Assessment 116
- Semi-Quantitative and Quantitative Approach to Benefit-Risk Assessment 117
- Option Analysis 122
- Decision-Making 123

10. Crisis Management in Pharmacovigilance 127
Renu Agarwal, Puneet Agarwal
- "Crisis": Definition 127
- The Key Characteristics of a Crisis 127
- "Crisis" in Pharmacovigilance 128
- Stakeholders 128
- The Threat Sources for Crisis in Pharmacovigilance 129
- Crisis Management 129
- Crisis Management Cycle 130
- Crisis Management Model 131
- Planning for Crisis Management 133

- Additional Activities that Favor "Crisis Prepared" Organizational Structures 138
- Crisis Prevention Principles 139

11. WHO Pharmacovigilance: Programme for Global Drug Monitoring   141
Sushma Srivastava, SK Gupta
- Role of WHO Programme for International Drug Monitoring 143
- Global Pharmacovigilance 147
- Joining the WHO Programme for International Drug Monitoring 148

12. Pharmacovigilance of Herbal Drugs   150
Rajani Mathur, SK Gupta
- Introduction: What are Herbal Medicines? 150
- Herbal Medicines: Are they Really Safe? 152
- Challenges Relating to the Safety Monitoring of Herbal Drugs 153
- Mechanisms Underlying ADR due to Herbal Drugs 155
- Pharmacovigilance of Herbal Medicines: Definitions, Goals and Need 157
- Adverse Event Reporting 158
- Adverse Event Reporting: The UK Lead 160
- Traditional Chinese Medicines: Boon or Bane? 161
- Measures to Improve the Pharmacovigilance of Herbal Medicines 161

13. Medical Dictionary for Regulatory Activities: An Overview   165
Sanjeev Miglani, Arun Gupta, Mugdha Chopra
- Objectives of MedDRA 165
- Applications of MedDRA 165
- Regulatory Status/Historical Overview 166
- MedDRA Structure 166
- MedDRA Rules 168
- Criteria for Term Selection 168
- MedDRA Versioning 172
- Standardized MedDRA Queries (SMQs) 172
- MedDRA and SMQ in Signal Detection 172

14. Pharmacogenetics and Pharmacovigilance   174
Rajani Mathur
- Adverse Drug Reactions: A Clinical Problem 174
- Why ADRs do not Affect Everybody Equally? 174
- Polymorphism in Genes Encoding Pharmacokinetic Parameters and ADRs 175
- Polymorphism in Genes 176
- Encoding Pharmacodynamic Parameters and ADRs 176
- Practical Challenges of Pharmacogenomics 177
- The Way Forward 177

15. Pharmacovigilance Regulations in Various Countries   180
Sushma Srivastava, SK Gupta, Mohit Hans
- Pharmacovigilance in Europe 180
- Process of Regulatory Pharmacovigilance 182

- United Kingdom 184
- France 188
- Brazil 190
- India 190
- China 193
- Japan 195
- Australia 196
- Canada 197
- United States of America 198

16. Pharmacoepidemiology and Pharmacovigilance 209
SK Gupta, Mohit Hans, Sushma Srivastava
- Methodologies in Pharmacoepidemiologic Studies 211
- Pharmacoepidemiology in Drug Development 214

17. Hospitalization due to Adverse Drug Reactions and its Economic Burden 216
SK Gupta, Mohit Hans, Sushma Srivastava
- Economic Burden of ADRs 219
- Types of Cost 221
- Cost of ADRs 222

18. Vigilance Systems for Medical Devices 225
SK Gupta, Sushma Srivastava, Mohit Hans
- Medical Device Regulations and Need for Harmonization 240
- Medical Device Regulations 243
- Medical Device Market: Focusing BRICS 247

19. Data Mangement in Pharmacovigilance 251
Kamal Akhtar, Manoj Sharma
- Role of Software/Computer-based Systems 251
- Methods of Safety Data Analysis 254
- Informatics in Pharmacovigilance—A New Paradigm 255
- Emerging Technologies/Computer-based Tools for Pharmacovigilance 259
- WebSDM™ for Analysis of Premarketing Safety Data 260
- MGPS and HBLR for Analysis of Postmarketing Data 260
- Drug Safety Technology Vendors 261
- Vendor Profile—ARIS GLOBAL 261
- ARIS GLOBAL Total Safety Suite 261
- Vendor Profile – Galt Associates Inc 263
- Vendor Profile – Insightful 263
- Vendor Profile – Oracle Corp 264
- Vendor Profile – Phase Forward 264
- Vendor Profile – Relsys Inc. 265
- Vendor Profile – eResearch Technologies (eRT) 265
- Vendor Profile – SAIC 266

- Vendor Profile - SAS 266
- Case Studies 267
- Data Mining and Signal Detection 268
- Uppsala Monitoring Center 269

Annexures
- **Annexure 1A and B:** ADR Forms: India 271
- **Annexure 2A and B:** Yellow Card: MHRA 275
- **Annexure 3A to C:** MedWatch Forms (US-FDA 3500, 3500A & 3500B) 279
- **Annexure 4:** First Information Report (FIR) 299
- **Annexure 5:** Preliminary Investigation Report (PIR) 302
- **Annexure 6:** Detailed Investigation Report (DIR) 309
- **Annexure 7:** AEFI- Laboratory Requisition Form (LRF) 314
- **Annexure 8:** Good Vigilance Practices Guidelines 316
- **Annexure 9:** ADR Report Form in English: China 596
- **Annexure 10:** Blue Card: Australia 598
- **Annexure 11A to C:** ADR Forms: Canada 600

Index 611

1

Key Definitions in Pharmacovigilance

Renu Agarwal, SK Gupta

Pharmacovigilance is an important tool for monitoring drug-related problems after market authorization in "real world setting". For an effective development pharmacovigilance system, a uniform set of definitions is of paramount importance. This chapter presents an alphabetical list of formal scientific definitions commonly used in pharmacovigilance. This list of definitions is also available in the Uppsala Monitoring Centre (UMC)/ Council for International Organizations of Medical Sciences (CIOMS) Monograph.

Absolute risk: Risk in a population of exposed persons; the probability of an event affecting members of a particular population (e.g. 1 in 1,000). Absolute risk can be measured over time (*incidence*) or at a given time (*prevalence*).

See also attributable risk and relative risk.

Adverse event: Any untoward medical occurrence that may present during treatment with a pharmaceutical product but which does not necessarily have a causal relationship with this treatment.

Synonym: adverse experience

Adverse event of special interest (AESI): A noteworthy event for the particular product or class of products that a sponsor may wish to monitor carefully. It could be serious or non-serious (e.g. hair loss, loss of taste, impotence), and could include events that might be potential precursors or prodromes for more serious medical conditions in susceptible individuals. Such events should be described in protocols or protocol amendments, and instructions provided for investigators as to how and when they should be reported to the sponsor.

Adverse drug reaction (ADR): A response which is noxious and unintended, and which occurs at doses normally used in humans for the prophylaxis, diagnosis, or therapy of disease, or for the modification of physiological function. An adverse drug reaction, contrary to an adverse event, is characterized by the suspicion of a causal relationship between the drug and the occurrence, i.e. judged as being at least possibly related to treatment by the reporting or a reviewing health professional.

Allopathy: Non-traditional, western scientific therapy, usually using synthesized ingredients, but may also contain a purified active ingredient extracted from a plant or other natural source; usually in opposition to the disease.

Compare *homeopathy*.

Association: Events associated in time but not necessarily linked as cause and effect.

Attributable risk: Difference between the risk in an exposed population (*absolute risk*) and the risk in an unexposed population (*reference risk*). Also referred to as excess risk. Attributable risk is the result of an absolute comparison between outcome frequency measurements, such as incidence.

Examples: If the exposed persons with a particular outcome are A, the exposed persons without the outcome are B, the unexposed persons with the outcome are C and the unexposed persons with the outcome are D, then the attributable risk is calculated as: $[A/(A + B)] - [C/(C + D)]$. If, during the same time period, the incidence of rash in a population treated with medicine X is $35/1,500 = 0.023$, and the incidence of rash in a population not treated with X is $5/2,000 = 0.0025$, the attributable risk is $(35/1,500) - (5/2,000) = 0.0205$.

Benefit: An estimated gain for an individual or population.

See also *Effectiveness/Risk*.

Benefit-risk analysis: Examination of the favorable (beneficial) and unfavorable results of undertaking a specific course of action. (While this phrase is still commonly used, the more logical pairings of benefit-harm and effectiveness-risk are slowly replacing it).

Biological products: Medical products prepared from biological material of human, animal or microbiologic origin (such as blood products, vaccines, insulin).

Case control studies: Studies that compare cases with a disease to controls without the disease, looking for differences in antecedent exposures.

Case reports: Reports of the experience of single patient. As used in pharmacoepidemiology, a case report describes a single patient who was exposed to a drug and experiences a particular outcome, usually an adverse event.

Case series: Reports of collections of patients, all of whom have a common exposure, examining what their clinical outcomes were. Alternatively, case series can be reports of patients who have a common disease, examining what their antecedent exposures were. No control group is present.

Causality assessment: The evaluation of the likelihood that a medicine was the causative agent of an observed adverse reaction. Causality assessment is usually made according established algorithms.

Caveat document: The formal advisory warning accompanying data release from the WHO Database: it specifies the conditions and reservations applying to interpretations and use of the data.

Clinical trial: A systematic study on pharmaceutical products in human subjects (including patients and other volunteers) in order to discover or verify the effects of and/or identify any adverse reaction to investigational products, and/or to study the absorption, distribution, metabolism and excretion of the products with the objective of ascertaining their efficacy and safety.

Cohort studies: Studies that identify defined populations and follow them forward in time, examining their rates of disease. Cohort studies generally identify and compare exposed patients to unexposed patients or to patients who receive a different exposure.

Combinations database: Quarterly report of all drug-ADR associations produced by the Bayesian confidence propagation neural network (BCPNN) scan.

Common: In pharmacovigilance, an event with a frequency between 1 in 100 and 1 in 10.

Compliance: Faithful adherence by the patient to the prescriber's instructions.

Control group: The comparison group in drug-trials not being given the studied drug.

Critical terms: Some of the terms in WHO-ART are marked as 'Critical Terms'. These terms either refer to or might be indicative of serious disease states, and warrant special attention, because of their possible association with the risk of serious illness which may lead to more decisive action than reports on other terms.

See Serious adverse event or reaction.

Cross-sectional studies: These examine exposures and outcomes in populations at one point in time; they have no time sense.

Data-mining: At the UMC, the use of an automated tool, based on Bayesian logic, for the scanning of the WHO database (*Vigibase*) in the process of detecting drug-adverse reaction associations: the BCPNN. Knowledge-detection is the preferred term for the process.

Dechallenge: The withdrawal of a drug from a patient; the point at which the continuity, reduction or disappearance of adverse effects may be observed.

Descriptive studies: Studies that do not have control groups, namely case reports, case series, and analyses of secular trends. They contrast with analytic studies.

Development safety update report (DSUR): A periodic summary of safety information for regulators, including any changes in the benefit-risk relationship, for a drug, biologic or vaccine under development, prepared by the sponsor of all its clinical trials.

Drug utilization research: The marketing, distribution, prescription and use of drugs in a society, with special emphasis on the resulting medical, social, and economic consequences.

Effectiveness/risk: The balance between the rate of effectiveness of a medicine versus the risk of harm is a quantitative assessment of the merit of a medicine used in routine clinical practice. Comparative information between therapies is most useful. This is more useful than the efficacy and hazard predictions from pre-marketing information that is limited and based on selected subjects.

Efficacy: The ability of a drug to produce the intended effect as determined by scientific methods, for example in pre-clinical research conditions (opposite of hazard).

See also absolute risk, reference risk, attributable risk and relative risk.

Epidemiology: The science concerned with the study of the factors determining and influencing the frequency and distribution of disease, injury and other health-related events and their causes in a defined human population for the purpose of establishing programmes to prevent and control their development and spread (Dorland's Illustrated Medical Dictionary).

See also pharmacoepidemiology

Essential medicines: Essential medicines are those that satisfy the priority health care needs of the population.

They are selected with due regard to public health relevance, evidence on efficacy and safety, and comparative cost-effectiveness.

See www.who.int/medicines/default.shtml.

EudraVigilance: The European Union data-processing network and management system, established by the European Medicines Agency (EMEA) to support the electronic exchange, management, and scientific evaluation of Individual Case Safety Reports related to all medicinal products authorized in the European Economic Area (EEA). EudraVigilance also incorporates data analysis facilities.

Excipients: All materials included to make a pharmaceutical formulation (e.g. a tablet) except the active drug substance(s).

Expected adverse drug reaction: One for which its nature or severity is consistent with that included in the appropriate reference safety information (e.g. Investigator's brochure for an unapproved investigational product or package insert/summary of product characteristics for an approved product).

Formulary: A listing of medicinal drugs with their uses, methods of administration, available dose forms, side effects, etc. sometimes including their formulas and methods of preparation.

Generic (multisource product): The term 'generic product' has somewhat different meanings in different jurisdictions.

Generic products may be marketed either under the non-proprietary approved name or under a new brand (proprietary) name. They are usually intended to be interchangeable with the innovator product, which is usually manufactured without a license from the innovator company and marketed after the expiry of patent or other exclusivity rights.

Good clinical practice (GCP): A standard for the design, conduct, performance, monitoring, auditing, recording, analyses, and reporting of clinical trials that provides assurance that the data and reported results are credible and accurate, and that the rights, integrity, and confidentiality of trial subjects are protected.

Good pharmacovigilance practice: A set of guidelines for the conduct of pharmacovigilance in the EU, drawn up based on Article 108a of Directive 2001/83/EC, by the European Medicines Agency in cooperation with competent authorities in Member States and interested parties, and applying to marketing authorization holders in the EU, the Agency and competent authorities in Member States.

Harm: The nature and extent of actual damage that could be caused by a drug. Not to be confused with risk.

Hazard: The inherent capability of an intervention to cause harm (and a hazard as a potential source of harm).

Herbal medicine: Includes herbs, herbal materials, herbal preparations and finished herbal products.

Homeopathy: Homeopathy is a therapeutic system which works on the principle that 'like treats like'. An illness is treated with a medicine which could produce similar symptoms in a healthy person. The active ingredients are given in highly diluted form to avoid toxicity. Homeopathic remedies are virtually 100% safe.

Compare *Allopathy*.

Incidence: The extent or rate of occurrence, especially the number of new cases of a disease in a population over a period of time.

Individual case safety report (ICSR): A report that contains 'information describing a suspected adverse drug reaction related to the administration of one or more medicinal products to an individual patient'.

(*Volume 9 of the Rules Governing Medicinal Products for Human and Veterinary Use in the European Union*).

Investigator brochure (IB): A compilation of the clinical and nonclinical data on the investigational product(s) that is relevant to the study of the investigational product(s) in human subjects.

Investigational product: A pharmaceutical form of an active ingredient or placebo being tested or used as a reference in a clinical trials, including a product with a marketing authorization when used or assembled (formulated or packaged) in a way different form the approved form, or when used for an unapproved indication, or when used to gain further information about an approved use.

Knowledge-detection: Preferred term as the alternative to data mining; searching for combinations and patterns using BCPNN.

Marketing authorization holder (MAH): MAH is usually an organization to whom permission has been granted for marketing the medicinal product(s) for specified indication. It has an appropriate system of pharmacovigilance in place in order to assure responsibility and liability for its products on the market and to ensure that appropriate action can be taken, when necessary. The European Agency for the evaluation of medicinal products, 1999.

Martindale: One of the prime reference sources for information about drugs throughout the world. Published by the Pharmaceutical Press, UK.

Medical error: "An unintended act (either of omission or commission) or one that does not achieve its intended outcomes." Leape, Lucien. Error in Medicine. *Journal of the American Medical Association* 1994;272(23): 1851-57.

Member countries: Countries which comply with the criteria for, and have joined the WHO Programme for International Drug Monitoring.

National pharmacovigilance centres: Organizations recognized by governments to represent their country in the WHO Programme (usually the drug regulatory agency). A single, governmentally recognized centre (or integrated system) within a country with the clinical and scientific expertise to collect, collate, analyse and give advice on all information related to drug safety.

Neural network: A type of artificial intelligence used in the BCPNN to scan the WHO ADR database (*Vigibase*).

Over the counter (OTC): Medicines which are available for purchase without prescription.

Pharmacoeconomics: Economic evaluation which is concerned with identifying, measuring and valuing inputs (i.e. estimating cost) and outputs (benefits) of a drug therapy or health care programme as compared to alternative course of action or, if realistic, 'doing nothing'. An assessment is made as to the collective improvement in the welfare of individuals relative to status quo, i.e. current normal practice.

Pharmacoepidemiology: Study of the use and effects of drugs in large populations. See also *epidemiology*.

Pharmacogenetics: Study of genetic causes of individual variations in drug response.

Pharmacogenomics: Genome-wide analysis of the genetic determinants of drug efficacy and toxicity.

Pharmacology: Study of the uses, effects and modes of action of drugs.

Pharmacovigilance: The science and activities relating to the detection, assessment, understanding and prevention of adverse effects or any other drug-related problem.

Phocomelia: Characteristic deformity caused by exposure to thalidomide in the womb, also very rarely occurring spontaneously. Meaning: limbs like a seal.

Phytotherapy: Western-style, scientific treatment using plant extracts or materials.

Placebo: An inactive substance (often called a sugar pill) given to a group being studied to compare results with the effects of the active drug.

Polypharmacy: The concomitant use of more than one drug, sometimes prescribed by different practitioners.

Post-marketing: The stage when a drug is generally available on the market.

Predisposing factors: Any aspect of the patient's history (other than the drug) which might explain reported adverse events (genetic factors, diet, alcohol consumption, disease history, polypharmacy or use of herbal medicines, for example).

Pre-marketing: The stage before a drug is available for prescription or sale to the public.

Prescription event monitoring (PEM): System created to monitor adverse drug events in a population. Prescribers are requested to report all events, regardless of whether they are suspected adverse events, for identified patients receiving a specified drug. Also more accurately named 'cohort-event monitoring'.

Prescription only medicine (POM): Medicinal product available to the public only on prescription.

Prophylaxis: Prevention or protection.

Prospective study: A study in which the subjects are identified and followed in time to watch for outcomes, such as the development of a disease, during the study period.

Randomized controlled trial (RCT): A study where the investigator randomly assigns patients to different therapies/study arms.

Rare: In pharmacovigilance an event with a probability between 1 in 10,000 and 1 in 1,000.

Rational drug use: An ideal of therapeutic practice in which drugs are prescribed and used in exact accordance with the best understanding of their appropriateness for the indication and the particular patient, and of their benefit, harm effectiveness and risk.

Rechallenge: The point at which a drug is again given to a patient after its previous withdrawal – see *dechallenge*.

Record linkage: Method of assembling information contained in two or more records, e.g. in different sets of medical charts, and in vital records such as birth and death certificates. This makes it possible to relate significant health events that are remote from one another in time and place.

Reference risk: Risk in a population of unexposed persons; also called baseline risk. Reference risk can be measured over time (*incidence*) or at a given time (*prevalence*). The unexposed population refers to a reference population, as closely comparable to the exposed population as possible, apart from the exposure.

Regulatory authority: The legal authority in any country with the responsibility of regulating all matters relating to drugs.

Examples: Drug Controller general of India (DCGI) for India, Food and Drug Administration (FDA) for USA, Medicines and Healthcare products Regulatory Agency (MHRA) for UK, Bundesinstitut für Arzneimittel und Medizinprodukte (BfArM for Germany), French Health Product Safety Agency (AFSSAPS) for France, Therapeutic goods administration (TGA) for Australia.

Relative risk: Ratio of the risk in an exposed population (*absolute risk*) and the risk in an unexposed population (*reference risk*). Relative risk is the result of a relative comparison between outcome frequency measurements, e.g. incidences.

Example: If the exposed persons with an outcome are A, the exposed persons without the outcome are B, the unexposed persons with the outcome are C, and the unexposed persons without the outcome are D, the relative risk is calculated as $[A/(A + B)]/[C/(C + D)]$. If the incidence of rash in a population treated with medicine X is $35/1{,}500 = 0.023$, and the incidence of rash in a population which is not treated with X, during the same time period, is $5/2{,}000 = 0.0025$, the relative risk is $(35/1{,}500)/(5/2{,}000) = 9.3$.

Risk: The probability of harm being caused; the probability (chance, odds) of an occurrence.

Risk minimization: This is a set of activities directed to reduce the probability of the occurrence or severity of an adverse reaction.

Risk management: The pharmacovigilance activities that aim to identify, characterize, prevent or minimize risks relating to medicinal product(s). This also includes the assessment of the effectiveness of the medicinal product(s).

Retrospective study: A retrospective study looks backwards and examines exposures to suspected risk or protection factors in relation to an outcome that is established at the start of the study. The study is usually done using medical records and interviews with patients.

Serious adverse event or reaction: A serious adverse event or reaction is any untoward medical occurrence that at any dose:
- results in death
- requires inpatient hospitalization or prolongation of existing hospitalization

- results in persistent or significant disability/incapacity
- is life-threatening.

To ensure no confusion or misunderstanding of the difference between the terms 'serious' and 'severe', the following note of clarification is provided: The term 'severe' is not synonymous with serious. In the English language, 'severe' is used to describe the intensity (severity) of a specific event (as in mild, moderate or severe); the event itself, however, may be of relatively minor medical significance (such as severe headache).

Seriousness (not severity), which is based on patient/event outcome or action criteria serves as guide for defining regulatory reporting obligations.

Side effect: Any unintended effect of a pharmaceutical product occurring at normal dosage which is related to the pharmacological properties of the drug.

Signal: Reported information on a possible causal relationship between an adverse event and a drug, the relationship being unknown or incompletely documented previously. Usually more than a single report is required to generate a signal, depending upon the seriousness of the event and the quality of the information. The publication of a signal usually implies the need for some kind of review or action.

Spontaneous reporting: System whereby case reports of adverse drug events are voluntarily submitted from health professionals and pharmaceutical manufacturers to the national regulatory authority.

See ICSR.

Suspected unexpected serious adverse reaction (SUSAR): A reaction which is both unexpected and serious in nature.

Thalidomide: Drug prescribed in the 1950s as a mild sleeping pill and remedy for morning-sickness for pregnant women. Led to serious birth defects. Returning to favor as a treatment for leprosy.

Traditional medicines: Traditional medicine is the sum total of the knowledge, skills, and practices based on the theories, beliefs, and experiences indigenous to different cultures, whether explicable or not, used in the maintenance of health as well as in the prevention, diagnosis, improvement or treatment of physical and mental illness.

See also allopathic medicine.

Uncommon: In pharmacovigilance an event with a frequency between 1 in 1.000 and 1 in 100.

Unexpected adverse reaction: An adverse reaction, the nature or severity of which is not consistent with domestic labeling or market authorization, or expected from characteristics of the drug.

VigiBase: The name for the WHO International ADR Database.

VigiFlow: VigiFlow (formerly called Vigibase Online) is a sophisticated case report management system created by the UMC, complying with GxP requirements.

Vigisearch: This is a custom search service offered by the UMC to third-party inquirers for which several types of standard presentation are available.

Vigimed: E-mail conferencing facility, exclusive to member countries of the WHO Programme for International Drug Monitoring.

SOURCES

1. Clinical safety data management: definitions and standards for expedited reporting E2A. International Conference on Harmonisation of Technical Requirements for Registration of Pharmaceuticals for Human Use (ICH) 1994.
2. Management of safety information from clinical trials. Council for International Organizations of Medical Sciences (CIOMS) Working Group VI, Geneva. 2005.

3. Strom BL. Pharmacoepidemiology. 4th edition. Chichester, England: John Wiley & Sons; 2005.
4. Guideline for good clinical practice E6 (R1). International Conference on Harmonisation of Technical Requirements for Registration of Pharmaceuticals for Human Use (ICH). 1996.
5. Guidelines on good pharmacovigilance practices (GVP) EMA/501523/2015.
6. The selection of essential drugs: report of a WHO expert committee. Geneva. 1977.
7. The importance of pharmacovigilance: safety reporting of medicinal products. Geneva: World Health Organization. 2002.
8. Pharmacovigilance planning E2E. International Conference on Harmonisation of Technical Requirements for Registration of Pharmaceuticals for Human Use (ICH). 2004.
9. Uppsala Monitoring centre (http://www.who-umc.org/).

2

Pharmacovigilance: Historical Perspective

Renu Agarwal, SK Gupta

Pharmacovigilance is the science of detection, assessment, understanding and prevention of adverse drug effects or any other possible drug-related problems.[1] Man must have experienced the adverse drug reactions when he first started using plants as medication and evidences of awareness of adverse drug effects can be observed in literature. This chapter gives an anecdotal view of historical aspects of awareness and systematic reporting of adverse drug reactions.

PHARMACOVIGILANCE BEFORE 18TH CENTURY

The study of literature from before 18th century reveals evidences of man's awareness towards the possibilities of harmful effects of drugs and therapeutic procedures undertaken for healing various ailments. Few such examples are mentioned here.

In 1780 BC the Babylonian Code of Hammurabi gives details of punishment for harm done by medical procedures. According to this description: *"If a physician make a large incision with the operating knife, and kill him, or open a tumor with the operating knife, and cut out the eye, his hands shall be cut off."*

In 10th century the Salerno medical School was empowered to inspect drugs for possible adulteration and severe penalties were imposed: *"whosoever shall have or sell any poison or noxious drug not useful or necessary to his art, let him be hanged".*

In 13th century the Oath of Apothecaries in Basle, Switzerland, mentions the following about use of drugs by physicians: *"drugs should be of such good quality and of such usefulness that he knows, upon his oath, that it will be good and useful for the confection what the physician is making".*

In 1599 a charter was issued to make provisions for the supervision of sales of drugs and poison by King James VI of Scotland. William Spang was the first inspector appointed and he took the responsibility of approving drugs for sale in Glasgow.

All the above mentioned evidences from literature clearly indicate the keen interest of man in taking steps to eliminate the adverse effects associated with therapeutic procedures. However, the measures taken were localized to small group of people and organized efforts to involve wider population did not exist.

PHARMACOVIGILANCE IN 18TH CENTURY

People in 18th century started putting more efforts to deal with the issue of safety-related to use of drugs as more alarming adverse drug reactions were revealed by physicians at that time. There are several examples of systematic attention given to the adverse effects of drugs during 18th century, some are discussed here.

An English physician William Withering (1741–1799) published his extensive work on foxglove in 1785 (Fig. 2.1). This work was later recognized as the first systematic paper on a medicinal drug with detailed description of adverse effects associated with digitalis treatment.

In his book entitled "An account of the Foxglove and Some of Its Medicinal Uses: with Practical Remarks on Dropsy and Other Diseases" Withering gives a detailed account of methods for the synthesis of digitalis from Foxglove in a standardized way, animal tests using turkeys, details of therapeutic effects and symptoms associated with digitalis overdoses. According to this description Foxglove when given in large and repeated doses leads to vomiting, purging, giddiness, altered vision, increased urination, increased frequency of motion, slow pulse, cold sweats, convulsions, syncope and death. He emphasized on the importance of proper measurement of doses. Today the knowledge of pharmacological properties of digitalis has increased significantly but the basic symptomatology associated with overdoses still remains the same. The Royal College of Physicians commemorates the achievements of William Withering in annual lecture named after him.[2,3]

In 1789, Wouter van Doeveren (Fig. 2.2), Professor of Medicine at Leiden University and a critic of the medical practice of that time, discussed in his academic lecture named Remedio Morbi, the diseases or ailments which often affect people as a result of administration of remedies for therapeutic purposes.[4-6] In his lecture van Doeveren mentioned that the treating physicians often consider the treatment-related problems as either essential or hazardous and are seldom moderate in their judgment. He also pointed out the hazards associated with the commonly used therapeutic methods at that time such as bloodletting and perspiration-inducing drugs for acute fever and concluded that many illnesses may result from inappropriate treatments administered without proper diagnosis. He warned that a second ailment may be added to the first or perhaps the death may result as a consequence of empirical treatment. This lecture indicates emerging scientific interest in adverse drug reactions in 18th century.

In 18th century Calomel (mercurous chloride) was widely used in America for the treatment of outbreaks of yellow fever. Treatment lead to mercurialism characterized by intense salivation, loosening of the teeth,

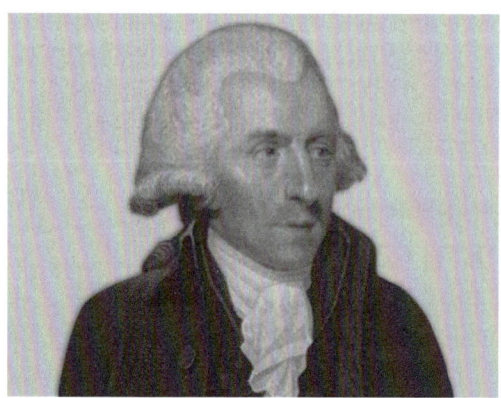

Fig. 2.1: William Withering (1741-1799)

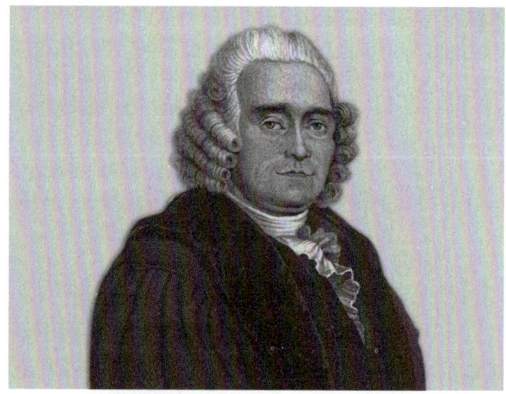

Fig. 2.2: Wouter van Doeveren (1730-1783)

ulceration, gangrene of the mouth and cheeks and osteomyelitis of the mandible. In spite of the adverse effects physicians continued to use Calomel. Later Oliver Wendall Holmes in 1861 said *"if the whole materia medica, as it is used now, could be sunk to the bottom of the sea, it would be all the better for mankind—and all the worse for the fishes."*

Although the adverse effects associated with administration of drugs must have been noted by others also but could not be pointed out strongly due to lack of sufficient corroborative evidence. The 18th century literature indicates even greater awareness of people especially the academicians and physicians, who started communicating by various means such as lectures and publications, with regard to the issues-related to safe use of drugs.

PHARMACOVIGILANCE IN 19TH CENTURY

The records of systematic reporting of adverse effects associated with therapeutic measures are available from early 19th century. One such example of systematic reporting involving cowpox vaccine is described here. The cowpox vaccination started as early as 1718 and in spite of claims put forth regarding its efficacy and safety, the cowpox vaccination was not generally accepted. A positive response was only observed after the publication of the work of Edward Jenner on variolae vaccines in 1798. Further with the help of Royal College of Physicians a campaign was launched in Netherlands for cowpox vaccination in 1808 with emphasis on collection of information in relation to effects of cowpox vaccine and any other peculiarities that may have been observed. The process not only proved the benefits of the vaccine but also demonstrated the safety.

In 1848 death of a 15-year-old girl as a result of chloroform anesthesia administered for ingrown toenail was reported. In response to more deaths following chloroform anesthesia Glasgow Committee was appointed by British Medical Association for inquiry in 1880. The committee concluded that *"Chloroform was injurious to the heart and in comparison more dangerous than ether".* Later in 1888 in Hyderabad, Edward Lawrie claimed safe use of chloroform in 40000 people without any fatality. As a result 'First Hyderabad Chloroform Commission' was appointed to verify the claim and after conducting experiments in 141 animals the commission concluded that chloroform could be safely used for anesthesia if the respiration is carefully monitored. This report was not accepted in England and a 'Second Hyderabad Chloroform Commission' was formed to reinvestigate. The second commission also included a representative from Lancet. Again the experiments were carried out in 430 animals and 54 humans. The second commission confirmed the findings of Glasgow Committee.[7]

In a similar development in 1848 in America a statute was passed to control the quality of drugs when the quinine imported for US army was found adulterated.

Systematic recording of illnesses associated with pharmacotherapy started much later and a book in this regard was published by L Lewin in 1881 (Fig. 2.3).

PHARMACOVIGILANCE IN 20TH CENTURY: PRETHALIDOMIDE ERA

During 20th century evidences show the beginning of participation of authorities for supervision of drug manufacturing. The food and drug administration (FDA) was established in 1906 to impose quality criteria for drug manufacturing and Pharmacopoeias were established. The 1938 was the landmark year when more stringent safety requirements were initiated and legislated in response to sulfanilamide disaster.[8] In 1937 the sulfa compounds were considered the 'miracle drugs' as they killed a wide range of harmful

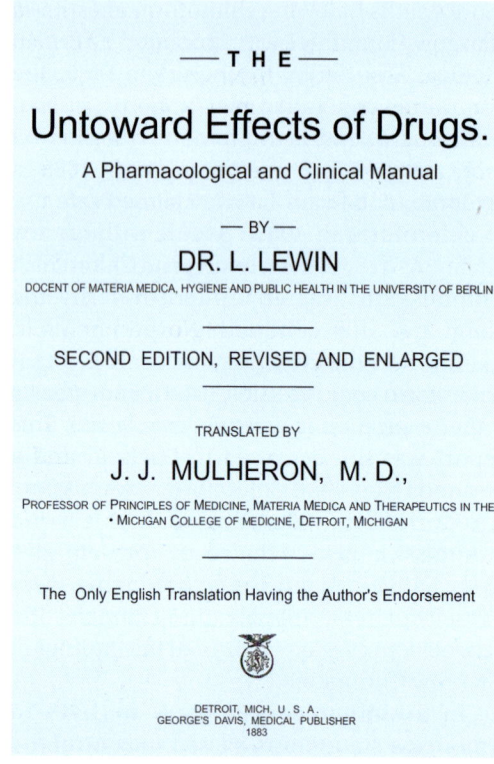

Fig. 2.3: First book on adverse Drug Reaction by Dr L Lewin

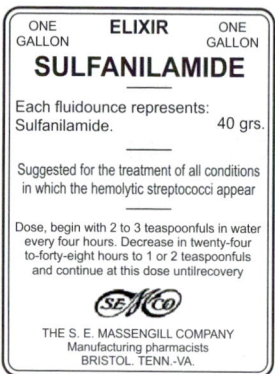

Fig. 2.4: Sulfanilamide Elixir containing solvent diethylene glycol killed 107 people

bacteria. One of the manufacturers in 1938 prepared an elixir of sulfanilamide by dissolving the drug in diethylene glycol. Subsequently, 107 people including 100 children were killed following use of this elixir of sulfanilamide, which was prepared in a poisonous solvent (diethylene glycol)(Fig. 2.4).

In June 1938, the Federal Food, Drug and Cosmetic Act was signed in USA. The new law required the safety testing of new drugs before marketing and it became essential that new drug application (NDA) incorporates the safety data. The law also required the adequate labeling of drugs for safe use. A similar response to enforce safety requirements was seen in 1950 with the set-up of a blood dyscrasia registry by Council on drugs of the American Medical Association following reports of association of aplastic anemia with the use of chloramphenicol.[9,10]

The efforts to address the concerns about adverse drug reactions were also evidenced by publication of a number of articles related to adverse drug reactions. In this regard an overview of the available literature was published by L Meyler in Dutch in 1951. Soon after in 1952 the English translation entitled 'Side Effects of Drugs' was also published and subsequently translation was done in other languages.[11,12] Later a number of publications followed and one such publication in 1955 by HL Alexander was entitled 'Reactions with Drug Therapy'. Also in 1955 an article published by Barr in JAMA reported that 5% of the patients admitted to the hospital suffer from major toxic reactions and accidents. A number of reports published later also mentioned similar figures.

The study of literature from books, journal articles and discussions during academic meetings shows gradual evolution of the science of pharmacovigilance with firm scientific basis during early part of 20th century. In 1961 thalidomide disaster brought about significant changes in the pharmacovigilance system world over with active participation from regulatory authorities, industry and health care workers.

PHARMACOVIGILANCE IN 20TH CENTURY: THALIDOMIDE DISASTER AND POST-THALIDOMIDE ERA

The thalidomide which was first synthesized in 1953 was extensively promoted in 1956 under various brand names in Germany, England and other countries and was available both as prescription and over-the-counter drug. An Australian physician McBride first observed a correlation between maternal use of thalidomide and congenital malformation in newborns and he sent a letter to Lancet in this regard in June 1961, which got published in December 1961.[13] In November during the same year, Dr Lenz from Germany discussed the association of congenital malformation with maternal use of thalidomide during a pediatric conference. As this association of thalidomide with congenital anomalies got more and more attention, the manufacturer Chemie Grünenthal withdrew thalidomide from the market on 25th November 1961. Later it was reported that nearly 6000–12000 children had congenital anomalies due to maternal use of thalidomide and majority of them were born in Germany (Fig. 2.5).[14,15]

THALIDOMIDE AND CONGENITAL ABNORMALITIES

Sir,
Congenital abnormalities are present in approximately 1.5% of babies. In recent months I have observed that the incidence of multiple severe abnormalities in babies delivered of women who were given the drug thalidomide ('Distaval') during pregnancy, as an antiemetic or as a sedative, to be almost 20%.

These abnormalities are present in structures developed from mesenchyme, i.e. the bones and musculature of the gut. Bony development seems to be affected in a very striking manner, resulting in polydactyly, syndactyly, and failure of development of long bones (abnormally short femora and radii).

Have any of your readers seen similar abnormalities in babies delivered of women who have taken this drug during pregnancy?

Hurstville, New South Wales. WG McBride. ∴ In our issue of December 2 we included a statement from the Distillers Company (Biochemicals) Ltd. referring to "reports from two overseas sources possibly associating thalidomide ('Distaval') with harmful effects on the fetus in early pregnancy". Pending further investigation, the company decided to withdraw from the market all its preparations containing thalidomide.

McBride's famous letter to the Lancet
—Ed.L.

McBRIDE'S FAMOUS LETTER TO THE LANCET THALIDOMIDE INFANT

Thalidomide tragedy led to the introduction of some very stringent measures in many countries. FDA started systematic collection of reports on all types of adverse drug reactions. In many other countries along with efficacy the safety of drugs was emphasized and standards were set which the new drugs were required to meet before getting authorization for marketing. Government organizations were instructed to set-up a post marketing surveillance system so as to pick up the

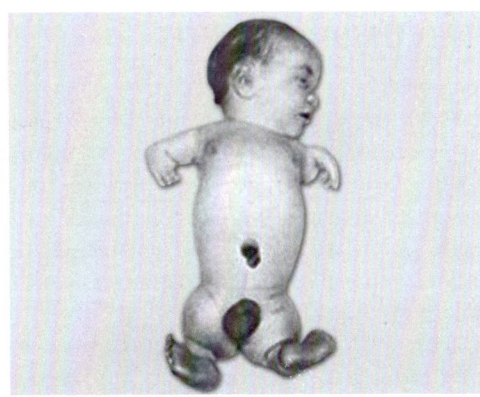

Fig. 2.5: Thalidomide infant

adverse drug reactions as early as possible and prevent similar tragedies in future. In 1968, a collaborative effort was made by 10 countries to cooperate with WHO for International drug safety monitoring.

As a result of increasing efforts and awareness to promote safe use of drugs many adverse drug reactions started getting noticed by treating physicians. In 1969, a major digitalis related disaster was unveiled in the Dutch town of Veenendaal. The Physician Mr AH Lely discovered the development of serious symptoms of digitalis toxicity over a period of about 2-3 months. Subsequently, it was revealed that due to production error the dispensed tablets were composed of digitoxin 0.20 mg and digoxin 0.05 mg instead of recommended digoxin 0.25 mg. At least 19 deaths were attributed to this production error.[16] One particular aspect of this tragedy to notice is the ability of the physician to closely observe the symptoms related to overdose and communicate them to others. It is also noticeable that other physicians who also must have observed the similar symptoms, failed to bring them to the notice of others either because they were not aware of the symptoms or simply did not inform others. Knowledge, keen observation and efficient reporting still form the basics of pharmacovigilance.

PHARMACOVIGILANCE: THE CURRENT STATUS

The foundation of World Health Organization (WHO) International Drug Monitoring Programme was laid in 1971 during 20th World Health Assembly. The current international system of pharmacovigilance is based on a report published in 1972 and accordingly the national pharmacovigilance centres work in collaboration with WHO.[17-19]

The WHO Collaborating Centre for International Drug Monitoring in based in Uppsala, Sweden (The Uppsala Monitoring Centre) and supports and coordinates the WHO International Drug Monitoring Programme. The WHO centre provides active support to the pharmacovigilance centres in developing countries. The Centre collects the pharmacovigilance data from national pharmacovigilance centres, maintains an international database, evaluates the efficiency and problems of ongoing national pharmacovigilance programmes and takes measures to further strengthen them with technical and financial support. In 2000 WHO Uppsala Monitoring Centre has provided guidelines for setting up and running a pharmacovigilance centre. In 2002 WHO publication 'The importance of Pharmacovigilance' provided the guidelines for implementation of pharmacovigilance programme at international level. The efforts of developing and implementing new legislation and qualitative requirements have led to the establishment of The Council for International Organizations of Medical Sciences (CIOMS) and International Conference on Harmonization (ICH). These organizations along with national regulatory authorities and pharmaceutical industry have been instrumental in development of pharmacovigilance.

PHARMACOVIGILANCE: THE CURRENT SYSTEM IN INDIA

A formal drug safety monitoring system was proposed for the first time in India in 1986. The proposal of adverse drug reaction monitoring system of 1986 consisted of 12 regional centres each covering a population of 50 million. More concrete efforts of drug safety monitoring in India began in 1997 in cooperation with WHO Uppasala Monitoring Centre. Under this programme three adverse drug reaction monitoring centres were identified including a National Pharmacovigilance Centre at All India Institute of Medical Sciences (AIIMS),

New Delhi and two WHO special centres at Mumbai and Aligarh. This programme could not succeed due to multiple reasons leading to launch of a more ambitious National Pharmacovigilance Programme (NPP) sponsored by WHO and funded by World bank on 1st January, 2005. The objectives of NPP are to involve a large number of health care professionals in the process, inculcate the culture of reporting adverse drug reactions and to be a benchmark for global drug monitoring. The NPP particularly solicits reports of:

- All adverse events suspected to have been caused by new drugs and 'drugs of current interest' (List published by CDSCO from time to time)
- All suspected drug interactions
- Reactions to any other drugs which are suspected of significantly affecting a patient's management, including reactions suspected of causing:
  - Death
  - Life-threatening reactions (real risk of dying)
  - Hospitalization (initial or prolonged)
  - Disability (significant, persistent or permanent)
  - Congenital anomaly
  - Required intervention to prevent permanent impairment or damage.

The NPP consists of a Pharmacovigilance Advisory Committee located at Central Drugs Standard Control Organization (CDSCO), New Delhi Government of India initiated a nation-wide pharmacovigilance programme in July, 2010, with establishment of National Coordinating Centre (NCC), AIIMS, New Delhi for monitoring adverse drug reactions (ADR) in the country. In 2010, a total of 22 ADR monitoring centres (AMCs) including AIIMS, New Delhi were set-up under this programme. Later in April, 2011, the NCC was shifted from the AIIMS, New Delhi to the Indian Pharmacopoeia Commission (IPC), Ghaziabad (Uttar Pradesh). Under NPP, implementation of Schedule Y has made it mandatory to report all serious adverse events (SAEs) including suspected unexpected serious adverse reactions (SUSARs) from clinical trials. Despite the ongoing efforts much needs to be accomplished for the success of NPP in India especially with regard to the reporting of ADRs from post marketed drugs.

CONCLUSION

The world has witnessed horrific disasters following use of drugs for prophylactic, diagnostic and therapeutic purposes since time immemorial. A comprehensive history of the evolution of the science of pharmacovigilance is still to be written. The literature from large number of sources such as scientific books and research papers provides evidences showing significant changes in awareness and methods of drug safety monitoring, especially after 1960 following thalidomide disaster. Currently, WHO Collaboration Centre for International Drug Monitoring, Uppsala is playing a central role by collaborating with national pharmacovigilance centres around the world for collecting, compiling and disseminating information related to drug safety monitoring. Integrated efforts from regulatory authorities, pharmaceutical industry and health care workers are mandatory for the success for national and international pharmacovigilance programmes. Therefore, it is important that the knowledge related to importance and methods of the science of pharmacovigilance spreads not only to the people participating actively in the programme but also to the people at large. Subsequent chapters will present a detailed account of various aspects of pharmacovigilance.

REFERENCES

1. WHO. The Importance of Pharmacovigilance, Safety Monitoring of medical products. WHO Geneva. 2002.
2. Withering W. An account of the foxglove and some of its medicinal uses. CGJ and J Robinson. London. 1785.
3. Rawlins MD. Pharmacovigilance: paradise lost, regained or postponed. The William Withering Lecture 1994. J Royal Coll Phys London. 1995; 29:41-9.
4. Doeveren W van. Sermo academicus de remedio morbo, sive de malis, quae hominibus a remedies, sanandi causa adhibitis, saepenumero accidere solent. Academic speech of February 8, 1779. Manuscript in University Library Amsterdam. 1779.
5. Meyler L, Woord vooraf. In: Meyler L, Schadelijke nevenwerkingen van geneesmiddelen, Supplement II. Van Gorcum. Assen. 1958.
6. Meyler L. Introduction drug-induced diseases. In: Meyler L, Peck MH (Eds). Drug-induced diseases. Van Gorcum. Assen. 1962.
7. Commission on Anaesthetics. Lancet. 1893; i:629-38.
8. Geiling EMK, Cannon PR. Pathogenic effects of elixir of sulfanilamide (diethylene glycol) poisoning. JAMA. 1938;111:919.
9. Rich ML. Fatal case of aplastic anaemia following chloramphenicol therapy. Ann Intern Med. 1950;33:1459.
10. Wallerstein RO, Condit PK, Kasper CK, Brown JW, Morrison FR. Statewide study of chloramphenicol therapy and fatal aplastic anemia. JAMA. 1969;208:2045.
11. Meyler L. Schadelijke nevenwerkingen van geneesmiddelen. Elsevier Publishing Company. Amsterdam. 1951.
12. Meyler L. Side Effects of Drugs. Excerpta Medica Foundation. Amsterdam. 1952.
13. McBride WG. Thalidomide and congenital abnormalities. Lancet. 1961;11:1358.
14. Wade OL. The dawn of concern. In: Adverse reactions to drugs: 1-10. Acford Ltd. Chichester. 1970.
15. Randell T. Thalidomide's back in the news, but in more favorable circumstances. JAMA. 1990;263:467-8.
16. Lely AH. Digitalisintoxicatie, waarnemingen betreffende een massale digitoxine-intoxicatie te Veenendaal. Thesis. State University of Groningen. Stafleu. Leiden. 1971.
17. WHO. Handbook of resolutions and decisions of the World Health Assembly and Executive Board, 11th edition. Geneva, World Health Organization, 1972. WHA 20.51. 1971.
18. WHO. International Drug Monitoring: The Role of National Centres. Technical Report Series. Geneva. 1972.
19. Olsson S. The Role of the WHO Programme on International Drug Monitoring in Coordinating Worldwide Drug Safety Efforts. Drug Saf; 1998;19:1-10.

3

Pharmacovigilance: Need and Objectives

Renu Agarwal

Pharmacovigilance is the science and activities relating to the detection, assessment, understanding and prevention of adverse effects or any other possible drug-related problems. The pharmacovigilance and all issues related to safe use of drugs are relevant for everyone whose life is affected by medical interventions.

NEED FOR PHARMACOVIGILANCE AND WIDENING HORIZONS

Today, the need for an efficient pharmacovigilance system is more than ever before to ensure safe use of drugs. There are multiple reasons for this increasing necessity for pharmacovigilance and some are discussed here (Box 3.1).

Unreliability of Preclinical Safety Data

When the drug is marketed for the first time the experiences with regard to safety and efficacy are mainly based on the results of clinical trials. As the clinical trials are usually conducted under well-controlled conditions it is extremely difficult to predict the actual efficacy, adverse effects and total benefit-risk-ratio under actual clinical setting. During the process of drug development, the research mainly focuses on evaluation of efficacy of drugs. Although, the adverse effects are also discovered but their value in real life situations is limited. Preclinical drug development process involves the evaluation of drug safety and efficacy in animal experiments and often it may not be appropriate to extrapolate the results of animal experiment to human. The clinical trials involving human volunteers are usually done under strictly controlled conditions involving a small sample size (rarely the sample size is more than 3000). The

Box 3.1: Need for pharmacovigilance

1. *Unreliability of preclinical safety data*
   - Well-controlled conditions
   - Small and specified sample size
   - Pressure from various groups to reduce time to approval
2. *Changing pharmaceutical marketing strategies*
   - Aggressive marketing
   - Direct to consumer advertising
   - Launch in many countries at a time
3. *Changing physician and patient preferences*
   - Increasing use of newer drugs
   - Increasing use of drugs to improve quality of life
   - Shift of supervised to self-administered therapy
4. *Easy accessibility*
   - Increasing conversion of prescription drugs to OTC drugs
   - Easy access by internet
   - Easy availability of complementary medicines
   - Easy availability of substandard drugs

data collected is selective and confidential. The clinical trials usually do not involve special groups of people (children, elderly, pregnant) and are not done under the conditions usually encountered in clinical practice. This makes it difficult to predict the occurrence of adverse drug effects in special group of people and in special circumstances such as coadministration with other drugs or in disease conditions (Box 3.2).

The premarketing safety evaluation of drugs often may not be as reliable as expected because of pressure from patient groups, pharmaceutical industry management, political groups and regulatory authorities to reduce the time taken for approval. As the time to approval decreases possibilities of detecting unexpected adverse drug reactions also decreases.

Changing Pharmaceutical Marketing Strategies

Aggressive marketing strategies and efforts to launch new products simultaneously in many countries by pharmaceutical companies has increased the possibility of a comparatively larger population to be exposed to newly launched understudied drugs and accordingly a large population is at risk of experiencing adverse drug reactions. Moreover direct to consumer advertising puts pressure on the physician to prescribe new drugs.

Changing Physician and Patient Preferences

The physicians as well as the patients are now eager to use new products without sufficiently studying the benefits of new medication over the established preparations. Often the drugs are used to improve the quality of life rather than the actual clinical conditions. Moreover as the population of educated and informed patients is increasing they have started playing more active role in therapeutic management. As a result usual hospital-based medically supervised therapy is shifting towards home-based self-administered therapy. This shift further makes it difficult to identify the occurrence, frequency, severity and actual character of adverse drug reaction by trained personnel. As the newer drugs with more complicated mechanisms of action are being developed, the adverse reactions too are expected to be complex making the observations necessary by trained personnel.

Easy Accessibility

Trend to convert more and more prescription only drugs to over-the-counter drugs has excluded the involvement of physicians and pharmacist sometimes therefore making the assessment and reporting of adverse drug reactions very difficult. Access to new drugs by using internet across the national boundaries has further made the accessibility to drugs much easier. The use of complementary medicines is becoming very popular and as the complementary medicines largely escape the official requirements of approval and quality control, they are easily available and it becomes difficult to understand the precise cause of drug-related adverse effects. Increasing penetration of market by substandard drugs in recent years further

---

Box 3.2: Limitations of clinical trial

1. *Homogenous population sample*
   - Strict inclusion/exclusion criteria
   - Subjects usually have single disease
   - Specific groups of children, elderly and pregnant are excluded
2. *Small sample size*
   - Detection of rare disease is difficult
3. *Short duration of trial*
   - Limits the detection of long-term adverse effects
4. *Inability to detect ADRs under real conditions*
   - Drug interaction
   - Drug food interactions
   - Large number of other unpredictable conditions
   - Detection of risk factors

PURPOSE OF PHARMACOVIGILANCE

Until recently, pharmacovigilance was mainly concerned with the detection of adverse drug events that were previously either unknown or poorly understood. Its particular purpose was to contribute to a scientific understanding of the safety profile of a rather small number of drugs and to advice national regulatory authorities.[4] During the last decade, the scope of pharmacovigilance has extended beyond the strict confines of detecting new signals and new kinds of safety concerns have now been realized worldwide. Recently, the concerns of pharmacovigilance have been widened to include:[5-8]

- Herbals
- Traditional and complementary medicines
- Blood products
- Biologicals
- Medical devices
- Vaccines

With the inclusion of such wide range of therapeutic and diagnostic modalities for monitoring, the potential of pharmacovigilance programme to serve a higher priority within public health has been realized. Many other issues that are also of relevance to the science of pharmacovigilance include:[9]

- Substandard medicines
- Medication errors
- Lack of efficacy reports
- Use of medicines for indications that are not approved and for which there is inadequate scientific basis
- Case reports of acute and chronic poisoning
- Assessment of drug-related mortality
- Abuse and misuse of medicines
- Adverse interactions of medicines with chemicals, other medicines and food.

SPECIFIC AIMS OF PHARMACOVIGILANCE IN VIEW OF WIDENING HORIZONS

As outlined above, the scope of pharmacovigilance continues to broaden and it is now not confined to the area of drug safety monitoring but includes a wide range of therapeutics and diagnostics. Therefore, pharmacovigilance is expected to play a major role in public health. Keeping in view the widening horizons WHO has outlined the following specific aims of pharmacovigilance in 2002 bulletin:[9]

- Improve patient care and safety in relation to the use of medicines and all medical and paramedical interventions.
- Improve public health and safety in relation to the use of medicines.
- Contribute to the assessment of benefit, harm, effectiveness and risk of medicines, encouraging their safe, rational and more effective (including cost-effective) use.
- Promote understanding, education and clinical training in pharmacovigilance and its effective communication to the public.

PRIORITY AREAS OF PHARMACOVIGILANCE

The discipline of pharmacovigilance has developed considerably since the 1972 WHO technical report and it remains a dynamic clinical and scientific discipline. Currently, the priority areas in this discipline that need to be addressed at national and international level have been outlined by WHO and include the following:[9]

Detection of Adverse Drug Reactions

- Improve detection and accurate diagnosis of adverse drug reactions (ADRs) by healthcare providers and patients

- Encourage active surveillance of specific drug safety concerns through epidemiological methods such as case control studies, record linkage and epidemiological studies
- Consider special activities and expertise required for the detection of safety concerns related to vaccines, biological, veterinary medicines, herbal medicines, biotechnology products and investigational drugs
- Improve signal detection systems by facilitating the rapid availability of ADR data that may have international relevance
- Revisit the definitions of terms used within the field of pharmacovigilance including the definitions of specific ADRs to ensure reliability and universal understanding of data obtained through ADR reporting systems
- Develop and implement ADR detection systems that could benefit populations with restricted access to health care.

Assessment of ADRs

- Further development of automated signal detection systems used in spontaneous monitoring programmes
- Improvements in assessment of drug safety concerns that are of international relevance
- Foster collaborative links both at local and international level that could allow countries to assess and respond appropriately to drug safety crises
- Consider methods by which information on local patterns of drug use can be integrated with pharmacovigilance information during assessment of benefit and harm at a national level.

Prevention of ADRs

- Improves access to reliable and unbiased drug information at all levels of health care
- Improves access to safer and more effective medicines for neglected diseases prevalent in developing communities
- Integrate pharmacovigilance activities into rational drug use among health professionals and the public
- Integrate pharmacovigilance activities into national drug policies and the activities arising from these (e.g. standard treatment guidelines, essential drugs lists, etc.)
- Further incorporation of pharmacovigilance principles into clinical practice and academic medicine
- Encourage the principles of product stewardship among the various partners in health care
- Improve regulation and pharmacovigilance of traditional and herbal medicines
- Develop systems which assess the impact of preventive actions taken in response to drug safety problems.

Communication

- Improve communication and collaboration between key partners in pharmacovigilance both locally and internationally
- The principles of good communication practice in pharmacovigilance and drug regulation should be encouraged, and the resources and expertise to deliver co-opted. Different solutions are likely to be developed in different countries and regions, and the experience should be shared
- Develop a better understanding of patients, their expectations of medicines and their perception of risk associated with the use of medicines in order to facilitate programmes that will better inform the public on the benefit and harm associated with medicine.
- Develop sustained and active relationships with the media in order to facilitate effective and accurate communication of drug information to the public

- Encourage harmonization of drug regulatory and pharmacovigilance activities by incorporating the wider international community in the development of harmonization policies.

Outcomes and Impact

- Conduct ongoing research to assess the cost-effectiveness of contemporary pharmacovigilance systems in contributing to patient welfare and public health
- Consider the sensitivity and specificity of current signal detection and assessment methods and the extent to which contemporary pharmacovigilance systems have been successful in detecting and preventing potential disasters while avoiding the premature withdrawal of safe and useful medicines from the market.

OUTCOME AND IMPACT OF CURRENT SYSTEM

The national and international pharmacovigilance programmes already in place have given encouraging results by identifying potentially dangerous adverse drug reactions and steps have been taken in the past by not only taking measures to effectively deal with the adverse drug reaction but also by withdrawing the potentially harmful drugs from the market. One such example of drug withdrawal from the market is described here.

The VIOXX Saga

Nonsteroidal anti-inflammatory drugs (NSAIDs) like aspirin and ibuprofen act primarily by inhibiting the cyclooxygenase I and II (COX I and COX II) enzymes thereby inhibiting the prostaglandin synthesis. COX I is a constitutively present enzyme which is required for a variety of body functions such as protection of gastric mucosa whereas COX II plays important role in inflammation. With the identification of two separate COX enzymes and their functions it was realized that any drug that can selectively inhibit COX II will be devoid of adverse effects so commonly associated with non-selective COX inhibitors like aspirin. Hence, the birth of Rofecoxib, popularly known as 'Vioxx', a selective COX II inhibitor, which at its inception held the promise of pain relief in osteoarthritis, rheumatoid arthritis, acute pain and primary dysmenorrhea without the dreaded adverse effects of non-selective COX inhibitors. Extensive human clinical trials, including a systematic evaluation of more than 8,000 patients demonstrated that Vioxx could provide therapeutic efficacy without gastrotoxicity. Considering that more than 16,500 people in the US, alone, die each year from NSAID related gastrointestinal bleeding, this discovery was of great significance and as a result all the shareholders of Merck & Co. reaped the benefits. However, on September 30, 2004 Merck & Co. announced voluntary withdrawal of Vioxx which was based on new data from a clinical trial 'Adenomatous Polyp Prevention on Vioxx' (Approve). It was a rigorous, multicentre, randomized, placebo-controlled double-blind study involving 2,600 patients for over 3 years. The trial was designed to evaluate efficacy of Vioxx 25 mg in preventing the recurrence of colorectal polyps in patients with a history of colorectal adenomas. The study was terminated prematurely when an increase in the relative risk for cardiovascular events such as myocardial infarction and stroke was noted. The important fact to notice from this clinical trial is that results from first 18 months did not show an increase in relative risk of cardiovascular events in Vioxx treated patients as compared to placebo treated patients. It was only after long-term treatment the increased risk was identified.

This story of Vioxx clearly reveals the importance of regular surveillance during post-marketing period. A list of some drugs withdrawn from market during last 10 years is shown in Table 3.1. Clearly, with a systematic and robust pharmacovigilance programme in place, the severity and frequency of drug-related problems can be estimated and benefit risk ratio associated with the use of a particular drugs in comparison with alternative treatment approaches can be done. Accordingly the health professionals and patients can be advised about the treatment choices. At least a quarter of adverse drug reactions and half to one-third drug-related deaths can be avoided by effective implementation of pharmacovigilance programme.[1-3]

WITHDRAWN, a resource for withdrawn and discontinued drugs is now publicly accessible at http://cheminfo.charite.de/withdrawn. This database comprises 578 withdrawn or discontinued drugs, their structures, important physico-chemical properties, protein targets and relevant signaling pathways.[10] Some of the withdrawn drugs are listed in Table 3.1.

Table 3.1: Drugs withdrawn from market since 1997 due to adverse drug reactions

Drug	Type of drug	Date withdrawn	Primary health risk
Pondimin (fenfluramine hydrochloride)	Appetite suppressant	9/15/1997	Valvular heart disease
Redux (dexfenfluramine hydrochloride)	Appetite suppressant	9/15/1997	Valvular heart disease
Seldane (terfenadine)	Antihistamine	2/27/1998	Torsades de pointes (potentially fatal irregular heartbeat)
Posicor (mibefradil dihydrochloride)	Cardiovascular	6/8/1998	Lowered heart rate in elderly women and adverse reactions with 26 other drugs
Duract (bromfenac sodium)	Analgesic and anesthetic	6/22/1998	Liver failure
Hismanal (astemizole)	Antihistamine	6/18/1999	Torsades de pointes
Raxar (grepafloxacin hydrochloride)	Antibiotic	11/1/1999	Torsades de pointes
Rezulin (troglitazone)	Antidiabetic	3/21/2000	Liver failure
Propulsid (cisapride monohydrate)	Gastrointestinal	7/14/2000	Torsades de pointes
Lotronex (alosetron hydrochloride)	Gastrointestinal	11/28/2000	Ischemic colitis
Propagest, Dexatrim (Phenylpropanolamine)	Appetite suppressant	22/12/2005	Stroke
Cerivastatin	Lipid lowering	08/08/2001	Rhabdomyolysis
Rapacuronium	Neuromuscular blocker	03/27/2001	Fatal bronchospasm
Vioxx (Rofecoxib)	Anti-inflammatory	09/30/2004	Myocardial infarction

Contd...

Pharmacovigilance: Need and Objectives

Contd...

Drug	Type of drug	Date withdrawn	Primary health risk
Adderall XR Mixed amphetamine salts	Attention deficit hyperactivity disorder	02/09/2005	Stroke
Palladone (Extended release hydromorphan)	Opioid analgesic	07/13/2005	Accidental overdose with alcohol
Cylert (Pemoline)	Narcolepsy	03/27/2005	Hepatotoxicity
Baxtra (Valdecoxib)	Anti-inflammtory	04/07/2005	Cardiovascular malfunction, severe rash
Tysabri (Natalizumab)	Multiple sclerosis, Crohn's disease	2005-2006, returned to market in July, 2006	Progressive multifocal leukoencephalopathy
Quinine containing preparations	Malaria	02/13/2007	Cardiac arrhythmia, thrombocytopenia, hypersensitivity
Tigan (trimethobenzamide suppositories)	Relief of nausea	04/07/2007	Lack of substantial evidence of effectiveness
Zelnorm	Irritable bowel syndrome	03/30/2007	Cardiovascular accidents
Permax (Pergolide)	Anti-Parkinsonism	03/29/2007	Heart valve damage
Trasylol (Aprotinin)	To control bleeding during heart surgery	11/06/2007	Increased mortality
Prexige (lumiracoxib)	Osteoarthritis	11/20/2007	Hepatotoxicity

CONCLUSION

The drug safety monitoring is an essential element for the effective use of medicines and for high quality medical care. It has the potential to inspire confidence and trust among patients and health professionals in medicines and contributes to raising standards of medical practice. Besides, the adverse drug reactions significantly diminish the quality of life, increase the rate and duration of hospitalization thus increasing the mortality and morbidity. The financial burden on health care authorities increases enormously. As the newer discoveries are becoming available to the needy population at a faster rate due to several recent trends in approval and regulation, the drug-related adverse reactions are also becoming more common, more severe and more complex. Clearly the formulation and implementation of a highly efficient pharmacovigilance programme, which can meet the required objectives is of prime importance at national and international level.

REFERENCES

1. Gandhi TK, Weingart SN, Borus J, et al. Adverse drug events in ambulatory care. N Engl J Med. 2003;348:1556-64.
2. Gurwitz JH, Field TS, Harrold LR, et al. Incidence and preventability of adverse drug events among older persons in the ambulatory setting. JAMA. 2003;289:1107-16.
3. Bates DW, Cullen DJ, Laird N, et al. Incidence of adverse drug events and potential adverse drug events. JAMA. 1995;274:29-34.
4. Pharmacovigilance and international health. The importance of pharmacovigilance, safety monitoring of medicinal products. WHO Bulletin, 2002.
5. Meyboom RHB, Egberts ACG, Gribnau FWJ, Hekster YA. Pharmacovigilance in perspective. Drug Safety. 1999;21(6):429-47.

6. Abbing HDCR. Legal aspects of medical devices: Study on regulatory mechanisms for safety control. Health services Research. IOS Press. 1993.pp.358-361.
7. Fracchia GN, Theofilatou M (eds); Mehta U, Milstien JB, Duclos P, Folbe Pl. Developing a national system for dealing with adverse events following immunization. Bull World Health Organ. 2000;78(2);170-7.
8. Craven BM, Stewart GT, Khan M, Chan TYK. Monitoring the safety of herbal medicines. Drug Safety. 1997;17(4):209-15.
9. A short history of involvement in drug safety monitoring by WHO. The importance of pharmacovigilance, safety monitoring of medicinal products. WHO Bulletin, 2002.
10. Siramshetty VB, Nickel J, Omieczynski C, Gohlke BO, Drwal MN, Preissner R. WITHDRAWN—a resource for withdrawn and discontinued drugs. Nucleic Acids Res. 2016;44(D1):D1080-6.

4

Current Methods of Pharmacovigilance

Arani Chatterjee, Manoj Sharma, SK Gupta

Information for the readers for their better understanding on various methods adopted for the conduct of Post Marketing Surveillance has been provided in the chapter entitled "Post Marketing Surveillance". This chapter envisages in providing further detailed information on various methods used to conduct pharmacovigilance.

Here, it should be noted that the term Pharmacovigilance is an umbrella term and covers the "Post Marketing Surveillance" also.

Pharmacovigilance is defined by the World Health Organization (WHO) as 'the science and activities relating to the detection, assessment, understanding and prevention of adverse effects or any other possible drug-related problems'.

The role of pharmacovigilance can be divided into three main areas:
- To identify, quantify and document drug-related problems
- To contribute to reduce the risk of drug-related problems in healthcare systems
- To increase knowledge and understanding of factors and mechanisms which are responsible for drug-related injuries.

PHARMACOVIGILANCE METHODS

As per the ICH-E2E[1] guidelines the pharmacovigilance method can be categorized as:
- Passive surveillance
  - Spontaneous reporting
  - Case series
- Stimulated reporting
- Active surveillance
  - Sentinel sites
  - Drug event monitoring
  - Registries
- Comparative observational studies
  - Cross-sectional study (survey)
  - Case-control study
  - Cohort study
- Targeted clinical investigations
- Descriptive studies
  - Natural history of disease
  - Drug utilization study.

Pharmacoepidemiological *(Pharmacoepidemiology is the science concerned with the benefit and risk of drugs used in populations and the analysis of the outcomes of drug therapies)* methods are also used as tools in pharmacovigilance for generating initial suspicions (Hypothesis generation methods) or testing hypotheses (Hypothesis testing methods) about changes in adverse effect profiles of medicines. The details of these two methods is provided as below:
- Hypothesis-generating methods
  - Spontaneous ADR reporting
  - Prescription event monitoring (PEM)

Hypothesis-generating studies, with a recently marketed drug, aim to provide unexpected ADRs.

- Hypothesis-testing methods
  - Case control studies
  - Cohort studies
  - Randomized controlled trials

Hypothesis-testing studies aim to prove whether any suspicions that may have been raised are justified.

Passive Surveillance

Spontaneous Reports

"A spontaneous report is an **unsolicited** communication by healthcare professionals or consumers to a company, regulatory authority or other organization (e.g. WHO, Regional Centres, Poison Control Centre) that describes one or more adverse drug reactions in a patient who was given one or more medicinal products and that does not derive from a study or any organized data collection scheme.[1] *This type of report is voluntary in nature (voluntary reporting), i.e. it may be initiated by the health care professionals or consumers as and when they become suspicious of any adverse reaction by any medication.*

Doctors (prescribers) or other health care professionals (e.g. pharmacists, nurses) are provided with a form (*see* annexures 1,2,3,4 for the suspected ADR reporting forms) for filling the details of the suspected ADR experienced by the patient along with the details of the suspected medication, patient details and the details of the doctor (or prescriber). These forms are generated by the concerned regulatory authority or the organizations working under the aegis of the government regulatory authorities; these are either provided on the websites or distributed to the health care professional through various training programmes conducted by the personals working in the area of pharmacovigilance or distributed by the sponsors which in most of the cases is a pharmaceutical company or a medical device manufacturing company. These filled forms are then notified to the central authority (country's governmental body) which is usually the drug regulatory authority (e.g. DCGI i.e. Drug Controller General India for India; USFDA for United States of America; TGA, i.e. Therapeutic and Goods Administration for Australia; MHRA for UK; BfARM for Germany; AFFSAPS for France, etc.).

In India, the form used for the spontaneous reporting is known as "Suspected Adverse Drug Reaction Reporting Form (Annexures 1A and 1B)" generated by CDSCO (Central Drug Standard Control Organization) working under the aegis of Directorate General of Health Services (DGHS), Government of India.

In the United Kingdom the form used for the spontaneous reporting is known as "Yellow Card". This has been used for the purpose of spontaneous reporting since 1964. The form is available separately for the **patients (patient reporting form)** and for the **health care professionals (health care professional reporting form)** (*see* Annexures 2A and 2B).

In the United States, the "Med Watch" form (Annexures 3A and 3B) is used in two different categories:

- **Form FDA 3500-Voluntary Reporting:** For use by health professionals, consumers and patients.
- **Form FDA 3500A-Mandatory Reporting:** For use by IND reporters, manufacturers, distributors, importers, user facilities personnel.

Similar forms are provided in the FP10 prescriptions pads, the British National Formulary, and other sources.

Although physicians and other health care professionals are encouraged to report new and unusual adverse drug reactions to the FDA, the system relies heavily on pharmaceutical manufacturers, whose field representatives and headquarters regulatory personnel are often the first to identify a potential reportable event. Here it should be noted that a pharmaceutical manufacturer is legally required to report serious unlabeled (not mentioned in the package insert or summary of product characteristic) adverse reactions to the Food and Drug Administration (FDA) with in 15 working days (or as per the applicable regulatory procedures) of learning of adverse reactions. Approximately, 80% of spontaneous reports about adverse drug reactions come to the FDA through drug companies.

Reporting of adverse reactions fluctuates with the length of time the drug has been on the market. The marketing of a new drug usually involves a slow release onto the market, which causes a slow rise in ADR reports. According to Weber,[2] the total number of ADR report increases until two year after the introduction and declines thereafter.

Spontaneous reports play a major role in the identification of safety signals once a drug is marketed. This has the potential to capture rare, unexpected adverse reactions more quickly than other study designs. In many instances, a company can be alerted to rare adverse events that were not detected in earlier clinical trials or other pre-marketing studies. Spontaneous reports can also provide important information on at-risk groups, risk factors, and clinical features of known serious adverse drug reactions. Caution should be exercised in evaluating spontaneous reports, especially when comparing drugs. The data accompanying spontaneous reports are often incomplete, and the rate at which cases are reported is dependent on many factors including the time since launch, pharmacovigilance-related regulatory activity, media attention, and the indication for use of the drug (Box 4.1).[3-6]

The various strengths and weaknesses of a spontaneous reporting system has been dealt in a separate chapter on "Postmarketing Surveillance"

Case Series

Case report describes the particular outcome or experience of a person who has been exposed to a drug. These reports are useful for generating hypotheses about the effects of the drug, and may lead to further studies to test these hypotheses. A case series, reports on two or more people with common exposure to a drug, or a common outcome.

Series of case reports can provide evidence of an association between a drug and an adverse event, but they are generally more useful for generating hypotheses than for verifying an association between drug exposure and outcome. There are certain distinct adverse events known to be associated

Box 4.1: Methods for the evaluation of spontaneous reports

More recently, systematic methods for the detection of safety signals from spontaneous reports have been used. Many of these techniques are still in development and their usefulness for identifying safety signals is being evaluated. These methods include the calculation of the proportional reporting ratio, as well as the use of Bayesian and other techniques for signal detection.[7-8] Data mining techniques have also been used to examine drug-drug interactions.[7-8] Data mining techniques should always be used in conjunction with, and not in place of, analyzes of single case reports. Data mining techniques facilitate the evaluation of spontaneous reports by using statistical methods to detect potential signals for further evaluation. This tool does not quantify the magnitude of risk, and caution should be exercised when comparing drugs. Further, when using data mining techniques, consideration should be given to the threshold established for detecting signals, since this will have implications for the sensitivity and specificity of the method (a high threshold is associated with high specificity and low sensitivity). Confounding factors that influence spontaneous adverse event reporting are not removed by data mining. Results of data mining should be interpreted with the knowledge of the weaknesses of the spontaneous reporting system and, more specifically, the large differences in the ADR reporting rate among different drugs and the many potential biases inherent in spontaneous reporting. All signals should be evaluated recognizing the possibility of false positives. In addition, the absence of a signal does not mean that a problem does not exist.

False positives: *A test result that shows evidence of a disease or an abnormal condition although it (the condition being tested for) is not present. In statistics it is also known as type I error or α-error.*

more frequently with drug therapy, such as anaphylaxis, plastic anemia, toxic epidermal necrolysis and Stevens-Johnson syndrome.[10,11] Therefore, when events such as these are spontaneously reported, sponsors should place more emphasis on these reports for detailed and rapid follow-up.

Example of Case Series:

For the evaluation of the preliminary efficacy and safety of alefacept in the treatment of moderate to severe mucosal lichen planus (LP)[12] seven subjects were randomly selected to receive either alefacept 15 mg or placebo every week for 12 weeks. Endpoints of the case series were the Physician Global Assessment (PGA) of disease severity, mucosal pain (MP) severity, and itch severity (IS). Two of the subjects receiving alefacept achieved significant improvement during the study. There were no serious adverse events during the course of the study period. In this small case series, alefacept may have conferred a modest therapeutic response in erosive LP. It was concluded that larger multicentric prospective studies will be needed to determine whether alefacept can improve erosive LP in a statistically significant way.

Stimulated Reporting

Stimulated reports are those that may have been motivated, prompted or induced and can occur in certain situations, such as notification by a Health Care Professional Communication (HCPC), public advisory, literature report, publication in the press, or questioning of health care professionals by MAH representatives. These reports should be considered unsolicited in nature and as a form of spontaneous reporting. Data obtained from stimulated reporting cannot be used to generate accurate incidence rates, but can be used to estimate reporting rates. Several methods have been used to encourage and facilitate reporting by health professionals in specific situations (e.g. in-hospital settings) for new products or for limited time periods.[13] Such methods include on-line reporting of adverse events and systematic stimulation of reporting of adverse events based on a pre-designed method. Although, these methods have been shown to improve reporting, they are not devoid of the limitations of passive surveillance, especially selective reporting and incomplete information.

During the early postmarketing phase, companies might actively provide health professionals with safety information and at the same time encourage cautious use of new products and the submission of spontaneous reports when an adverse event is identified. A plan can be developed before the product is launched (e.g. through site visits by company representatives, by direct mailings or faxes, etc.). Stimulated adverse event reporting in the early postmarketing phase can lead companies to notify healthcare professionals of new therapies and provide safety information early in use by the general population [e.g. early postmarketing phase vigilance (EPPV) in Japan].

Active Surveillance

Active surveillance, in contrast to passive surveillance, seeks to ascertain completely the number of adverse events via a continuous preorganised process. An example of active surveillance is the follow-up of patients treated with a particular drug through a risk management programme. Patients who fill a prescription for this drug may be asked to complete a brief survey form and give permission for later contact.[13] In general, it is more feasible to get comprehensive data (complete or widespread data) on individual adverse event reports through an active surveillance system rather than through a passive surveillance system. The various methods to get the comprehensive data through active surveillance are depicted below.

Sentinel Sites

Active surveillance can be achieved by reviewing medical records or interviewing patients and/or physicians in a sample of sentinel sites to ensure complete and accurate data on reported adverse events from these sites. The selected sites can provide information, such as data from specific patient subgroups that would not be availal le in a passive spontaneous reporting system. Further, information on the use of a drug, such as abuse, can be targeted at selected sentinel sites.[14] Some of the major weaknesses of sentinel sites are problems with selection bias, small numbers of patients, and increased costs. Active surveillance with sentinel sites is most efficient for those drugs used mainly in institutional settings such as hospitals, nursing homes, hemodialysis centres, etc. Institutional settings can have a greater frequency of use for certain drug products and can provide an infrastructure for dedicated reporting. In addition, automatic detection of abnormal laboratory values from computerized laboratory reports in certain clinical settings can provide an efficient active surveillance system. Intensive monitoring of sentinel sites can also be helpful in identifying risks among patients taking orphan drugs.

Drug Event Monitoring

Drug event monitoring is a method of active pharmacovigilance surveillance. In drug event monitoring, patients might be identified from electronic prescription data or automated health insurance claims. A follow-up questionnaire can then be sent to each prescribing physician or patient at pre-specified intervals to obtain outcome information. Information on patient demographics, indication for treatment, duration of therapy (including start dates), dosage, clinical events, and reasons for discontinuation can be included in the questionnaire.[15-18]

Limitations of drug event monitoring may include:
- Poor physician and patient response rates
- Unfocused nature of data collection, which can obscure important signals.

In addition to the above mentioned limitations maintenance of patient confidentiality might be a concern. On the other hand, more detailed information on adverse events from a large number of physicians and/or patients might be collected.

Registries

A registry is a list of patients presenting with the same characteristic(s). This characteristic can be a disease (disease registry) or a specific exposure (drug registry). Both types of registries, which only differ by the type of patient data of interest, can collect a battery of information using standardized questionnaires in a prospective fashion. Disease registries, such as registries for blood dyscrasias, severe cutaneous reactions, or congenital malformations can help collect data on drug exposure and other factors associated with a clinical condition. A disease registry might also be used as a base for a case-control study comparing the drug exposure of cases identified from the registry and controls selected from either patients with another condition within the registry, or patients outside the registry.

Exposure (drug) registries address populations exposed to drugs of interest (e.g. registry of rheumatoid arthritis patients exposed to biological therapies) to determine if a drug has a special impact on this group of patients. Some exposure (drug) registries address drug exposures in specific populations, such as pregnant women. Patients can be followed over time and included in a cohort study to collect data on adverse events using standardized questionnaires. Single cohort studies can measure incidence, but, without a comparison group, cannot provide proof of association. However, they can be useful for signal amplification, particularly for rare outcomes. This type of registry can be very valuable when examining the safety of an orphan drug indicated for a specific condition.

Example of registry:

Survival trends between the years 2000 and 2004 for 20 common cancers based on follow-up data from **12 cancer registries** *(disease registry)* from diverse areas of Europe using model-based period analysis techniques were examined.[19] Between 2000 and 2004, marked rises were seen in 5-year relative survival amongst patients with prostate, breast and colorectal cancer, which were statistically significant in 10, 8 and 7 of the 12 participating cancer registries, respectively. For cancer sites amenable to effective early detection and treatment, major geographical differences in patient prognosis still persisted, with a lower survival generally observed in Eastern European countries. It was concluded that model-based period analysis enables the timely monitoring of recent trends in population-based cancer survival. For colorectal and breast cancers, the identified rises in survival are probably (at least partly) explained by the improvements in clinical care and the management of the disease. Nevertheless, persisting geographic differences do point to the potential for a further reduction in the burden of cancer throughout Europe, towards which improvements in diverse areas of care, including secondary prevention, access to advances in treatment as well as subspecialization and regionalization of oncologic care may all contribute.

Comparative Observational Studies

Traditional epidemiologic methods are a key component in the evaluation of adverse events. There are a number of observational study designs that are useful in validating signals from spontaneous reports or case series. Major types of these designs are cross-sectional studies, case-control studies, and cohort studies (both retrospective and prospective).[15,16]

Cross-sectional Study (Survey)

Data collected on a population of patients at a single point in time (or interval of time) regardless of exposure or disease status constitute a cross-sectional study. These types of studies are primarily used to gather data for surveys or for ecological analyses. The major drawback of cross-sectional studies is that the temporal relationship between exposure and outcome cannot be directly addressed. These studies are best used to examine the prevalence of a disease at one time point or to examine trends over time, when data for serial time points can be captured. These studies can also be used to examine the crude association between exposure and outcome in ecologic analyses. Cross-sectional studies are best utilized when exposures do not change over time.

Case-control Study

In a case-control study, cases of disease (or events) are identified. Controls, or patients without the disease or event of interest, are then selected from the source population that gave rise to the cases. The controls should be selected in such a way that the prevalence of exposure among the controls represents the prevalence of exposure in the source population. The exposure status of the two groups is then compared using the **odds ratio**, which is **an estimate of the relative risk of disease in the two groups**. Patients can be identified from an existing database or using data collected specifically for the purpose of the study of interest. If safety information is sought for special populations, the cases and controls can be stratified according to the population of interest (the elderly, children, pregnant women, etc.). For rare adverse events, existing large population-based databases are a useful and efficient means of providing

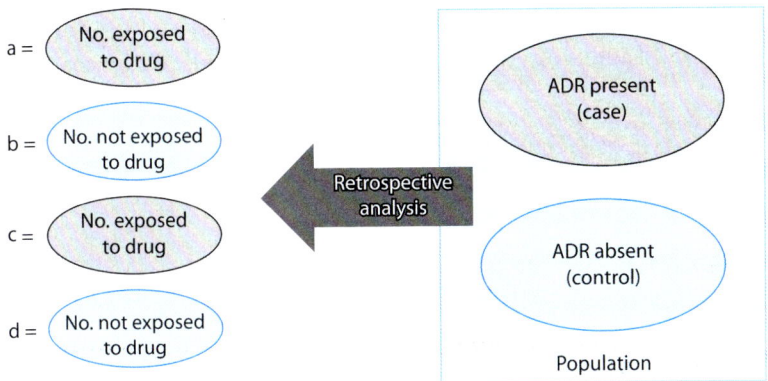

The odds ratio (OR) is a measure of the strength of association between the risk factor (exposure to the drug) and the disease or outcome (presence of a suspected adverse reaction), and is measured as odds or exposure among the cases against the odds of exposure among the controls

$$OR = \frac{a/(a+c)/c(a+c)}{b/(b+d)/d(b+d)} = \frac{ad}{bc}$$

Fig. 4.1: Retrospective case-control study

needed drug exposure and medical outcome data in a relatively short period of time. Case-control studies are particularly useful when the goal is to investigate whether there is an association between a drug (or drugs) and one specific rare adverse event, as well as to identify risk factors for adverse events. Risk factors can include conditions such as renal and hepatic dysfunction that might modify the relationship between the drug exposure and the adverse event. Under specific conditions, a case-control study can provide the absolute incidence rate of the event. If all cases of interest (or a well-defined fraction of cases) in the catchment area are captured and the fraction of controls from the source population is known, an incidence rate can be calculated (Fig. 4.1).

Cohort Study

In a cohort study, a population-at-risk for the disease (or event) is followed over time for the occurrence of the disease (or event). Information on exposure status is known throughout the follow-up period for each patient. A patient might be exposed to a drug at one time during follow-up, but non-exposed at another time point. Since, the population exposure during follow-up is known, incidence rates can be calculated. In many cohort studies involving drug exposure, comparison cohorts of interest are selected on the basis of drug use and followed over time. Cohort studies are useful when there is a need to know the incidence rates of adverse events in addition to the relative risks of adverse events. Multiple adverse events can also be investigated using the same data source in a cohort study (Fig. 4.2). However, it can be difficult to recruit sufficient numbers of patients who are exposed to a drug of interest (such as an orphan drug) or to study very rare outcomes. Like case-control studies, the identification of patients for cohort studies can come from large automated databases or from data collected specifically for the study at hand. In addition, cohort studies can be used to examine safety issues in special populations (the elderly, children, patients with comorbid conditions, pregnant women) through over-sampling of these patients or by stratifying the cohort if sufficient numbers of patients exist. There are several automated databases available for pharmacoepidemiologic studies.[15,16,20]

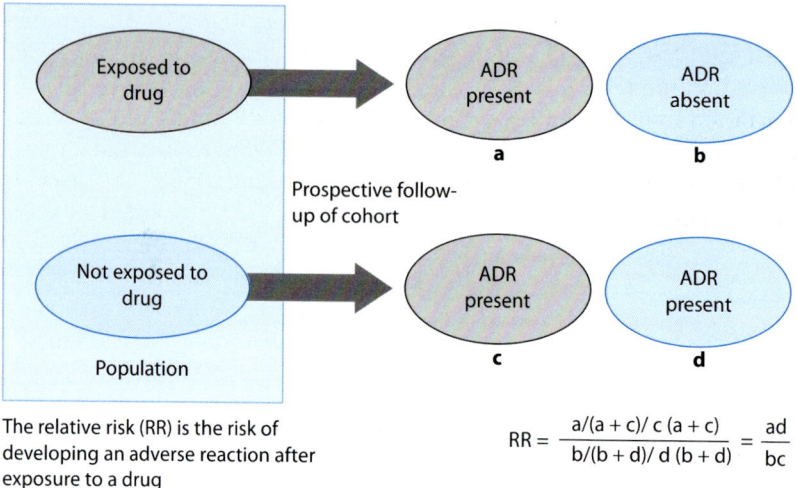

Fig. 4.2: Cohort study

They include databases which contain automated medical records or automated accounting/billing systems. Databases that are created from accounting/billing systems might be linked to pharmacy claims and medical claims databases. These datasets might include millions of patients. Since, they are created for administrative or billing purposes, they might not have the detailed and accurate information needed for some research, such as validated diagnostic information or laboratory data. Although, medical records can be used to ascertain and validate test results and medical diagnoses, one should be cognizant of the privacy and confidentiality regulations that apply to patient medical records.

Targeted Clinical Investigations

When significant risks are identified from pre-approval clinical trials, further clinical studies might be called for to evaluate the mechanism of action for the adverse reaction. In some instances, pharmacodynamic and pharmacokinetic studies might be conducted to determine whether a particular dosing instruction can put patients at an increased risk of adverse events. Genetic testing can also provide clues about which group of patients might be at an increased risk of adverse reactions. Furthermore, based on the pharmacological properties and the expected use of the drug in general practice, conducting specific studies to investigate potential drug-drug interactions and food-drug interactions might be called for. These studies can include population pharmacokinetic studies and drug concentration monitoring in patients and normal volunteers. Sometimes, potential risks or unforeseen benefits in special populations might be identified from pre-approval clinical trials, but cannot be fully quantified due to small sample sizes or the exclusion of subpopulations of patients from these clinical studies. These populations might include the elderly, children, or patients with renal or hepatic disorder. Children, the elderly, and patients with comorbid conditions might metabolise drugs differently than patients typically enrolled in clinical trials. Further clinical trials might be used to determine and to quantify the magnitude of the risk (or benefit) in such populations. To elucidate the benefit-risk profile of a drug outside of the formal/traditional clinical trial setting and/or to fully quantify the risk of a critical but relatively rare adverse event, a large simplified trial might be conducted. Patients enrolled in a large simplified trial are usually randomized to avoid selection bias. In this type of trial, though, the event of interest will be focused to ensure a convenient and practical study. One limitation of this method is that the outcome measure might be too simplified and this might have an impact on the quality and ultimate usefulness of the trial. Large, simplified trials are also resource-intensive.

Descriptive Studies

Descriptive studies are an important component of pharmacovigilance, although not for the detection or verification of adverse events associated with drug exposures. These studies are primarily used to obtain the background rate of outcome events and/or establish the prevalence of the use of drugs in specified populations.

Natural History of Disease

The science of epidemiology originally focused on the natural history of disease, including the characteristics of diseased patients and the distribution of disease in selected populations, as well as estimating the incidence and prevalence of potential outcomes of interest. These outcomes of interest now include a description of disease treatment patterns and adverse events. Studies that examine specific aspects of adverse events, such as the background incidence rate of or risk factors for the adverse event of interest can be used to assist in putting spontaneous reports into perspective.[16] For example, an epidemiologic study can be conducted using a disease registry to understand the frequency at which the event of interest might occur in specific subgroups, such as patients with concomitant illnesses.

Drug Utilization Study

Drug utilization studies (DUSs) describe how a drug is marketed, prescribed, and used in a population, and how these factors influence outcomes, including clinical, social, and economic outcomes.[15] These studies provide data on specific populations, such as the elderly, children, or patients with hepatic or renal dysfunction, often stratified by age, gender, concomitant medication, and other characteristics. DUS can be used to determine if a product is being used in these populations. From these studies denominator data can be developed for use in determining rates of adverse drug reactions. DUS have been used to describe the effect of regulatory actions and media attention on the use of drugs, as well as to develop estimates of the economic burden of the cost of drugs. DUS can be used to examine the relationship between recommended and actual clinical practice. These studies can help to determine whether a drug has the potential for drug abuse by examining whether patients are taking escalating dose regimens or whether there is evidence of inappropriate repeat prescribing. Important limitations of these studies can include a lack of clinical outcome data or information of the indication for use of a product.

It should be noted that the best method to address a specific situation can vary depending on the product, the indication, the population being treated and the issue to be addressed. The method chosen can also depend on whether an identified risk, potential risk or missing information is the issue and whether signal detection, evaluation or safety demonstration is the main objective of further study. When choosing a method to address a safety concern, the most appropriate design should be employed.

METHODS FOR VACCINE SAFETY[21-23]

A vaccine is a biological preparation that improves immunity to a particular disease. A vaccine typically contains an agent that resembles a disease-causing microorganism, and is often made from weakened or killed forms of the microbe, its toxins or one of its surface proteins. The agent stimulates the body's immune system to recognize the agent as foreign, destroy it, and "remember" it, so that the immune system can more easily recognize and destroy any of these microorganisms that it later encounters.

Each year, vaccines prevent more than 2.5 million child deaths globally. Although, vaccines used in national immunization programmes (NIPs) are considered as safe and effective when used correctly, however vaccines are not risk-free as adverse events will occasionally occur following vaccination.

Although most adverse events are minor (e.g. redness at injection site, fever), more serious reactions (e.g. seizures, anaphylaxis) can occur at a very low frequency.

The general public has low tolerance to any adverse events following vaccination because vaccines are given to healthy persons to prevent disease. For this reason, a higher standard of safety is expected of immunizations compared with medications that are used to treat people who are sick (e.g. antibiotics, insulin). This lower tolerance for risks from vaccines translates into a greater need to detect and investigate any adverse event following immunization (AEFI) than is generally expected for other pharmaceutical products.

An AEFI is defined as a medical incident that takes place after an immunization, causes concern, and is believed to be caused by immunization.

Types of AEFI

AEFIs can be classified into five types:[21]
1. Vaccine reaction
2. Programme error
3. Coincidental reactions
4. Injection reaction
5. Unknown

Isolated and Clusters of AEFI[21]

Isolated AEFI

This is a solitary medical incident that takes place after immunization, causes concern and is believed to be caused by immunization.

Table 4.1: Types of AEFIs[21]

Type	Definition	Example
	1. Vaccine reaction: An event caused or precipitated by the active component or one of the other components of the vaccine (e.g. adjuvant, preservative and stabilizer). This is due to the inherent properties of the vaccine	• High-grade fever following DPT vaccination • Anaphylaxis
	2. Programme error: An event caused by an error in vaccine preparation, handling or administration	Bacterial abscess due to unsterile injection/wrong diluent
	3. Coincidental. An event that occurs after immunization but is not caused by the vaccine. This is due to a chance temporal association	Pneumonia after oral polio vaccine administration
	4. Injection reaction: Event caused by anxiety about, or pain from the injection itself rather than the vaccine	Fainting spell after immunization
	5. Unknown The cause of the event cannot be determined	Does not fit into any of the above four types

Current Methods of Pharmacovigilance 35

Table 4.2 : Common programme errors leading to AEFIs[21]

Programme errors		Possible AEFI
Non-sterile injection		
	• Contact of needle with unsterile surface e.g. finger, swab, table, etc. • Contaminated vaccine or diluent Administering injection over clothes • Improper handling of vaccine vials like touching of septum	Infection, e.g. local abscess at site of injection, sepsis
	• Use of reconstituted vaccines beyond the stipulated time (4 hours for BCG and measles, 2 hours for Japanese encephalitis) • Reuse of reconstituted vaccine at subsequent sessions	Toxic shock syndrome or death
	• Reuse of disposable syringe and needle • Improper storage and handling of syringes and needles leading to loss of sterility. • Syringes and needles used after expiry date	
		Blood-borne infections, e.g. Hep B, HIV, Hep C, etc. Abscess
Reconstitution error/ Wrong vaccine preparation		
	• Reconstitution with incorrect diluent • Reuse of the reconstitution syringe • Use of expired vaccine or diluents • Drug substituted for diluent • Inadequate shaking of T-series vaccines	• Less vaccine effectiveness • Drug reaction; Death • Local abscess
Injection at incorrect site/route		
	Injection into gluteal region (buttocks)	Sciatic nerve damage, paralysis
	BCG/T series vaccine given subcutaneously	Local reaction or abscess
Vaccine transportation/storage incorrect		
	Improper storage of vaccines like freezing of T-series vaccines and subsequent administration of frozen and thawed freeze-sensitive vaccine	Increased local reaction such as sterile abscess Less vaccine effectiveness
Contraindications ignored		
	DPT2 given after history of convulsions with DPT1	More severe convulsions

Cluster AEFI

A cluster is defined as two or more cases of the same or similar event, which is related in time, and has occurred within the same district or geographical unit, or associated with the same vaccine, same batch number administered or same vaccinator.

Vaccine Adverse Event Reporting System (VAERS),[24] is the national postmarketing safety monitoring system that accepts reports about adverse events that occur after administration of US licensed vaccines.

In India, Ministry of Health and Family Welfare Government of India has developed Standard Operating Procedures for Investigation of Adverse Event Following Immunization (AEFI).[21] The details of reporting system of AEFI has been provided in the National AEFI Surveillance and response Operational Guidelines, 2010. The non-serious AEFI should be reported "routinely" on a monthly basis and the serious AEFI should be reported immediately and also included in the monthly report and the line list

There are two channels of reporting AEFIs:
1. Monthly routine reporting
2. Immediate serious AEFI reporting

Monthly Routine Reporting

This includes reporting of all non-serious and serious AEFIs from the level of Health worker (Auxiliary Nurse Midwife or ANM) up to the National level (coordinated by the district) through monthly progress reports using existing immunization monthly progress reports/forms (vary from state to state). It is necessary for the ANM to submit "Nil" report in case no AEFI case detected from her area during the month. This information is collated and compiled by health workers in monthly reporting formats under the heading of "Any untoward reactions or reportable AEFIs" and forwarded to the next level. These include:
1. Deaths
2. Injection site abscesses
3. High-grade fever (>102° F)
4. Persistent inconsolable screaming (>3 hours)
5. Seizure
6. Hypotonic hyporesponsive episode (HHE)
7. Other complications (including the cases not listed above such as severe local reaction, brachial neuritis, thrombocytopenia, lymphadenitis, disseminated BCG infection, osteitis/osteomyelitis and any untoward incident that the vaccinator, ANM, Medical Officer think is a result of immunization.

Immediate Notification of Serious AEFI

The serious AEFI is defined as "any untoward medical occurrence that results in death, hospitalization or prolongation of hospitalization, persistent or significant disability/incapacity, or is life-threatening". All serious AEFI are to be immediately notified by the first person who identifies the event. This 'first' person should notify the case to the nearest government Primary Health Centre (PHC), Community Health Centre (CHC) and or the District Immunization Officer (DIO)/ by quickest means of communication, e.g. telephone, messenger, etc. All persons involved in reporting AEFI should be aware of the timeline and channels of reporting. Notification should be followed up with a First Information Report (FIR) as mentioned in Annexure 4.

The Process of Reporting Serious AEFIs

In India, the following reporting reports are used to guide AEFI investigation and causality assessment.
1. First Information Report (FIR): Annexure 4.
2. Preliminary Investigation Report (PIR): Annexure 5.
3. Detailed Investigation Report (DIR): Annexure 6.
4. AEFI- Laboratory Requisition Form: Annexure 7

The case definitions of some reportable adverse events are mentioned in Table 4.3.

These events are an emergency and need to be immediately investigated, managed and reported on standardized AEFI formats. Each serious event(s) should be followed up to determine the cause for its occurrence (causality assessment).

Table 4.3: Case definitions of some reportable adverse events[21]

AEFI	Case definition	Vaccine
Vaccine associated paralytic poliomyelitis (presenting as AFP)	An acute flaccid paralysis 4–30 days following receipt of OPV, or within 4–75 day after contact with a recipient of OPV, with neurological deficits remaining 60 days after onset, of death	OPV
Anaphylactoid reaction (acute hypersensitivity reaction)	Exaggerated acute allergic reaction, occurring within 2 hours after immunization, characterized by one or more of the following: • Wheezing and shortness of breath due to bronchospasm • Laryngospasm/laryngeal edema • One or more skin manifestation, e.g. hives, facial edema, or generalized edema Do not report less severe allergic reactions	All
Anaphylaxis	Severe immediate (within 1 hour) allergic reaction leading to circulatory failure with or without bronchospasm and/or laryngospasm/laryngeal edema	All
Disseminated BCG infections	Widespread infection occurring within 1 to 12 months after BCG vaccination of confirmed by isolation of *Mycobacterium bovis* BCG strain. Usually in immunecompromised individuals	BCG
Encephalopathy	Acute onset of major illness characterized by any two of the following three conditions: • Seizures • Severe alteration in level consciousness lasting for one day or more • Distinct change in behavior lasting one day or more. Needs to occur within 48 hours of DPT vaccine of from 7 to 12 days after measles vaccine, to be related to immunization	Measles, pertussis
Fever	The fever can be classified (based on temperature) such as • Mild fever: 100.4°F to 102°F (38 to 38.9°C) • High fever: 102°F to 104.7° (39 to 40.4°C) • Extreme fever: 104.7°F or higher (> 40.5°C)	All
Hypotonic, hyporesponsive episode (HHE or shock-collapse)	Event of sudden onset occurring within 48 [usually less than 12] hours of vaccination and lasting from one minute to several hours, in children younger than 10 years of age. All of the following must be present: • Limpness (hypotonic) • Reduced responsiveness (hyporesponsive) • Pallor or cyanosis or failure to observe/recall	Mainly DPT, rarely others
Injection site abscess	• Fluctuant or draining fluid filled lesion at the site of injection • Bacterial if evidence of infection (e.g. purulent, inflammatory signs, fever, culture), sterile abscess if no evidence of bacterial infection on culture. Sterile abscesses are usually due to the inherent properties of the vaccine	All injectable vaccines
Lymphadenitis (includes suppurative lymphadenitis)	• Either at least one lymph nodes enlarged to >1.5 cm in size (one adult finger width) or a draining sinus over a lymph node • Almost exclusively caused by BCG and then occurring within 2 to 6 months after receipt of BCG vaccine, on the same side as inoculation (mostly axillary)	BCG
Osteitis/Osteomyelitis	Inflammation of the bone with isolation of *Mycobacterium bovis* BCG stain	BCG
Persistent inconsolable screaming	Inconsolable continuous crying lasting 3 hours or longer accompanied by high pitched screaming	DPT, pertussis

Contd...

Contd...

AEFI	Case definition	Vaccine
Seizures	Occurrence of generalized convulsion that are not accompanied by focal neurological signs or symptoms. Febrile seizures: if temperature elevated >100.4°F or 38°C (rectal) Afebrile seizures: If temperature is normal	All, especially pertussis, measles
Sepsis	Acute onset of severe generalized illness due to bacterial infection and confirmed (if possible) by positive blood culture. Needs to be reported as possible indicator of programme error	All injectable vaccines
Severe local reaction	Redness and/or swelling centred at the site of injection and one or more of the following: • Swelling beyond the nearest joint • Pain, redness, and swelling of more than 3 days • Requires hospitalization Local reactions of lesser intensity occur commonly and are trivial and do not need to be reported	All injectable vaccines
TSS	Abrupt onset of fever, vomiting and watery diarrhea within a few hours of immunization. Often leading to death within 24 to 48 hours. Report as a possible indicator of programme error.	All injectable vaccines

Abbreviations: BCG, Bacillus-Calmette-Guerin; OPV, oral polio vaccine; DPT, diphtheria, pertussis tetanus; TSS, toxic shock syndrome

REFERENCES

1. ICH Topic E2E Pharmacovigilance Planning (Pvp) June 2005 CPMP/ICH/5716/03.
2. Weber JCP. Epidemiology of adverse reactions to non steroid anti-inflammatory drugs. Advances in Inflammation Research, Volume 6. New York: Raven Press; 1984.
3. Pinkston V, Swain EJ. Management of adverse drug reactions and adverse event data through collection, storage, and retrieval. In: Stephens MDB, Talbot JCC, Routledge PA. (Eds.) Detection of New Adverse Drug Reactions. 4th edition. 1998; MacMillan Reference Ltd, London. p. 282.
4. Goldman SA. Limitations and strengths of spontaneous reports data. Clinical Therapeutics. 1998; 20 (Suppl C):C40-C44.
5. Faich GA. US adverse drug reaction surveillance 1989-1994. Pharmacoepidemiol Drug Saf. 1996;393-8.
6. Hartmann K, Doser AK, Kuhn M, Postmarketing safety information: how useful are spontaneous reports. Pharmacoepidemiol Drug Saf. 1999;8:S65-S71.
7. DuMouchel W. Bayesian data mining in large frequency tables, with an application to the FDA Spontaneous Reporting system. Am Stat. 1999;53:177-90.
8. Bate A, Lindquist M, Edwards IR. A Bayesian neural network method for adverse drug reaction signal generation. Eur J Clin Pharmacology. 1998;54:315-21.
9. Van Puijenbroek E, Egberts ACG, Heerdink ER, Leufkens HGM. Detecting drug-drug interactions using a database for spontaneous adverse drug reactions: an example with diuretics and non-steroidal anti-inflammatory drugs. Eur J Clin Pharmacol. 2000;56:733-8.
10. Venning GR. Identification of adverse reactions to new drugs. III: Alerting processes and early warning systems. BMJ. 1983;286:458-60.
11. Edwards IR. The management of adverse drug reactions: From diagnosis to signal. Thérapie 2001;56:727-33.
12. Chang AL, Badger J, Rehmus W, Kimball AB. Alefacept for erosive lichen planus: a case series. J Drugs Dermatol. 2008;7(4):379-83.
13. Mitchell AA, Van Bennekom CM, Louik C. A pregnancy-prevention program in women of childbearing age receiving isotretinoin. N Engl J Med. 1995;333(2):101-6.
14. Task Force on Risk Management. Report to the FDA Commissioner. Managing the risks from medical product use: Creating a risk management framework. Part 3. How does

FDA conduct postmarketing surveillance and risk assessment. 1999.
15. Strom BL (Ed.). Pharmacoepidemiology, 3rd edition. 2002; John Wiley and Sons, Ltd, New York, NY.
16. Mann RD, Andrews EB (Eds.). Pharmacovigilance 2002, John Wiley and Sons, Ltd, West Sussex, England.
17. Coulter DM. The New Zealand intensive medicines monitoring programme in pro-active safety surveillance. Pharmacoepidemiol Drug Saf. 2000;9: 273-80.
18. Mackay FJ, Post-marketing studies. The work of the Drug Safety Research Unit. Drug Saf. 1998;19:343-53.
19. Gondos A, Bray F, Brewster DH, Coebergh JW, Hakulinen T, Janssen-Heijnen ML, et al. The EUNICE Survival Working Group. Recent trends in cancer survival across Europe between 2000 and 2004: A model-based period analysis from 12 cancer registries. Eur J Cancer. 2008;44(10):1463-75. Epub 2008 Apr 30.
20. Garcia Rodriguez LA, Perez Gutthann S. Use of the UK General Practice Research Database for Pharmacoepidemiology. Br J Clin Pharmacol. 1998; 45:419-25.
21. Adverse Event Following Immunization. Standard Operating Procedure. Ministry of Health and Family Welfare, Govt. of India, New Delhi. 2010. p. 1-40.
22. Pillai RK. Epidemiological Methods for Pharmacovigilance. The case of Vaccine Safety. J Pharmacovigilance. 2015;3(3). http://dx.doi.org/10.4172/2329-6887.1000164.
23. http://vaccine-safety-training.org/Importance-of-immunization-programmes.html. Accessed on 03 Aug 2017.
24. https://www.cdc.gov/vaccinesafety/ensuringsafety/monitoring/vaers/index.html. Accessed on 03 Aug 2017.

5

Adverse Drug Reactions: Classification, Mechanism and Interaction

SK Gupta, Manoj Sharma, Arani Chatterjee

"Doctors are men who prescribe medicines of which they know little, to cure diseases of which they know less, in human being whom they know nothing."

—*Voltaire*

The World Health Organization (WHO) defines a drug/medicine as "any substance in a pharmaceutical product that is used to modify or explore physiological systems or pathological states for the benefit of the recipient." The term drug/medicinal product is used in a wider sense to include the whole formulated and registered product, including the presentation and packaging, and the accompanying information. As per WHO following are the definitions for adverse event/adverse experience (AE) and adverse drug reaction (ADR).

ADVERSE EVENT (OR ADVERSE EXPERIENCE)

'Any untoward medical occurrence that may appear during treatment with a pharmaceutical product but which does not necessarily have a causal relationship with the treatment.'

An adverse event (AE) can therefore be any unfavorable and unintended sign (including an abnormal laboratory finding, for example), symptom, or disease temporally associated with the use of a medicinal product, whether or not considered related to the medicinal product.

ADVERSE DRUG REACTION (ADR)

'A response to a drug which is noxious and unintended, and which occurs at doses normally used in man for the prophylaxis, diagnosis, or therapy of disease, or for the modification of physiological function.' This definition is a well accepted definition for the marketed products.

International Council for Harmonisation of Technical Requirements for Pharmaceuticals for Human Use (ICH) guidelines on Clinical Safety Data Management (E2A guidelines) further elaborates the definition of adverse drug reactions during the pre-approval (before marketing of the pharmaceutical product) phase. As per the ICH E2A[1] guidelines:

In the pre-approval clinical experience with a new medicinal product or its new usages, particularly as the therapeutic dose(s) may not be established: all noxious and unintended responses to a medicinal product related to any dose should be considered adverse drug reactions.

For the purpose of the recording or reporting, it is important that all adverse medical events rather than ADR or side effects are collected, as the term 'ADR' imply that the adverse medical event was caused by drug and, if the recorder is not certain whether the event was caused by a drug then it would not be recorded. The term 'adverse event' or 'adverse experience' is preferable and should be used in clinical trials[2-4] and post marketing.[5-6]

ADVERSE DRUG REACTIONS: IMPORTANCE

As evident from many clinical studies, adverse drug reactions are a major clinical problem. The studies have shown that they account for about 2–6% of all hospital admissions.[7-12] A meta-analysis have suggested that adverse drug reactions were between the fourth and sixth commonest cause of death in United States.[13] Surveys conducted recently have also shown that adverse drug events are associated with an increased length of stay in hospital of 2 days, thereby leading to an increased cost of approximately $2500 per patient. In addition to the above mentioned reasons adverse drug reactions may have many other indirect effects, which also provide their importance. The various **direct and indirect effects of adverse drug reactions** are given below:

- Adverse affect on patient quality of life
- Admission to hospitals or attendance in primary health centre
- Length of hospital stay gets increased (prolongation of inpatient hospitalization)
- Cost of patient care gets increased
- Patient may lose confidence in their treating doctor
- Adverse reactions may mimic disease and result in unnecessary investigations and/or delay in treatment procedures
- Adverse reactions may lead to death/permanent disability/congenital anomaly or birth defects.

The history of classification of adverse drug reactions based on dose relatedness and time course is shown in Table 5.1.

Table 5.1: The history of classification of adverse drug reactions

Year	Classification based on dose relatedness	Classification based on time course
1958[13]	Predictable effects ('toxic effects......related to the main action of the drug or to its side effects) and unpredictable effects (not related to the main or subsidiary pharmacological action of drug) were distinguished	
1973[14]	Dose related reactions (idiosyncratic and toxic) and non-dose related reactions (allergic) were distinguished	Acute, subacute and chronic toxic reactions
1976[15]	Dose related effects and non-dose related effects were distinguished	Long term and teratogenic effects
1977[16]	Two type of reactions *viz.* type A and type B were proposed	
1981[17]	Addition of a *mnemonic* to type A *(augmented)* and type B *(bizarre)*	
1984[18]	Further classification of type A and type B reactions as dose related and non-dose related reactions	Long term and delayed.
1990[19]		Acute, subacute and latent allergic reactions
1992[20,21]		Type C (long-term) and Type D (delayed) reactions Type C into two types: Type C (continuous) and Type E (End of use)

Contd...

Contd...

Year	Classification based on dose relatedness	Classification based on time course.
1997[22]		Five different patterns of time course that are useful in diagnosing adverse reactions were distinguished
2000[23]	Type F (Failure of therapy)	
2002[24]	Type G (genetic/genomic)	
2003[25]	Three types of dose related reactions (toxic, collateral and hypersusceptibility reactions)	Time dependent and time independent reactions with important subtypes were distinguished

RISK FACTORS FOR ADVERSE DRUG REACTIONS[26]

There is an effect of certain factors on the occurrence of adverse drug reactions. These factors mainly include:
I. Patient related factors
   a. Age
   b. Gender
   c. Maternity Status
   d. Fetal development status
   e. Creatinine clearance
   f. Allergic condition
   g. Fat distribution and body weight.
II. Social factors
   a. Race and Ethnicity
   b. Smoking
   c. Alcohol drinking
III. Drug related factors
   a. Drug Dose and Frequency
   b. Polypharmacy
IV. Disease related factors

Patient Related Factors

a. **Age:** Age is an important factor which affects the occurrence of ADRs. Elderly and pediatric patients are particularly vulnerable to ADRs because drugs are less likely to be studied in these age groups. Also drug absorption and metabolism is more variable and less predictable in both of these groups. In elderly, the factors like multiple drugs, multiple medical problems, reduced capacity to eliminate drugs make elderly patients more susceptible to adverse drug reactions. Infants and very young children are at high risk of ADRs because their capacity to metabolize the drug is not fully evaluated.

b. **Gender:** Gender plays an important role as there exist biological differences in terms of body weight, body composition, gastrointestinal tract factors, liver metabolism and renal function. Females have lower body weight, organ size, lower glomerular filtration rate (GFR) and more body fat, different gastric motility in comparison to male. These factors alter the pharmacokinetics and pharmacodynamics of the drugs including drug absorption, distribution, metabolism and elimination.

c. **Maternity status:** The physiologic changes during pregnancy mainly affect drug pharmacokinetics and pharmacodynamics. The renally excreted drugs would have an increased rate of excretion as there is an increase in renal plasma flow, increase in GFR during pregnancy. Also, motility, acidity and GIT tone are decreased during pregnancy which might interfere with drug absorption or excretion and finally drug metabolism.

d. **Fetal development:** The effect of drugs on each trimester is different depending on the degree of fetal development. Drug effect is determined by the type of drug and amount of drug exposed, duration of exposure and the level of fetal growth and development. Drug teratogenicity is mostly reported when drugs are taken during the first trimester of pregnancy. In case when drug is taken during the second and third trimesters, ADRs get manifested in the neonate (birth to 1 month) or infant (1 month to 1 year) as retardation in growth, respiratory problems, infection or bleeding.

e. **Creatinine clearance:** The function of kidneys in excretion of drugs is determined by the creatinine clearance. The drug toxicity may increase or the therapeutic effect may decrease depending on change in the renal profile. The renal disease increases the possibility of appearance of ADRs in such patients.

f. **Allergy:** A drug allergy gets manifested due to drug independent cross–reactive antigens which induces sensitization. After primary sensitization, a second exposure causes affected T cells and antibodies to elicit type I to IV immune reactions (Gell and Coombs Classification). The immune reactions mainly include, Type I (IgE-mediated), Type II (cytotoxic), Type III (immune complex), Type IV (delayed, cell mediated).

g. **Fat distribution and body weight:** Drug distribution also varies from person to person. Obese people may store large amounts of fat soluble drug whereas very thin people may store relatively little amount.

Social Factors

a. **Race and ethnicity:** Ethnicity is an important demographic variable as ethnic background elicits a substantial influence on the drug response and action. The interindividual differences arise due to polymorphism in genes encoding drug metabolizing enzymes, drug transporters and receptors. A study on epidemiological risk factors for hypersensitivity reactions to Abacavir found the Caucasian race as risk factors for ADRs. In another cohort study, African Americans were found to be more susceptible to ACE-related angioedema than other ethnic groups. The risk of cough was three times higher in East Asian patients as compared to white patients.

b. **Smoking:** Smoking affects the metabolic process by affecting liver enzymes. It is one of the risk factors for diseases like cancer, cardiovascular disease and peptic ulcer. Cigarette smoking increases the rate of heparin clearance because of the smoking related activation of thrombosis with increases of heparin binding to antithrombin III.

Drug Related Factors

a. **Drug dose and frequency:** Drug dosing and frequency is also a factor affecting the development of ADRs. For example, Bisphosphonates taken at bed time may cause esophagitis. Aspirin when taken in evening elicits more potent antiplatelet effect than in the morning.

b. **Polypharmacy:** Polypharmacy is the prescription of too many medications for a particular patient. The number and severity of ADRs increases disproportionately as the number of drugs taken increases. In a study[28] conducted in Taiwan it was observed that the risk of dementia increases steadily with the number of medications used. As the polypharmacy triggers the modulation of the pharmacologic activity of one drug with the prior or concomitantly administered drug, it can result into drug interaction. The addition of non-prescription medications play a very important role in causing ADRs. Studies[28] conducted in patients aged >65 years indicate that patients in this age group use on average 2–6 prescribed medications, and 1-3 non-prescribed medications. A drug combination may sometimes cause synergistic toxicity, which is greater than the sum of the risks of toxicity of either agent used alone. For example, the risk of peptic ulcer disease is 15 times greater in patients receiving corticosteroids and NSAIDs than that of nonusers of either drugs.[28]

Disease Related Factors

Patients become more vulnerable to ADRs due to presence of many diseases and the use of many drugs. For example, if hypertension is accompanied with other diseases, these diseases might have an impact on the response of the body to antihypertensive drugs. In patients with peptic ulcer disease, the drugs including NSAIDs when prescribed may lead to serious problems. Multiple diseases leads to drug-disease interactions and ADRs.

Adverse reactions can be classified in seven different ways. These classifications are necessary for different purposes. Further classifications are also available for each different class as mentioned below:

PHARMACOLOGICAL CLASSIFICATION[12]

Type –A (Augmented)

This is the commonest type (up to 70%) of ADR which is predictable by the pharmacological mechanisms, e.g. hypotension by beta-blockers, hypoglycemia caused by insulins or oral hypoglycemics, or NSAID-induced gastric ulcers. These type of adverse drug reactions are dose dependent henceforth severity increases with dose. Such ADRs are preventable in most part by slow introduction of low dosages. Sometimes referred to as Type 1 ADRs (Table 5.2).

Type–B (Bizzare)

This type of ADR is not expected from the known pharmacological mechanisms, e.g. hepatitis caused by halothane, aplastic anemia caused by chloramphenicol, neuroleptic malignant syndrome caused by some anesthetics and antipsychotics. Such ADRs are unrelated to dose. Sometimes referred to as Type 2 ADRs (Table 5.2).

Table 5.2: Characteristics of Type A and B reactions[29]

Characteristic	Type A (Augmented) or Type 1	Type B (Bizarre) or Type 2
Mechanism	Pharmacological	Idiosyncratic or Hypersensitive
Predictability	Predictable	Unpredictable
Dose relationship	Related	Not related
Frequency	Common	Uncommon, Rare
Severity	Variable, usually mild	Variable, proportionately more severe than type A
Morbidity	High	High
Mortality	Low	High
First detection	Majority of ADRs become known before marketing (Phase I-III)	Majority of ADRs become known after marketing, i.e. usually phase IV, occasionally phase III
Proportion of adverse drug reaction	80%	20%
Host Factors	Genetic factors may be important	Dependent on (usually uncharacterized) host factors
Animal Models	Usually reproducible in animals	Animal models not known

Type-C (Continuous Drug Use)

This type of ADR occurs as a result of continuous drug use. Such type of ADR may be irreversible, unexpected, unpredictable, e.g. tardive dyskinesias by antipsychotics, dementia by anticholinergic medications.

Type-D (Delayed)

This type of ADR is characterized by the delayed occurrence even after the cessation of treatment, e.g. corneal opacities after thioridazine, ophthalmopathy after chloroquine, or pulmonary/peritoneal fibrosis by methyserzide.

Type-E (End of Dose)

This type of ADR is usually characterized by withdrawal reactions. Such ADRs occur typically with the depressant drugs, e.g. hypertension and restlessness in opiate abstainer, seizures on alcohol or benzodiazepines withdrawal; first dose hypotension caused by alpha-blockers (Prazosin) or ACE inhibitors.

Type-F (Failure of Therapy)

This type of ADR results from the ineffective treatment, e.g. accelerated hypertension because of inefficient control. This may also be called as lack of efficacy.

According to WHO definition this was previously excluded from analysis.

Note: Reports of lack of efficacy[27-30] should not normally be reported on expedited basis, but should be discussed in the relevant Periodic Safety Update Report. However, in certain circumstances reports of lack of efficacy should be treated as expedited cases (15 days) for reporting purposes. Medicinal products used for the treatment of life-threatening diseases, vaccines and contraceptives are examples of classes of medicinal products where lack of efficacy should be considered as cases requiring expedited reporting. Judgement should be used in reporting, considering if other cases qualify for reporting. For example, antibiotics used in life-threatening situations where the medicinal product was not in fact appropriate for the infective agent should not be reported. However, a life threatening infection where the lack of efficacy seems to be due to the development of a newly resistant strain of a bacterium previously regarded as susceptible should be reported on an expedited basis.

CAUSALITY CLASSIFICATION (WHO-UMC CLASSIFICATION)[31]

Certain

A clinical event, including laboratory test abnormality, occurring in a plausible time relationship to drug administration, and which cannot be explained by concurrent disease or other drugs or chemicals. The response to withdrawal of the drug (dechallenge) should be clinically plausible. The event must be definitive pharmacologically or phenomenologically, using a satisfactory rechallenge procedure if necessary.

Comment

It is recognized that this stringent definition will lead to very few reports meeting the criteria, but this is useful because of the special value of such reports. It is considered that time relationships between drug administration and the onset and course of the adverse event are important in causality analysis. So also is the consideration of confounding features, but due weight must placed on the known pharmacological and other characteristics of the drug product being considered. Sometimes, the clinical phenomena described will also be sufficiently specific to allow a confident causality assessment in the absence of confounding features and with appropriate time relationships, e.g. penicillin anaphylaxis.

Probable/Likely

A clinical event, including laboratory test abnormality, with a reasonable time sequence to administration of the drug, unlikely to be attributed to concurrent disease or other drugs or chemicals, and which follows a clinically reasonable response on withdrawal (dechallenge). Rechallenge information is not required to fulfil this definition.

Comment

This definition has less stringent wording than for "certain" and does not necessitate prior knowledge of drug characteristics or clinical adverse reaction phenomena. As stated no rechallenge information is needed, but confounding drug administration underlying disease must be absent.

Possible

A clinical event, including laboratory test abnormality, with a reasonable time sequence to administration of the drug, but which could also be explained by concurrent disease or other drugs or chemicals. Information on drug withdrawal may be lacking or unclear.

Comment

This is the definition to be used when drug causality is one of other possible causes for the described clinical event.

Unlikely

A clinical event, including laboratory test abnormality, with a temporal relationship to drug administration which makes a causal relationship improbable, and in which other drugs, chemicals or underlying disease provide plausible explanations.

Comment

This definition is intended to be used when the exclusion of drug causality of a clinical event seems most plausible.

Conditional/Unclassified

A clinical event, including laboratory test abnormality, reported as an adverse reaction, about which more data is essential for a proper assessment or the additional data are under examination.

Inaccessible/Unclassifiable

A report suggesting an adverse reaction which cannot be judged because information is insufficient or contradictory, and which cannot be supplemented or verified.

Another causality classification as put forward by Karch and Lasagna[32] in 1975 is given below:

Definite

A reaction that follows a reasonable temporal sequence from administration of the drug or in which the drug level has been established in body fluids or tissues; that follows a known response pattern to the suspected drug and that is confirmed on stopping the drug (dechallenge) and reappearance of the reaction on repeated exposure (rechallenge).

Probable

A reaction that follows a reasonable temporal sequence from administration of the drug; that follows a known response to the suspected drug; that is confirmed by dechallenge and that could not be reasonably explained by the known characteristics of the patient's clinical state.

Possible

A reaction that follows a reasonable temporal sequence from administration of the drug; that follows a known response to the suspected drug but that could have been produced by the patient's clinical state or other modes of therapy administered to the patient.

Conditional

A reaction that follows a reasonable temporal sequence from administration of the drug; that does not follow a known response pattern to the suspected drug but that could reasonably be explained by the known characteristics of the patients clinical state.

Doubtful

Any reaction that does not meet any of the above criteria is known as doubtful.

SEVERITY CLASSIFICATION[33]

Mild/Minor

No antidote, therapy or prolongation of hospitalization is required.

Moderate

Requires a change in drug therapy, specific treatment, or an increase in hospitalization by at least one day.

Severe

Potentially life threatening, causing permanent damage or requiring intensive medical care.

SERIOUSNESS CLASSIFICATION[34]

A serious adverse event (experience) or reaction (SAE/SAR) is any untoward medical occurrence that at any dose:
- results in death
- is life-threatening
  (*Note:* The term "life-threatening" in the definition of "serious" refers to an event/a reaction in which the patient was at risk of death at the time of the event/reaction; it does not refer to an event/a reaction which hypothetically might have caused death if it was more severe),
- requires inpatient hospitalization* or prolongation of existing hospitalization
- results in persistent or significant disability/incapacity, or
- is a congenital anomaly/birth defect
- is an important medical events or reaction, that may jeopardize the patient or subject and may require medical or surgical intervention to prevent one of the outcomes listed above.

For the purpose of reporting to the concerned regulatory authorities the SAE/SAR is further classified as: suspected unexpected serious adverse reaction (SUSAR) and suspected serious adverse reaction (SSAR).For the better understanding of above mentioned terms, i.e. SUSAR and SSAR, it should be noted that from the perspective of previously observed adverse reactions (well evident by documentation in the product labeling/package insert or summary of product characteristics for the marketed products or in the investigator brochure for investigational product relating to the trial in question) the ADRs are further classified as unexpected adverse reaction and expected adverse reaction.

Unexpected ADR

An ADR whose nature, severity, specificity, or outcome *is not consistent* with the term or description used in the local /regional product labeling (e.g. Package Insert or Summary of Product Characteristics for the marketed or licensed product) or investigator's brochure

---

* *Hospitalization is defined as an inpatient admission, regardless of length of stay.*

(for an unapproved investigational medicinal product relating to the trial in question).

Expected ADR

An ADR whose nature, severity, specificity, or outcome is consistent with the term or description used in the local /regional product labeling (e.g. Package Insert or Summary of Product Characteristics for the marketed or licensed product) or investigator's brochure (for an unapproved investigational medicinal product relating to the trial in question).

Henceforth, SUSAR means that the adverse reaction term which has led to the seriousness of the reaction is not consistent with the information as set out in the summary of product characteristics (SmPC) or package insert/product labeling (in case of marketed product) or in the investigator's brochure (in case of unapproved investigational medicinal product relating to the trial in question).

In pharmaceutical companies though the SAE/SAR are always reported in the expedited manner (as per the company standard operating procedure), however only the SUSARs should be reported in the expedited manner as per the country specific regulatory guidelines. *[e.g. As per the schedule Y of drugs and cosmetics act "any unexpected serious adverse event (SAE) (as defined in GCP Guidelines) occurring during a clinical trial should be communicated promptly (within 14 calendar days) by the Sponsor to the Licensing Authority and to the other investigator(s) participating in the study"].*

To ensure no confusion or misunderstanding that exist between the terms "serious" and "severe," which are not synonymous, the following note of clarification is provided:

The term "severe" is often used to describe the intensity (severity) of a specific event (as in mild, moderate, or severe myocardial infarction); the event itself, however, may be of relatively minor medical significance (such as severe headache). This is not the same as "serious," which is based on patient/event outcome or action criteria usually associated with events that pose a threat to a patient's life or functioning. *Seriousness (not severity) serves as a guide for defining regulatory reporting obligations.*

FREQUENCY CLASSIFICATION

The frequency of adverse drugs reaction is calculated on the basis of number of events (numerator) occurring in a particular number of population (denominator). Based on the frequency of occurrence of adverse reactions the classification is given as follows:

Very common	≥1/10	(≥10%)
Common (frequent)	≥1/100 and <1/10	(≥1% and <10%)
Uncommon (infrequent)	≥1/1,000 and <1/100	(≥0.1% and <1 %)
Rare	≥1/10,000 and <1,000	(≥0.01% and <0.1%)
Very rare	<1/10,000	(<0.01%)

Source: National Pharmacovigilance Protocol Ministry of Health and Family Welfare, Government of India

MECHANISM CLASSIFICATION[35]

Karch and Lasagna described various mechanisms for adverse drug reactions. These mechanisms are related to the pharmacologic or pharmacodynamic aspects of drugs and can be used to classify the type of reactions that occurs.

Idiosyncracy

An uncharacteristic response of a patient to a drug, usually not occurring on administration.

Hypersensitivity

A reaction not explained by the pharmacological effects of the drug caused by an altered reactivity of the patient and generally considered to be an allergic phenomenon.

Intolerance

A characteristic pharmacological effect of a drug produced by an unusually small dose so that the usual dose tends to induce a massive overaction. It indicates a low threshold of the individual to the action of a drug. In some patient, for example, ataxia may be caused due to carbamazepine.

Drug Interaction

An unusual pharmacological response which cannot be explained by the action of a single drug but may be caused by two or more drugs.

Pharmacologic

A known inherent pharmacological effect of the drug directly related to dose. This includes:
- *Overdose:* Occurring on administration of a dose larger than normally administered dose of drug.
- *Unavoidable side effect:* Occurring with average, normal dose of a drug.

STATISTICAL CLASSIFICATION

Specific

When the ADR has no known natural occurrence.

Non-specific

An ADR which either simulates or increases the incidence of naturally occurring diseases.

MECHANISM OF ADVERSE DRUG REACTIONS

The separation of adverse effects of drugs into Type A and Type B reactions is useful in diagnosis and management of adverse reactions as well as in understanding underlying mechanisms (Figs. 5.1 and 5.2). Factors responsible for Type A (pharmacological adverse reactions) reactions mainly include drug dose, pharmaceutical variation in drug formulation, pharmacokinetic or pharmacodynamic abnormalities and drug-drug interactions (Table 5.3).

Type A Reactions

Pharmaceutical Causes

The pharmaceutical cause for the occurrence of these reactions usually involve alteration in the quantity of drug available for systemic absorption or an influence in the release rate so as to produce a local toxicity at the site of absorption.

The availability of drug for systemic absorption is influenced by the various

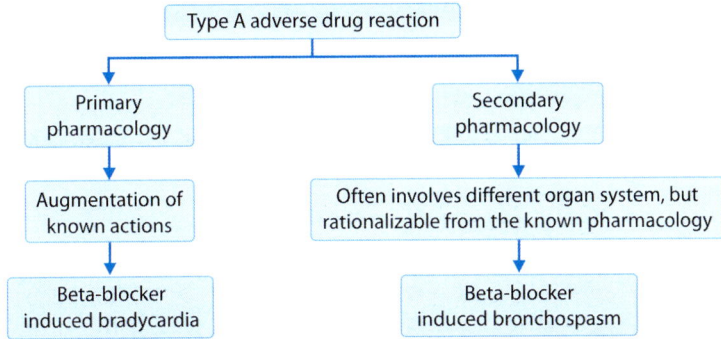

Fig. 5.1: Type A adverse drug reactions can be due to the primary and/or secondary pharmacological characteristics of the drug[29]

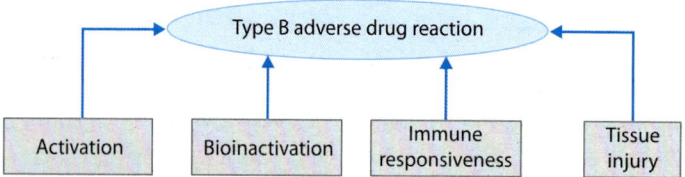

Fig. 5.2: Multifactorial etiology for Type B or idiosyncratic reactions[29]

Table 5.3: Responsible factors for Type A adverse drug reactions

Type (Causes)	Example	Toxicity	Mechanism
Pharmaceutical	Phenytoin	Phenytoin toxicity (ataxia, nystagmus, etc)	Increase in bioavailability as a consequence of change in formulation
Pharmacokinetic (involves absorption, distribution, metabolism and excretion)	Digoxin	Digoxin toxicity (nausea, arrhythmias, etc.)	Decreased elimination as a consequence of impaired renal function
Pharmacodynamic	Indomethacin	Left ventricular failure	Water and sodium retention
Genetic	Nortryptyline	Confusion	Reduced hepatic elimination as a consequence of CYP2D6
Drug-Drug interaction	Lithium-NSAIDs	Lithium toxicity	Inhibition of excretion of lithium

factors *viz.* particle size in the particular pharmaceutical preparation (e.g. tablet, capsule, injection, suspension, emulsion, creams, lotions, etc.), the nature and quantity of excipients *(an excipient is defined as any material other than the therapeutically active substances, present in a pharmaceutical formulation)*, coating materials. Any alteration in the systemic absorption will lead to an altered intensity of drug action. Toxicity may be seen where the drug absorption is increased.

Altered release rate of the drug at the site of absorption may lead to toxicity. This is important in case drugs producing their irritant effect on the gastrointestinal tract. Those formulations which permit an irritant drug to come into prolonged contact with a small area of the gastrointestinal tract lead to gastric hemorrhage, ulceration and perforation, e.g. potassium chloride tablets[36] and matrix preparation of nonsteroidal anti-inflammatory drugs (NSAIDs).

Pharmacokinetic Causes

Pharmacokinetic is the study of absorption, distribution, metabolism and excretion of drugs. Henceforth any alteration in absorption, distribution and elimination may produce Type A reactions.

Absorption

Drug absorption is defined as the process of movement of unchanged drug from the site of administration to systemic circulation. A drug that is completely but slowly absorbed may fail to show therapeutic response as the plasma concentration for desired effect is never achieved. On the contrary, a rapidly absorbed drug attains the therapeutic level easily to elicit pharmacologic effect. Thus, both the rate and the extent of drug absorption are important. The oral route of drug administration is the most common for systemically acting drugs and therefore more emphasis is given to gastrointestinal absorption of drugs as the absorption occurs along the entire length of the gastrointestinal tract. The rate and extent of drug's absorption from the gut is determined by its pharmaceutical and physicochemical characteristics. Changes in gastrointestinal motility can influence the extent of absorption through its effect on gastric emptying or on small intestinal motility. Drugs that are unstable in the acid environment of the stomach (e.g. penicillins) may undergo degradation when gastric emptying is prolonged. In the small intestine, reduced motility may increase the duration of time available for a drug to undergo absorption. For drugs which undergo incomplete absorption across the gastrointestinal tract an increased 'residence time' with in the small intestinal lumen may enhance absorption. For example: bioavailability of digoxin gets increased when propanthelin is administered at the same time.

Distribution

Distribution is reversible transfer of a drug between the blood and the extravascular fluids and tissues.

As soon as the drug reaches the general circulation its extravascular distribution is dependent on various factors such as:
- physicochemical characteristics,
- regional blood flow,
- tissue binding,
- plasma protein binding and
- active transport.

Tissue binding of drugs (tissue localization of drugs) is known to be responsible for the pathogenesis of some adverse reactions and this mechanism is of wider importance. Tissue drug binding results in localization of a drug at a specific site in the body (with a subsequent increase in biological half life). A number of drugs bind irreversibly with the tissues (contrast to plasma protein binding); for example, oxidation products of paracetamol, phenacetin, chloroform, carbon tetrachloride and bromobenzene bind covalently to hepatic tissues. For majority of drugs that bind to extravascular tissues, the order of binding is: liver>kidney>lung>muscle. The examples of extravascular tissue-drug binding are:

1. **Liver:** Epoxides of a number of halogenated hydrocarbons and paracetamol bind irreversibly to liver tissues resulting in hepatotoxicity.
2. **Kidneys:** Metallothionein, a protein present in kidneys binds to heavy metals and results their accumulation and toxicity.
3. **Lungs:** Drugs like imipramine, chlorpromazine and antihistamines accumulate in lungs.
4. **Skin:** Chloroquine and phenothiazines accumulate in skin by interacting with melanin.
5. **Eye:** The retinal pigments of the eye also contain melanin. Binding of chloroquine and phenothiazines to it is responsible for retinopathy.
6. **Hairs:** Arsenicals, chloroquine and phenothiazines are reported to deposit in hair shafts.
7. **Bones:** Tetracycline is an excellent of a drug that binds to bones and teeth. Administration of this antibiotic to infants or children during odontogenesis results in permanent brown–yellow discoloration of teeth. Lead is known to replace calcium from bones and cause their brittleness.
8. **Fats:** Lipophilic drugs like thiopental and the pesticide DDT accumulate in the adipose tissues by partitioning into it.
9. **Nucleic acids:** Molecular components of cells such as DNA interact strongly with drugs like chloroquine and quinacrine resulting in distortion of its double helical structure. Another example is carcinogenicity of alkylating agents such as cyclophosphamide, azathioprine, and chlorambucil which is related to their binding to DNA.

Metabolism

It is the conversion of drug from one chemical form to another. The term metabolism is used synonymously with biotransformation. The chemical changes are usually affected enzymically in the body and thus, the definition excludes chemical instability of a drug within the body; for e.g., conversion of penicillin to penicilloic acid by the bacterial penicillinase and mammalian enzymes is metabolism but its degradation by the stomach acid to penicillanic acid is chemical instability.

Although a number of organs including the kidney, lung, skin and gut, have some drug metabolizing capacity, the liver is the primary site for metabolism of almost all the drugs because of its relative richness in possessing a large variety of enzymes in large amounts. The decreasing order of drug metabolizing ability of various organs is: liver>lungs>kidneys>intestine>placenta>adrenals>skin.

The most important pathway of biotransformation of drugs through liver is oxidation by cytochrome P-450 group of isoenzymes. Drugs which undergo metabolism by this route include oral anticoagulants, phenothiazines, tricyclic antidepressants, many anticonvulsants, benzodiazepines and most barbiturates.

Differences observed in the metabolism of a drug among different races are called as ethnic variations. Such a variation may be monomorphic or polymorphic. When a unimodal frequency distribution is observed in the entire population, the variations are called as continuous or monomorphic; for example, the entire human race acetylate para amino benzoic acid (PABA) and para aminosalisylic acid (PAS) to only a small extent. A polymodal distribution is indicative of discontinuous variation (polymorphism). An example of polymorphism is the acetylation of isoniazid (INH) in humans. A bimodal population distribution was observed comprising of slow acetylator or inactivator phenotypes (metabolize INH slowly) and rapid acetylator or inactivator phenotypes (metabolize INH rapidly)(Table 5.4).

Approximately equal percent of slow and rapid acetylators are found among whites and blacks whereas the slow acetylators dominate Japanese and Eskimo populations. Dose adjustments are therefore necessary

In the latter group since high levels of INH may cause peripheral neuritis. Other drugs known to exhibit pharmacogenetic differences in metabolism are debrisoquine, succinyl choline, phenytoin, dapsone and sulfadimidine.

Recently the role of genetic variation in the metabolism of warfarin (anticoagulant) by CYP2C9 has attracted a great attention. The major risk of warfarin treatment is hemorrhage with an incidence of 8–26 per 100 patient years.[38] Minimization of the risk of bleeding depends on accurate clinical prediction of dosage requirements during warfarin therapy.

There are differences in the rate of drug metabolism in different age groups (neonates, young, adults and elderly) because of variations in the enzyme content, enzyme activity and hemodynamics. In neonates (upto 2 months), the microsomal enzyme system is not fully developed and many drugs are metabolized or biotransformed slowly for example, caffeine has a half life of 4 days in neonates in comparison to 4 hours in adults. A major portion of this drug is excreted unchanged in urine by the neonates. Conjugation with sulfate is well developed (Paracetamol is excreted mainly as sulfate) but glucuronidation occurs to a very small extent. As a result, hyperbilirubinemia precipitates kernicterus and chloramphenicol leads to cyanosis or Gray baby syndrome in newborn. Similarly sulfonamides cause renal toxicity and paracetamol causes hepatotoxicity. Infants (between 2 months and one year) show almost a similar profile as neonates in metabolizing

Table 5.4: Ethnic variation in the N-acetylation of Isoniazid[37]

Ethnic group	% Slow acetylator	% Rapid acteylator
Whites (USA and Canada)	45	55
Blacks (USA)	48	52
Latin Americans	67	33
American Indians	79	21
Japanese	87	13
Eskimos	95	05

drugs with improvement in the capacity as age advances and enzyme activity increases. Children (between one year and 12 years) and older infants metabolize several drugs more rapidly than adults as the rate of metabolism reaches a maximum somewhere between 6 months and 12 years of age. As a result they require large mg/kg doses in comparison to adults; for example, the theophylline half life in children is two-third of that in adults. In very elderly persons, the liver size is reduced; the microsomal enzyme activity is decreased and hepatic blood flow also declines as a result of reduced cardiac output all of which contribute to decreased metabolism of drugs.

As liver is the primary site for metabolism of most drugs, all pathologic conditions associated with it result in enhanced half lives of almost all drugs. Thus, a reduction in hepatic drug metabolizing ability is apparent in conditions such as hepatic carcinoma hepatitis, cirrhosis, obstructive jaundice, etc. Biotransformations such as glycine conjugation of salicylates, oxidation of vitamin D and hydrolysis of procaine which occur in kidney, are impaired in renal diseases. Congestive cardiac failure and myocardial infarction which result in a decrease in the blood flow to the liver, impair metabolism of drugs having high hepatic extraction ratio, e.g. propranolol and lidocaine. In diabetes, glucuronidation is reduced due to decreased availability of uridine diphosphoglucuronic acid (UDPGA).

Drug Elimination or Drug Excretion

Drugs and/or their metabolites are removed from the body by excretion. Excretion is defined as the process whereby drugs and/or metabolites are irreversibly transferred from internal environment to external environment. Excretion of unchanged or intact drug is important in the termination of its pharmacologic action. Although the principal organs of excretion are kidneys, the drug may be removed from the body through bile or by metabolism by the liver to metabolites which are then excreted. Differences between individuals in the drug elimination rates are a major cause of Type A reactions, since reduced elimination leads to increased drug plasma concentration and toxicity. Conversely, enhanced rates, resulting in low plasma and tissue drug concentrations, may cause therapeutic failure.

Drug interactions: Patients on polytherapy are more likely to have Type A reactions. The likelihood of developing an adverse interaction increases with the number of drugs prescribed.[36-39] An Australian study showed that 4.4% of all adverse drug reactions resulting in hospital admission were due to drug interactions.[40] Drug interactions due to effects on metabolic pathways may either be due to enzyme induction or enzyme inhibition.[38] Enzyme induction usually leads to increased metabolism of the drug and thus increases drug clearance. This will lead to reduced drug efficacy rather than drug toxicity (unless the adverse reaction is due to a metabolite rather than to the parent drug). Enzyme inhibition, on the other hand, is more likely to lead to type A reaction since the clearance of the affected drug is reduced; this is particularly likely when the affected drug has narrow therapeutic index.[38-41] An important recent example was the interaction between the CYP3A4 inhibitors ketoconazole and erythromycin and the non-sedating antihistamin terfenadine (Fig. 5.1).

The identification of the role of drug transporters in the disposition of drugs has led to a new mechanism of drug interaction. Many drug transport proteins are present on membranes, some of which are responsible for drug influx and drug efflux, while others can transport in both directions. One of the protein P-glycoprotein (P-gp) is encoded by the MDR1 gene. Over expression of P-gp is one of the mechanisms responsible for resistance of tumors to chemotherapy.[42] P-gp is also responsible for the transport of a number of other drugs including digoxin. Digoxin does not undergo any significant degree of metabolism, but is known to interact with drugs such as quinidine, verapamil and amiodarone, all of which can precipitate digoxin toxicity. A recent study has shown that the mechanism of this interaction involves inhibition of P-gp, thereby reducing the efflux of digoxin from the gut and kidney.[43]

Pharmacodynamic Causes

The actions of most drugs occur within the setting of complex physiological control systems. Intercurrent diseases also unmask pharmacological effects that are not apparent in normal individuals. Hemorrhage or perforation of peptic ulcers in association with administration of nonsteroidal anti-inflammatory drugs or corticosteroids are a typical example. Others include broncho-constriction in association with beta blockers in patients with obstructive airways disease and neuromuscular blockade precipitated by aminoglycoside antibiotics in individuals with myasthenia gravis or in patients who have recently been given muscle relaxants.

Type B Adverse Reactions

The various causes for the occurrence of Type B reactions *viz.* pharmaceutical, pharmacokinetic or pharmacodynamic are given below

Pharmaceutical Causes

The main pharmaceutical causes of Type B adverse reactions include decomposition of the active constituents, toxic effects of excipients, and effects produced by byproducts of the active constituents of the preparation. Though some drugs are remarkably stable, many undergo degradation during prolonged storage or in adverse climatic conditions. Administration of a decomposed drug is most likely to result in therapeutic failure when the products are devoid of pharmacological properties. However, in few cases, decomposition products may be toxic, for e.g. paraldehyde and tetracycline.

In pharmaceutical preparations excipients may also cause toxicity, for example additives such as propylene glycol, carboxymethylcellulose, and tartrazine may cause hypersensitivity reactions in man.[44,45] Certain drugs of low solubility (prepared for intravenous injection) may be formulated with polyethoxylated castor oil. This solvent is probably responsible for the anaphylactoid reactions reported with the anesthetic agent alphaxalone. Similar reactions to preparations of diazepam and vitamin K made up in this solvent have also been reported. Other formulations containing polyethoxylated castor oil, when given to patients over several days can lead to hyperlipidemia and hematological changes.

Pharmacokinetic Causes

Drug metabolism can be considered to be a detoxication process in that it converts therapeutically active compounds to inactive metabolites, which can then be excreted harmlessly from the body. In certain circumstances, the drug-metabolizing enzymes can convert a drug to a toxic, chemically reactive metabolite (CRM), a process known as bioactivation.

Bioactivation or toxicological activation is the formation of highly reactive metabolites (from relatively inert chemical compounds) which interact with the tissues to precipitate one or more of the several forms of toxicities such as carcinogenesis and teratogenesis. For a number of drugs that undergo metabolism, CRM will be formed irrespective of the dose of the drug. When a drug is taken in therapeutic dosage any toxic metabolite formed will be detoxified by normal enzymatic or non enzymatic cellular defense mechanisms. An imbalance between bioactivation and bioinactivation leading to toxicity may be created by taking a drug overdosage. This leads to the formation of large amounts of chemically reactive metabolites and leading to cell damage. An excellent example is paracetamol which causes hepatotoxicity when taken in overdosage.

In therapeutic dosage, paracetamol is largely metabolized by phase II processes (glucuronidation and sulphation) to stable metabolites, but between 5% to 10% also undergoes P450 metabolism to the toxic N-acetyl p-benzoquinoneimine (NAPOI) metabolite.[46] This is detoxified by cellular glutathione. In overdosage, saturation of the phase II metabolic pathways results in greater proportion of the drug undergoing bioactivation. This ultimately leads to depletion of cellular glutathione, and allows the toxic metabolite to bind to hepatic proteins resulting in hepatocellular damage. The use of N-acetylcysteine in the treatment of paracetamol overdosage illustrates the important point that elucidation of the mechanism of drug toxicity can lead to the development of rational therapies that will prevent the toxicity. [*Generation of reactive metabolites is indicated by modification in enzyme activities, formation of glutathione conjugates (or mercapturic acids) and depletion in tissue levels of glutathione. Since the availability of glutathione in the body determine the threshold for toxic response, thiols (e.g. N-acetyl cysteine) can be used to treat poisoning by drugs such as paracetamol that yield reactive metabolites.*]

Alcoholics show increased susceptibility to paracetamol overdosages because excess alcohol consumption results in depletion of glutathione and induction of the P450 isoform CYP2EII.

Table 5.5 lists some of the compounds whose metabolites are tissue reactive.

Table 5.5: Compounds and their metabolic reaction that generate toxic intermediates

Compounds	Metabolic Pathway	Toxicity
Paracetamol	P450	hepatotoxicity
Benzo(a) pyrene	Aromatic epoxidation	Lung cancer
Aflatoxin B1	Olefin epoxidation	Hepatic cancer
Thalidomide	Hydrolytic cleavage of lactam	Teratogenesis
Chlorinated hydrocarbon e.g CHCl3	Oxidative dehalogenation	Nephrotoxicity

Pharmacodynamic Causes

Type B adverse reactions may develop as a consequence of pharmacodynamic differences between individuals. The reactions may be genetic, immunological, or neoplastic and teratogenic in origin.

A classical example for the genetic basis of occurrence of type B reactions is hemolysis in patients with the deficiency of glucose 6-phosphate dehydrogenase in their red blood cells.

The example for immunological basis of occurrence of type B reaction include penicillin induced anaphylaxis.

Further, the possible mechanisms[47] for Type B adverse reactions are given in Table 5.6.

Incidence of ADRs

Assessment for the incidence of ADRs in the community, in hospitals, and as a cause of

Table 5.6: The mechanisms of type B or idiosyncratic adverse drug reactions

Mechanism	Example
Pharmaceutical variation	Eosinophilia-myalgia syndrome with L-tryptophan
Receptor abnormality	Malignant hyperthermia with general anesthetics
Immunological	Penicillin induced anaphylaxis
Drug-Drug interaction	Increased incidence of isoniazid hepatitis with concomitant administration of rifampicin
Multifactorial	Halothane hepatitis

hospital admissions have been made in many studies.[48-57]

Because of differences in the methodology for collection of adverse reaction data and difficulty in detecting and validating adverse drug reactions estimates of such reactions in these studies have varied very widely from as low as 1% or less to as high as 28%. There are smaller reported differences between figures for the proportion of total hospital admissions attributed to adverse reactions ranging from 3% to 6%.[52-56]

Most surveys[57] have shown that deaths of hospital inpatients from adverse drug reactions fall into the range of 0-0.31%. A study on the intensive monitoring for adverse drug effects in patients discharged from medical wards have shown that 2.5% of consultations are concerned with the ill effects of drugs. A study conducted on adverse drug reactions in general practice in England have shown that more than 40% of patients undergoing drug therapy are upset by their treatment.[58]

ADVERSE DRUG INTERACTIONS

Adverse drug interactions are said to occur when the pharmacologic activity of a drug is altered by the concomitant use of another drug or by the presence of food, drink or environmental chemicals. *The drug whose activity is affected by such an interaction is called as the object drug (prime drug) and the agent which causes or precipitates such an interaction is referred as the precipitant (interacting agent).* Drug interactions are generally quantitative whereby the intensity of effect is changed (for example, an increase or decrease). Most of the adverse drug interactions are specific type with altered efficacy of the drug, for example an enhanced pharmacologic activity (e.g. hemorrhagic tendency of warfarin when phenylbutazone is given subsequently) or a decrease in the therapeutic activity resulting in loss of efficacy; for example concomitant administration of tetracyclenes with food, antacids or mineral supplements containing heavy metal ions results in loss of efficacy.

Classification of Adverse Drug Interactions

Adverse interactions are broadly classified as:
- pharmacodynamic interactions
- pharmacokinetic interactions
- pharmaceutical interactions

Pharmacodynamic Interactions

These are the interactions in which the activity of the prime drug (object drug) is altered by the precipitant at its site of action. Such interactions are may be direct or indirect. A direct pharmacodynamic interaction is the one in which drugs having similar or opposing pharmacologic effects are used concurrently. The three consequences of **direct interaction** are:

Antagonism: The interacting drugs have opposing actions; for example:
- Acetyl choline and noradrenaline have opposing effects on heart rate.
- The effect of warfarin can be reversed by vitamin K.
- Inhibition of ulcer healing properties of carbenoxolone by spironolactones.
- Inhibition of hypnotic effects of the barbiturates by caffeine.

Addition or Summation: The interacting drugs have similar actions and the resultant effect is the sum of individual drug responses, e.g. CNS depressants like sedatives, hypnotics, etc.

Synergism or Potentiation: It is enhancement of action of one drug by another; for example:
- Alcohol enhances the analgesic activity of aspirin.
- Sedatives, hypnotics, antihistamines, analgesics, tranquillizers, antidepressants, antinauseants, anticonvulsants and alcohol when used together cause enhanced CNS depression.

- Increase in the ototoxicity of gentamicin by frusemide in patients with renal failure.
- Serious myocardial depression by the concomitant use of verapamil and beta blocking drugs.
- Hyperkalemia because of the administration of potassium supplements to patients taking potassium sparing diuretics, e.g. spironolactone.
- Gangrene because of the combined vasoconstrictor effects of dopamine and ergometrine.

Indirect Pharmacodynamic Interactions

These are the interactions in which both the object (prime drug) and the precipitant drugs (interacting agent) have unrelated effects but the precipitant drug in some way alters the effects of the former, for example, salicylates decrease the ability of the platelets to aggregate thus impairing the hemostasis if warfarin induced bleeding occurs. The other example include rise in the serum levels of lithium because of the use of a diuretic which alters the loss of sodium ions by the kidney tubules.

Another type of indirect interaction occurs if the interacting drug alters the structure of a tissue or organ, such as those drugs which can cause gastrointestinal bleeding, and therefore enhance the actions of concurrently administered anticoagulants.[59]

Pharmacokinetic Interactions

All pharmacokinetic interactions result due to alteration in the rate of absorption, distribution, metabolism or excretion of drugs (and therefore called as **ADME interactions**). All factors which influence the ADME of a drug affect its pharmacokinetics.

Interactions due to Absorption of Drugs

Since the majority of drugs are administered orally, hence altered absorption is very common after oral administration. This interaction may result in a change in the rate of absorption (an increase or decrease), a change in the amount of drug absorbed (an increase or decrease) or both. Several mechanisms may be involved in the alteration of drug absorption from the GIT. In general, drugs that are not absorbed completely/rapidly are more susceptible to changes in GI absorption.

An alteration in parentral drug absorption is rare but can occur when an adrenergic agent such as adrenaline or a cholinergic drug such as methacholine is extravascularly injected concomitantly with another drug. Table 5.7 lists some of the important absorption interactions:

Interactions due to Distribution of Drugs

Irrespective of the fact whether drug is being taken orally or parenterally, drugs are distributed to the body by the general circulation. This distribution of the drugs takes place through binding of the drugs to the plasma proteins (particularly the albumin fraction). It is only the free (non-protein bound) fraction remaining in the plasma water that possesses pharmacological activity. Clinically significant interactions may occur due to competition between drugs for binding to proteins/tissues and displacement of one drug by the other. Competitive displacement which results when two drugs are capable of binding to the same site on the protein causes the most significant interactions. Greater risks of interactions exists when the displaced drug is highly protein bound (more than 95%), has a small volume of distribution and has a narrow therapeutic index (e.g. tolbutamide, warfarin and phenytoin), and when the displacer drug has a high degree of affinity than the drug to be displaced. In such situations, displacement of even a small percent of drug results in a tremendous increase in the free form of the drug which precipitates increased therapeutic or toxic effects.

Drugs may also be displaced from binding sites in tissues. An interesting example of this is oral hypoglycemics such as sulfonylureas

Table 5.7: Absorption interactions

Object drug(s)/Prime drug(s)	Precipitant drug(s)/Interacting drug	Effect on the object drug(s)/Prime drug(s)
1. Complexation and Adsorption		
Tetracycline, penicillamine	Antacids, food and mineral supplements containing Al,Mg,Fe,Zn,Bi and Ca ions	Formation of poorly soluble and unabsorbable complex
Ciprofloxacine, norfloxacine	Antacids containing Al,Mg and Ca and sucralfate	Reduced absorption due to complex formation
Cephalexin, sulfamethoxazole, trimethoprim, warfarin and thyroxine	Cholestyramine	Reduced absorption due to adsorption and binding
2. Alteration of GI pH		
Sulfonamides, aspirin	Antacids	Enhanced dissolution and absorption rate
Ferrous sulfate	Sodium bicarbonate, calcium carbonate	Decreased dissolution and hence absorption
Ketoconazole, tetracycline, atenolol	Antacids	Decreased dissolution and bioavailability
3. Alteration of Gut Motility		
Aspirin, diazepam, levodopa, lithium carbonate, paracetamol	Metoclopramide	Rapid gastric emptying; increased rate of absorption
Levodopa, lithium carbonate, mexiletine	Anticholinergics	Delayed gastric emptying; decreased rate of absorption

Source: Brahmankar DM, Jaiswal SB. Biopharmaceutics and Pharmacokinetics. 'A Treatise" Vallabh Prakashan, 2nd edition (2009); 1-352.

Table 5.8: Distribution interactions

Object drug(s)/Prime drug(s)	Precipitant drug(s)/Interacting drug	Effect on the object drug(s)/Prime drug(s)
Displaced drug(s)	Displacer(s)	
Anticoagulants (warfarin)	Phenylbutazone, chloral hydrate, salicylates	Increased clotting time; increased risk of hemorrhage
Tolbutamide (long acting)	Sulfonamides	Increased hypoglycemic effect
Methotrexate	Sulfonamides, salicylic acid	Increased methotrexate toxicity
Phenytoin	Valproic acid	Phenytoin toxicity

Source: Brahmankar DM, Jaiswal SB. Biopharmaceutics and Pharmacokinetics. 'A Treatise" Vallabh Prakashan, 2nd edition (2009); 1-352.

(tolbutamide, glibenclamide,etc.). These agents exert their therapeutic effects by displacing insulin from protein binding sites in pancreas, plasma and other regions resulting in its elevated levels. Table 5.8 lists some of the important distribution interactions.

Interactions due to Metabolism of Drugs

The most important and the most common cause of pharmacokinetic interactions is alteration in the rate of biotransformation of drugs. Some drugs slow or inhibit the metabolism of others so that their effects are prolonged and toxicity may develop. Drugs with well recognized enzyme inhibitor activity include the sulphonamides, dicoumarol, disulfiram, chloramphenicol, metronidazole and isoniazid.

A deliberately exploited inhibition interaction occurs with disulfiram which by inhibiting the activity of acetaldehyde dehydrogenase, allows the accumulation of acetaldehyde within the body. This results in the unpleasant disulfiram (or antabuse) reaction and is used to deter alcoholics from continuing to drink. Other drugs and chemical agents that induce the same reaction by the same mechanism include metronidazole, dimethylformamide and some of the cephalosporin antibiotics.

The clinical significance of many of the enzyme inhibition interactions depends on the extent to which the serum levels of the drug rise. If the serum level remains within the therapeutic range, the interaction may prove to be advantageous. If not, the interaction becomes adverse as the serum levels come in the toxic range. Table 5.9 lists some of the important metabolism interactions.

Interactions due to Excretion of Drugs

The clearance of drugs is affected by passive as well as active excretory mechanism. Clinically significant renal excretion interactions occur when an appreciable amount of drug or its active metabolite(s) are eliminated in the urine. Excretion pattern can be affected by alteration in GFR, renal blood flow, passive tubular reabsorption, active tubular secretion and urine pH. An interesting pharmacokinetic interaction that results due to the pharmacodynamic drug effect is between thiazide diuretics and lithium. Due to the influence of the thiazide diuretics on the renal tubular transport of sodium the lithium ions are retained in the body resulting in its toxicity. Table 5.10 lists some of the important excretion interactions.

Pharmaceutical Interaction

It is a physiological interaction that occurs when drugs are mixed in intravenous infusions causing precipitation or inactivation of the active principles. These interactions are also called as the incompatibilities, for example ampicillin, chlorpromazine and barbiturates interact with dextran in solutions and are broken down or form chemical complexes.

Table 5.9: Metabolism interactions

Object drug(s)/Prime drug(s)	Precipitant drug(s)/Interacting drug	Effect on the object drug(s)/Prime drug(s)
1. Enzyme Induction		
Corticosteroids, oral contraceptives, coumarins, phenytoin, tolbutamide, tricyclics	Barbiturates	decreased plasma levels, decreased efficacy of object drugs
Corticosteroids, oral contraceptives, theophylline, cyclosporine	Phenytoin	-do-
Oral contraceptives, oral hypoglycemics, coumarins	Rifampicin	-do-
2. Enzyme Inhibition		
Tricyclic antidepressants	Chlorpromazine, haloperidol	Increased plasma half life ($t_{1/2}$) of tricyclics; increased risk of sudden death from cardiac disease in such patients
Coumarins	Metronidazole, phenyl butazone	Increased anticoagulant activity; risk of hemorrhage
Azathioprine, mercaptopurine	Xanthine oxidase inhibitors (allopurinol)	Increased toxicity of antineoplastics
Alcohol	Disulfiram, metronidazole, tinidazole	Disulfiram like reactions due to increase in plasma acetaldehyde levels

Source: Brahmankar DM, Jaiswal SB. Biopharmaceutics and Pharmacokinetics. 'A Treatise" Vallabh Prakashan, 2nd edition (2009); 1-352.

Table 5.10: Excretion interactions

Object drug(s)/Prime drug(s)	Precipitant drug(s)/Interacting drug	Effect on the object drug(s)/Prime drug(s)
1. Changes in active tubular secretion		
Penicillin, cephalosporin, nalidixic acid, methotrexate, dapsone	Probenecid (acid)	Elevated plasma levels of acidic drugs; risk of toxic reactions
Acetohexamide	Phenylbutazone	Increased hypoglycemic effect
Procainamide, ranitidine	Cimetidine (base)	Risk of toxicity
2. Changes in urine pH		
Amphetamine, tetracycline, quinidine	Antacids, thiazides, acetazolamide	Increased toxicity
3. Changes in renal blood flow		
Lithium	NSAIDs	Decreased renal clearance of lithium; risk of toxicity

Source: Brahmankar DM, Jaiswal SB. Biopharmaceutics and Pharmacokinetics. 'A Treatise" Vallabh Prakashan, 2nd edition (2009); 1-352.

REFERENCES

1. http://www.ich.org (accessed on: 23 Dec 2017.
2. Skegg DCG, Doll R. The case for recording events in clinical trials. Br Med J. 1977;2:1523-4.
3. Weintraub M. Recording events in clinical trials. Br Med J. 1978;i:581.
4. Simpson RJ, Tiplady B, Skegg DCG. Event recording in a clinical trial of a new medicine. Br Med J. 1980;280:1133-4.
5. Anon. Lessons from the benoxaprofen affair. Lancet, 1982;529.
6. Seventh European Symposium on Clinical Pharmacological Evaluation in Drug Control, Deidesheim, 1978. WHO Euro Reports and Studies, WHO, Copenhegen, 13.
7. Einarson TR. Drug related hospital admissions. Ann Pharmacotherapy. 1993;27:832-40.
8. Bates DW, Boyle DL, Viliet MVV, Schenieder J, Leapse L. Relationship between medications errors and adverse drug events. J Gen Intern Med. 1995a;10:199-205.
9. Bates DW, Cullen DJ, Laird N, Petersen LA, Small SD, Servi D, et al. Incidence of adverse drug events–implications for prevention. J Am Med Assoc. 1995b;274:29-34.
10. Bates DW, Spell N, Culen DJ, Burdick E, Laird N, Petersen LA, et al. The cost of adverse drug events in hospitalized patients. J Am Med Assoc. 1997;277:307-11.
11. Clasen DC, Pestotnik SL, Evans RS, Lloyds JF, Burke JP. Adverse drug events in hospitalized patients. Excess length of stay, extra costs, and attributable mortality. J Am Med Assoc. 1997;277:301-6.
12. Dhikav V, Singh S, Anand KS. Adverse Drug Reaction Monitoring in India. JIACM. 2004; 5(1):27-33.
13. Wayne EJ. Problems of toxicity in clinical medicine. In Walpole AL. Spinks A (Eds). The Evaluation of Drug Toxicity. London: J&A Churchill Ltd. 1958;1-11.
14. Levine RR. Factors modifying the effects of drugs in individuals. In Pharmacology: Drug Actions and Reactions. Boston (MA): Little Brown and Co. 1973;261-9.
15. Wade OL, Beeley L. Adverse Reactions to Drugs (2nd edn). London: Wiliams Heinemann Medical Books Ltd. 1976: Chapter II.
16. Rawlins MD, Thompsons JW. Pathogenesis of adverse drug reactions. In: Davies DM. (Ed). Textbook of Adverse Drug Reactions. 2nd edn. Oxford University Press 1977;44.
17. Rawlins MD, Thompsons JW. Pathogenesis of adverse drug reactions. In: Davies DM (Ed). Textbook of Adverse Drug Reactions (2nd edn). Oxford University Press. 1981;II.
18. Grahame-Smith DG, Aronson JK. The Oxford Textbook of Clinical Pharmacology and Drug Therapy. Oxford: Oxford University Press. 1984;134.
19. Hogne R, Jaeger MD, Wymann R, et. al. Time pattern of allergic reactions to drugs. Agents Actions Suppl. 1990;29:39-58.

20. Park BK, Pirmohammad M, Kitteringham NR. Idiosyncratic drug reaction; a mechanistic evaluation of risk factors. Br J Clin Pharmacology. 1992;34:377-95.
21. Lawrence DR, Bennett PN. Clinical pharmacology. Edinburgh: Churchill Livingstone. 1992;121-2.
22. Femer R, Mann RD. Drug safety and pharmacovigilance. In: Curtis MJ, Sutter MC, et al. (Eds). Integrated Pharmacology (1st edn). London: Mosby, 1997;83-90.
23. Hartigan-Go KY, Wong JQ. Inclusion of therapeutic failures of adverse drug reactions. In: Aronson JK (Ed). Side Effects of Drugs. Annual 23. Amsterdam: Elsevier, 2000: xxvii-xxxiii.
24. Aronson JK. Evidence based medicine and principles of drug therapy; Chapter 2. In: Hasslett C, Chivers ER, Boon NA, et. al. (Eds). Davidsons Textbook of Medicine; Edinburgh; Churchill Livingstone, 2002.
25. Aronson JK, Femer RE. Joining the DoTS: Classifying adverse reactions by dose responsiveness, time course and susceptibility. BMJ. 2003;327:1222-5.
26. Alomar MJ. Factors affecting the development of adverse drug reactions (Review Article). Saudi Pharmaceutical Journal. 2014;(22):83-94.
27. Lai SW, Lin CH, et al. Association between polypharmacy and dementia in older people: A population based case control study in Taiwan. Geriatri Gerontol Int. 2012;12(3):491-8.
28. Routledge PA, O'mahony MS, Woodhouse KW. Adverse drug reactions in elderly patients. BJCP. 2003;57(2):121-6.
29. Munir Pirmohamed, B. Kevin Park. Metabolic Mechanisms. In Basis of Pharmacovigilance (Edn). R.D. Mann and E.B. Andrews), 2002, p.57-77.
30. Guideline on good pharmacovigilance (GVP) Module VI – Collection, management and submission of reports of suspected adverse reactions to medicinal products. 28 July 2017. EMA/873138/2011 Rev (2).
31. http://www.who.int/medicines/areas/quality_safety/safety_efficacy/WHOcausality_assessment.pdf [Accessed on 23 Dec 2017].
32. Karch FE, Lasagna L. Adverse drug reactions. JAMA. 1975;234(12):1236.
33. Gregory PJ, Keir KL. Medication misadventures: adverse drug reactions and medication errors. In Drug Information: A Guide for Pharmacists McGraw-Hill Professional, 2000,pp.487-518.
34. Post-Approval Safety Data Management: Definitions and Standards for Expedited Reporting. ICH E2D. Current step 4 version dated November 2003.
35. Karch FE, Lasagna L. Towards the operational identification of adverse drug reactions. Clin Pharmacol Therapeutics. 1977;21:247-54.
36. Boley SJ, Allen AC, Schultz L, Schwartz S. Potassium-induced lesions of the small bowel. Clinical aspects. JAMA. 1965;193:997-1000.
37. Kalow W. Pharmacogenetics: Heredity and the response to drugs. Saunders. Philadelphia. 1962.
38. Petty GW, Brown RD Jr, Whisnant JP, Sicks JD, O'Fallon WM, Wiebers DO. Frequency of major complications of aspirin, warfarin, and intravenous heparin for secondary stroke prevention. A population-based study. Ann Intern Med. 1999;130(1):14-22.
39. D'Arcy PF. Epidemiological aspects of iatrogenic disease.In:D'Arcy PF,Griffin JP. (Eds). Iatrogenic Diseases. Oxford: Oxford University Press, 1986; 29-58.
40. Stanton LA, Peterson GM, Rumble RH, Cooper GM, Polack AE. Drug related admissions to an Australian Hospital. J Clin Pharm Therapeut. 1994;19:341-7.
41. Brodie M, Feely J. Adverse drug interactions. In: Feely J, (Ed). New Drugs. Londo: BMJ, pp.29-39.
42. Germann UA. P-glycoprotein a mediator of multidrug resistance in tumour cells. Eur J Cancer. 1996;32A:927-44.
43. Fromm MF, Kim RB, Stein CM, Wilkinson GR, Roden DM. Inhibition of P-glycoprotein-mediated drug transport: A unifying mechanism to explain the interaction between digoxin and quinidine. Circulation. 1999;99(4):472-4
44. Schneider CHde, Breck AL, Stanble E. Carboxymethylcellulose additives in penicillins and the elicitation of anaphylactic reactions. Experimentia 27,167-78.
45. Wilkinson DS. Sensitivity to pharmaceutical additives. In: Mechanisms of Drug Allergy. Dash, CH, Jones HEH (Eds). Churchill, Livingstone, Edinburgh, London. 1972.
46. Nelson SD. Molecular mechanisms of the hepatotoxicity caused by acetaminophen. Semin Liver Dis. 1990 Nov;10(4):267-78.

47. Park BK, Pirmohamed M, Kitteringham NR. Idiosyncratic drug reactions: a mechanistic evaluation of risk factors. Br J Clin Pharmacol. 1992;34(5):377-95.
48. Barr DP. Hazards of modern diagnosis and therapy-the price we pay. JAMA. 1955:159; 1452-6.
49. Mcdonald MG, Mackay BR. Adverse drug reactions. JAMA. 1964;190:1071-174.
50. Schimmel EM. The hazards of hospitalization. Ann Intern Med. 1964;60:100-10.
51. Reidenberg MM. Registry of adverse drug reactions. JAMA. 1968;203:31-4.
52. Seidl LG, Thornton GF, Cluff LE. Epidemiology studies of adverse drug reactions. Am J Pub Hlth. 1965;55:1170-5.
53. Hurwitz N. Admissions to hospital due to drugs. Br Med J. 1969 Mar 1;1(5643):539-40.
54. Gardner P, Watson LJ. Adverse reactions: a pharmacist-based monitoring system. Clin Pharmacol Ther. 1970 Nov-Dec;11(6):802-7.
55. Miller RR. Hospital admissions due to adverse drug reactions. A report from the Boston Collaborative Surveillance Program. Arch Intern Med. 1974;134219-223.
56. Caranasos GJ, May FE, Stewart RB, Cluff LE. Drug-associated deaths of medical inpatients. Arch Intern Med. 1976;136(8):872-5.
57. Karch F, Iasagna L. Adverse drug reactions in the United States: An Analysis of the Scope of the problem and recommendations for future approaches. Report for medicine in the public interest. Inc. Washington 1974.
58. Martys CR. Adverse reactions to drugs in general practice. Br Med J. 1979;2(6199):1194-7.
59. O'Reilly RA, Sahna MA, Ageller PM. Impact of aspirin and chloathalidone on the pharmacodynamics of oral anticoagulant drugs in man. Ann Ny Acad Sci. 1971 Jul;179:173-86.

6

Signal Detection in Pharmacovigilance

Renu Agarwal, Puneet Agarwal

INTRODUCTION

New drug development is a challenging and costly process as it involves focus on quality, efficacy as well as safety. In relation to safety issues thorough evaluation of drug-related adverse drug reactions (ADRs) is indispensable. Some of the ADRs can be predicted based upon the previous experience with the pharmacologically similar drugs and others are detected during clinical trials. For detection of ADRs the clinical trials usually provide limited information as they are conducted under strictly controlled conditions and largely focus on efficacy evaluation. Some of the ADRs can be detected only after long-term use in a large population and in specific patient groups due to specific concomitant medications or disease. Such ADRs are difficult to detect at early stages and can only be detected after the drug is marketed. The visual field defects during vigabatrin therapy and valve defects following fenfluramine-phentermine therapy are few such examples when ADRs were detected after the drug was marketed. Therefore, early recognition of previously unknown adverse effects of medicines during post-marketing period is the primary objective of pharmacovigilance. The early warning of the possible occurrence of an adverse drug reaction, i.e. signal detection consists of a hypothesis, which is relevant to the safe use of drugs and is based upon a set of data. The data constituting the hypothesis can be epidemiological, pharmacological or pathological. Meyboom (1997) defined a signal as a set of data constituting a hypothesis that is relevant to the rational and safe use of a drug in humans. World Health Organization has defined a pharmcovigilance signal as "reported information on a possible causal association between an adverse event and a drug, the relationship being unclear or incompletely documented previously". According to Council for International Organizations of Medical Sciences (CIOMS) (2010) a pharmacovigilance signal is defined as "information that arises from one or multiple sources (including observations and experiments), which suggest a new potentially causal association, or a new aspect of a known association, between an intervention and an event or set of related events, either adverse or beneficial, that is judged to be of sufficient likelihood to justify verificatory action."

The process of signal detection is not restricted to detecting association of newly detected ADR with the drug but also involves detection of drug-drug interaction, drug-food interaction, drug-related syndromes and risk factors. The process helps in identification of unknown associations, quantification of associations and causality assessment. After a signal has been detected other methods are

utilized to either confirm or disapprove it, to determine its incidence and identify the high-risk population. The process of signal detection involves a step-wise approach consisting of:
- Signal generation
- Signal strengthening
- Signal testing, evaluation and explanation.

Signal Generation

Signal generation consists of formulation of a hypothesis suggesting a possible association between exposure to drug and appearance of ADR. Thus, the signal generation is a method of highlighting potential adverse reactions and safety issues related to the use of a particular drug that need further investigations. The possibility of new ADR to a medicinal product, i.e. signal generation may be difficult to identify often because most of the adverse drug effects are not new clinical entities and new signal often concerns with new cause of an old disease. A causal relationship between the drug and adverse reaction is difficult to establish as a particular drug can cause multiple ADRs and a particular ADR can be caused by multiple drugs. Moreover, the frequency and severity of a particular ADR in response to a drug can vary in different population groups depending upon age, sex, race, indication for use, etc. Various situations either favor or hinder the signal generation. A summary is presented in Table 6.1.

Signal Strengthening

The signal generation and hypothesis formulation is followed by preliminary assessment of available data also known as signal strengthening. The available preliminary data can be qualitative derived from clinical observations or quantitative derived from epidemiological studies, case-reports, experiments, etc. Only in exceptional cases a single report may be sufficient to indicate that the signal is valid. In most of the cases assessment of a larger qualitative/quantitative data from a number of case-reports along with supportive evidence is required. In cases where data is quantitative simple calculations are done to find the relative risk and higher the relative risk stronger is the signal. While calculating relative risk, the data required is relatively large and it is often difficult to rule out the confounding factors. The methods of signal detection such as follow-up studies, intensive hospital monitoring and prescription event monitoring that combine the qualitative and quantitative data also have limited applicability, as their sensitivity of detecting ADR is low. In spite of limitations, the preliminary data assessment leads to improved knowledge about the suspected ADR not only from scientific perspective but also the public health perspective by indicating alteration in benefit/risk ratio and need for early warning and regulatory intervention.

Table 6.1: Factors accelerating and hindering signal generation

Situations accelerating signal generation	Situations hindering signal generation
1. Cluster of symptoms, which usually have low natural frequency	1. Very high background frequency of suspected drug effect
2. The signs and symptoms are unusually characteristic or can be explained on the basis of pharmacological mechanisms	2. Very low frequency of suspected ADR
3. Similar effects related to drug intake appearing with high frequency in one type of population	3. Very low frequency of drug exposure
4. The observed adverse reaction is a known drug related effect	4. No time and dose relationship
5. High frequency of drug exposure or high frequency of adverse drug reaction	5. The observed drug effect unrelated to usual pharmacological effects
6. A close time and dose relationship	

Signal Testing, Evaluation and Explanation

Once a signal is generated and is found to be of sufficient strength after preliminary data assessment it requires further testing and evaluation to provide explanations especially in relation to strength of association and causal relationship. Based upon the Henle-Koch's postulates, Evans in 1976 proposed that to establish a causative relationship between the exposure and disease it is important that (i) the disease occurs with increased frequency in exposed population, (ii) The diseased population has higher rate of exposure and (iii) in the absence of exposure the incidence of disease reduces. Further Meyboom et al. (1997) have proposed that a very careful and aggregated assessment of all available data from different sources is essential to understand the drug-ADR association and a framework suggested for data assessment is as follows:

- Quantitative data needs to be evaluated statistically for the strength of association as indicated by the number of case reports showing occurrence of ADR following exposure to drugs
- Qualitative data needs to be evaluated for:
  - Consistency of frequency and pattern of presence of a characteristic feature and absence of features suggesting the opposite
  - Exposure-response relationship in terms of site of reaction, timing, dose and reversibility
  - Explanation to the occurrence of specific ADR available based on pharmacological and pathological mechanisms
  - Evidences from experiments and laboratory investigations suggesting a definite association/causation such as a positive dechallenge (events after stopping the drug) rechallenge (events appearing after re-exposure), high tissue and blood concentrations of drug, its metabolites or drug-dependent antibodies
  - The ADR known to be a drug-related reaction or similar reaction observed following exposure to related drugs
  - Final assessment for causality depends upon the accuracy and validity of data from all sources.

It is important to realize that the framework suggested above differs for different types of reactions such as immunological reactions, teratogenicity, cancer, etc. Moreover, as none of the currently available system is fully validated for assessing the causal relationship the choice of most suitable method is based on prevailing situation.

SOURCES AND METHODS OF SIGNAL DETECTION

Signals are usually derived either from patients or population groups. Different types of signals require different types of detection methods. Each time a new signal is detected there are differences from the previous experiences and according to prevailing situations the methods of signal detection need to be modified. The methods of signal detection include spontaneous reporting system, intensive hospital-based surveillance system, prescription event monitoring, case reports in literature and epidemiological studies.

Spontaneous Reporting System

The spontaneous reporting system (SRS) is the oldest, most productive and cost-effective method of ADR reporting. Effective use of the system requires a well-established national and international network for reporting by the concerned participants. The SRS involves the voluntary participation of health professionals, pharmacist, nurses and patients themselves for reporting the observations related to ADRs. The health professionals can use the report form to give all relevant data related to drug and suspected ADR. The experts review the reports on a case-by-case basis and try to evaluate if there is a pattern representing the possible signal. Often a single report may not be conclusive and a cluster of spontaneous reports from independent observers is required to generate a signal. Further studies will be required to either confirm or disapprove the signal as it is only a warning and not the actual evidence of possible association.

SRS is useful in detecting type B effects (those effects that are often allergic or idiosyncratic reactions, characteristically occurring in only a minority of patients and usually unrelated to dosage and that are serious, unexpected and unpredictable) and unusual type A effects (those effects that are related to the pharmacological effects of the drug and are dosage-related). Type C effects (those effects related to an increased frequency of 'spontaneous' disease) are difficult to study, however, and continue to pose a pharmacoepidemiological challenge.

As the reporting system is spontaneous it has some very important limitations and the most noticeable is the under-reporting. All the ADRs observed by health professionals are not reported and also the specific ADR may be under-reported leading to decreased sensitivity of the system. Sometimes the ADRs are not even suspected either due to difficulty in relating the ADR with the drug clinically or because no such reactions have previously been described or because of long time lag between exposure and event. Besides, the reporting rate is also influenced by a number of factors such as type of drug, type of ADR, inherent toxicity of drug, duration for which the drug is present in the market, publicity of the drug, availability in combinations, place where the drug is used, etc. Some degree of under-reporting is unavoidable and the extent of under-reporting is hard to measure. Thus, the data generated only on the basis of spontaneous reporting cannot be used to estimate the rate of occurrence of suspected ADR and the frequency of ADRs is often underestimated. However, a hypothesis can be formulated for further investigation. Other sensitive methods are required to further support the signal detection especially when the number of reported cases is very small. In spite of all its limitations, the method is a widely used system and is relatively fast and efficient in generating signals. It is easy to use and covers all the drugs and patient population including the special groups such as pregnant, children, etc. The method is non-interventional and therefore takes into account the situations like ADRs due to inappropriate prescription and overdoses as that cannot be studied due to ethical reasons. The database generated by SRS is utilized for detecting association between the suspected ADR and drug use, drug-drug interaction, drug-associated syndromes and identification of risk factors.

The establishment of causality relationship only on the basis of spontaneously reported cases is difficult but at times a strong possibility is considered such as when there are reports of rechallenge cases or when the ADR has no background incidence of disease and there are no signs of confounding. Despite the limitations of SRS the decision to withdraw the drug from the market may have to be taken on the basis of spontaneously reported cases to avoid the risk of exposure of large population to suspected drug as there can be considerable delay before the results of confirmatory studies become available.

Intensive Hospital-based Drug Surveillance System

This is the hospital-based drug surveillance system. In-patient record is maintained with details of drug used, indication, dose, route of administration, the date of starting and stopping treatment and reasons for stopping treatment. Any adverse event such as rash, fever, nausea, vomiting, gastrointestinal (GI) bleeding, convulsions alteration in biochemical parameters, etc. occurring while the patient is on drug are also recorded. Although, the method is expensive and time-consuming, the availability of sophisticated software has made it easy to analyze the data quickly to find association between a suspected ADR and the drug. The system requires a big hospital set-up with support from experts in various fields such as clinicians, pharmacologists, pharmacists, nurses, biostatisticians and IT professionals. The method is useful for estimating rate of occurrence of ADR, detecting unrecognized new ADRs. This method of surveillance is the most comprehensive method with no under-reporting.

The hospital-based system of drug surveillance can also be based on outpatient records of first and subsequent visits. The patients can also be contacted telephonically to collect information related to suspected ADRs.

Prescription-event Monitoring

Prescription-event monitoring (PEM) is used as a large-scale post-marketing surveillance method in UK. All National Health Service prescriptions issued by general practitioners are analyzed centrally. The system identifies the patients who are receiving a particular drug and the doctor who prescribed the drug. A follow-up questionnaire is sent to the treating physician at the end of the first year of initial prescription. The doctors are required to sent all information related to the use of drug especially the details of adverse events which the patient may have suffered while on treatment. Attempt is made to study all new chemical entities along with old suspected drugs. The analysis can be made by case-by-case analysis to identify drug-ADR association. In addition quantitative methods can be applied to the database to recognize potential signals. The signals generated from the entire PEM database are further subjected to confirmatory studies.

Case Reports in Literature

The case reports by observant physicians contribute significantly in signal detection. Although, a single report by itself may not generate a signal it can stimulate others to be watchful for the same. Later repeated appearance of reports showing similar drug-related event generate a signal, which needs further confirmation. Case reports are the major source of information used to withdraw a drug from market for safety reasons.

Epidemiological Studies

These are carefully designed studies specifically directed to study adverse effects related to the use of a particular drug. The cohort or prospective studies follow a group of patients over a period of time following exposure to drug in question. These studies are time-consuming and expensive but are useful in identifying the specific ADR rate. The case-control studies estimate the frequency of exposure to a drug in a group of people experiencing similar events. These are retrospective studies used to establish association between the ADR and drug use.

The epidemiological studies do not take into account the other associated factors such as concomitant use of other drugs or disease conditions and do not detect all ADRs related to a specific drug. The epidemiological studies primarily test the hypothesis of suspected or known ADR.

National Pharmacovigilance Centres

The National Pharmacovigilance Centres are the organizations designated by the ministries of health (or equivalent) of member countries as responsible for the collection and processing of ADR reports. National Pharmacovigilance Centres of member countries work in cooperation with UMC and send ADR reports, which are the source of data in WHO database. The National Pharmacovigilance Centres receive input from regional centres. The number of member countries has gone up to 75 in 2004 from 10 in 1968. The National Pharmacovigilance centres in different member countries vary considerably in size, resources, support structure and scope of activities. The core activity of national centres remains the collection and assessment of spontaneous reports of suspected ADRs. The scope of activities of national centres also includes the following:

- To communicate about the risks and benefits to patients, prescribers and public
- To undertake active surveillance depending upon the availability of support system
- To provide training to health care providers about the ADR reporting procedures
- To communicate drug-related information to national regulatory authorities which in turn communicate with other national regulatory authorities to discuss the safety data
- To raise the public awareness of drug safety and contribute to development of public health policy.

At National Pharmacovigilance Centres the reports are analyzed by trained professionals on a case-by-case basis for detection of possible signals. Further a systematic continuous review of database for detection of drug ADR combination is essential to optimize the primary goal of pharmacovigilance, i.e. detection of unexpected or unknown ADR. With increasing volume of data during past few years automated signal detection methods have been developed to supplement the qualitative methods. These methods are important supplementary tools and utilize the clinical trial database and observational databases to evaluate the strength of association of a suspected adverse effect with the use of drug. Although, a number of different methods are used, the primary aim is to find the extent to which the number of observed cases differ from number of expected cases, i.e. a measure of disproportionality. The pharmacovigilance data from national centres is communicated to WHO-ADR database (VigiBase) where further analysis is done to either confirm or disprove the signal and decide accordingly for the necessary action (Fig. 6.1).

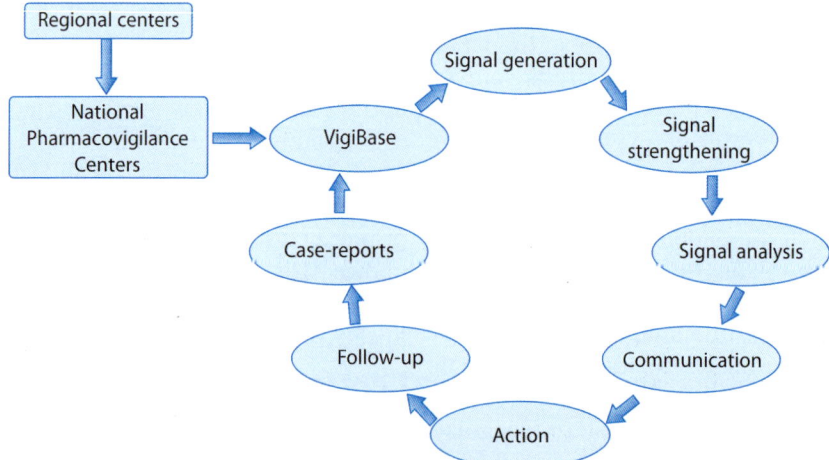

Fig. 6.1: Signal detection with international collaboration with safe and rational use of medicines

AUTOMATED QUANTITATIVE SIGNAL DETECTION

As a result of increasing volume of data the traditional method of case-by-case analysis is no longer feasible and computer-based automated screening programmes are used for rapidly detecting signals of interest in large electronic database. These programmes statistically compare the frequency of occurrence of a particular ADR in combination with the drug against the background frequency in the database. Such computer-based evaluation can be done quickly on a large database, which is then reduced to a smaller one of specific interest. Besides being quick, the method offers great advantage of being objective, transparent, reproducible and is not influenced by previous knowledge and bias. The method also suffers from drawbacks as the clinical and pharmacological factors are not taken into account and secondly even if a serious ADR has true association but does not show statistical significance, may be overlooked.

WHO Adverse drug reaction database—VigiBase

Maintaining and developing the ADR database particularly for signal detection is the core responsibility of UMC. VigiBase is the working name of the WHO database, which consists of ADR reports received from member countries. The system was started in 1978 and until 2002 it was based on old WHO standard form for ADR reporting and was known as International Drug Information System (INTDIS). Due to increasing demands of international community on pharmacovigilance, access to new technology and increasing volume of data, the INTDIS has been replaced by much more sophisticated system known as VigiBase. The system was introduced on the recommendations of CIOMS 1A working group (1995) and International Conference on Harmonization (ICH E2B EWG). The VigiBase uses internationally accepted codes as described in:

1. WHO Drug dictionary (WHO-DD)
2. WHO Adverse Reaction Terminology (WHO-ART)
3. ICH medical dictionary for regulatory affairs (MedDRA)
4. International Classification of Diseases (ICD).

Although, old WHO standard format for reporting is still accepted, most of the national centres have started using E2B-format database. Some national centres use VigiBase Online for ADR reporting. UMC provides information about the coding system to be used by national centres. The incoming reports in VigiBase are processed as shown in Figure 6.2.

The reports held in VigiBase are individual cases of spontaneous ADR reports bearing unique case-record number, which is also retained in VigiBase. All case-reports to be accepted by VigiBase must contain a set of data including reporting country, a unique report number, a suspected drug and an adverse reaction. The national centres are responsible for verifying the authenticity of reports and are encouraged to ensure that data is as complete as possible. Before the data is accepted in VigiBase it undergoes extensive quality control procedures involving syntax check, inter-field coherence check, check for drug names, ADR terms and duplication of reports. The professionals working for data input at UMC are pharmacists with special training in medical terminology and are capable of doing necessary corrections of inappropriate terminology. After being accepted in VigiBase the case-reports are automatically assigned a grade according to predefined criteria relating to data quality. Besides grading each case-report the system also screens data to provide information on indication for which drug was used, causality assessment, dechallenge and rechallenge. Further the system also checks for duplication of reports, helps in correcting

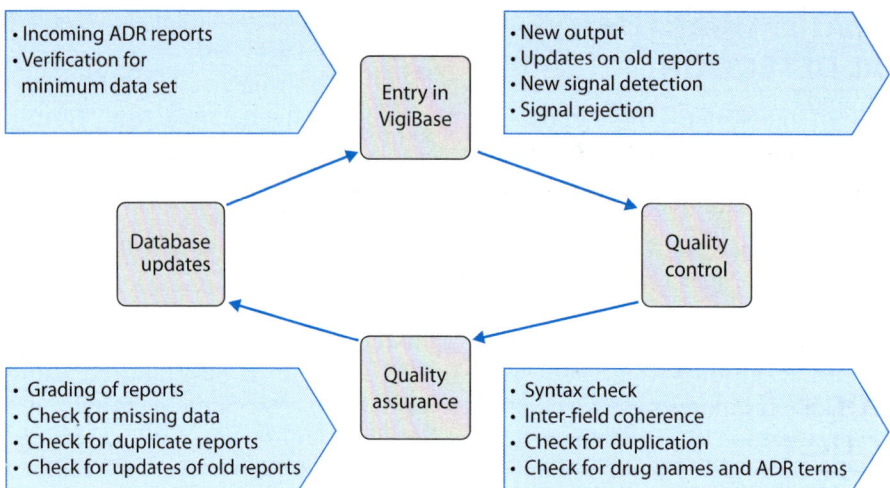

Fig. 6.2: Processing of reports in VigiBase

incomplete and incorrect reports, produces reporting statistics and sends acknowledgment of receipt to reporting centres. The VigiBase database is updated as soon as reports are received on a daily basis (Fig. 6.2).

A signal in pharmacovigilance must not be viewed simply as a statistical association but it consists of a hypothesis, relevant data and possible explanations. Once the automated signal detection process picks up a particular drug-ADR combination, the decision has to be taken about its significance as a true signal and requirement for further investigations. The criteria for selection of a signal as a potential one have been described by Meyboom et al. and include—an unknown and unexpected event, an expected but unlabelled event, highly characteristic and definitive drug-related event with low background frequency and of sufficient severity. In addition the potential relevance of the drug-ADR combination plays an important part in selecting the signal for further evaluation. The detection of new ADR is highly relevant when it is expected to be a potential threat to public health and therefore requires early warning and possibly regulatory action. This kind of situation prevails when the drug in question is extensively used, is used for very serious indication, the resultant ADR is very serious and large number of cases start emerging post drug exposure. Further evaluation of a signal may also be required in the absence of threat to public health when it is likely to explain a previously unknown pharmacological activity and thereby is likely to contribute significantly to scientific knowledge about the drug.

Once a relevant signal has been generated by automated signal detection method further observations of the database are required to assess its strength and evolution with time. In case of a signal of adequate strength absolute number of cases reported increases with time as a larger population is exposed. The next step is to analyze the data statistically to find consistency in the pattern of reporting and characteristics of ADR when larger population is using the drug over a longer time period. A characteristic and consistent pattern of reported events from different countries is a strong argument in favor of drug-ADR connection. Further supportive evidences are gathered by a variety of comparisons keeping in view the hypothesis such as comparison among different populations, different drug groups and different drug combinations. A nested case-control study using the same database can also be done to get a better picture. Use of data from all other sources including the experimental observations provides further support for signal strengthening as well as for possible explanations to newly discovered ADR. The signal follow-up with a combined approach using individual case-reports as well as the aggregate data is the mainstay in determining the signal strength as well as its relevance for individual user and for the public at large.

APPLICATION OF QUANTITATIVE METHODS FOR SIGNAL DETECTION

Quantitative signal detection involves application of numerical methods to pharmacovigilance. With the help of computer-assisted programmes various statistical methods can be applied to the data generated by the systems described above. Despite differences in methodology used, all statistical methods primarily aim to search the database for disproportionality and detect:

- The extent to which the number of observed cases differs from the number of expected cases.
- The extent to which the reported ADR is associated with the suspected drug as compared to other drugs in the database.

Based upon the observations in literature and dataset of SRS, a hypothesis is formulated stating the possibility of an association between the drug and ADR. This process of assessing drug-ADR association is subjective. The quantitative methods evaluate the associations objectively and results can be presented as point estimate with confidence interval. Although quantitative signal detection methods are very useful tools but it is important to note that statistically significant results do not conclusively establish an association and statistically not significant results do not disapprove the association completely.

Bayesian Confidence Propagation Neural Network

Bayesian confidence propagation neural network (BCPNN) is a semi-automated knowledge-detection technique that helps to find new drug-ADR associations likely to be potential signals by quantitative data filtration in VigiBase. The technique is based on Bayesian theorem first proposed by an English clergyman and mathematician, Thomas Bayes (1702-1761). The Bayesian theorem is a branch of logic applied to decision-making and inferential statistics that deals with probability inference and is used to predict the future events based upon the knowledge of previous events. The original theorem has now undergone modifications and the currently used method at uppsala monitoring centre (UMC) has been developed in collaboration with the Royal Institute of Technology, Sweden.

The BCPNN methodology can manage large databases and is robust in handling very incomplete data. The method can be used to find patterns of information within datasets with complex dependencies. The method can identify the drug-ADR combinations occurring with high frequency as against the background frequency, unexpected patterns and variations in patterns over time. The measure of disproportionality as calculated by BCPNN is expressed as Information Component (IC). The IC value indicates the strength of quantitative dependency between a drug and an ADR but does not give evidence of causality. For the assessment of causality individual case reports must be studied. A positive IC value is indicative of higher occurrence of drug-ADR association than expected, a negative value indicates that the association is observed less frequently than expected statistically and a zero IC value indicates that there is no quantitative dependency between drug and ADR. However, it is very important to remember that a positive

IC value by itself does not necessarily mean that the drug-ADR combination represents a signal and a negative IC value does not always indicates absence of potential signal. The IC value is based on:
- Total number of reports
- Total number of reports with drug-ADR association
- Total number of reports showing use of drug
- Total number of reports showing ADR

As more and more data is added the IC value may increase or decrease. Larger the data used for calculation of IC, narrower will be the standard deviations and less will be the chance of variations when new data is added. The method is highly objective, picks up the associations early and also indicates the strength of association based on IC value. The use of BCPNN methodology has further been extended to detect dependencies between several variables. The method is thus useful in detecting new syndromes, age groups affected, population groups at high-risk and dose relations. The method also provides information about variations in ADR patterns among different countries.

VIGI METHODS AND TOOLS

Uppsala monitoring centre has developed a numbers of methods and tools to facilitate use of large database in VigiBase. These tools help in faster signal detection by expediting search and analysis of data.

VigiGrade is a tool that measures the amount of clinically relevant information in individual ICSR stored in VigiBase. VigiGrade highlights quality issues and gives a completeness score to each ICSR. Grading by this tool does not take into account the causality association between drug and ADR. However, a number of other fields such as time to onset, indication, outcome, age sex, dose, country, primary reporter, report type and comments have been included in calculating the completeness score. A score is given to each field if it has information and a penalty is imposed for missing information. The individual field scores are weighted and combined into a score for the whole ICSR. The maximum score is 1.0. Primarily VigiGrade helps in communicating with member countries with regards to data quality. However, it has also proven to be an indicator of true signal.

VigiMatch is another method developed by UMC. It is a probabilistic record matching method and identifies unexpectedly similar record pairs in large databases. It computes a match score for each pair by rewarding the matching information and penalizing the mismatch. The match score is a reflection of probability that the two records relate to the same underlying entity or that they are duplicates.

VigiRank is predictive model that ranks pharmacovigilance safety signals according to multiple aspects of strength of evidence. Parameters that make up the VigiRank are Disproportionate reporting (IC_{025}), Recent reporting, Geographic spread ($N_{Country}$), Informative reports (VigiGrade completeness score as N_{comp09}) and Narratives. The VigiRank has been successfully implemented in UMC's signal detection since 2014.

VigiPoint identifies and pinpoints key features in a subset of data in contrast to a broader dataset such as ages, sex, co-reported drugs and adverse reactions.

VigiLyze is a powerful search and analysis tool that provides access to VigiBase data on conventional medicines, traditional medicines (herbals), as well as biological medicines including vaccines. It is available to all member countries. VigiLyze enables international comparison with national spontaneous reporting data, as well as gives access to ADR information on drugs that are not yet on national market.

VigiFlow is a web-based ICSR management system that is specially designed for use by national centres in the WHO Programme for

International Drug Monitoring. It is based on and compliant with the ICH E2B standard. ICSR data can be manually entered into VigiFlow and built-in error checks help to enter the data correctly.

VigiMine provides statistical data regarding the case reports in VigiBase. The system incorporates the WHO Drug Dictionary and ATC structure, as well as both the MedDRA and WHO-ART terminologies. It gives access to statistical data on all drug-ADR pairs reported to VigiBase. It also allows filtering of the results by statistical criteria and stratification by age, sex, country, and year of reporting. VigiMine also shows the change in the statistical values over time. VigiMine data can be used to compare with statistics in a national database and as an independent aid in the detection of new signals.

THE UMC SIGNALING PROCESS

Currently, the UMC scans the data received from national centres quarterly using BCPNN methodology. The results are presented in a computerized table called the combinations database. This database contains a comprehensive listing of all suspected drug-ADR combinations as well as the separate total counts for the drug and ADR in question. For each combination the statistical figures generated by BCPNN such as IC and its standard deviation are also reported. The combinations database is sent to the national centres every quarter to help them review the international contents of relevance. The signal detection process at UMC is complementary to the ongoing work at national centres. Any drug-ADR combination with a positive value of the lower 95% confidence limit of the IC, which is IC minus two standard deviation (IC-2sd), is highlighted for clinical review. Besides this statistical criterion, other criteria are also taken into account to filter the data and select important combinations requiring further investigation. The filtering process known as triage logic applies certain predefined algorithms to narrow down the number of combinations and allow focus on important and manageable number of combinations. The algorithm used in UMC signaling triage is shown in Box 6.1.

The next stage in triage process is to check for already available information on drug-ADR combinations of importance from all available sources of published product information. For combinations where complete information is not available the case-reports are retrieved from VigiBase and are sent to appropriate experts in the review panel. The UMC expert review panel consists of around 30 consultants from 20 countries. The reviewers assess the case-reports using the available data from literature, their clinical experiences and knowledge of pharmacology.

The causality assessment in a drug-ADR combination depends upon a number of factors. A causal relationship is 'certain' if an ADR (clinical event or a laboratory test) is observed within a reasonable time sequence to administration of drug, cannot be explained by concurrent disease/drug or chemical use

Box 6.1: Algorithm used in UMC signaling triage

Serious ADR and new drug
- Drug first entered into the database in the last one or two years
- The 'reaction' is a critical term
- There is at least one report having fatal outcome
- The drug-ADR combination exceeds the statistical threshold for review, i.e. it has a lower 95% confidence limit of the IC above zero
- Few reports for the combination

Rapid reporting increase
- The drug-ADR combination exceeds the statistical threshold for review
- The IC has increased by 2 points or more on the scale since the last quarter

Special interest reactions
- Stevens-Johnson syndrome or Lyell's syndrome
- Agranulocytosis
- Rhabdomyolysis
- Other important and typically drug related reactions

Source: Viewpoint, Part 2, The Uppsala Monitoring Centre

and dechallenge and rechallenge procedures can be explained pharmacologically. A causal relationship is 'likely' if the ADR is within a reasonable time sequence, unlikely to be explained by concurrent disease/drug or chemical use and shows clinically reasonable dechallenge response. A causal relationship is said to be 'possible' when ADR occurs within a reasonable time sequence but could be explained by concurrent disease/drug or chemical use and information on dechallenge is lacking. A causal relationship is 'unlikely' when ADR is not within a reasonable time sequence and concurrent disease/drug and chemical use provides plausible explanations. When a reported ADR requires more data for proper explanation or the additional data is under examination the event remains 'unclassified'. If a reported ADR cannot be assessed properly due to insufficient or contradictory information and further varification is not possible it is said to be 'unclassifiable'.

The reviewers at UMC make a final assessment and a judgment is made about the causal association of drug and ADR and the strength of association. A short report is drafted and after an internal review at UMC if the signal is considered worth notifying it is included in the SIGNAL document, which is distributed to national centres.

The SIGNAL document is an UMC publication that includes signals with varying characteristics and levels of suspicion (Fig. 6.3). The document is distributed to national centres, regulatory authorities and pharmaceutical industry. Single international market authorization holders may be given opportunity of pre-publication comments on signals related to their products before license expiry. The SIGNAL document plays an important role in signal detection by national centres and thus has a direct impact on drug safety related issues handled by member countries. Although some of the countries may be self-sufficient in handling drug safety issues due to strong national pharmacovigilance system, international data holds prime importance for better characterization of previously detected hazards and new emerging potential hazards which have not yet come to attention in one country.

WHO AND UMC LEADERSHIP IN SIGNAL DETECTION

The WHO Centre in Uppsala is playing an important role in signal detection. The national pharmacovigilance data from various countries is pooled and then analyzed to detect the signals, which were not picked up earlier by the national centres. When only a few cases are reported to national pharmacovigilance centres they may not be sufficient to generate a signal but after pooling multiple national data the potential signals can be recognized easily (Lindquist 1999). The WHO receives reports from member countries on a reporting format. Although, the reports are accepted even if some

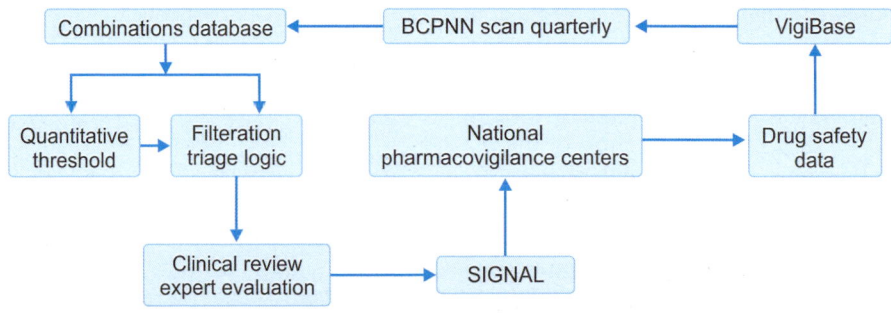

Fig. 6.3: The UMC signaling process

of the data is missing but information such as unique ID and name of country, drug and ADR is essential. The member countries differ from each other in the methods of collecting reports. Some have a centralized system while other depend upon the regional centres for data collection. In some countries the reporting is voluntary, in some mandatory and in others both voluntary and mandatory depending upon the reporter. Some countries like US encourage adverse event reporting while other countries require suspected adverse reactions. Some countries receive reports via pharmaceutical companies while others receive from health professionals. The countries also differ in the preferred professional groups identified for reporting such as physicians, nurses, pharmacist, etc.

The method of case by case analysis with clinical consideration can be done applied to national database but for huge WHO database quantitative methods are required to screen all drug-ADR combinations, to select combinations for further review and possibly provide quantitative aid to signal detection. The high degree of heterogeneity of WHO data should be kept in mind while making assessment for potential signals. The signals detected at Uppsala Centre are presented by clinical review experts in the WHO document known as 'Signal' document. The signal document is made available to all member countries WHO Programme for International Drug Monitoring (Meyboom et al. 1997).

CONCLUSION

The signal detection is the first step in the process of risk-benefit assessment. A large number of methods are available for data collection but the spontaneous reporting system remains the backbone of the pharmacovigilance systems worldwide for signal generation. Further studies using most appropriate method (epidemiological, pharmacological and pathological) are required to test the hypothesis suggesting a potential signal. Whatever may be the method used, the primary aim is to detect previously unknown ADRs as soon as possible after the drug is marketed, calculate their incidence rates, to understand their nature and the population at risk and provide updates as more and more information becomes available. It is important to realize that quantitative methods with the use of power of computer are extremely useful tools in supporting and enhancing signal generation in pharmacovigilance but clinical evaluation continues to remain the key process. In pharmacovigilance, while weighing the credibility of the signal it is important to assess the balance between all the evidences in favor and against the suspicion and accordingly decide its importance for individual user as well as for public health, the measures required and consequences if the signal proves false.

The detection of a pharmacological signal may require a variety of actions depending upon its relevance to individual and public health and may range from a simple communication to scientific publication and regulatory action. The decision-making as to the action required may take place before the results of confirmatory studies become available to avoid exposure of larger population to potentially harmful drugs.

BIBLIOGRAPHY

1. ADR reporting systems and signal detection. Viewpoint, Part 2, the Uppsala Monitoring Centre. 2005.
2. Almenoff JS, LaCroix KK, Yuen NA, Fram D, DuMouchel W. Comparative performance of two quantitative safety signalling methods: implications for use in a pharmacovigilance department. Drug Saf. 2006;29(10):875-87.
3. Alvarez-Requejo A, Carvajal A, Begaud B, Moride Y, Vega T, Arias LH. Under-reporting of adverse drug reactions. Estimate based on a spontaneous reporting scheme and a sentinel system. Eur J Clin Pharmacol. 1998;54:483-8.

4. Arnaiz JA, et al. The use of evidence in pharmacovigilance. Case reports as the reference source for drug withdrawals. Eur J Clin Pharmacol. 2001;57(1):89-91.
5. Begaud B, Miremont F, Tubert-Bitter P. Expected number of adverse reactions in a sample. Post Marketing Surveillance. 1993;799-118.
6. Edwards IR, Aronson JK. Adverse drug reactions: definitions, diagnosis, and management. Lancet. 2000;356:1255-9.
7. Egberts TC. Signal detection: Historical background. Drug Safety. 2007;30(7):607-9.
8. Finney DJ. Systematic signalling of adverse reactions to drugs. Methods of Information in Medicine. 1974;13(1):1-10 .
9. Griffin C. The Advanced Theory of Statistics. London: 1995.
10. Hauben M. A brief primer on automated signal detection. Ann Pharmacother. 2003;37(7-8): 1117-23.
11. Hauben M. Signal detection in the pharmaceutical industry: integrating clinical and computational approaches. Drug Saf. 2007; 30(7): 627-30.
12. http://who-umc2010.phosdev.se/DynPage.aspx?id=97220&mn1=7347&mn2=7252&mn3=7254 Accessed on 05/07/2017
13. https://www.who-umc.org/vigibase/vigilyze/vigimethods/ Accessed on 05/07/2017
14. Introduction to Categorial Statistics. In: Greenland S, Rothman KJ. Greenland S, Rothman KJ (Eds). Modern Epidemiology. Philadelphia: Lippincott-Raven. 2001;231-52.
15. Ioannidis JP, Contopoulos-Ioannidis DG. Reporting of safety data from randomised trials. Lancet. 1998;352:1752-3.
16. Lindquist M, et al. From Association to Alert-a revised approach to International Signal Analysis. Pharmacoepidemiology and Drug Safety. 1999;8:S15-S25.
17. Matsushita Y, Kuroda Y, Niwa S, Sonehara S, Hamada C, Yoshimura I. Criteria revision and performance comparison of three methods of signal detection applied to the spontaneous reporting database of a pharmaceutical manufacturer. Drug Saf. 2007;30(8):715-26.
18. Meyboom RH, Egberts AC, Edwards IR, Hekster YA, de Koning FH, Gribnau FW. Principles of signal detection in pharmacovigilance. Drug Saf. 1997;16(6):355-65.
19. Meyboom RHB, Lindquist M, Egberts ACG, Edwards IR. Signal selection and follow-up in pharmacovigilance. Drug Saf. 2002;25(6): 459-65.
20. Orre R, Lansner A, Bate A, Lindquist M. Bayesian neural networks with confidence estimations applied to data mining. Comput Stat Data Anal. 2000;34:473-93.
21. Rawlins MD. Spontaneous reporting of adverse drug reactions. I: the data. British Journal of Clinical Pharmacology. 1988;26(1):1-5.
22. Stephens MDB. The pre-marketing establishment of the side-effect profile of a new drug. In: Stephens MDB, Talbot JCC, Routledge PA (Eds). Detection of new adverse drug reactions. New York: Grove's dictionaries inc. 1998;197-253.
23. Stricker BHCh, Tijssen JGP. Serum sickness-like reactions to cefaclor. J Clin Epidemiol. 1992;45:1177-84.
24. Wiholm B-E, et al. Spontaneous reporting systems outside the US. In: Pharmacoepidemiology. Strom BL (Ed). Churchill Livingstone: New York. 1994,pp.139-57.

7
Postmarketing Surveillance

Manoj Sharma, SK Gupta

"There are three actions of a drug: the one you want, the one you don't want, and the one you don't know about"

—DJP BARKER

The drug development process includes the continuum from the identification of a potential pharmaceutical agent to research on possible efficacy and safety through regulatory approval (Fig. 7.1).The drug approval process mainly involves phase I, II, III and postmarketing trials (sometimes referred to as phase IV trials). Premarketing studies (Phase I, II, and III trials) necessarily take place in controlled situations with selected groups of people. Though a new drug appears to be safe in these studies, unseen adverse effects can occur when a drug is released for use in general population.[1]

Postmarketing surveillance (PMS) is a general term used to describe the research and studies associated with product safety evaluation after a drug has been approved for marketing.[2]

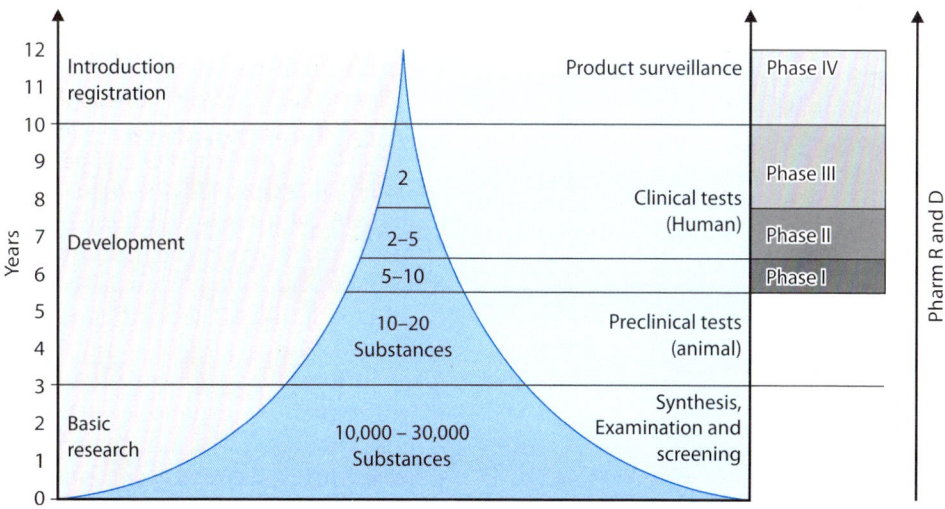

Fig. 7.1: Drug development process

It aims to monitor the use of a drug in a large number of patients after marketing (Post Approval) to evaluate adverse events (AEs)/adverse drug reaction (ADRs) in order to continuously analyze its benefit/risk ratio.

PMS activities usually include the collection, reporting, and evaluation of adverse experience reports: the analysis of drug use data to calculate reporting rates; and the conduct of epidemiologic and other studies to better quantitate the public health importance of these events. The overall purpose of postmarketing surveillance is to develop new safety information on a drug as it is used in the market place in real world clinical practice.[3]

NEED OF POSTMARKETING SURVEILLANCE: WHY

Clinical trials are the backbone of the drug approval process and are designed to determine drug efficacy and toxicity. Postmarketing surveillance complements premarketing clinical trials. It should be noted that both clinical trials and postmarketing surveillance contribute for the understanding of drug safety. The various characteristics of clinical trial methodology are highlighted in Box 7.1. These characteristics have been discussed in detail with more focus on the fact that how postmarketing surveillance provides complimentary data (i.e, how postmarketing surveillance complements premarketing clinical trials). These include size (sample size, i.e. no of patients), clinical trial duration, patient selection, drug indications, concomitant drugs and patient compliance.[3,4]

Size, i.e. Number of Patients

It is well evident that the number of patients exposed (administered/prescribed) during the premarketing phases of clinical trial (i.e. phase I, phase II and phase III) is very less (may be less than 5,000) as compared to the number of patients which are exposed to the drug after getting the marketing approval, i.e. during postmarketing phase from the concerned regulatory. Because many adverse events are rare and occur at the rate of 1 in 2000 to 1 in 100,000 persons exposed, the more rare events would not usually be detected in clinical trials.

Based on the fact that a large number of patient population is exposed during the postmarketing period it is anticipated that the unrecognized adverse events that occur at an extremely low frequency can be discovered. Often safety signals, not recognized during premarketing phases, can be identified using postmarketing spontaneous reporting. Theoretically, spontaneous reporting could capture the events affecting all of these patients; unfortunately, in practice, many events are not recognized and fewer are still reported. Lack of a control or other comparison group also limits the value of spontaneous reports.

Clinical Trial Duration

One of the important factor to be considered in the clinical trials is their time limit. Since clinical trials are time limited, patient treatment and follow-up usually continue for only a period of weeks to months. Once approved and available many drugs are taken intermittently or regularly for a period of years. Adverse experiences that require a long "incubation" or latency period from time of drug exposure to event and those that occur only after chronic exposure to a drug are difficult to recognize in clinical trials.

Box 7.1: Characteristics of clinical trials

- Specified number of participants, i.e. number of patients
- Short duration
- Non-representative patient selection (elderly, pregnant women and children are usually excluded)
- Narrow drug indications or limited indications
- Limited concomitant drug use
- Higher level of patient compliance

These events can also be difficult to identify from spontaneous reports, although epidemiologic studies can sometimes identify them.

The use of postmarketing epidemiological studies have successfully identified and recognized the link between vaginal carcinoma and maternal intrauterine exposure to diethylstilbestrol (DES). The association between carcinoma and DES was discovered through retrospective epidemiologic studies of women with vaginal carcinoma. It was found that mothers of these women had taken DES 15 to 25 years before while they were pregnant.

Non-representative Patient Selection

In a clinical trial study patients are selected based on the various exclusion and inclusion criteria (selection criteria) as defined in the protocol for that study. Henceforth, patients meet stringent criteria for acceptance into a study. These criteria are usually formulated to minimize the diversity within the group. The more homogenous the group and the less confounding variables there are, the more efficient data analysis can be. Thus, patients in clinical trials may not be representative of those using the drug after approval regarding extent of disease, age, gender, and other variables. These patient variables can affect the adverse event profile associated with a given drug.

A frequent selection factor in clinical trials involves age. Most patients in clinical trials are drawn from restricted age groups. The very young and the very old are often underrepresented (or sometimes not included). The reasons for not including the elderly may include concomitant disease, medication, and various other factors. The elderly however, may respond to a drug differently from younger adults because increase in age is associated with pharmacodynamic changes due to factors including decreased renal functions and alterations in the relative proportions of body fat, muscle and water.

Table 7.1: Pregnancy categories used in drug labelling

Pregnancy category	Animal studies	Data from human female drug exposure
A	-	-
B	-	No studies
B	+	-
C	+	No studies
C	No studies	No studies
D*	No studies	+
X †	+	+

* Drug is labeled in the "warnings" section. The potential benefits from the use of the drug in pregnant women may be acceptable despite its potential risk.
† Drug is labeled in the "contraindications" section. The risk of the use of the drug in pregnant women clearly outweighs any possible benefit.
- = Data show negative teratogenic results.
+ = Data show positive teratogenic results.
(*Source:* 21 CFR201.57 {f} {6}.)

The exclusion of children form clinical trials is also very frequent except when pediatric indications for a drug are specifically being studied. The inclusion of children in clinical trials can introduce complex ethical issues such as complicated informed consent requirements and uncertainty about the effects of the medication on child's growth, development and overall long-term health. These issues can complicate study design.

Pregnant women are excluded from most of the clinical trials because of the risk of teratogenic and mutagenic effects. Although determination of a pregnancy category "(including categories A through D, and X as defined in Table 7.1). For drugs not specifically indicated in pregnancy, the pregnancy categories are often determined from animal studies that assess teratogenicity and mutagenicity. For many drugs adequate data are not available at the time of approval to comprehensively determine the drug's safety in each of the trimesters of pregnancy.

Limited Indications

In clinical trials the indications for which a drug is intended to be used is often narrow (usually only one indication) and well-defined. This is done to limit the variables in assessing the efficacy. It is statistically much simpler to document efficacy if all study patients have equivalent disease, and the drug is used for clearly specified indications.

Once a drug is marketed, however, it may be used for patients with various conditions. Some drugs may be prescribed for indications not in the labeling, the so called "unlabelled indications" or prescribing "off label". Other drugs gain approval for expanded indications after initial approval for selected indications. For example, propranolol was initially marketed as an antiarrhythmic drug, but it is currently approved for several indications, including its use in stable postmyocardial infarction, in angina pectoris due to coronary atherosclerosis, and as a prophylactic agent for common migraine headache. Carbamezepine was approved as an antiepileptic but is now commonly used for the treatment of manic depressive disorder.

The use of the drug in indications other than the labeled indications may change the risk-benefit profile. For example, if a drug has potentially severe hematologic effects, it may be appropriate to use it in life-threatening or terminal disease because the benefit is obvious and the risk of hematologic disease becomes relatively less serious. To use that same drug prophylactically for a minor disease, however, would change the risk-benefit profile because the potential benefit would not be as great, although the risk may be the same.

Concomitant Medications or Limited Concomitant Drug Use

In clinical trials patients are selected for a specific stage of a specific disease and thus concomitant medications are limited. For this reason drug interactions often remain undetected. On the contrary when a drug is marketed patients may be taking that drug and numerous other drugs concomitantly. These drugs may interact to affect various processes such as absorption, protein binding, hepatic metabolism and renal excretion and may also produce additive pharmacologic effects. Therefore, it is during the postmarketing phase that additional drug interactions may be recognized.

Patient Compliance

In clinical trials patients are more compliant than other patients because of the intensive monitoring associated with the clinical study participation. Furthermore, in clinical trial patients the medication and medical care is often provided at no charge there by eliminating financial barriers associated with compliance.

POSTMARKETING SURVEILLANCE METHODOLOGIES

Many methods are used to monitor drugs after FDA (applicable regulatory authority) approval. These methods include:
- Spontaneous reporting system
- Case reports
- Case control studies
- Cohort studies
- Randomized clinical trials
- Database research and monitoring
- Meta-analyses.

Spontaneous Reporting Systems

Before going to the details of the functioning of spontaneous reporting system let us first understand what a spontaneous report is:

A spontaneous report is an unsolicited communication by healthcare professionals or consumers to a company, regulatory authority or other organization (e.g. WHO, regional centres, poison control centre) that describes one or more adverse drug reactions in a patient who was given one or more medicinal products and that does not derive from a study or any organized data collection scheme.[5]

If a practitioner (e.g. pharmacist, physician, nurse) suspects that a particular medication is associated with an adverse event observed during the course of caring for a patient, then he or she reports the adverse drug reaction to a formal reporting system. When several practitioners report adverse drug reactions to a central location, the data can then be reviewed and analyzed for trends. One practitioner observing one adverse drug reaction associated with a particular drug may not consider the adverse drug reaction to be significant or common, but several practitioners reporting the same adverse drug reaction to a central locale allows for the determination of its extent and seriousness.

The spontaneous reports database is widely used for detecting signals*of ADRs related to the drug interactions.[6]

An excellent example of the functioning of spontaneous reporting system can be best understood from the French pharmacovigilance system which is based on a network of 31 regional centres located in teaching hospitals and coordinated by the French Medicines Agency ["Agence Française de Sécurité Sanitaire des Produits de Santé" (AFSSAPs)]. A study [7]was conducted to describe the characteristics of the reports and the reporting trends in the French pharmacovigilance spontaneous reporting database from 1986 to 2001. Since 1984, they have shared a common database of adverse drug reactions (ADRs) that are spontaneously reported by healthcare professionals. All the reports from January 1986 to December 2001 were included. Drugs and ADRs were translated to anatomical therapeutic chemical (ATC) codes and MedDRA classifications, respectively. The total number of reports was 197 580 over the 16-year period, with linearly increase over time. The median [interquartile range (IQR)] age of the patients was 53 (34–70) and the male/female ratio was 0.82. The median (IQR) time between the date of occurrence of the ADR and the date of report was 73 days (34–166). The reporter was a specialist in 74% of the reports and a general practitioner in 17%. The annual rate of reporting according to medical demography strongly increased for the specialists, especially since 1994. At least one ADR was considered as serious in 44.8% of the reports. The ADRs were most frequently related to nervous system drugs (23%), followed by cardiovascular drugs (19%) and systemic anti-infective (17%). The latter class had the fastest progression mostly due to antiretroviral therapy since 1996. According to the Medical Dictionary for Regulatory Activities (MedDRA) coding, the system organ most often reported was skin and subcutaneous tissue disorders (29%), followed by nervous system disorders (19%), gastrointestinal disorders (12%), blood and lymphatic system disorders (12%), vascular disorders (12%) and general disorders and administration site conditions (12%). This first description of the data of the French pharmacovigilance database involving all drugs and ADRs showed an increasing tendency to reporting over time, especially in specialists and for anti-infective drugs.

The consequences drawn from the spontaneous reporting are taken into account by the prescribers and the regulators for the prescriptions. This can be easily understood by a study[8] carried out in Italy. The results analyzed from the spontaneous reporting database were taken into account by physicians before prescribing amoxicillin/clavulanic

---

*A signal is defined as a possible relationship between an adverse event and a drug, the relationship being unknown or incompletely documented previously. Usually more than a single report is required to generate a signal, depending upon the seriousness of the event and the quality of the information. The publication of a signal usually implies the need for some kind of review or action as the reported information on a possible causal relationship

acid to patients. In this study adverse drug reactions related to amoxicillin alone and in association with clavulanic acid were analyzed from database of spontaneous reporting of suspected adverse drug reactions. The analysis was made to compare the safety profile of amoxicillin and amoxicillin/clavulanic acid. Data were retrieved from the spontaneous reports collected by six Italian regions (the GIF database) from January 1988 to June 2005. Drug utilization data were also available for the two drugs. The comparison between amoxicillin and amoxicillin/clavulanic acid was made using the Chi (2) or Student's t-test, when appropriate. Disproportionality in reporting of adverse events was assessed using reporting odds ratio methodology. Up to June 2005, the GIF database collected 37,906 reports, of which 1088 were related to amoxicillin/clavulanic acid and 1095 to amoxicillin. The percentage of skin reactions was statistically higher for amoxicillin (82%) than for amoxicillin/clavulanic acid (76%); on the contrary, the percentage of gastrointestinal, hepatic and hematological reactions was significantly higher for amoxicillin/clavulanic acid (13%, 4% and 2%, respectively) than for amoxicillin (7%, 1% and 1%, respectively). Amoxicillin/clavulanic acid seemed to be associated with a higher risk of Stevens-Johnson syndrome, purpura and hepatitis than amoxicillin alone. In particular, the reporting rate of hepatitis was on average 9-fold higher for amoxicillin/clavulanic acid than for amoxicillin. This analysis showed a different safety profile for the two selected drugs. Since, the combination of amoxicillin/clavulanic acid has been increasingly used in Italy and now represents the most frequently antibiotic prescribed by Italian general practitioners these results are taken into account by physicians before prescribing amoxicillin/clavulanic acid to patients.

Spontaneous reporting systems can be found at local, regional, and national levels. It is the responsibility of all practitioners to report suspected adverse drug reactions; however, the responsibility for the creation and maintenance of the reporting systems in health care institutions typically falls under the purview of the pharmacy department. The various reporting systems known include:

- WHO International system
- US FDA "MedWatch"
- UK 'Yellow Card' System
- Pharmacovigilance Programme of India.

WHO International System[9]

The WHO Programme for International Drug Monitoring provides a forum for WHO member states to collaborate in the monitoring of drug safety. Within the Program, individual case reports of suspected adverse drug reactions are collected and stored in a common database, presently containing over 3.7 million case reports. In each of the countries participating in the Program, the government has designated a National Centre for pharmacovigilance.

The WHO Program, which was established in 1968, consists of a network of the National Centres, WHO Headquarters, Geneva and the WHO Collaborating Centre for International Drug Monitoring, the Uppsala Monitoring Centre, in Uppsala, Sweden. As of December 2007, 84 countries (Table 7.2) had joined the WHO Drug Monitoring Program, and in addition, 23 countries (Table 7.3) were considered 'associate members' awaiting compatibility between the national and international reporting formats.

The administration of the WHO Programme is shared. In accordance with an agreement between WHO and the Government of Sweden, WHO Headquarters is responsible for policy issues, while the operational responsibility rests with the Uppsala Monitoring Centre (UMC). Functions of the WHO Programme for International Drug Monitoring include:

- Identification and analysis of new adverse reaction signals from the case report information submitted to the

Postmarketing Surveillance

Table 7.2: Official member countries and their year of entering the Programme

- Argentina (1994)
- Armenia (2001)
- Australia (1968)
- Austria (1991)
- Belarus (2006)
- Belgium (1977)
- Brazil (2001)
- Brunei Darussalam (2005)
- Bulgaria (1975)
- Canada (1968)
- Chile (1996)
- China (1998)
- Colombia (2004)
- Costa Rica (1991)
- Croatia (1992)
- Cuba (1994)
- Cyprus (2000)
- Czech Republic (1992)
- Denmark (1968)
- Egypt (2001)
- Estonia (1998)
- Fiji (1999)
- Finland (1974)
- France (1986)
- Germany (1968)
- Ghana (2001)
- Greece (1990)
- Guatemala (2002)
- Hungary (1990)
- Iceland (1990)
- India (1998)
- Indonesia (1990)
- Ireland (1968)
- Islamic Republic of Iran (1998)
- Israel (1973)
- Italy (1975)
- Japan (1972)
- Jordan (2002)
- Korea, Rep of (1992)
- Kyrgyzstan (2003)
- Latvia (2002)
- Lithuania (2005)
- The Former Yugoslav Republic of Macedonia (2000)
- Malaysia (1990)
- Malta (2004)
- Mexico (1999)
- Republic of Moldova (2003)
- Morocco (1992)
- Mozambique (2005)
- Nepal (2006)
- Netherlands (1968)
- New Zealand (1968)
- Nigeria (2004)
- Norway (1971)
- Oman (1995)
- Peru (2002)
- Philippines (1995)
- Poland (1972)
- Portugal (1993)
- Romania (1976)
- Russian Federation (1998)
- Serbia (2000)
- Singapore (1993)
- Slovakia (1993)
- South Africa (1992)
- Spain (1984)
- Sri Lanka (2000)
- Suriname (2007)
- Sweden (1968)
- Switzerland (1991)
- United Republic of Tanzania (1993)
- Thailand (1984)
- Togo (2007)
- Tunisia (1993)
- Turkey (1987)
- Uganda (2007)
- Ukraine (2002)
- United Kingdom (1968)
- Uruguay (2001)
- USA (1968)
- Uzbekistan (2006)
- Venezuela (1995)
- Vietnam (1999)
- Zimbabwe (1998)

Table 7.3: Associate member countries

- Algeria
- Andorra
- Bahrain
- Barbados
- Benin
- Bhutan
- Botswana
- Cameroon
- Côte d'Ivoire
- Dem Rep of Congo
- Eritrea
- Ethiopia
- Georgia
- Kazakhstan
- Kenya
- Madagascar
- Mongolia
- Pakistan
- Panama
- Sierra Leone
- Sudan
- Zambia
- Zanzibar

National Centres, and from them to the WHO database. A data-mining approach (BCPNN) is used at the UMC to support the clinical analysis made by a panel of signal reviewers

- Provision of the WHO database as a reference source for signal strengthening and ad hoc investigations. Web-based search facilities and customized services are available
- Information exchange between WHO and National Centres, mainly through 'VigiMed', an e-mail information exchange system
- Publication of periodical newsletters, (WHO Pharmaceuticals Newsletter and Uppsala Reports), guidelines and books in the pharmacovigilance and risk management area.
- Supply of tools for management of clinical information including adverse drug reaction case reports. The main products are the WHO Drug Dictionary and the WHO Adverse Reaction Terminology.
- Provision of training and consultancy support to National Centres and countries establishing pharmacovigilance systems.
- Computer software for case report management designed to suit the needs of National Centres (VigiFlow).

- Annual meetings for representatives of National Centres at which scientific and organizational matters are discussed.
- Methodological research for the development of pharmacovigilance as a science.

US FDA "MedWatch"

MedWatch is the US FDA Safety Information and Adverse Event Reporting Program. This serves both healthcare professionals and the medical product-using public. MedWatch provides important and timely clinical information about safety issues involving medical products, including prescription and over-the-counter drugs, biologics, medical and radiation-emitting devices, and special nutritional products (e.g. medical foods, dietary supplements and infant formulas).

Medical product safety alerts, recalls, withdrawals, and important labeling changes that may affect the health of all Americans are quickly disseminated to the medical community and the general public.

MedWatch allows healthcare professionals and consumers to report serious problems that they suspect are associated with the drugs and medical devices they prescribe, dispense, or use. Reporting can be done on line, by phone, or by submitting the MedWatch 3500 form by mail or fax. The MedWatch program, like all spontaneous systems, solicits information's on potentially confounding factors as well as the suspected drug and adverse drug reactions. Confounding information typically collected by spontaneous reporting systems includes, age gender, weight, race, allergies, past medical history, medication history and social medication history. All confounding factors should be considered when determining the likelihood that the suspect drug actually caused the adverse drug reaction. When the Medwatch programme receives a sufficient number of adverse drug reactions attributed to a particular drug, several enforcement options are available to the FDA. The agency can mandate the addition of information describing the newly detected adverse drug reaction to the drug's label or package insert. The FDA can also require the manufacturer to distribute letters to all registered physician and pharmacist informing them about the newly identified adverse drug reactions. These letters typically include a description of the adverse drug reactions, its frequency of occurrence, risk factors, and instruction for the monitoring the adverse drug reactions. Finally, the FDA can require the manufacturer to develop a formal surveillance programme to monitor the rate and extent of the adverse drug occurrence; however, this step is uncommon and is typically suggested at the time of the drug approval. If the drugs risks are determined to outweigh the benefits of the drug then the FDA can suggest withdrawal of the drug from the market.

UK 'Yellow Card' System[10]

In the UK, the system for spontaneous reporting is the "Yellow Card Scheme" (YCS). The tragic events surrounding the use of Thalidomide by pregnant women led to the introduction of the Committee on Safety of Drugs (CSD). This commitee was charged with collecting and disseminating information relating to adverse effects of drugs. To achieve these objectives, Sir Derrick Dunlop, the chairman of the CSD announced the launch of the UK's Spontaeneous Reporting Scheme in 1964, when he made it the (voluntary) remit of "**every member of the medical and dental profession in the UK...**" to report "**...promptly the details of any untoward condition in a patient which might be the result of drug treatment...**"

The principles of this reporting scheme were such that:
- *Suspected adverse reactions* should be reported, with no establishment of causality
- It was a *responsibility* of all doctors and dentists to report suspected adverse reactions

- The report should be *prompt*
- All reports are treated *in confidence*.

The coincidental abundance of yellow paper at the time of sending out the first samples of the reporting cards resulted in the eponymous reference to the scheme. The total annual reports received since the inception of the Yellow Card Scheme till year 2002 are shown in Figure 7.2.

This system in the UK has had numerous successes which are enlisted below:
- Halothane- Jaundice[11,12]
- Oestrogens and thromboembolism[13,14]
- Protriptyline-photosensitivity[15]
- Nalidixic acid—CNS effects[16]
- Ibufenac and liver damage[17]
- Mianserin-induced arthropathy[18]
- Amiodarone-induced hepatitis[18]
- Piroxicam-induced congestive cardiac failure[18]
- Methyldopa and hepatitis[12]
- Metoclopramide and extrapyramidal side effects[12]

This system has had its failures as enlisted below:
- Practolol oculomucocutaneous syndrome[12]
- Incorrect identification of erythromycine estolate as being a more important cause of jaundice than other esters.
- Benoxaprofen.

Pharmacovigilance Program of India[19-21]

The Ministry of Health and Family Welfare (MoHFW), Government of India launched the nationwide Pharmacovigilance Programme of India (PvPI) in the year 2010. The programme was launched to inspire confidence and trust among patients and healthcare professionals with respect to medicines safety in India. Indian Pharmacopoeia Commission (IPC) under the MoHFW has been functioning as the National Coordination Centre (NCC) for PvPI since April 2011. Teaching hospitals and

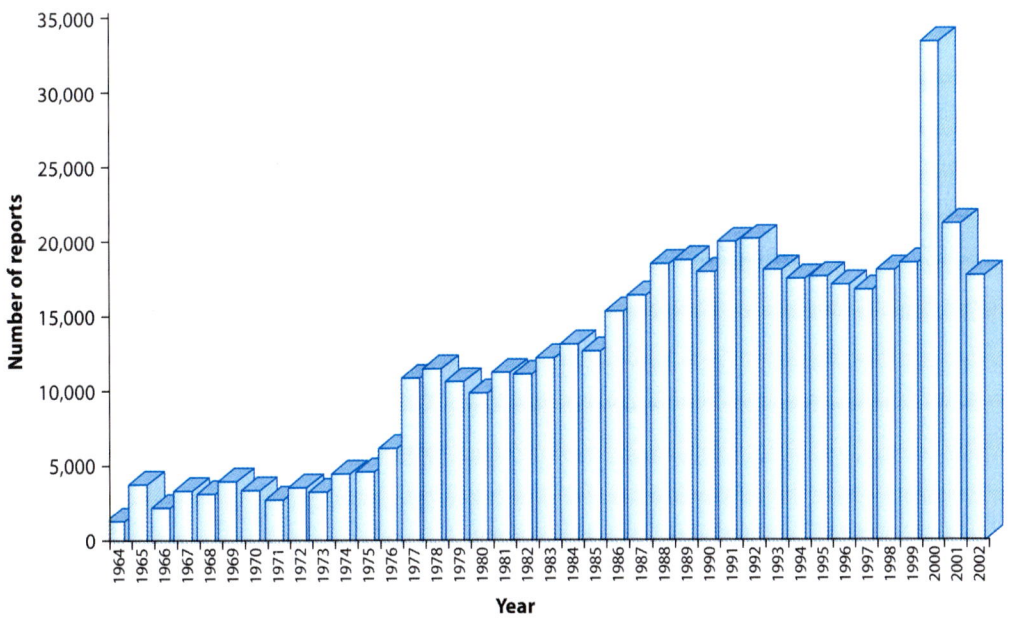

Fig. 7.2: Number of Yellow Card reports received between 1964-2002

corporate hospitals approved by Medical Council of India have been identified as ADRs Monitoring Centres (AMCs) across the country. These centres are covered in four zonal offices of Central Drugs Standard Control Organization (CDSCO) for administrative and logistic purpose. These AMCs are connected with international networking [reporting through VigiFlow; WHO-Uppsala Monitoring Centre (UMC) software]. These AMCs report ADRs to NCC through VigiFlow, the software owned by WHO-UMC, (Sweden). Over 5 years, the NCC has played a significant role in creating awareness among healthcare professionals about reporting ADRs that saw more than 1,49,000 ADRs reported till December 2015. Currently, the contribution of India to the WHO global Individual Case Safety Reports (ICSRs) database is 3%. The healthcare professionals are encouraged to report through feedback and Newsletters.

A helpline number (toll free), i.e. 1800 180 3024 facility for reporting adverse events was launched to enhance the participation of patients, healthcare professionals, and the pharmaceutical industry in enhancing medicines safety by reporting suspected ADRs to the NCC-PvPI. This may be one of the innovative methods to create awareness and to reach every corner of the country for the pharmacovigilance activity. This facility will be useful for the healthcare professionals those who are working in tertiary healthcare system to report ADRs. Adverse events-related information which received at NCC will be communicated to nearest AMCs for validating the reports. Since sending timely feedback or acknowledgment will build public confidence. Recently this facility has been upgraded by sending short message service feedback/ acknowledgment to the ADRs reporters.

Under PvPI program, the drugs have been kept under scanner and quarterly drug safety alerts on suspected unexpected serious adverse reactions (SUSARs) are issued to health care professionals via News letters (Table 7.1). Based upon PvPI database, Indian manufacturers have been instructed to include Steven-Johnson syndrome (SJS) in package insert of product containing carbamazepine and physicians have been advised to screen the patients for HLA-B*1502 allele before initiating treatment with carbamazepine.

In the 9th signal review panel (SRP) meeting of PvPI held on 29 October 2016 at CDSCO west zonal office Mumbai, the review panel recommended new signals, drug safety label change and the drug alerts for the following pharmaceutical products which are marketed in India (Table 7.6).

Table 7.4: SUSARs reported during 2011-2013

Sl. No	Suspected drug	Adverse drug reaction	SUSAR's in PvPI database	SUSARs in WHO VigiBase
1.	Sodium valproate	Slurred speech	11	14
2.	Streptokinase	Hepatitis	4	18
3.	Bupivacaine	Confusional state	2	13
4.	Omeprazole	Hypokalemia	1	49
5.	Metronidazole	Thrombophlebitis	1	2
6.	Gentamicin	Thrombophlebitis	1	1
7.	Tramadol	Renal and urinary tract neoplasm	1	5
8.	Amphotericin-B	Hypernatremia	1	6
9.	Nitrofurantion	Lipedema	1	9

Table 7.5: Recommendations of Signal Review Panel

Sl. No.	Drugs	Adverse drug reactions	Recommendations
1.	Furosemide	Dermatitis lichenoid	Signal
2.	Itraconazole	Acute generalized exanthematous pustulosis	Signal
3.	Lithium carbonate	Drug reaction with eosinophilia and systemic symptoms (DRESS)	Signal
4.	BCG vaccine	Lymphadenopathy	Drug safety label change
5.	Docetaxel	Candidiasis	Drug safety label change
6.	Phenytoin	Acute generalised exanthematous pustulosis	Drug safety label change
7.	Meropenem	Hypokalemia	Drug alert
8.	Montelukast	Hypokalemia	Drug alert

Table 7.6: Drug safety alerts from PvPI database

Sl. No.	Drug	Indication	Adverse drug reaction
1.	Cabergoline	Hyperprolactinemia and inhibition of lactation	Steven-Johnson syndrome
2.	Amlodipine	Angina, hypertension, coronary artery disease	Alopecia
3.	Nitrofurantoin	Urinary tract infection, cystitis	DRESS (Drug reaction with eosinophilia and systemic syndrome)
4.	Atenolol	Angina, myocardial infarction, arrhythmias, hypertension, migraine prophylaxis	Dermatitis lichenoid
5.	Cefixime	Otitis media, uncomplicated UTIs, effective against infections caused by *enterobacteriaceae*, *H. influenza* species	Anal ulcer
6.	Olanzapine	Schizophrenia, and other psychotic disorders, mania/mixed episodes, psychomotor agitation, violent behavior	DRESS
7.	Montelukast	Prophylaxis of mild to moderate asthma	Tinnitus

Hemovigilance Program of India (HvPI)

Hemovigilance is a set of surveillance procedures covering the whole transfusion chain from the collection of blood and its components to the follow-up of its recipients intended to collect and assess information on unexpected or undesirable effects resulting from the therapeutic use of labile blood products and to prevent their occurrence and recurrence. It is an important tool for improving safe blood transfusion practices in a country.

The Hemovigilance Programme of India (HvPI) was launched on 10th December, 2012 in the country.

Textbook of Pharmacovigilance

Table 7.7: Comparative status of global drug alerts with PvPI database

Sl. No.	Name of drug	Risk	International Status (Global Drug Alerts)	India Status (PvPI Database)
1.	Atypical antipsychotics	Sleep apnea	Health Canada had carried out a safety review to investigate risk of sleep apnea with the use of atypical antipsychotics. It recommends that current product labels for atypical antipsychotics (aripiprazole, asenapine, clozapine, lurasidone, olanzapine, paliperidone, quetiapine, risperidone and ziprasidone) are updated to include the risk of sleep apnea	A total of 3 reports were received on atypical antipsychotics for the risk of sleep apnea
2.	BCR-ABL Tyrosine kinase inhibitors	Hepatitis B virus reactivation	Therapeutic good administration (TGA), Australia worked with manufacturers to update the product information documents of BCR-ABL Tyrosine kinase inhibitors (TKIs) such as Imatinib, Nilotinib, Dasatinib and Ponatinib by including a precautionary statement about the risk of HBV reactivation. The Ministry of Health, Labor and Welfare (MHLW) and Pharmaceutical and Medical Devices Agency (PMDA), Japan announced that package inserts for BCR-ABL TKIs (imatinib, nilotinib, dasatinib and bosutinib) have been updated to include the risk of reactivation of HBV as an important precaution. The Health Science Authority (HSA), Singapore stated that local package inserts for BCR-ABL TKIs (dasatinib, imatinib and nilotinib) updated to include the risk of HBV reactivation	Two cases of hepatitis B virus reactivation were received for Imatinib
3.	Etanercept	Potential harm due to in utero exposure during pregnancy	Health Canada's safety review noted that taking Etanercept during pregnancy associated with potential risk of experiencing a miscarriage. It is also working with the manufacturer of etanercept on updating the product safety information on the risks of birth defects due to in utero exposure during pregnancy	One case of abortion due to etanercept was reported
4.	Metoclopramide containing products	Restriction on dose and duration of use due to neurological and cardiovascular adverse effects	European Union review confirmed a relationship between high doses or long-term use of metoclopramide and an increase in the risk of neurological and serious cardiovascular adverse reaction (IV route). HSA noted that nearly one in five neurological adverse report associated with metoclopramide from 1993 to August 2014 were reported in children. Hence, HSA had recommended that the package inserts for metoclopramide containing products are updated to include restrictions on dose and duration of use	Multiple report of neurological ADR and two report of cardiovascular ADR due to metoclopramide administration were documented in PvPI
5.	Natalizumab	Progressive multifocal leukoencephalopathy, granule cell neuronopathy and acute retinal necrosis	MHLW and PMDA, Japan had announced that package insert for natalizumab (Tysabri®) updated to include the risk of progressive multifocal leukoencephalopathy (PML), granule cell neuronopathy and acute retinal necrosis in patients as clinically significant adverse reactions	One case of PML was reported to NCC

Contd...

Contd...

Sl. No.	Name of drug	Risk	International Status (Global Drug Alerts)	India Status (PvPI Database)
6.	Olanzapine	Drug induced hypersensitivity syndrome (DIHS)	MHLW and PMDA, Japan had announced that package inserts for Olanzapine (Zyprexa® and others) updated to include the risk of drug-induced hypersensitivity syndrome (DIHS) as a clinically significant adverse reaction	Two cases of DIHS were reported to NCC
7.	Allopurinol	Serious cutaneous adverse reactions (SCAR) and role of genotyping	HSA found evidence of a strong association between HLAB*5801 allele and allopurinol –induced SCAR (100 times high risk) compared to others. This is consistent with international data. Hence, HSA issued advice to health care professionals about cautions required with the use of allopurinol to minimize risk of allopurinol-induced SCAR	44 cases of SCAR (SJS and TEN) were reported to NCC
8.	Isotretinoin	Psychiatric adverse event	Isotretinoin (Roaccutane® and generics) is indicated for the treatment of severe cystic acne. Therapeutic Goods Administration (TGA), Australia stated that psychiatric adverse reactions, including depression and suicidality are a known risk associated with the use of isotretinoin. TGA advised healthcare professionals to perform careful psychological assessment before and during treatment with isotretinoin	NCC-PvPI received six cases of psychiatric disorders with the use of isotretinoin

Major Strengths and Weaknesses of Spontaneous Reporting System see Table 7.8

Table 7.8: The strengths and weaknesses of a spontaneous reporting system

Strengths	Weaknesses
Low set-up and running cost	Under-reporting is a major problem
Allows for perpetual monitoring of all drugs after marketing	There is no direct information on incidence
May generate rapid alerts and stimulate follow-up	Sensitive to selective reporting and other influential factors
Does not limit monitoring to specific patient groups	Quality of information can vary greatly, and can prevent proper clinical evaluation
Least likely to influence prescribing behavior	Depends on reporters to identify an event as a reaction to a drug

An interesting note for the readers

Weber effect: The marketing of a new drug usually involves a slow release onto the market, which causes a slow rise in ADR reports. According to Weber, the total number of ADR report increases until two years after the introduction and declines thereafter.

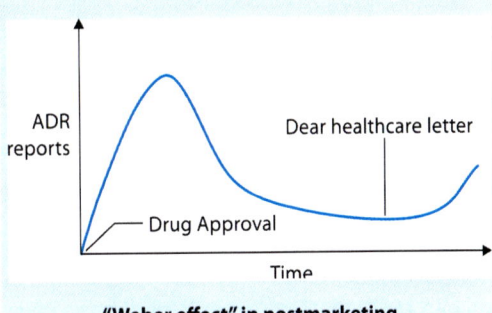

"Weber effect" in postmarketing

Source: Weber JCP. Epidemiology of adverse reactions to non steroid anti-inflammatory drugs. In: Advances in inflammation Research, Volume 6. New York: Raven Press, 1984

Case Reports

Case reports and case series allow practitioners to share their individual experiences in published medical literature. These play a vital role in communicating previously unidentified uses and dangers of drugs. Case reports can serve the same role as spontaneous reports and warn practitioners of suspected adverse drug reactions. These also offer the sharing of new medications or applications for drugs.

A best example for the application of case reports and case series in the PMS is the experience with the anorexant drug combination, phentermine/fenfluramine (phen-fen) in the United States. The phen-fen combination actually comprises of two separate drugs phentermine and fenfluramine. These are prescribed together to promote weigh loss. Phentermine was approved by the FDA in 1971, and fenfluramine was approved in 1973. During the 20 years following approval, the drugs were prescribed individually, and patients received one drug or the other. Neither drug was widely used during this time period. Then, in the mid-1990s, it was determined that the combination use of the two drugs showed significant benefit in weight reduction.[22] Phen-fen usage of the two drugs showed significant benefits in weight reduction. Phen-fen usage increased dramatically, thereafter. In 1996, more than 18,000,000 prescriptions were filled for the Phen-fen combination.[16]

Connolly and colleagues had published[23] a case series describing 24 young, overweight women with no prior history of cardiac disease who were diagnosed with valvular heart disease while taking then phen-fen combination. Eight of the women in the case series also had pulmonary hypertension. Many of the women required surgical intervention. These cases alarmed practitioners, patients, and regulatory agencies. On September 5, 1997, fenfluramine was withdrawn from the market.

Case series as mentioned above has shown to be very powerful tool. The Phen-fen case series changed medical practice instantaneously. Practitioners began to screen patients using anorexant drugs for signs and signs and symptoms of valvular heart disease and primary pulmonary hypertension. Practitioners also began eliciting information on cardiac on cardiac risk factors before initiating anorexant-associated adverse drug reactions to the FDA, and more case reports were published in the medical literature.

Case-control Studies[24]

The case-control design is an analytical, retrospective study comparing people with the disease to a sample of people without the disease (controls) with respect to exposure or characteristics of interest. In a case-control study, cases of disease (or events) are identified. Controls, or patients without the disease or event of interest, are then selected from the source population that gave rise to the cases. The controls should be selected in such a way that the prevalence of exposure among the controls represents the prevalence of exposure in the source population. The exposure status of the two groups is then compared using the odds ratio, which is an estimate of the relative risk of disease in the two groups. Patients can be identified from an existing database or using data collected especifically for the purpose of the study of interest. If safety information is sought for special populations, the cases and controls can be stratified according to the population of interest (the elderly, children, pregnant women, etc.). For rare adverse events, existing large population-based databases are a useful and efficient means of providing needed drug exposure and medical outcome data in a relatively short period of time. Case-control studies are particularly useful when the goal is to investigate whether there is an association between a drug (or drugs) and one specific rare adverse event, as well as to identify risk factors for adverse events. Risk factors can include conditions such as renal and hepatic dysfunction that might modify the relationship between the drug exposure and the adverse event. Under specific conditions, a case-control study can provide the absolute incidence rate of the event. If all cases of interest (or a well-defined fraction of cases) in the catchment area are captured and the fraction of controls from the source population is known, an incidence rate can be calculated.

Example of Case-control study

A retrospective, matched case-control study[25] using California Medicaid claims data study was conducted to determine the difference in risk of hepatotoxicity in patients receiving doxycycline or tetracycline. The cases were defined as recipients who had at least one diagnosis of hepatotoxicity any time from 1 July 1999 to 31 December 2001. One control was identified for each case, matched on age, gender and race. Logistic regression was used to determine the adjusted odds ratio (OR) and 95% confidence intervals for current users and past users of tetracycline and doxycycline. Covariates controlled for in the analysis were age, use of other hepatotoxic drugs, renal dysfunction, pregnancy, and alcohol or illicit drug use. A total of 3,377 cases of hepatotoxicity were identified. Current users and past users of tetracycline had a statistically significant increased risk of developing hepatotoxicity (current use OR 3.70, 95% CI 1.19-11.45; past use OR 2.72, 95% CI 1.26-5.85). Current users or past users of doxycycline did not have an increased risk of developing hepatotoxicity (current use OR 1.49, 95% CI 0.61-3.62; past use OR 1.74, 95% CI 0.99-3.06). Tetracycline was commonly used for acne, acute bronchitis and upper respiratory infections. Doxycycline was commonly used for acute bronchitis, vaginitis and acne. From this study it was concluded that Doxycycline was potentially less hepatotoxic than tetracycline. Also, Doxycycline could potentially be a safe substitute for tetracycline, when appropriate.

The major advantage of case control design are that it can often be used with study populations of relatively smaller size than prospective cohort studies or clinical trials ,and at a somewhat lower cost. This efficiency of size and cost is particularly advantageous for studying rare conditions or conditions that appear after long latency periods. A classic small definitive case-control study consisting of only 8 cases and 32 controls was responsible for definitively establishing the link between maternal diethylstilbestrol therapy and adenocarcinoma of the vagina in daughters.[26]

The major problem in conducting a case control study relate to selecting cases and controls, collecting valid retrospective data from records or relying on recall, and interpreting the result to remove the effects of confounding factors (factors associated with the disease or adverse reaction under study); sex, age, education level, and socioeconomic status are often related to drug selection and access to medical care.

Cross-sectional Studies[24,27]

A cross-sectional study or survey is an observational study in which drug exposure and disease status or symptoms are determined at a single point in time (or interval of time) (Fig. 7.3). These are also called as prevalence studies as these are usually conducted to estimate the prevalence of the outcome of interest for a given population, commonly for the purposes of public health planning. In these studies data is usually collected on a population of patients regardless of exposure or disease status. Data can also be collected on individual characteristics, including exposure to risk factors, alongside information about the outcome. In this way cross-sectional studies provide a 'snapshot' of the outcome and the characteristics associated with it, at a specific point in time. These studies are primarily used to gather data for surveys or for ecological analyses.

A cross-sectional study design is used when the purpose of the study is:
- Descriptive often in the form of a survey
- To find the prevalence of the outcome of interest, for the population or subgroups within the population at a given timepoint.

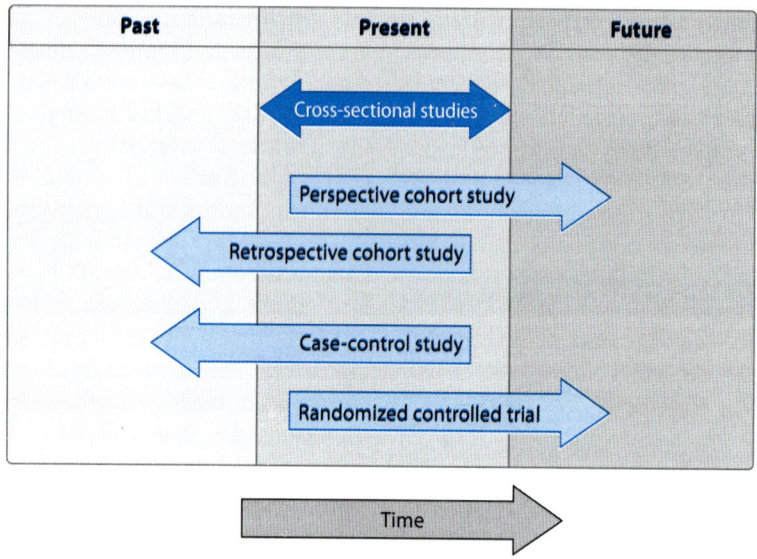

Fig. 7.3: Cross-sectional studies

Advantages of Cross-sectional Studies

- Relatively inexpensive and takes up little time to conduct
- Prevalence of outcome of interest can be estimated since sample is usually taken from the whole population
- Assessment of many outcomes and risk factors
- Useful for public health planning, understanding disease etiology and for the generation of hypotheses
- There is no loss to follow-up.

Disadvantages of Cross-sectional Studies

- Difficult to make causal inference
- Only a snapshot: The situation may provide differing results if another time-frame had been chosen;
- Associated with prevalence—incidence bias (also called Neyman bias). Especially in the case of longer-lasting diseases, any risk factor that results in death will be under-represented among those with the disease.

Example of Cross-Sectional study

Prevalence of overweight and obesity in East and West German children in the decade after reunification was measured using a population-based series of cross-sectional studies.[28]

The aim of the study was to analyze time trends in overweight and obesity from 1991 to 2000 in samples of German children and to test the hypothesis of a trend difference between the samples from East and West Germany during this time period using data of 35,434 five to seven-year-old children from school entry examinations in several rural and urban areas in East and West Germany. Since the main outcome measures were overweight and obesity so weight and height were measured and body mass index was calculated. International cut-off points were used to classify overweight and obesity. From 1991 to 2000, the prevalence of overweight increased from 10.0% to 17.5% in the East and from 14.8% to 22.2% in the West. The prevalence of obesity increased from 2.1% to 5.7% in the East and from 3.6% to 7.6% in the West. All increases were significant. There was no evidence of a trend difference between the East and the West German samples.

Conclusion: Unlike in other countries in transition, prevalence of childhood overweight and obesity were increasing in samples of East German children after reunification in 1990, possibly as a result of the rapid adoption of a western lifestyle in the East. Although, prevalence were generally higher in the West German samples, there was no evidence that the increase was leveling off in the West. Overall, trends were similar in the East and West German samples.

Cohort Studies

In cohort studies groups of individuals (cohorts) are identified, characterized, and followed over time to determine the incidence of some predetermined outcome or outcome. Controlled cohort studies with one cohort characterized by exposure to the drug being evaluated and a second cohort untreated or exposed to an alternative drug are scientifically preferable to uncontrolled cohort studies in which there is no control group. Cohort studies may be conducted either prospectively or retrospectively.

In a prospective cohort study, a cohort may be selected for reasons of convenience (e.g. medical records are available, volunteers) or because the group is known to have experienced an exposure of interest (e.g. the first 1000 prescriptions to receive a prescription for a newly marketed drug). The major advantages and disadvantages of the prospective cohort study are discussed below:

Advantages

- The characteristics of the cohort can be determined (e.g. drug exposure, smoking, compliance) prior to knowing whether a disease outcome or an adverse drug reaction has occurred
- The investigator can determine in advance what information to collect
- Calculation of adverse reaction incidence rates and comparison of the difference of incidence between cohorts (attributable risk).

Disadvantages

- The cost and the difficulty of guarding against inherent biases (e.g. physician and patient selection of treatment, selection of alternative therapies, and of enrolling representative volunteers)
- Prospective cohort studies are not large enough to detect rare adverse reactions
- Requirement of large cohorts when the disease of interest has a low incidence.

Examples of the Cohort Studies

- Framingham Heart Study[29]
- Physician's and Nurses Health Study[30]
- Collaborative perinatal project, sponsored by the National Institute of Neurological and Communicative Disorders of the National Institute of Health.

The Framingham Heart Study

In 1948, the Framingham Heart Study—under the direction of the National Heart Institute (now known as the National Heart, Lung, and Blood Institute; NHLBI)—embarked on an ambitious project in health research to determine risk factors associated with the development of cardiovascular disease. Since 1971, the Framingham Heart Study has been conducted in collaboration with Boston University. The cohort in this study comprises of original cohort, offspring cohort and the generation III cohort.

Original cohort
The researchers recruited 5,209 men and women between the ages of 30 and 62 (initial cohort) from the town of Framingham, Massachusetts, (and began the first round of extensive physical examinations and lifestyle interviews that they would later analyze for common patterns related to CVD development). Since 1948, the subjects have continued to return to the study every two years for a detailed medical history, physical examination, and laboratory tests.

Offspring Cohort

In 1971, the study enrolled a second-generation group—5,124 of the original participants' adult children and their spouses—to participate in similar examinations.

Generation III Cohort

A Third Generation (the children of the Offspring Cohort) is currently being recruited and examined, seeking to further understand how genetic factors relate to cardiovascular disease. These participants are being given an extensive cardiovascular examination similar to their parents and grandparents. The goal is to recruit and examine 3,500 grandchildren of the original cohort.

Over the years, careful monitoring of the Framingham Study population has led to the identification of the major CVD risk factors—high blood pressure, high blood cholesterol, smoking, obesity, diabetes, and physical inactivity—as well as a great deal of valuable information on the effects of related factors such as blood triglyceride and HDL cholesterol levels, age, gender, and psychosocial issues. Although, the Framingham cohort is primarily white, the importance of the major CVD risk factors identified in this group have been shown in other studies to apply almost universally among racial and ethnic groups, even though the patterns of distribution may vary from group to group. Since its inception, the study has produced approximately 1,200 articles in leading medical journals.

Physician's and Nurse's Health Study

The physician's and nurses health studies are cohort studies similar to Framingham Heart Study; however subjects in these cohort studies were chosen based on profession rather than geographic location. The Nurse's Health Study began in 1976 and enrolled 12,1700 female registered nurses from 30 to 55 year old. Information in this study is obtained via questionnaires on enrollment and every 2 years thereafter.

Collaborative Perinatal Project, Sponsored by the National Institute of Neurological and Communicative Disorders of the National Institute of Health

This project enrolled 50,282 mother child pairs in 12 medical centres between the year 1959 and 1965. Although this study did not identify any "new thalidomides", new methods to analyze the enormous amount of information that is collected in large prospective cohort studies were developed.

Randomized Clinical Trials

A controlled clinical trial is a prospective study that involves two or more treatment groups and controls who may be treated with an active drug, a placebo or both. The purpose of conducting a controlled clinical drug trial is to assess the effectiveness of drug therapy in either preventing disease (prophylactic trials) or treatment established disease (therapeutic trials).

A randomized controlled clinical trial is characterized by assignment of participants to treatment or control groups in a random and unbiased fashion. The most stringent clinical trial methodologies involve double blind techniques where neither the patient nor the physician knows which therapy the patient is receiving and triple blind techniques where the epidemiologist/statistician also is unaware of the patient's therapy.

Though the randomized clinical trials are considered the gold standard in epidemiological research, there are certain limitations (disadvantages) associated with the clinical trials in regard to adverse events.

Limitations of Clinical Trials

- **Controlled situation of clinical trials:** Clinical trials are conducted in the controlled situation as per the protocol ICH

GCP guidelines, by the clinicians trained in this area, consequently these cannot monitor adverse effects that may occur due to the consequence of inadequate prescribing, use for the wrong indications, or over – or under prescribing.
- **Duration and cost:** Clinical trials are expensive and time bound. They do not provide follow upon of patients with chronic diseases and drugs administered over a long period of time.
- **Observations at specified intervals in clinical trials:** In clinical trials observations are recorded and analyzed at repeated time intervals as defined in the protocol. These repeated observations and testing of the same cohort causes special problems in statistical methodology.
- **Sample size:** This is the most limiting factor for the side effects which occur with a low frequency. Very large numbers of patients are then needed to obtain any useful degree of statistical power.

Database Research and Monitoring

The past several decades have gained the popularity for database research. Many health care organizations have automated all health care records such that outpatient visits, pharmacy records, and hospital admissions all are stored in one data base. These data bases can be used to evaluate associations between drug exposures and outcomes, there by providing all of the necessary information as recorded accurately in the databases.

Computerized databases that link drug histories with medical care records allow pharmacoepidemiologists to design and implement cost-effective studies.

Major Strengths of Database

- Efficiency in identifying large numbers of people who were exposed to a drug or who developed a disease
- Provides additional information in analyzing a temporal relationship for the disease or the adverse events
- Computerized databases that are useful for pharmacoepidemiological studies fit into three broad categories: Databases containing information on disease only, databases including information on drugs and disease, and clinical databases that contain drug and disease histories and pertinent laboratory values
- When patients and/or medical records are accessible, large automated databases provide a cost-effective ideal method for identifying patients of interest for either case control or cohort studies.

Limitations of Database Research

- Databases needs the verification for the accuracy of data. The verification can be conducted by validation of some of the cases. This validation is performed by taking a random sample (e.g. 10%) of cases generated by the computer and following up with either the patient or the practitioner to validate whether the computer records are accurate and the patient truly has been diagnosed with the outcome of interest.
- Investigator does not know what factors may have affected the phycision's decision to prescribe a drug or whether the diagnosis was accurate and complete (confounding factors).

Meta-Analyses

These are the studies that combine the results of two or more individual studies into one large study. They are also referred as systemic reviews. These studies are useful when conflicting results are obtained in different studies or when studies had inadequate sample size.

Example of Meta-analysis[31]

A meta-analysis was conducted to evaluate the association between green tea consumption and the risk of gastric cancer. Electronic search of the Cochrane Library, MEDLINE, EMBASE and Chinese Bio-medicine Database, which have articles published between (1966 and 2006), was conducted to select studies for this meta-analysis. This included 14 epidemiologic studies, with a total number of 6123 gastric cancer cases and 1,34,006 controls. The combined results based on all studies showed that green tea consumption was not associated with the risk of gastric cancer [odds ratio (OR) = 0.98, 95% confidence interval (CI) = 0.77-1.24]. The summary OR from all population-based case-control studies showed a minor inverse association between green tea consumption and risk of gastric cancer (OR = 0.68, 95% CI = 0.49-0.92), while no associations were noted from hospital-based case-control studies (OR = 1.12, 95% CI = 0.70-1.77) and cohort studies (OR = 1.56, 95% CI = 0.93-2.60). No associations were noted both in males (OR = 1.10, 95% CI = 0.76-1.60) and females (OR = 0.99, 95% CI = 0.64-1.51). The summary OR from seven studies suggest that the highest consumption level of green tea was more than 5 cups per day and no associations were noted (OR = 0.99, 95% CI = 0.78-1.27). The results of this meta-analysis indicated that there is no clear epidemiological evidence to support the suggestion that green tea plays a role in the prevention of gastric cancer.

An Interesting Note for the Readers

The US Food and Drug Administration's Adverse Event Reporting System is the primary surveillance database used for the identification of safety problems of marketed drugs. Despite the limitations of under-reporting, differential reporting, and uneven quality, submitted reports often allow the identification of serious adverse events that are added to the product labeling information. In rare instances, additional regulations, up to and including market removal, have been required. Physicians, pharmacists, other healthcare professionals, and patients are encouraged to continue to report serious suspected and known adverse drug reactions to manufacturers and the Food and Drug Administration.

A work flow in receiving, maintaining database and analyses of adverse drug events is provided for further reading and better understanding of the process.[32]

Disagreements between manufacturers and the FDA may be resolved through formal dispute resolution and the use of an Advisory Committee. Title 21 of the Code of Federal Regulations (e.g. Sections 2.5, 7.1-7.87, 314.150, and 314.151) describe regulatory actions that can be taken for the removal of a drug for safety reasons. These include recall procedures (usually for lot specific problems), declaration of the drug as an imminent hazard (invoked only once for phenformin and lactic acidosis), and notification of a judicial hearing. In most situations after important safety problems become evident, drugs are voluntarily withdrawn by the market authorization holder.

In September 2004, Merck & Co, Inc, voluntarily withdrew rofecoxib (Vioxx) from the global market because of an increased risk of cardiovascular events. Two months later, the FDA announced that manufacturers of isotretinoin will obtain registration of prescribers of isotretinoin, dispensing pharmacies, and patients who are prescribed the drug.[33] The agency also announced the requirement of documentation of a negative pregancy test result before isotretinoin is given to women capable of becoming pregnant. In April 2005, valdecoxib (Bextra) was withdrawn from the market because of serious dermatological conditions and an unfavorable risk vs benefit profile.

In 1994, the FDA established that any over-the-counter drug products (e.g. quinine sulfate) for the treatment and/or prevention of nocturnal leg cramps is not generally recognized as safe and effective and is misbranded.[34] In 1998, the FDA established that over-the-counter drug products containing quinine for the treatment and/or prevention of malaria are not generally recognized as safe and are misbranded.[35]

| The Office of Drug Safety (formerly the Office of Post-Marketing Drug Risk Assessment) of the FDA receives reports of adverse drug events primarily from physicians and pharmacists who submit them on a standardized form (referred to as the MedWatch form) indirectly through pharmaceutical companies or directly to the FDA |

↓

| Each report is entered into the AERS computerized database using a coding thesaurus of adverse reaction terms used for searching and retrieval purposes |

↓

| **Beginning of the process for identifying adverse events and for initiating regulatory action for drug safety problems |

Note: Health practitioners and patients may also report adverse drug events by telephone or by accessing the MedWatch Internet site. Published reports of adverse drug reactions also may be submitted

Note: Reports are entered manually; in late 1997, the system was redesigned to begin accepting a growing number of electronic reports submitted by pharmaceutical

**The various steps involved in the process for identifying adverse events and for initiating regulatory action for drug safety problems are as follows:
- FDA safety staff (primarily pharmacists) receive AERS reports daily and review them for possible drug causality
- After a sufficient number of convincing reports and/or other data (including published studies and case reports) have accumulated implicating the drug with a reaction, pharmacists and epidemiologists present the evidence in writing to the division that reviewed and approved the drug
- If the reviewing division agrees that the data are compelling enough to require regulatory action (e.g. a change in the product information), it notifies the manufacturer and requests the action.

CONCLUSION

Postmarketing surveillance plays an important role in identifying and measuring the effects and uses of drugs in clinical practice. It is clear that no single method can be used to investigate all responses and reactions in the wide variety of settings under which PMS studies needs to be conducted. In a postmarketing setting, spontaneous reporting is a mode of surveillance of adverse effects possibly related to the use of medicines in a well-defined geographic region. It is achieved by physicians who voluntarily report any effect they believe to be attributable to a drug "taken by the patient". Communication among practitioners via case reports and case series also facilitate the dissemination of information regarding new uses and dangers of drugs. No single method can be relied upon to answer all questions that may be posed. Each method answers a particular need and each has its own advantages and disadvantages.

REFERENCES

1. Lamarque V, Plétan Y. The pharmaceutical industry and the adverse effects of the drugs. Ann Pharm Fr. 2007; 65(5):308-14.
2. Hartzema AG, Porta MS, Tilson H. Introduction to pharmacoepidemiology. Drug Intelli Clin Pharm. 1987:21:739-40.
3. Faich G. Adverse Drug reaction Monitoring. N Engl J Med. 1986:314(24):1589-92.
4. Rogers AS. Adverse drug events. Identification and attribution. Drug Intelli Clin Pharm. 1987:21:741-7.
5. ICH Guidance E2D; Post-approval Safety Data Management: Definitions and Standards for Expedited Reporting. November 2003.
6. Thakrar BT, Grundschober SB, Doessegger L. Detecting signals of drug-drug interactions in a spontaneous reports database. Br J Clin Pharmacol. 2007;64(4):489-95.

7. Thiessard F, Roux E, Miremont-Salamé G, Fourrier-Réglat A, Haramburu F, Tubert-Bitter P, et al. Trends in spontaneous adverse drug reaction reports to the French pharmacovigilance system (1986-2001). Drug Saf. 2005; 28(8):731-40.
8. Salvo F, Polimeni G, Moretti U, Conforti A, Leone R, Leoni O, et al. Adverse drug reactions related to amoxicillin alone and in association with clavulanic acid: data from spontaneous reporting in Italy. J Antimicrob Chemother. 2007; 60(1):121-6.
9. http://www.who-umc.org. Accessed on January 2008.
10. http://www.liv.ac.uk/pharmacovigilance/pages/pharmuk.html. Accessed on January 2008.
11. Inman WHW, Mustrin WW. Jaundice after repeated exposure to Hlothane: an analysis of reports to the committee on safety of medicines. Br Med J. 1974;1(5):10.
12. Griffin JP. Post marketing surveillance of licensed medicinal and other products. Health Trends. 1981;13:85-8.
13. Inman WHW, Vessey MP. Investigations of deaths from pulmonary, coronary and cerebral thrombosis and embolism in women of childbearing age. Br Med J. 1968;2:193-9.
14. Inman WHW, Vessey MP, Westerholm B, Engelind A. Thromboembolic disease and the steroidal content of oral contraceptives. Br Med J. 1970;2:203.
15. Inman WHW. Monitoring by voluntary reporting at national level. In: Richards DJ, Rondel RK (Eds). Adverse Drug Reactions. Churchill Livingstone, 1972.
16. Cahal DA. Adverse reaction to nalidixic acid. Lancet. 1965:1:441.
17. Wade GL. In: Richards DJ, Rondel RK (Eds). Adverse Drug Reactions. Churchill Livingstone: Edinburgh, 1972, pp.52.
18. Anon. How the yellow card system might be improved. Pharm J. 1983;231:160.
19. Kalaiselvan V, Thota P, Singh GN. Pharmacovigilance Programme of India: Recent developments and future perspectives. Indian J Pharmacol. 2016;48:624-8.
20. Lihite RJ, Lahkar M. An update on the Pharmacovigilance programme of India. Frontiers in Pharmacology. 2015. Volume 6. Article 194.
21. Newsletter. Pharmacovigilance Programme of India. 2016;6(17).
22. Langreth R. Critics claim diet clinics misuse obesity drugs. Wall Street Journal. 1997:B8.
23. Connolly HM, Crary JL, McGoon MD, et al. Valvular heart disease associated with fenfluramine-phentermine. New Engl J Med.1997;337(9): 581-8.
24. Guidance for Industry: E2E Pharmacovigilance Planning. US Department of Health and Human Services. Food and Drug Administration. Center for Drug Evaluation and Research (CDER).Center for Biologics Evaluation and Research (CBER) April 2005.
25. Heaton PC, Fenwick SR, Brewer DE. Association between tetracycline or doxycycline and hepatotoxicity: a population based case-control study. J Clin Pharm Ther. 2007;32(5):483-7.
26. Herbst AL, Ulfelder H, Poskanzer DC. Adenocarcinoma of the vagina: association of maternal stillbestrol therapy with tumor appearance in young women. N Engl J Med 1971; 284:878-91.
27. Levin KA. Study design III: Cross-sectional studies evidence-based dentistry. 2006;7: 24-5.
28. Apfelbacher CJ, Cairns J, Bruckner T, Möhrenschlager M, Behrendt H, Ring J, et al. Prevalence of overweight and obesity in East and West German children in the decade after reunification: population-based series of cross-sectional studies. J Epidemiol Community Health. 2008;62(2):125-30.
29. http://www.nhlbi.nih.gov/about/framingham/index.html. Accessed on January 2008
30. Willett WC, Stampfer MJ, Colidtz GA, Rosner BA, Hennekens CH, Speizer FE. Dietary fat and the risk of breast cancer. N Engl J Med.1987; 316: 22-8.
31. Zhou Y, Li N, Zhuang W, Liu G, Wu T, Yao X, et al. Green tea and gastric cancer risk: meta-analysis of epidemiologic studies. Asia Pac J Clin Nutr. 2008; 17(1):159-65.
32. Wysowski DK, Swartz L. Adverse Drug Event Surveillance and Drug Withdrawals in the United States, 1969-2002. The Importance of

Reporting Suspected Reactions. Arch Intern Med. 2005; 165:1363-9.
33. US Food and Drug Administration. FDA Talk Paper: November 23, 2004: FDA announces enhancement to isotretinoin risk management program. Available at: http://www.fda.gov/bbs/topics/ANSWERS/2004/ANS01328.html.
34. US Food amd Drug Administration. Drug products for the treatment and/or prevention of nocturnal leg muscle cramps for over-the-counter human use: FDA: final rule. Fed Regist. 1994; 59:43234-43252.
35. US Food and Drug Administration. Drug products containing quinine for the treatment and/or prevention of malaria for over-the-counter human use: FDA: final rule. Fed Regist. 1998; 63:13526-9.

Setting up of A Pharmacovigilance Centre

Sushma Srivastava

INTRODUCTION

The advent of a large number of drug molecules has made pertinent to have an effective pharmacovigilance system in the country, which can protect the patients from the noxious effects of the drugs. World Health Organization (WHO) initiated a Programme on International Drug Monitoring on the basis of a resolution taken by the Twentieth World Health Assembly decades back to initiate a project on the feasibility of an international system of monitoring adverse drug reactions (ADRs) in which more than fifty countries participated.

WHO Programme of International Drug Monitoring (PIDM) was started after thalidomide tragedy and the Uppsala Monitoring Centre (UMC) in Sweden is carrying it out since 1978. The programmes started with 10 participating countries and now includes more than 150 countries, 29 countries are awaiting full membership. It was considered by the WHO that the pharmacovigilance system must be backed by the drug regulatory body of the country, which is effective and can take proper regulatory measures.

The data of ADRs are collected by the UMC from all over the world, especially from the member countries. The number of countries willing to participate gradually increased. These countries expressed their wish to receive support from WHO and made efforts to develop and strengthen their national drug programmes. Almost all developed countries have joined the programme while new requests are being received from the developing countries.

The information on marketed therapeutic drugs is scarce. The data on possible adverse reactions prior to marketing is not sufficient. The preclinical researches are done on animals and these tests cannot totally extrapolate human safety. During a clinical trial, a limited number of volunteers are selected, the conditions of trial differ with the actual conditions of use of these drugs. The data on rare but serious adverse reaction or chronic toxicity; use in special groups such as children, pregnant or elderly women is usually lacking. The post marketing monitoring data is also limited. There are region- and country-wise variations in the occurrence of adverse drug reactions and other drug related issues which may be due to drug production, distribution and use; food habits and traditions of the people; the quality and composition of the local pharmaceutical products and the use of herbal medicines. All this necessitated the need of pharmacovigilance at national and international level.

It is also true that the data generated in one country may not be relevant for other countries or regions due to differences in the situation. The international monitoring can provide compiled information on possible safety issues for the benefit of the individual countries for its use. Pharmacovigilance can help in reducing the agony of people, caused by the drugs, and can avoid the unnecessary financial burden associated with unexpected adverse reactions of the drugs.

The pharmacovigilance system at the national level is centralized or decentralized. The centralized system was the original model that had a strongly centralized National Centre that collected the reports from health professionals from all over the country. Now a decentralized system is preferred by many nations that consists of a National Coordination Centre and different regional and local centres. The National Coordination Centre functions as a focal point for these regional/local centres. There are countries, which are starting their system according to this model, and some countries having long existing drug monitoring programmes are also making efforts for developing a decentralized programme.

Pharmacovigilance provides detection, assessment and prevention of adverse reactions to drugs and aims at early detection of adverse reactions and interactions, frequency of adverse reactions, identification of risk factors for adverse reaction with its possible mechanisms, quantitative analysis of the benefits/risks and dissemination of information required to improve the prescription of drugs and related regulations. Pharmacovigilance also aims at the rational use of medicines and all medical and paramedical interventions, assesses the risks and benefits of the marketed drugs, communicates the information to the people, patients, health professionals, regulatory authorities thereby creating awareness among one and all.

Reporting of suspected adverse drug reaction from any part of the country is the pre-requisite of pharmacovigilance. In order to receive such reports, from the periphery to the central agencies at the earliest, a system of reporting is needed.

INITIATION OF DRUG MONITORING CENTRES

To strengthen and streamline the pharmacovigilance in the country, i.e. continuous monitoring of the medicines available in the market, there is a need for a pharmacovigilance centre.

The process of starting a pharmacovigilance centre involves the preliminary phase. It can be started on a very small scale with only one part time professional. It can become an established and effective centre very soon with the help of the dedicated and enthusiastic staff. The centre should have experts and dedicated personnel and the process of having such centre requires time and vision.

The location of the centre can be decided after considering the health care system of the country and the local issues. The various suitable options for pharmacovigilance centre would be government department/hospital or a space in academic institutions dealing in clinical pharmacology, clinical pharmacy, clinical toxicology or epidemiology. The process may start by reporting the adverse drug reactions associated with medicinal products, known as Individual Case Safety Reports (ICSRs) in one hospital, which can subsequently be extended to other hospitals. Later on, the compilation of such reports can be activated at the national level. The communication of such information would be the major issue while starting such centre and IT-based networking may be most useful.

The support of drug regulating agencies/governmental support would be most important for sustaining the pharmacovigilance centre. The coordination among the health functionaries, medical institutions and hospitals will have to be established for the fruitful pharmacovigilance and its further use.

PRACTICALITIES IN THE ORGANIZATION OF A PHARMACOVIGILANCE CENTRE

WHO has published guidelines for setting up a Pharmacovigilance Centre (WHO 2000). Various steps should be considered while establishing a pharmacovigilance centre:
- Human resource
- Infrastructure
  - Equipments
  - Database
  - Location
- Continuity
- Advisory committee
- Services provided
  - Information services
  - ADR reporting
  - Assessment of reports
  - Use of data
- Communication
- Funding
- International association

Human Resource

A new centre is initiated usually with a part time physician or pharmacist supported by a secretarial staff. As the activities of the centre increases a full time expert becomes essential to look up the functioning of the centre. In order to run a pharmacovigilance centre an expertise is needed in the fields of clinical medicine, pharmacology, toxicology and epidemiology. The experts having combined expertise in clinical medicine, pharmacology, toxicology and epidemiology do the assessment of the adverse reaction case reports. The existing staff of the centre can be trained. Sometimes, the services of specialized consultants can also be taken. The expansion of the secretarial staff is also required once the centre becomes established. The number of the staff to be appointed is calculated on the basis of the average assessment time per case report, (about one hour).

Infrastructure

A drug-monitoring centre requires very minimal infrastructure initially.

Equipments

Very few basic equipments are needed initially, these include:
- **A multi-connection telephone** to receive more number of calls simultaneously. The multi-connection phone enables the reporter to communicate without any delay.
- **Computer system** with a software programme for the management of adverse reaction. The data can be managed manually during the initial stages of setting up of the centre, but as the centre becomes established manual management of case reports becomes inconvenient and time taking. A computer system helps in processing and retrieving the data according to suspected drugs and adverse reactions.
- **A printer** attached to the computer system
- **Internet connection** for communicating the information immediately and receiving the inputs from various sources
- **Fax**
- **Photocopier**

Database

A database, an administrative system for the storage and retrieval of data, should be established.

Location

The best location of a pharmacovigilance centre is in a government department. It can also be initiated in any of the departments of a hospital or an academic institute involved in the clinical pharmacology, clinical pharmacy, clinical toxicology or epidemiology. To begin with, reporting of ADR can start locally in one hospital and gradually can extend to other hospitals and private practitioners of the region. Professional bodies like National Medical Association can be a suitable home for the centre.

In conditions where the centre is part of a larger organization such as a poison control unit, a clinical pharmacology department, or a hospital pharmacy that provides administrative continuity then the centre can function even with one professional (a physician or a pharmacist) mainly responsible for pharmacovigilance.

Continuity

The service provided by the centre should be continuous and easily accessible. For this it must have a permanent office for receiving calls, mails and maintenance of database. The documentation of literature and coordination of various activities is maintained at the centre.

Advisory Committee

A multi-disciplinary advisory committee supports the pharmacovigilance centre in maintaining the quality of procedures in:
- Data collection and assessment
- The interpretation of the collected data
- The publication of information

The advisory committee is constituted with the members from the field of general medicine, pharmaceutics, clinical pharmacology, toxicology, epidemiology, pathology, drug information, drug regulation and quality assurance and phytotherapy. Experts from different specialization are also consulted. The benefit of the centre of being localized in a hospital includes the easy availability of such experts.

Services Provided

The pharmacovigilance centre caters various services including information dissemination, stimulation of reporting, ADR reporting, assessment of the case reports, using the data related to ADR reports, providing training, creating awareness, etc.

Information Services

The main responsibility of a drug-monitoring centre is to provide a high-class information service regarding adverse reactions of a drug to health professionals, public, etc. A comprehensive and upto-date literature information database is required for this purpose. The Uppsala Monitoring Centre (UMC) provides a list of relevant references that can be accessed easily by the drug-monitoring centre. If a centre is a part of a large hospital or an institute it has the added advantage of a library within reach. National centres also can have online access to the database of the UMC. These NPC are included in the mailing lists of ADR and drug bulletins of WHO and other national and regional centres all over the world.

ADR Reporting

Reporting of ADR is done mainly by spontaneous reporting—pharmacovigilance is primarily based on the information on suspected adverse drug reactions from regions/periphery. It should be cheap and easy as can be, as it takes the distribution of several thousands of forms to avail only few hundred case reports.

How to report?

The ADR are filled by the clinicians or health professionals in a ADR Reporting form which elicits the information regarding the details of the patient, adverse event, suspected drug, other drugs in use, etc. A reporting form, appropriately designed should be distributed to different departments of hospital and institutions, family practitioners, etc. in order to collect the case reports.

A case report in pharmacovigilance must at least contain the information about the patient, adverse reaction of the drug, details of the suspected drugs, including all other drugs used, risk factors and details of the reporter as described below:

- The patient:
  - Age
  - Sex
  - Brief medical history (when relevant).
  - Ethnic origin (required to be specified in some countries).
- Adverse event:
  - Description (nature, localization, severity, characteristics),
  - Results of investigations and tests,
  - Start date,
  - Course and
  - Outcome.
- Suspected drug(s):
  - Name (brand or ingredient name + manufacturer)
  - Dose
  - Route
  - Start/ stop dates
  - Indication for use (with particular drugs, e.g. vaccines, a batch number is important).
- All other drugs used (including self-medication):
  - Names
  - Doses
  - Routes
  - Start/stop dates.
- Risk factors (e.g. impaired renal function, previous exposure to the suspected drug, previous allergies, and social drug use).
- Name and address of reporter (should be confidential and used only for data verification, completion and case follow-up).

To achieve effective reporting special free-post or business reply reporting forms having above mentioned questions can be distributed to healthcare personnel throughout the target area at regular, making it easy and cost effective.

A yearly distribution of thousands of forms may result in getting only hundreds of case reports. Efforts made to include the reply paid reporting forms in the national formulary, drug bulletin or professional journals may increase the number of case reports. Besides telephone, fax and e-mail are also the convenient ways of reporting.

What to report?

In a newly established pharmacovigilance centre all suspected ADR reports are accepted in order to inculcate the habit of notification. The healthcare professionals should be guided to learn how and what to notify, and the staff of the pharmacovigilance centre may be trained in assessment, coding, and interpretation. However, in established pharmacovigilance systems for new drugs usually reporting of all suspected reactions is requested. Reporting of serious or unusual suspected adverse reactions is important for established drugs, whereas known and minor reactions are of less interest. Suspicion of increased frequency of a given reaction may also be notified.

The sudden splurge in the use of herbal drugs has led to the adverse events associated with it in spite of the myth that herbal drugs are free from side effects. Adverse drug reactions associated with herbal medicines should also be considered. Drug abuse and drug use in pregnancy (teratogenicity) and lactation are given more importance.

Lack of efficacy and other drug-related defects might be reported in case of possible manufacturing defects or counterfeit drugs.

Cosmetics contain obsolete or toxic ingredients like mercury, lead, arsenic, etc. therefore adverse reactions related to the use of cosmetics should also be reported.

Problems related to medical devices and equipment may also be taken up by a pharmacovigilance centre if no other organization in the country is dealing with the issues.

Reporting of adverse event during clinical trials is done as per GCP guidelines. Reporting of adverse events is voluntary in many countries but some have made it compulsory for the practitioners, however penalty is not being imposed upon the failure to report. In some countries, it has been made mandatory for the pharmaceutical companies to report any suspected ADR to the regulatory authorities.

Who will report?

Health care professionals are the most preferred source of information for collecting the data related to the ADR. Family physicians, dentists, medical specialists, pharmacists, midwives, nurses and other health workers also prescribe medicines and should report relevant experiences. Pharmacists and nurses can provide additional information on co-medication and previously used drugs. These can play a major role in stimulating the people for ADR reporting.

Drug manufacturers are mainly responsible for the safety of their products. Any contraindications should be clearly mentioned on the label while any observed postmarketing adverse reactions of their manufactured products should be reported by them to the competent authority.

Patients can also report adverse reactions directly to the local or national centre of Pharmacovigilance. In that case, their physicians can be consulted to receive additional information that may be useful.

Special issues in reporting

Centralized or decentralized reporting, stimulation of reporting and under-reporting are several issues which are important from the point of view of ADR reporting and making the programme a success.

- **Centralized or decentralized reporting:** Spontaneous reporting, which is the major system of monitoring the ADR at national level uses a single central database for obtaining the countrywide overview. However, if the data is generated regionally the number of reports obtained will be more and the quality of data will also be improved. These regional centres can easily communicate with the practitioners to stimulate the reporting and can improve the feedback. However, the regional centres should maintain a good liaison with the national centre in terms of data exchange. Decentralization reporting is more successful in case of countries with different regional cultural differences. But it is not economical, as it requires more facilities and staff.
- **Stimulation of reporting:** It takes a lot of motivation and stimulation to make people report adverse reactions of a drug or any therapeutic product. Stimulation for ADR reporting should be a continuous process, enabling the people or health professionals to develop a positive attitude towards pharmacovigilance in order to accept the ADR reporting in routine.

Integration of pharmacovigilance in the further development of clinical pharmacy and clinical pharmacology in the country can also stimulate reporting.

The reporting can be stimulated by easy access to prepaid reporting forms or other means of reporting. The multi-connection phone or internet connections are very useful in this regard as they are less time-consuming and convenient to many users. A personal letter or a phone call in acknowledgment of receipt of the ADR reports should be sent to the reporters. Articles published in journals, ADR reaction bulletins, or newsletters should be sent to the reporters as feedback. The staff of the drug monitoring centre should be engaged in postgraduate education and scientific meetings. Centre should have collaboration with local drug or pharmacovigilance committees and collaboration with professional associations or organizations is also desired.

Under-reporting: Another important issue is under-reporting of ADRs in almost all countries. This causes a delay in signal detection and in turn the problem is underestimated. Apart from the number of reports the quality of data and the relevance of the case reports are also important.

The reasons for under-reporting are:
- Non-availability of ADR forms
- Ignorance
- Fear of risk of litigation
- Fear of negative reflection of one's competence
- Doubts regarding the causal role of the drug
- Simple procedures and clarity of criteria for reporting along with the good motivational practice can improve the problem.

Review and Assessment of Reports

The specialized consultants and the Pharmacovigilance centre staff, who are trained to develop expertise for the same, assess the case reports. The combined expertise in clinical medicine, pharmacology, toxicology, and epidemiology is needed.

The review is based on the following:
1. *Documentation quality:* The data should contain the complete information regarding the details of the patients, adverse event, suspected drug, other drugs in use, risk factors and the reporter.
2. *Coding:* Name of the Drug should be registered systematically based on any standard classification. WHO Adverse Reaction Terminology (WHOAART) or another internationally accepted terminology (MedDRA) may be used for the coding of the adverse events.
3. *Relevance* of the reports in relation to the detection of new reactions, drug regulation, or scientific or educational value.
   The queries must be raised regarding:
   - Whether the drug is New?
   - Whether the reaction is Unknown?
   - Whether the reaction is Described in the literature?
   - Whether the reaction is Serious?
   (*See Chapter 1 for Definitions*)
4. *Identification of duplicate reports:* Sex, age or date of birth, dates of drug exposure, etc. may be used to identify duplicate reporting.
5. *Casualty assessment*: With few exceptions, case reports describe suspected adverse drug reactions. Various approaches have been developed for the structured determination of the likelihood of a casual relationship between drug exposure and adverse events, for example by the WHO Drug Monitoring Programme (*See Glossary*), the European Commission, and the French National Pharmacovigilance Programme. These systems are largely based on four considerations:
   - The association in time (or place) between drug administration and event
   - Pharmacology (including current knowledge of nature and frequency of adverse reactions)
   - Medical or pharmacological plausibility (signs and symptoms, laboratory tests, pathological findings, mechanism)
   - Likelihood or exclusion or other causes.

   The WHO causality category has the advantages of being internationally agreed and easy to use. Definitions for selected adverse reactions have been worked out and reached by international agreement. For some of these reactions, special causality algorithms have also been developed (Benichou, 1994).
6. *Data processing:* Case reports are managed by a computer system once the flow of case reports increases. So, that the data can be retrieved according to the suspected drug and adverse reactions promptly. The hierarchical drug file should be maintained in which the drugs may be recorded according to the product name, generic name, and therapeutic category.

The terminologies and classification of drugs used should be of international standards so that the comparison of results can be done at the international level and data can be shared globally. It is advisable to maintain the compatibility with the reporting requirements of WHO drug monitoring programme. In order to organize the entered data for submitting it to WHO database instructions are available from the uppsala monitoring centre (UMC). Instead of designing a system for management of adverse reaction reports it is advisable to go for a commercially available programmes that are cheaper and can be customized as per the local needs including languages.

Use of Data

Data collected after the review and assessment of ADR reports is utilized in many ways.

- **Hypothesis generation and strengthening:** Early detection of signals mainly the target of the pharmacovigilance. However, these signals may not necessarily be the definite signals. Prior to any regulatory action, this should be further explored. Hence, it is advisable to confirm it through the data available from other countries also.
- **Drug regulation:** Once a drug is approved for marketing it is continuously monitored by the regulatory authorities and the pharmaceutical company which produced it. It is advisable to adopt the approved product information such as new adverse effects, indications, and contraindications. Prior to approving a drug in one country, the experiences of other countries regarding that drug may also be shared. This can be achieved through collaborating with UMC, which is running the global drug monitoring programme.
- **Information:** The information gathered through all these ways can be spread among the interested practitioners, health care professionals through an adverse drug bulletin or a column in already existing medical and pharmaceutical journals. In case of utmost urgency, letters can be directed to the practitioners and pharmacists directly. However, this type of action is taken usually with the collaboration of the competent regulatory authority and the pharmaceutical company experts.
- **Education and feedback:** The information disseminated educates continuously healthcare professionals which is another important aim of the pharmacovigilance. It increases the awareness and knowledge of ADR and stimulates reporting.
- **Limitations of use of data:** There are various limitations of the data. It can be biased. Many times the signal received is not substantial and needs further confirmation before taking any regulatory actions. The centre has to ensure that the data received by the healthcare professionals are used carefully in a responsible manner. The spontaneous reporting system can detect ADRs that are specific or occur in a suggestive time relationship with the use of drug, however, it is not helpful in other types of ADRs such as cancer. Thus, its potential to determine the true frequency of a drug related ADR is limited. The confidentiality of the data should be maintained by the centre that includes the identity of patients, doctors, reporters, etc. Data management protocols should be adhered to.

Communication

An adverse drug bulletin or a regular column in medical/pharmaceutical journals is an excellent way of spreading the gathered information. Data sheet amendments should be done promptly. In emergency situations letters addressed as '*Dear Dr.*' may be sent to the practitioners to alert them.

Funding

The funding required for pharmacovigilance is calculated as a function of reporting required and size of population. The collection of good data both quantitatively and qualitatively has a price. The PV centre should also have a regular source of income to ensure the continuity of the work, which can be as drug registration fee or as a special mandatory pharmacovigilance contribution. This can be included in the budget of the drug regulatory authority.

1. Additional funding can also be done by approaching
2. Health insurance companies
3. University departments
4. Professional associations
5. Government departments interested in drug safety

The funding of pharmacovigilance should be guaranteed and not affected due to political changes or economic factors.

Associations

It is of utmost importance to develop a relationship with the local, state or national health authorities and with the local, regional or national institutions or groups working in the field of clinical medicine, pharmacology and toxicology. The sustenance of the pharmacovigilance centre depends upon the support from health authorities and the government. The importance of the project and its purposes should be explained to them in order to get national coordination, good collaboration, and financial as well as other support. It also prevents unnecessary competition and duplication.

The Drug Regulatory Authority should be informed in case of any serious adverse event without any delay or any interesting finding related to ADR or high/increasing frequency of ADR. The same information should be passed to the drug manufacturing company directly or through regulatory authority.

Professional medical and pharmaceutical associations should also be approached and the relationship between the centre and these organizations should be maintained as these can be approached in case of any emergency.

A pharmacovigilance centre can be initiated where there is already a poison control and drug information centre. The two have similarities in the organization as well as from a scientific point of view, hence their collaboration helps in curtailing the expenditures by sharing the facilities of a secretariat, computer resources, and library services, etc.

A newly established centre should contact *WHO Collaborating Centre for International Drug Monitoring* in Uppsala, Sweden. Apart from this, it is advisable to keep contact with the national centres of neighboring countries. These can be useful for training the staff of the lesser-experienced centre.

The association with academia, media, and consumer organizations helps in the general acceptance of the programme. Pharmacovigilance can be added in the curriculum of the postgraduate programme. Similarly, relationship with media, etc. can be helpful for the general public relationship and in case of acute problems help can be sought.

PHARMACOVIGILANCE CENTRES IN INDIA

India has the abundance of healthcare professionals and patients still the ADR reporting is in its formative years. The ADR Centres were being initiated by ICMR and DCGI in 1980s, but the people were unaware of the activities of these centres as their activities were limited to certain institutes. On 23rd November 2004 the central drug regulatory agency, the Central Drugs Standard Control Organization (CDSCO) launched the National Pharmacovigilance Programme under Ministry of Health & Family Welfare, Government of India, for creating awareness of pharmacovigilance in the country based on the WHO Guidelines for setting up and running a pharmacovigilance centre. The programme included centres at peripheral, regional and zonal levels besides National Pharmacovigilance Advisory Committee and the National Pharmacovigilance Centre (NPC) situated at CDSCO, New Delhi. ADRs were reported directly or through zonal or peripheral centres to NPC for a regulatory action.

PHARMACOVIGILANCE PROGRAMME OF INDIA (PVPI)

The CDSCO initiated a nationwide Pharmacovigilance Programme of India (PvPI) in July, 2010, with All India Institute of Medical Sciences (AIIMS), New Delhi as the National Coordinating Centre (NCC) for monitoring Adverse Drug Reactions (ADR) in the country. However, for implementing the programme more effectively the NCC was shifted to Indian Phamacopoeia Commission (IPC), Ghaziabad. Adverse Drug Reaction Monitoring Centres (AMCs) have been established in government and private hospitals to address the issue of under-reporting of adverse drug reactions. So far about 250 AMCs have been established throughout India. These AMCs are connected with international networking (reporting through VigiFlow; WHO- UMC software). These AMCs report ADRs to NCC through VigiFlow, the software owned by WHO-UMC, (Sweden). NCC-IPC receives the Individual Case Safety Reports (ICSRs) from its AMCs, identifies and analyses the new signals from reported cases. It uses the inferences to recommend informed regulatory interventions, besides communicating risks to healthcare professionals and the public.

Under-reporting of adverse drug reactions is a major concern in pharmacovigilance throughout the globe. The PvPI has taken several measures to promote reporting culture of adverse events and consequently developing confidence between the patients and healthcare professionals. Some of the achievements of PvPI are given below (Kalaiselvan et al. 2014, 2015, 2016):

- Currently, 250 AMCs have been established all over India.
- On October 11, 2013, PvPI launched a toll free helpline No. 18001803024 to encourage adverse events reporting by healthcare professionals as well as patient population.
- Along with the suspected ADR reporting form, PvPI developed a medicine side effect reporting form for consumers/patients in 10 regional languages Hindi, Kannada, Malayalam, Assamese, Bengali, Odiya, Tamil, Telugu, Gujarati, and Marathi to make the reporting easier.
- An Android Mobile Application was launched by the Secretary Health, MoHFW, Government of India, on May 22, 2015.
- PvPI has been associated with National Health Programmes of India to monitor the safety of drugs used in these programmes. such as Revised National Tuberculosis Control Programme (RNTCP), National Aids Control Organization (NACO), National Vector-Borne Disease Control Programme (NVBDCP), Adverse event following immunization (AEFI) of India's Universal Immunization Programme (UIP).
- Awareness about the programme is being created by social mobilization, publishing newsletters, articles in national and international journals.
- Training and education is given to healthcare providers, industry professionals, students etc.
- The contribution of India to the WHO global ICSRs database is 3% with the documentation grading and completeness score of 0.94 out of 1.0.

The PvPI is successfully striding towards its main goal of ensuring the patient safety and promoting the safe use of medicines in the country. To achieve this the PvPI is also working towards detection of medicines of substandard quality as well as prescribing, dispensing and administration errors, counterfeiting, antimicrobial resistance, etc.

BIBLIOGRAPHY

1. Bavdekar SB, Karande S. National Pharmacovigilance Program. Indian Pediatrics. 2006;43:27-32 .
2. Begaud B, Chaslerie A, Fourrier A, Haramburu F, Miremont G (Eds). Methodological approaches in pharmacoepidemiology. Applications to spontaneous reporting. Elsevier Science Publishers, Amsterdam, 1993. ISBN 0-444-81-577-5.
3. Benichou C (Ed). Adverse drug reactions. A practical guide to diagnosis and management. Wiley, Chichester, 1994. ISBN 0 471 94211.
4. Dikshit RK, Desai C, Desai MK. Pleasures and pains of running a pharmacovigilance centre. Indian J Pharmacol 2008; 40: 31-4
5. Griffin JP, Weber JCP. Voluntary systems of adverse reaction reporting. In: Griffin JP, D'Arcy PF, Harron DWG (Eds). Medicines: Regulation, Research and Risk. Greystone Books, Antrim, 1989.
6. http://www.ipc.gov.in/PvPI/pv_home.html
7. International Drug Monitoring: The Role of National Centres. WHO Technical Report Series, No. 498, Geneva, 1972.
8. Kalaiselvan V, Prakash J, Singh GN. Pharmacovigilance programme of India. Arch Pharm Pract. 2012;3:229-32.
9. Kalaiselvan V, Sharma S, Singh GN. Adverse reactions to contrast media: An analysis of spontaneous reports in the database of the pharmacovigilance programme of India. Drug Saf. 2014;37:703-10.[PubMed]
10. Kalaiselvan V, Thota P, Singh A. Current status of adverse drug reactions monitoring centres under pharmacovigilance programme of India. Indian J Pharm Pract. 2014;7:19-22.
11. Kalaiselvan V, Rishi K, Prasad T, Arunabh T, Singh GN. Status of documentation grading and completeness score for Indian individual case safety reports. Indian J Pharmacol. 2015;47(3): 325-7.
12. Kalaiselvan V, Thota P, Singh GN. Pharmacovigilance Programme of India: Recent developments and future perspectives. Indian J Pharmacol [serial online] 2016 [cited 2017 Sep 3];48:624-8. Available from: http://www.ijp-online.com/text.asp?2016/48/6/624/194855.
13. Olsson S (Ed). National Pharmacovigilance Systems. 2nd Edition 1999; WHO Collaborating Centre for International Drug Monitoring, Uppsala, Sweden. ISBN 91-630-7678-0.
14. Safety Monitoring of Medicinal Products: Guidelines for setting up and running a Pharmacovigilance Centre. 2000. The Uppsala Monitoring Centre (the UMC), WHO Collaborating Centre for International Drug Monitoring, Uppsala, Sweden. also available at apps.who.int/medicinedocs/en/d/Jh2934e/3.html
15. Strom B (Ed). Pharmacoepidemiology. 2nd edition. Wiley, Chichester, 1994.

9

Benefit-Risk Assessment in Pharmacovigilance

Renu Agarwal, SK Gupta

The use of drugs to treat human illness dates back to prehistoric times when man used plants as a source of drugs. Since those early days man knew the occurrence of undesired effects associated with the use of drugs. The drugs are an inevitable part of modern day life and become acceptable when the expected therapeutic benefits are higher than the risks. The overall benefit-risk assessment is essential before as well as after the drug is marketed. Some of the definitions related to risks and benefits are as follows:

DEFINITIONS

Risk

- The probability of an adverse health effect and the severity of that effect, consequential to (a) hazard(s) in that food (Codex Alimentarius Commission, 2005)
- The probability of an adverse effect in an organism, system or (sub)population caused under specified circumstances by exposure to an agent (IPCS, 2004).

Hazard

- A biological, chemical or physical agent in, or condition of, food, with the potential to cause an adverse health effect (Codex Alimentarius Commission, 2005).
- An inherent property of an agent or situation having the potential to cause adverse effects when an organism, system or (sub)population is exposed to that agent (IPCS, 2004).
- The inherent property of a nutrient or related substance to cause adverse health effects depending upon the level of intake (FAO/WHO, 2006).

Harm

Condition that inflicts injury, loss; the injury inflicted; hurt (Webster's Comprehensive Dictionary).

ADVERSE HEALTH EFFECT

A change in morphology, physiology, growth, development, reproduction or lifespan of an organism, system or (sub) population that results in an impairment of functional capacity, an impairment of the capacity to compensate for additional stress, or an increase in susceptibility to other influences (IPCS, 2004; FAO/WHO, 2006).

Benefit

"A reduction in the probability and/or severity of an adverse health effect and/or an increase in the probability and/or magnitude of a positive health effect in a group of individuals under defined conditions of exposure." According to another definition benefits is "the improvement attributable to the drug, in terms of human health, health-related quality of life, and/or economic benefit to the individual or group."

Benefit-risk analysis weighs in its assessment the probability of harm against the probability of benefit as a basis for management decisions and for communication to the public.

ACTUAL VERSUS PERCEIVED BENEFITS AND RISKS

The assessment of benefit-risk ratio is essential to ensure the safe use of drugs. Often the perceived risks are higher than the actual risk and for a drug to stay in market it is important that it has a high perceived benefits to risk ratio. The risks depend upon the occurrence of all negative effects and their frequency of occurrence. The benefits depend upon the severity of condition for which the drug is used, the efficacy and safety profile of drug as well as the efficacy and safety profile of other available treatment approaches. The overall acceptability of the involved risk as compared to benefits finally decides the presence of a drug in the market. In less severe conditions even a small risk may not be acceptable while comparatively higher risk become acceptable in very severe conditions. The benefit-risk assessments are often done at population levels but sometimes a drug showing obvious benefits in a population may not give the expected benefits in certain patient's subgroups or in an individual patient or a special patient group or an individual patient may show higher incidence of adverse effects therefore it is important to assess actual and perceived risks and benefits at population subgroups and individual levels. It is obvious that the major players in decision making about the benefit-risk balance include: regulatory authority, prescriber and patient himself (Fig. 9.1).

BENEFIT-RISK ASSESSMENT: A DYNAMIC PROCESS

The benefit-risk assessment is a dynamic process. When the drug is initially launched in the market the available safety data is mainly based on animal studies and clinical trials. As the clinical trials are conducted in

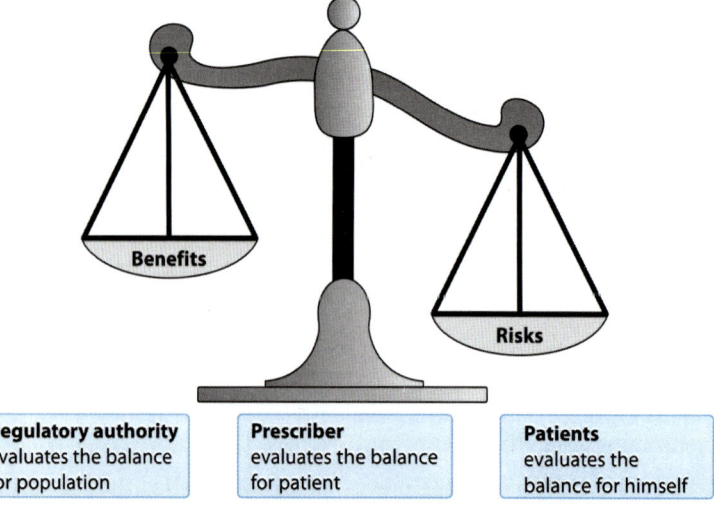

Fig. 9.1: Benefit-risk assessment

well-controlled conditions and focus largely on efficacy of the drug, the data generated from these clinical trials provides only a limited information and poor understanding of potential adverse reactions. As the drug is utilized by a larger population under varying conditions the understanding of benefits as well as risks increase. A good benefit to risk ratio indicated by data from early postmarketing surveillance ensures the presence of drug in the market. During late postmarketing phase, with increasing volume of data further knowledge is gained not only to strengthen the understanding of efficacy and safety of the drug but also for comparative evaluation with alternative treatment approaches. Subsequently, continued review in the light of increasing availability of data is essential for dynamic monitoring of benefit-risk balance (Fig. 9.2). The benefit-risk balance keeps on changing as more and more information becomes available in relation to new unexpected side effects of drug, availability of new treatment approaches with better benefit-risk profile or availability of new information on already available alternative treatment approaches. When the risks associated with the use of a drug outweigh the benefits it must be withdrawn from the market. In situation where the benefits of the drug outweigh the risks in special population subgroups, the use can be recommended in that special group only, however, the effective implementation in this case is very important.

Although, it seems easy to suggest that the drugs with large benefits and low risks must be selected for therapeutic purpose, the actual process of assessment of risks and benefits associated with the use of a drug is a very complex issue. The overall benefits of the use of a drug are related to the number of therapeutic indications, which is usually a single benefit for the patient, but the associated risks may be multiple. A large number of factors collectively influence the actual and perceived risks and benefits and therefore overall decision on the benefit-risk balance of a medicine is difficult to express with mathematical precision. Edwards et al. (1996) suggested the term merit assessment rather than the benefit-risk assessment as it indicates assessment of the worth of a medicine in a given context. A number of other assessment methods have been suggested to improve drug safety monitoring, pharmacovigilance and quality of public health.

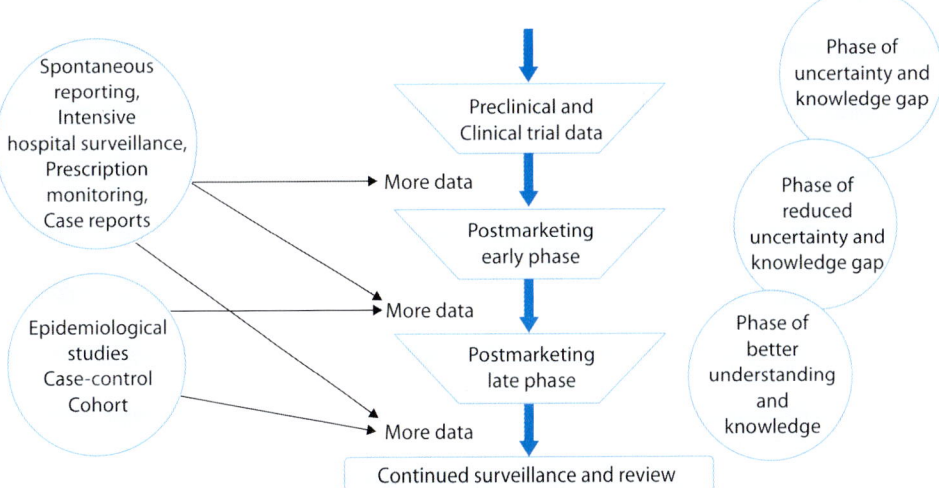

Fig. 9.2: The dynamic process of benefit-risk assessment with increasing use of drug

FACTORS AFFECTING BENEFIT-RISK BALANCE

Actual and perceived risks and benefits of a medicine are not the same and are susceptible to the context in which they occur. The benefit-risk assessment by regulatory authority, prescriber and patient is largely affected by three important factors that include: severity, duration and incidence (Fig. 9.3).

The decision about the overall benefit-risk balance by the prescriber depends upon his perception about the risk caused by the use of medicine and the risk due to the disease itself. In the event of a serious ADR during treatment of a trivial condition the prescriber may find himself causally responsible and therefore the situation makes him consider the risk associated with the use of drug very high. The perceived risk by the prescriber also depends upon the severity of condition, the magnitude of therapeutic benefit, duration of the therapeutic benefit as compared to time course of the disease and the frequency with which the therapeutic benefit is achieved in a patient population with similar indication as mentioned in literature or as per his own past experiences.

The benefit-risk balance as assessed by patients is also highly dependent on individual perceptions. Some of the patients anticipate high degree of benefits with the use of drug and have the misconception that the drugs are completely safe. In this context even mild drug reactions attract extra attention. However, if the disease under treatment is very serious even moderate to severe drug reactions are well-tolerated by patients. The duration of beneficial effect as compared to duration of symptoms and the frequency with which the beneficial effects are observed further influence the benefit-risk perception by the patients.

Introduction of new drugs in the market usually involves a cautious as the amount of safety data is limited and is generated primarily from clinical trials that are conducted under strictly controlled environment. After the launch of drug in the market more and more data becomes available from spontaneous

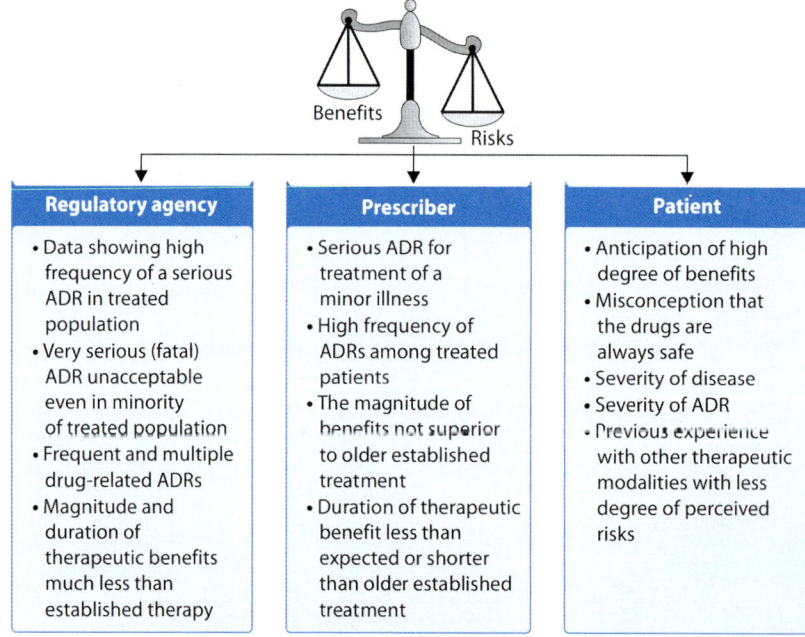

Fig. 9.3: Factors affecting benefit-risk assessment

reporting as well as case-control and cohort studies. Subsequent re-evaluations of the benefit-risk balance help in providing greater knowledge about the efficacy and adverse effects. The overall decision about the benefit-risk balance is made by regulatory authorities as well as by prescribers.

STEPWISE APPROACH TO BENEFIT-RISK ASSESSMENT

The process of assessment of benefit-risk profile of a medicine is a stepwise procedure that involves benefit/risk identification, benefit/risk evaluation, benefit/risk characterization and decision making. Following points are important while considering the benefit-risk assessment (Fig. 9.4).

- The efficacy of the drug is indicated by improvement in parameters indicating the degree of disability due to disease but at times the parameters monitored may not be directly correlated with the degree of disability. Therefore in some diseases a little improvement in parameters can result into great reduction in disability while in others great improvement in parameters is required to experience even a little change in degree of disability.
- The benefits of drug use are also assessed by degree of improvement of overall disease condition. The degree of improvement of disease condition may be due to significant changes in parameters like quality of life without showing much improvement in specific parameters indicating degree of illness.
- The drug treatment may provide benefits other than the improvement in primary condition for which the treatment was started.
- The risk identification initially is often based on data from animal and human studies indicating relationship of exposure with effect and the disease indicating biomarkers and pharmacokinetic profile of the drug.
- Dose-response relationship and exposure relationship are the important factors to assess in benefit-risk balance.
- The risk associated with the use of drug depends upon the severity of ADR as compared to the disease itself. The ADR may further add on the ongoing disease process thus making the situation unacceptable or it can be a minor effect as compared to the disease itself.
- The assessment of benefit-risk balance with public health perspective also takes into account the cost to be borne by community if the disease is left untreated and its consequences and the cost of treatment and its consequences.

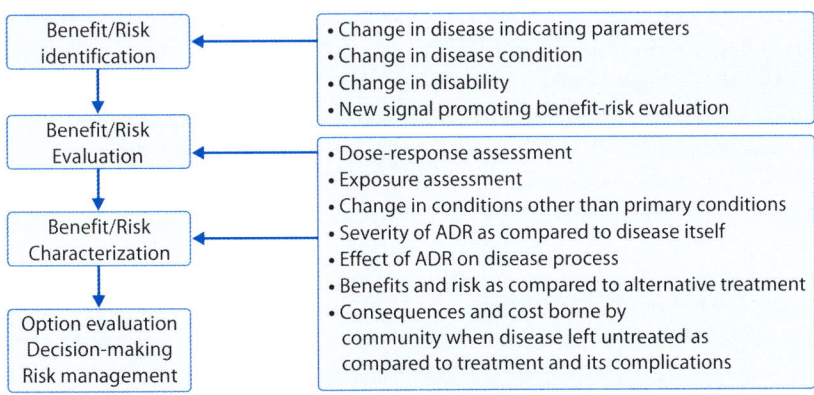

Fig. 9.4: Stepwise process of assessing the benefit-risk balance

- The risk characterization includes all aspects of potential ADRs (severity, duration, incidence) interactions, population at risk, factors modifying the ADR including concomitant diseases, no adverse effect level (NOAEL) and environmental influences.
- After a thorough assessment of benefit-risk balance careful analysis of all available options is done and accordingly the decisions on the actions to be taken should follow.
- The aim of this stepwise approach is to optimize the use of the product by maximizing its benefits and minimizing newly detected risks.

BENEFIT-RISK ASSESSMENT

Council for International Organizations of Medical Sciences (CIOMS) Working Group IV in their document entitled "Benefit-risk balance for marketed drugs: evaluating safety signals"[6] have described methods that can be used for benefit-risk assessment. Assessment of benefit-risk balance should begin with separate evaluation of both the benefits and risks associated with the therapeutic use of a drug.

Points to Consider in Benefit Evaluation

Benefits should be described and wherever possible quantified in a way that is comparable to the quantification of risks. Benefit (and risk) may be defined in terms of the individual being treated, of net benefits across individuals being treated or, as in the case of vaccines or antibiotics, of the net benefit to society. Evaluation of benefits must include following points:
- Prevalence and incidence of disease.
- Nature of disease: Fatal, disabling, self-limiting, associated morbidity and mortality.
- Purpose of therapy: disease prevention, treatment, cure, prevent disease progression, reduce risk for subsequent disease, reduce disabling symptoms and reduce/delay morbidity and mortality.
- Nature of therapy: First or second line therapy, orphan drug, reported adverse effects and therapeutic responses, duration of therapeutic benefits.
- Characteristics of population requiring treatment: High risk population if any, percentage of treated population showing positive therapeutic responses.
- Quality of data.

Points to Consider in Risk Evaluation

Drug-risk evaluation requires a multifactorial approach in order to determine the qualitative profiles of different adverse reactions, their frequency of occurrence, and, if possible, the one or more health outcomes common to different reactions. Important points to consider in risk evaluation include the following:
- Nature, severity and duration of ADR
- Dose and duration of treatment
- Preventability, predictability and reversibility of the reaction
- Possibility of a class effect
- Possible effect of concomitant treatment
- Possible correlations with factors like demographics and concomitant diseases
- Supporting evidence from clinical trials or animal studies.

The adverse reaction that dominates the overall risk profile (carries the most weight) is referred to as the risk driver or dominant risk. More signal may originate even after documentation of a risk driver therefore in addition to the data on ADR that prompted the risk evaluation, all other data related to adverse reaction specially the serious and frequent ADRs must also be taken into account while assessing the overall risk. Several methods have been suggested for quantification of risk however a universally acceptable standardized method still needs to be developed.

Points to Consider in Benefit-risk Evaluation

For benefit-risk evaluation no structures and harmonized approach is available that can serve as standard however some general points to be considered have been suggested by CIOMS Working Group IV and these include the following:

- Avoid the expression "benefit-risk ratio". Until adequate quantitative approaches are validated, the term conveys a misleading mathematical credibility and has little meaning relative to impact on the public health.
- Avoid the use of relative expressions of benefits and risks in isolation; they do not reflect the true medical impact, which is better expressed in absolute values. For example, a 33% relative risk reduction may mean a decrease from an incidence of 30% to 20%, or 3% to 2%, or 0.3% to 0.2%.
- Be wary of uncritical use of overall expression of risk or benefit. Benefit and risk are rarely evenly distributed over time, the population treated, or the use of a drug (e.g. indication- or dose-dependency).
- Always frame the issue and the results in the proper therapeutic context, as in the following examples:
  - Treatment of a fatal disease with drugs that can cause fatal adverse reactions (e.g. treatment of acute leukemia)
  - Prevention of a serious, possibly fatal, condition vs. risk of a serious, possibly fatal, adverse reaction (aspirin or ticlopidine in stroke prevention vs. risk of gastrointestinal or cerebrovascular hemorrhage or, in the case of ticlopidine, agranulocytosis)
  - Palliative treatment that improves quality of life vs. a serious, sometimes fatal reaction (disease-modifying antirheumatic drugs in rheumatoid arthritis)
  - Rrelief of symptoms in non-fatal, acute, self-limiting disease (aspirin for "flu", with risk of gastrointestinal bleeding; "cure worse than the disease?)"
  - Prevention of risks to an individual or others, as in vaccination (e.g. children vaccinated against rubella to protect pregnant women).

SEMI-QUANTITATIVE AND QUANTITATIVE APPROACH TO BENEFIT-RISK ASSESSMENT

Development of properly validated quantitative models for comparative benefit-risk evaluation is in its infancy and decisions are being made on a relatively informal basis. However, the semi-quantitative and quantitative methods can add a straightforward descriptive and transparent approach to the assessment of the relative merits of different therapies. Beckmann Model is a simple multi-criteria model, which scores benefits and risks in three aspects.[7] Benefit score is based on efficacy, response rate and evidence; while the risk score is based on seriousness, incidence and evidence. This model does not take into account relative importance of benefit and risk criteria. It does not integrate benefit and risk. Additionally, it does not readily incorporate statistical uncertainty in input data into the analysis. CIOMS Working Group IV proposed two simple frameworks to assist the decision-making in benefit-risk assessment, which are described here and include 'Principle of Three' and 'TURBO' models.

Principle of Three

The 'Principle of Three' is a grading system based on the concept of severity, duration and incidence in relation to disease indication, degree of improvement by drug and adverse

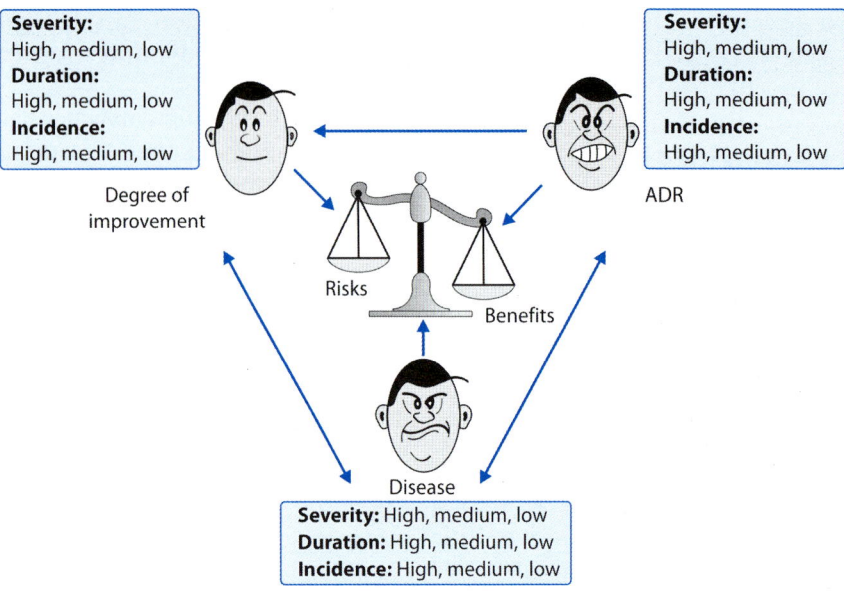

Fig. 9.5: "Principle of three" framework for decision-making in benefit-risk assessment

Table 9.1: Grading three parameters for disease, drug effectiveness and ADR

Property	High (3)	Medium (2)	Low (1)
Seriousness	Fatal	Disabling	Inconvenient
Duration	Permanent	Persistent (long-lasting)	Temporary (short-lived)
Incidence	Common	Infrequent (frequent)	Rare (occasional)

Table 9.2: Benefit-risk evaluation for felbamate

	Disease	Effectiveness of drug	Dominant reaction
Seriousness	3	3	3
Duration	3	3	3
Incidence	1	0	2
Total	7	6	8

effects ascribed to the drug (Fig. 9.5). All three parameters are graded at three levels essentially based on the visible weighing of the scores for the "level of improvement produced by the medicine" against the scores for "the adverse effects" criteria. A numerical scale is used for the qualitative terms (low = 1, medium = 2, high = 3)(Table 9.1). An simple example of the drug felbamate is described here.

Felbamate, an antiepileptic drug, is the only effective treatment available for management of Lennox-Gastaut epilepsy which is a rare intractable disease with high mortality. Treatment with felbamate does not cure the disease but markedly reduces the mortality and morbidity. Dominant risk associated with felbamate treatment is blood dyscrasia with aplastic anemia which is generally persistent, usually fatal and occurs in 1 in 4,000 treated patients. The results are shown in Table 9.2. The incidence of ADR may also be given a score of 3 since the "acceptable" incidence for serious adverse reactions is often perceived as being very small compared with disease.

The results shown above clearly indicate that risk profile of felbamate is only marginally worse than the disease and that too only for incidence. In this case as no effective treatment is available for such a serious disease, comparison of benefits and risks leads to the conclusion that felbamate can be used for this special population but is not suitable for general treatment of epilepsy.

If sufficient data on benefits and risks related to therapeutic use of a drug is available a more quantitative approach can be adapted using the same principle of three described above. An example of such an approach is described here.

An antibiotic used to treat acute-on-chronic bronchitis, which is a disabling disease, provides 40% cure rate. Of the treated patients 20% develop skin rash (lasting for 3 days after stopping the drug), 10% develop stomach upset (lasting for 1 day after stopping the drug), 5% develop diarrhea (lasting for 3 weeks and is prostrating in 0.05% cases), and 0.005% develop agranulocytosis with 10% fatality. For scoring benefit-risk properties a similar approach as described above is used with grading: low = 10, medium = 20, high = 30.

Benefit score

= cure rate × seriousness of the disease × chronicity/duration of the disease
= 0.4 × 30 (disabling disease) × 20 (acute-on-chronic)
= 240

Common adverse reactions (Mean score 13.3)
Skin-rash score = 0.2 × 10 ("low" seriousness) × 10 ("low" duration) = 20
Stomach-upset score = 0.1 × 10 × 10 = 10
Diarrhea score = 0.05 × 10 × 20 = 10

Rare adverse reactions (Mean score 0.078)
Prostrating diarrhea score
= 0.0005 × 20 × 20 = 0.2
Agranulocytosis score
= 0.00005 × 30 × 20 = 0.03
Fatal agranulocytosis score
= 0.000005 × 30 × 30 = 0.0045

An overall "benefit-risk ratio" (B/R) can be calculated by using the mean of all adverse-reaction scores [(13.3 + 0.078) /2 = 6.69]: B/R = 240/6.69 = 35.9

A number of drugs may be associated with the same or multiple different adverse reactions of different severity and frequency. Moreover, the signal event leading to a new benefit-risk evaluation may occur when the data sheet already contains a more "serious" adverse reaction recognized as the dominant risk ("risk -driver") in the overall risk profile. Also, it is likely that there is better evidence for causality and actual incidence of the most common and serious reactions. Therefore, to make a fair comparison of risks between therapies, the "principle of threes" can accommodate most situations: choose the three most serious and three most frequent adverse reactions (and benefits) for each drug in the comparison. The scores may be added across each drug and the totals compared to provide a crude relative ranking.

TURBO Model

The TURBO ("Transparent Uniform Risk Benefit Overview") model performs risk-benefit assessment by quantitative and graphical approach. The risks and benefits of a medicine for a given therapeutic indication are quantified and displayed on TURBO diagram. The risk factor "R" is defined as the sum of two risks: the risk associated with the most medically serious adverse effect (score from 1 to 5), and the risk associated with the second most serious adverse effect or the most frequent adverse effect (score from 0 to 2). The Benefit factor "B" is calculated in a similar way, as the sum of the primary benefit, and the ancillary benefit(s) (Tables 9.3 and 9.4). The R factor and B factor are placed in the TURBO diagram and a T-score expressing the intrinsic benefit risk analysis ranging from 1 to 7 is assigned (Table 9.5).

Multi-criteria decision analysis (MCDA) as mentioned in the report of the CHMP (Committee for medicinal products for human use) working group on benefit-risk assessment models and methods, uses an algorithm that combines value judgment along multiple dimensions (Fig. 9.6). The first step is to identify the relevant risk and benefit criteria. The option for each criterion is given a

Table 9.3: TURBO model. Calculating the R-score associated with the most serious adverse effect (R0)

Estimated attributable risk ↑	Frequency					
	Common					5
	Not uncommon				4	
	Rare			3		
	Very rare		2			
		1				
		Minor	Slight	Moderate	Severe	Very severe
	Estimated severity ──────────────────────────────────▶					

Severity = impact on health status and socioprofessional capabilities (definitions are tentative):
1 = some hindrance, but not really incapacitating
2 = temporarily/intermittently incapacitating
3 = incapacitating, but not life-threatening/-shortening
4 = life-shortening, but not life-threatening
5 = life-threatening

Source: Report of the CHMP working group on benefit-risk assessment models and methods. Doc Ref. EMEA/CHMP/15404/2007.

Table 9.4: TURBO model. Calculating the B-score associated with the benefit in the given indication (B0)

Probability of benefit ↑	Nearly always					5
	Frequent				4	
	Common			3		
	Not common		2			
	Rare	1				
		Minor	Slight	Moderate	Marked	Major
	Degree of benefit ──────────────────────────────────▶					

Benefit = impact on indication as reflected by change(s) in health status and socioprofessional capabilities (definitions are tentative):
1 = less hindering, but capabilities remain unchanged
2 = less frequently incapacitating or incapability lasts shorter
3 = less incapacitating, but no change in life expectancy
4 = less life-shortening
5 = less immediately life-threatening

Source: Report of the CHMP working group on benefit-risk assessment models and methods. Doc Ref. EMEA/CHMP/15404/2007.

Table 9.5: Intrinsic Benefit-Risk Balance: The TURBO diagram

R-Factor								
7	T= 1	T= 2	T= 3				T= 4	
6						T= 4		
5					T= 4		T= 7	
4				T= 4		T= 6		
3			T= 4		T= 5			
2		T= 4						
1	T= 4							
	1	2	3	4	5	6	7	B-Factor

Source: Report of the CHMP working group on benefit-risk assessment models and methods. Doc Ref. EMEA/CHMP/15404/2007.

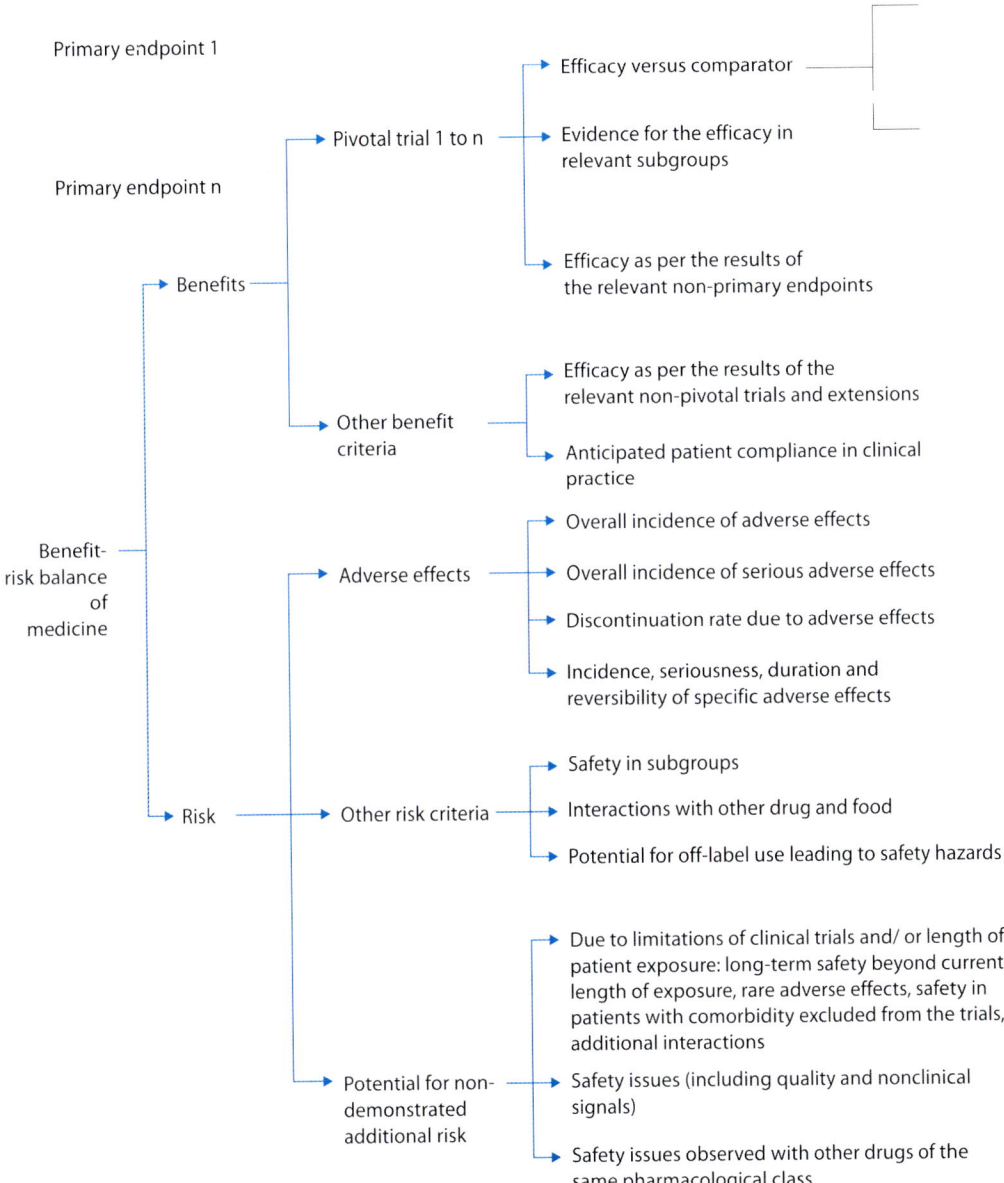

Fig. 9.6: Multi-criteria decision analysis (MCDA). Value tree for benefit-risk assessment[8]

numerical score between two reference points. Each criterion is assigned weight according to its importance in decision-making. The score for each option is multiplied with the weight of the respective criteria and the products for both risks and benefits are added. Next the computer added sensitivity analysis is done to compare the total score for risks and benefits.

The methods described above help to simplify the process, however it is important to screen the data logically before arriving at a decision about the grading of various parameters. The quality and completeness of the data are the key factors affecting overall assessment. The first two methods although useful in conveying the general idea about the risks and benefits and identifying areas demanding more research, does not allow the use of entire profile of benefits and ADR attributable to the drug. MCDA takes into account additional benefit and risk criteria and thus could be extended to comparable clinical situations. It allows discussions and before deciding for the weight for each criterion. Subsequent sensitivity analysis also allows comparison of benefit-risk balance between different treatment arms. As the method is based on numerical scoring and quantitative analysis using point estimates rather than confidence intervals, the subjective variations in assigning weights to relevant criteria is not taken into account for decision-making which can sometimes be misleading. As the method is largely quantitative the qualitative differences often get ignored. Besides, each situation requires building up of a complex model the method is time-consuming.

Besides the methods mentioned above for benefit-risk assessment a large number of other quantitative methods have also been developed in pharmacoepidemiology and pharmacoeconomics. Theses methods require assessment for validity and usefulness.

OPTION ANALYSIS

Once the assessment of benefit-risk balance is completed and outcomes are characterized it is important to analyze the available options so as to allow the appropriate decision making. The options available to regulators and manufacturers are similar but not necessarily identical, and they are not mutually exclusive; they are:

- Maintenance of the status quo if the original signal was found to be of no concern.
- In case the available data is insufficient to reach a valid conclusion, regulatory authority may not take an immediate action and manufacturer may need to continue careful monitoring and data collection
- Parallel action may sometimes be required pending the results of additional data collection. Additional data may be required to reach an appropriate decision however, a decision to go for collection of additional data will depend upon time required to collect the data and the nature and magnitude of safety concern. Manufacturer may consider designing additional studies, observation for more cases with ADR, analyzing comparative data on drugs with similar therapeutic use or pharmacological class or seeking additional expert opinion.
- Regulatory agency or the manufacturer may consider following modification of product, product information or its use.
  - Addition of new risk information
  - Change in words to emphasize, clarify or specify ADRs, restrictions or indications
  - Removal of information
  - To add a therapeutic recommendation for treating adverse reactions associated with the product
  - Selective restriction of the availability of a product to reduce risk of ADR or to allow close safety monitoring, e.g. reclassifying from non-prescription to prescription status
  - To limit distribution to patients enrolled in a "monitored release" programme (Europe) or in a compassionate use/named patient programme (North America/Europe), or to patients who have signed an informed-consent document
  - To impose limits on reimbursement in order to restrict product use to a particular patient population or to limit its duration.
  - To change the formulation or appearance of a product or the

manufacturing process so as to minimize or eliminate an identified risk (or a reduced benefit) related to the physico-chemical properties of a medicament, e.g. change in particle size, excipient, delivery system, etc.
- When the magnitude of safety concern is still under investigation, some regulatory authorities may chose to temporarily suspend the product license. When the safety issue is resolved manufacture may resume marketing without fresh new-drug-application.
- When it becomes clear that product's safety risks outweigh the benefits and new safety risk is an "imminent hazard" to drug users, product withdrawal is considered.
- Product withdrawal may also be considered in absence of clear characterization of benefit-risk balance if specific measures to reduce the risk have not been identified. Clozapine was withdrawn from some markets following reports of agranulocytosis from Finland. Later it was reintroduced with a restricted indication for schizophrenia refractory to other therapy; in addition, mandatory white-blood-cell monitoring is required wherever the drug is used.
- While considering the product withdrawal careful evaluation is required as to:
  - The severity of damage that the drug may cause if regular review or less immediate administrative procedures are followed
  - The magnitude of damage that withdrawal might cause to current users keeping in view the availability of alternative therapies and time required to adjust to them
  - Other approaches to protect public health
  - The likelihood of drug withdrawal after completion of customary review and administrative procedures.

Product withdrawal, whether voluntary by the manufacturer or mandated, necessitates consideration of a product recall to healthcare professionals and patients on a regional or global basis.

DECISION-MAKING

Decision-making means determining the actions to be taken, who should take them, and the order and methods of taking action; it also entails decisions on the best means of monitoring and follow-up, and of communicating the appropriate information to the parties concerned. As suggested by (CIOMS) Working Group IV decision-making should follow three principles: objectivity, equity and accountability.

Objectivity

The decision making must be unbiased and should be based on available data. Attempts should be made to generate scientifically based support especially in situations of external pressure from media, people or legal authorities in the absence of imminent hazard to avoid precipitous decision-making. According to Working Group the objectivity in decision-making relies on several attributes and these are:
- Data collection and analysis from all possible sources by all possible methods.
- Utilization of best available professional experts and advisors from all relevant fields.
- All involved experts must disclose the conflict of interest on all relevant occasions. If bias is probable, an expert may be asked to testify but not to make a recommendation or to vote.
- Use of computer-assisted algorithms in decision-making might be considered.
- Specific criteria may be established to assess the acceptability of a new drug found more efficacious than others of the same class but with greater toxicity.

Equity

Equity demands that all drugs and other therapeutic interventions be treated fairly by ensuring comparability in requirements for evidence, analytical approaches, professional expertise and decision-making rules. The standards that can be incorporated are:
- Every effort should be made to use the available evidence to render the best comparisons possible.
- All major stakeholders (at least manufacturer/sponsor) to take part in decision-making.
- Interagency coordination with full and open discussion on available evidences and conclusions. Working Group strongly recommends cross-national communication.
- Decision-making must be specific to the circumstances and the scientifically identified criteria on which the decision is based must be specified.
- Although, all benefit-risk decisions are made in the face of at least some degree of uncertainty, it is important to assess the level of uncertainty involved before decision-making. If it exceed the "acceptable uncertainty" for decisions in this group of drugs or risks, i.e. the uncertainty is too great, additional data may be required before a meaningful decision can be reached. The extent to which the society is ready to accept the limitations of science and technology is crucial to acceptance of decisions in the face of inevitable uncertainty.
- Maintaining transparency in the process of decision-making is important as the decisions taken by one member state affect materially all other member states. This can be achieved by expressing the processes involved in decision-making such as arguments among stakeholders, criteria applied and results of analysis, in a way that can help other to consider acceptability in different settings.

Accountability

Decisions are made at specific time based on the evidences available at that time and as the circumstances change the results of the actions taken cannot be predicted. Therefore, the accountability of decisions made can be assured to some extent by:
- Specifying or estimating the expected outcomes
- Establishing criteria for determining and assessing the effectiveness of the actions chosen
- Continued data collection as a part of ongoing safety monitoring accept in cases of drug withdrawal.

FDA and EMA Recommendations

The risk management strategy by FDA recommends optimization of risk-benefit balance of regulated products throughout the lifecycle of the product. FDA and the EMA both require proactive approaches for drug safety surveillance. To provide a basis and guidance for risk management, FDA issued 3 documents in 2005: Premarketing risk assessment, good pharmacovigilance practices and pharmacoepidemiologic assessment, and the development and use of risk minimization Action Plans (RiskMAPs). Subsequently, FDA formulated risk evaluation and mitigation strategies (REMS). REMS is a safety strategy for management of known or potential risks associated with the use of drugs or biological products. FDA Amendments Act (FDAAA) 2007 provides FDA the authority to require a REMS from manufacturers to ensure that the benefits of a drug or biological product outweigh its risks. A REMs may be required by the FDA as part of the approval of a new product, or for an approved product when new safety information arises. After marketing authorization, manufacturers are required to routinely assess the incorporated REMS programme at 18 months, 3 years, and

7 years. If necessary, FDA may stipulate shorter or longer intervals between assessments. The contents of REMS are required to include a timetable for submission of assessments. Other contents may include medication guide, patient package insert and a communication plan. Additionally, elements to ensure safe use may be included such as dispensing only by certified healthcare facility, pharmacist or practitioner; dispensing only with patient monitoring or dispensing only to patients enrolled in a registry.

EMA introduced the concept of risk management plans (RMPs) in 2005. Subsequently, guidelines on risk management systems, a template for an RMP, and new pharmacovigilance regulations were issued by EMA in 2008. Emphasis was made on putting a strong pharmacovigilance system in place particularly postmarketing. As per European Union (EU) legislation, when required, detailed EU-RMP should be submitted. Generally such requirement arises when routine pharmacovigilance is considered insufficient such as in case of known or potential serious risk associated with the use of a drug or biological product, a product with new active substance or significant change in indication. EU-RMP comprises of 2 parts. Part I includes information that helps to determine the adequacy of routine postmarketing pharmacovigilance and whether additional investigations are needed. It includes a summary of known and potential risks, population at risk, outstanding safety questions and missing information. Part II includes details of additional pharmacovigilance and risk minimization activities. Since, the risk minimization activities may vary from one case to another depending on the nature and seriousness of the risk, no specific guidelines are stated with regards to the type of activity to be undertaken under specific situation. One of the important risk minimization activities is by means of providing Summary of Product Characteristics (SPC), and patient information leaflets to prescribers and patients. Other activities may include conduct of educational programmes and dissemination of educational material to healthcare professionals and patients and update of documents based on new safety information.

CONCLUSION

Benefit-risk assessment is a dynamic process and continues to change as more information becomes available with time. The data from clinical trials largely provides extensive information regarding the efficacy of drug but the information on ADRs especially when infrequent and rare cannot be obtained. As the medicine is more widely used more ADRs get detected and at the same time more benefits may also be experienced. The wider use of medicine will also allow the comparison with alternative treatment approaches. The data showing benefits/adverse effects due to concomitant diseases and simultaneous use of other drugs becomes available only after the drug is marketed. Comparing the efficacy profile of a drug with the risk profile based on the data available from various sources is a difficult and complex process. A number of methods that have been suggested that are largely semi-quantitative or quantitative and none has been recognized as an ideal method. It is important to realize that quantitative methods cannot replace the qualitative evaluation and expert judgment remains the cornerstone of benefit-risk evaluation for authorization of medicinal products. When technicalities involved in benefit-risk assessment are completed all available options are evaluated and appropriate and scientifically-based decisions are made based all available data with participation of all stakeholders. The primary objective is to optimize the use of the product by maximizing its benefits and minimizing newly detected risks.

BIBLIOGRAPHY

1. Beckmann J. Basic Aspects of Risk-Benefit Analysis. Semin Thromb Hemost. 1999;25:89-95.
2. Beechinor JG. Principles of risk/benefit assessment of veterinary medicinal products. Irish Veterinary J. 2007; 60(5): 291-4.
3. CIOMS Working group IV. Benefit risk balance for marketed drugs: evaluating safety signals. 1998.
4. Edwards R, Wiholm B-E, Martinez C. Concepts in risk-benefit assessment: A simple merit analysis of a medicine? Drug Saf. 1996;15(1):1-7.
5. Hildegard P. Looking at both sides of the coin – Use of risk-benefit analysis. Scientific forum "From safe foods to healthy diets" Brussels. 2007;20-21.
6. Lis Y, Roberts MH, Kamble S, J Guo J, Raisch DW. Comparisons of Food and Drug Administration and European Medicines Agency risk management implementation for recent pharmaceutical approvals: report of the International Society for Pharmacoeconomics and outcomes research risk benefit management working group. Value Health. 2012;15(8):1108-18.
7. Lynd LD, O'Brien BJ. Taking calculated risks: advances in risk – benefit evaluation usingprobabilistic simulation methods. J Clin Epidemiol. 2004;57:795-803.
8. Report of the CHMP working group on benefit-risk assessment models and methods. Doc Ref. EMEA/CHMP/15404/2007.
9. US Department of Health and Human Services, Food and Drug Administration, Center for Drug Evaluation and Research (CDER), Center for Biologics Evaluation and Research (CBER). Guidance for industry: Development and Use of Risk Minimization Action Plans. March 2005. Available from: http://www.fda.gov/downloads/RegulatoryInformation/Guidances/UCM126830.pdf. [Accessed July 04, 2017].
10. Waller PC, Evans SJW. A model for the future conduct of pharmacovigilance. Pharmacoepidemiol Drug Saf. 2003;12:17-29.

10

Crisis Management in Pharmacovigilance

Renu Agarwal, Puneet Agarwal

"CRISIS": DEFINITION

A series of unexpected adverse events or adverse drug reactions (ADRs) occurring over a short period of time whose seriousness, if confirmed throws into question the risk/benefit ratio and creates a situation of crisis. Generally speaking a crisis is a period of trauma, distress and changes that are inevitable and often it is difficult to predict what brings about the crisis, although crisis certainly leads to changes –often for the worse. Few formal definitions of 'crisis' as described by WHO are as follows:

"A crisis is any unplanned event or a series of events, which leads to interruption, or destabilization of the normal operations or activities of an organization."

"An unplanned event, which triggers a real, perceived or possible threat to safety, health or environment, or to the organization, its reputation or credibility. A crisis has the potential to significantly impact the (organization's) operations or pose a significant environmental, economic, reputational or legal liability."

"A low probability high impact situation that is perceived by critical stakeholders to threaten the viability of the organization and that is subjectively experienced by these individuals as personally and socially threatening. Ambiguity of cause, effects and means of resolution of the organizational crisis will lead to disillusionment or loss of psychic and shared meaning, as well as to the shattering of commonly held beliefs and values and individual's basic assumptions. During the crisis, decision-making is pressed by perceived time constraints and colored by cognitive limitations."

THE KEY CHARACTERISTICS OF A CRISIS

Although each individual incidence of crisis is unique in terms of cause and effects it generates, some features that are commonly observed during most of the crisis situations are shown in Box 10.1.

The crisis can emerge suddenly without any warning or it might rumble unnoticed

Box 10.1: Characteristics of a "crisis"

- Appears suddenly or builds up over time
- Cause/effects largely uncertain or unknown
- Creates shock, surprise, disorientation and panic
- Offers little time for decision making
- Increasing demand for more information
- Increasing interference from outsiders
- Increasingly difficult communication
- Increasing pressure on routine business
- Increasing demand for relevant information
- Increasing demand for immediate decision and implementation
- Creates surprise, shock, disorientation and panic
- Sense of loss of control
- Urge to avoid confrontation, defense, excuse and find someone to blame

for sometime but has potential to escalate with serious consequences. In either case the cause and effects initially are very uncertain or unknown as the situation builds up unexpectedly. The situation often comes as a surprise and shock with little information. With escalating flow of events the members of organization might get disoriented and panic may prevail as the crisis may pose a major threat to effectiveness and survival of the organization and its stakeholders. Once the specific threats are identified the concerned authorities have little time to respond. Once the crisis comes to public notice the organization faces more and more external and internal scrutiny from media, government, regulatory agencies, activist groups, key stakeholders and the management team itself to reveal information about the crisis. The pressures build over time and the organization often gets a sense of loss of control and an urge to defend and excuse. During such incidences the communications become increasingly difficult, routine business gets affected, outsiders start interfering with more interest in the situation and the reputation of organization suffers. Under these situations the members of organization may panic leading to delay or complete paralysis of decision-making process and if attempts are made to avoid confrontation with the central issues, the crisis may inflict more damage on the organization.

To avoid delay in the process of decision making in larger public interest it is important to have a pre-defined threshold at which the organization formally recognizes the crisis situation and implements the crisis management plan.

"CRISIS" IN PHARMACOVIGILANCE

In relation to drug safety monitoring the "crisis" is defined as "the event which occurs when new information, which could have a serious impact on public health, is received for a marketed product and which requires an immediate action."

The new information leading to crisis is usually related to pharmacovigilance issues, i.e. urgent safety concerns. However, at times it may be related to both quality and safety concerns such as contamination of a product leading to safety concerns. The crisis is usually provoked by spontaneous reporting and this is most likely to occur in a country with a strong and well-developed pharmacovigilance system in place. At the time when crisis is identified the information may not be public however, if it becomes public handling of situation with effective communication is crucial as the public confidence is at risk. At times a crisis may be initiated in the absence of substantial information but excessive media exposure leads to public concerns about a product. As soon as the situation of crisis is evoked the concerned authorities must move into "crisis –management" mode. Immediate measures need to be taken to initiate a pharmacovigilance investigation to either confirm or disprove the signal. The results of such an investigation must be documented. Simultaneously, the health authorities have to interact with the manufacturers to prepare for possible legal actions and implementation of regulatory measures that may be required to ensure safe use of the drug. At times no regulatory action may be required and a clarification for such a situation must be recorded. The total time required to deal with the crisis situation will depend on the severity, magnitude and type of crisis however the proposed procedures should be flexible enough to allow the urgent safety measures to be implemented as per requirements. As a matter of principle, all concerned authorities and stakeholders must work in close cooperation in crisis management.

STAKEHOLDERS

All those who have stake, rights, legitimate interest or involvement in drug safety related issues are the stakeholders. In pharmacovigilance, people from various fields are

> **Box 10.2:** Stakeholders in pharmacovigilance
> - Pharmaceutical manufacturers
> - Drug distributors
> - Retail, hospital pharmacists, OTC sellers
> - Health professionals
> - Consumer, i.e. general and patient population
> - Government and regulatory authorities
> - International regulatory authorities
> - Scientists and researchers
> - Activist groups
> - Non-governmental and voluntary organizations
> - Media, politicians, and lawyers

> **Box 10.3:** Potential threat sources
> 1. Pharmaceutical manufacturing:
>   - Manufacturing errors
>   - Inadequate quality control
>   - False therapeutic claims
> 2. Health professionals and patients
>   - Error in diagnosis
>   - Error in prescription
>   - Poor patient compliance
>   - New ADR reports
> 3. Regulatory authorities
>   - Delayed decision and response
>   - Regulatory actions in other countries
> 4. Human errors
>   - Miscommunication
>   - Faulty administration of the drug
> 5. Human dishonesty
>   - Product tampering
>   - Counterfeit products
>   - Illegal imports
>   - Malpractice/incompetence
> 6. Pressures from various sources
>   - Media reports
>   - Patient and activist groups
>   - Accusations of/actual secrecy, bias, incompetence
>   - Media reports in other countries.

involved as stakeholders and some of these are enlisted in Box 10.2.

During the periods of crisis, involvement of all stakeholders in close cooperation to identify the possible source, causes and effects, to assess the severity and magnitude of the problem, to finalize and implement a plan for crisis management, to prepare for the after-shocks and to effectively communicate the facts to media and public, is crucial.

THE THREAT SOURCES FOR CRISIS IN PHARMACOVIGILANCE

As stated earlier each crisis situation is unique in itself and accordingly the sources of threat will vary. In general the potential sources of threat for the development of a crisis in pharmacovigilance are discussed in Box 10.3.

Various organizations usually identify their own potential sources of threat leading to crisis. This makes the identification of the crisis and its characteristics a little easier so that the crisis management plan can be implemented without undue delay.

CRISIS MANAGEMENT

As defined by WHO the crisis management is "a process through which organizations, in collaboration with external stakeholders prevent crisis or effectively manage those occur." All stakeholders usually work in cooperation so as to anticipate and avoid the crisis situation however when one is precipitated from any source a systematically planned operation is implemented to facilitate quick, efficient and effective response. The success of such an operation is judged by assessing the balance between the positive and negative outcomes. Thus, the objectives of a crisis management plan are:

- To anticipate and avoid crisis
- To achieve favorable balance between positive and negative outcomes
- To continue with the existing business capacity
- To learn lessons so as to effectively handle such situations in future.

Crisis management requires the skills and techniques to assess, understand and react to cope with any serious situation from the moment it first occurs to the point of recovery. The crisis management also involves establishing criteria to define a situation that constitutes crisis, to establish a trigger mechanism to initiate response and to establish effective communication during response phase. The framework of crisis management plan for immediate response, which primarily utilizes the existing organizational structures and management, should always be in place to encounter any unpredictable situation. Additional help from other internal and external organizations may arrive later. The multiple benefits of having a framework of systematic, efficient and effective crisis management plan include the following:

- Ability of the organization to assess the situation quickly
- Ability to utilize techniques at hand to limit the spread of damage
- Ability to continue with the ongoing business
- Ability to maintain compliance with regulatory and ethical requirements
- Ability of better management of serious incidents
- Improved awareness among staff as to their roles and responsibilities
- Increased ability, confidence and morale within organization
- Protected and enhanced reputation of the organization
- Reduced risk of post event litigation.

CRISIS MANAGEMENT CYCLE

Each crisis situation is unique and therefore requires a specialized approach to deal with it. However, based on general principles a universal model, applicable under most situations with modifications, can be created. This universal model must take into account various important elements as discussed below:

Pre-Crisis Conditions

The conditions and causes thought to be responsible to finally leading to an incidence of crisis are not only related to immediate events but to the overall culture and working environment of the organizations. This culture becomes an integral part of the working environment of the organization and may often be noticed by outsiders and insiders as the potential contributory cause of crisis. Some of the practices within an organization which often favor the precipitation of a crisis include:

- Inward-looking, immature and poor management
- Poor organizational skills of analysis and risk assessment
- Ignorance towards utilizing opinion and wisdom of people from outside and inside the organization
- Poor contacts with other related organizations, which play an important role in detecting and sending information on signals indicating upcoming crisis
- Not paying attention to reported adverse events
- Extreme secrecy leading to suspicion and loss of confidence in general public. This can also be a consequence of precipitation of a crisis
- Poor preparation to deal with the crisis leading to severe damage.

The pre-crisis conditions are the major players in deciding the course of action during crisis and post crisis impact. Thus, it is important that all organizations think widely well beyond their territory and establish good working relation and communication channels with other supporting organizations which can provide crucial help not only during detection of crisis but also in handling the situation.

Crisis: Intrinsic versus Perceived

The crisis is said to be *intrinsic crisis* when a truly neutral observer to whom complete facts related to situation are available assesses the objective situation. It is important to quickly determine the nature, extent and possible impact of the intrinsic crisis keeping in view the perceptions and feelings of all the stakeholders. The situation as experienced by different individuals as per their opinions is the *perceived crisis*. The extent, severity and impact of perceived crisis will depend upon the individual's own interpretation of the situation and the extent of personal and emotional involvement.

Crisis Response

An adequate, effective and mature immediate response to crisis plays big role in deciding the final outcome. At times if the pre-crisis conditions as outlined above dominate the working culture of an organization and preparedness to deal with the crisis is poor, an immature immediate response is seen due to surprise, shock, denial and defense on the part of organization. Further if the organization tries to take immediate measures based on the differently perceived crisis by many individuals, the outcomes are usually not only ineffective but also damaging. Therefore, it is important to educate, train and prepare the concerned staff to deal with the crisis and avoid immediate inappropriate reactions, however at times even the trained professionals can respond in inappropriate manner when exposed to real situations.

An immediate adequate, effective and mature crisis response in the form of first response to situation should always be incorporated in overall crisis management plan. The next step of crisis response is to recognize it and address it quickly with organization of a response team. The response team must formulate the plan of action and to begin with the most important aspect is the collection, analysis and processing of all relevant information. This is followed by mobilization of entire unit and implementation of the plan. It is important that the adequate communication is maintained within and outside the organizations during crisis management. No communication gap should exists between sources of decision-making and plan implementation and this can be achieved by keeping the communication chain as short as possible as this improves the rate and quality of performance with minimal chances of misperception. When exposed to a crisis, an immediate encounter with a mature immediate response is likely to settle down the acute manifestations and then a further plan to deal with the incidence can be formulated.

Post-Crisis

In the aftermath of the crisis it is important to review the process from the beginning and capture the positive and negative aspects of the course of action taken. Equally important is the documentation of the activities related to detection, immediate and delayed measures taken and post-crisis impacts. Further it is of utmost importance that the organizations learns lesson from the event and conveys it to all concerned so that effective preparatory and curative actions are well-documented and become an integral part of a management planning and training tool.

CRISIS MANAGEMENT MODEL

Designing an efficient, robust and flexible model for crisis management is essential to limit the impact and duration of an event and incorporates positive planning and response regimens. A crisis management model can be developed keeping in view various steps of crisis management cycle (Fig. 10.1).

Pre-Crisis Planning

Depending upon the level of preparedness to encounter the crisis the organizations can be either crisis prone, i.e. they are ill-prepared and are likely to handle the crisis badly or they can be well-prepared to face the crisis and are capable of reacting efficiently during emergencies. The collection of information and evidences as quickly as possible and its subsequent analysis is vital for the recognition

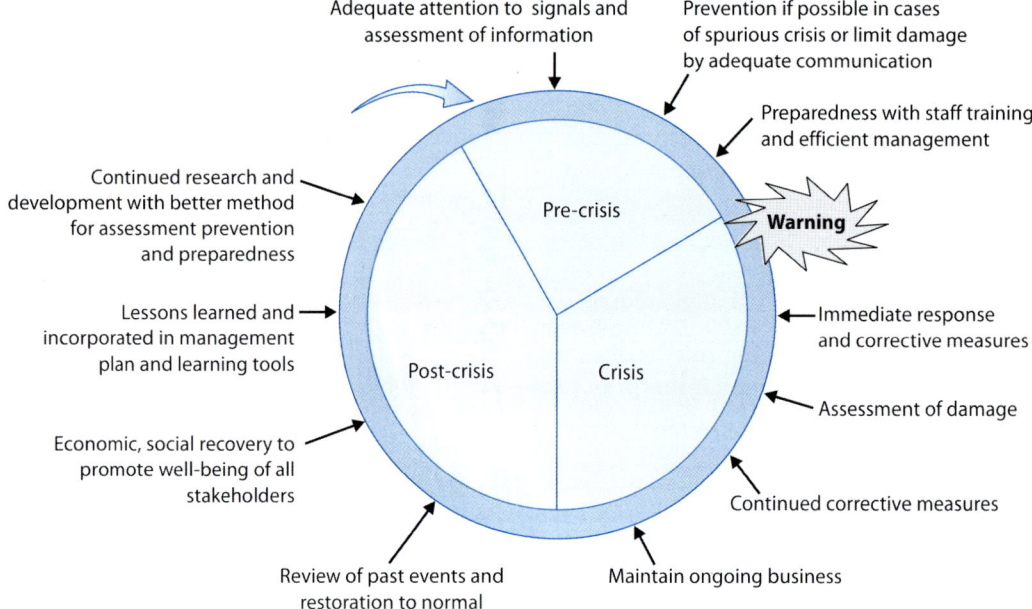

Fig. 10.1: Crisis management cycle

of an upcoming crisis. Therefore, adequate preparation and planning to facilitate early and accurate recognition of an upcoming event is the first step in the crisis management model. The organizations must equip themselves with:
- Availability of appropriate sources of information at all times
- Availability of efficient communication channels to obtain as much information as possible without delay
- Availability of staff, which is well-informed about their roles and responsibilities at all times, so as to channelize the information correctly
- Availability of a very efficient system of documentation of all information
- Availability of a group of trained managers for prioritizing, analyzing, assessing the information and quick risk identification
- Availability of set format for immediate response to avoid immature early response
- Availability of procedures to quickly mobilize the crisis management team to formulate and implement the plan to manage the crisis situation
- Availability of cooperation from all stakeholders
- Availability of efficient communication channels to ensure confidence among all stakeholders.

The primary aim of the pre-crisis planning is to create a working atmosphere which is sensitive enough to recognize the crisis as early as possible while keeping in view the rights, feelings and perceptions among stakeholders. In emotionally charged situations involving vulnerable population it becomes even more important to promote communication among parties and build confidence. It is important to learn lessons from previous mistakes rather than hiding them. Equally important is to promote high degree of transparency and honesty.

Continued measure to ensure the availability of the above mentioned planning requisites at all times is the key to be in a perfect state of preparedness to face the emergencies. Even though this requires huge amount of human and financial resources, lot of planning skills and time, the importance of all time preparedness must be stressed to safeguard the interests of stakeholders and reputation of organization before it is damaged beyond repair.

Crisis Handling

As soon as the crisis is recognized the crisis management team must take all measures to avoid an immature immediate response and then formulate and implement a detailed plan as quickly as possible. Planning and implementation of a crisis management plan although largely depends upon the nature of crisis, certain general rules can be followed:
- Making best possible use of all available human and financial sources
- Plans must be formulated and implemented in a sensitive manner so as to give adequate respect to the rights and feelings of all stakeholders
- The plan must be flexible enough to allow modifications, as the situation requires from time to time
- Maintain excellent communication and cooperation among the members of team to allow smooth implementation as per situation
- Maintain excellent communication of the team with other authorities within and outside the organization so as to avail necessary help whenever required
- Time to time review of the ongoing measures and take steps to modify for the better outcome.

In spite of planning and implementation of best possible plans according to situations, the negative outcomes will be there along with positives and trade-offs may have to made. At times the situations will be beyond rescue. However, such experiences should not undermine the investments of human and financial resources in preparedness and planning for crisis management.

Post-Crisis Review

It is important to review the entire process of preparation and planning of the crisis management plan once the situation resolves. The review must be done with genuineness and objectivity. This will help in outlining the mistakes during preparation and handling of the recent crisis, the additional measures which could have been taken to improve the outcome and the measures to be added in future planning. Case histories must be written which can be reviewed later by experienced professionals and their opinions can be utilized by making necessary amendments in the existing system or by adding new dimensions to the existing system. All possible technical skills must be utilized with utmost intelligence keeping in mind the emotional sensitivities and at no cost the importance of overall critical review can be undervalued.

PLANNING FOR CRISIS MANAGEMENT

Once the organizations are adequately prepared and have adapted measures to establish an efficient model of crisis management as outlined above, the complete process is expected to run smoothly in an organized and systematic manner. The primary objective of crisis management planning is to provide guidance and advice for the production of effective crisis management plans, or the successful review of existing arrangements. To fulfill the objectives it is important that the organization is ready with well-rehearsed plans, which can be put in practice at very short notice. Based upon the crisis management model discussed above various components of crisis management plan can be designed and implemented. Some of the important aspects of proper crisis management plan are discussed in Figure 10.2.

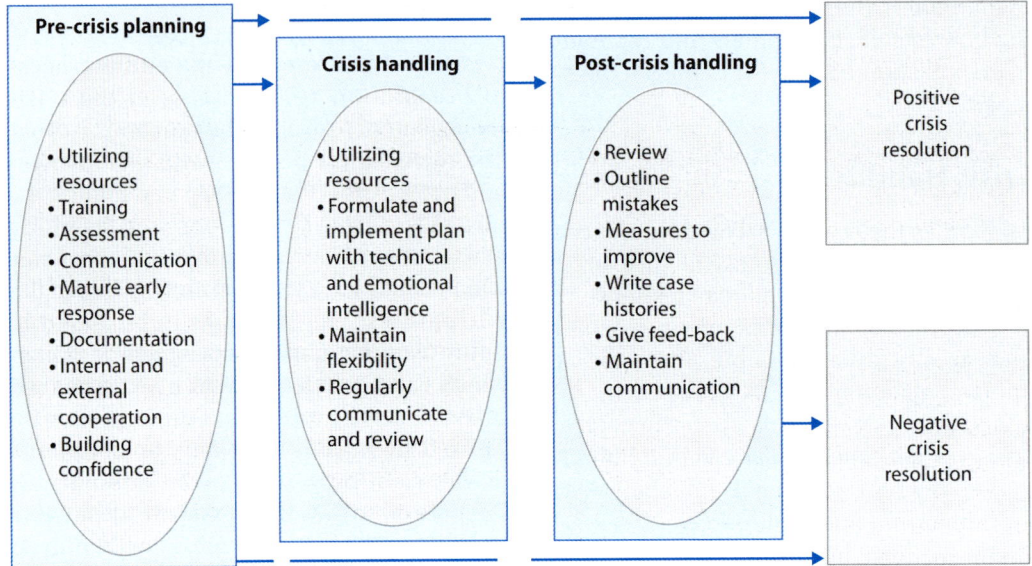

Fig. 10.2: Crisis management model

Establishing a Strategic Crisis Planning Team

A strategic crisis planning team, which is composed of a core group of managers, needs to be established. The team may include members other than managers. All individuals in the team belong to various sectors and levels within the organization. The team should have the executive authority of its activities and should report to Chief Executive or the Board. At times when the strategic crisis management team comprises of the usual Senior Management Team, meeting specifically called for issues related to crisis management are essential. It may not be wise to get over the crisis management issues during the meetings called for other management issues. The functions of this team include the following:

Scanning the Existing Structure

A complete and thorough scan of the existing organizational structure for preparedness to face emergency situation. Institute of crisis management has devised a questionnaire, which can be utilized for this purpose. The questionnaire provides a thorough screening by asking questions related to following issues:

- Time required for the management team to assemble in response to crisis appearing beyond office hours
- The details of emergency plan in relation to appropriateness, problems encountered during rehearsals, positives and negatives in comparison with the similar plans of other organizations
- State of awareness among staff for their roles and responsibilities
- Internal organizational problems, which can surface at the time of crisis and interfere with the performance of the plan and damage the business. The impact of such a situation and the remedial measures if planned
- The current state of information channels both for the incoming and outgoing information. Existing guidelines for how much information to reveal, how to reveal, who will communicate and how much time it will take

- Existing guidelines about deputing specific people to communicate with media, ability to handle tough questions from public and media
- Specific guidelines as to how and when to approach other organizations and stakeholders to communicate current situation, ask for help and reassurance and the time required for the same
- State of confidence among people, media and all other stakeholders.

Gathering information: In the initial stages of planning it is important to ask as many as questions as possible and collect relevant information to reinforce corrective measures and strengthen the planning. Some of the questions are enlisted in the uppsala monitoring centre (UMC) management manual and are presented in Figure 10.3.

The scope of collecting information can further be extended to better understand:
- The potential sources of threat
- The names and contact details of all concerned individuals and groups
- The key interests, sensitivities and concerns of all those affected by crisis
- The entire range of possible risks in relation to magnitude, severity and impact
- The relationship of possible risks with management actions

As far as possible the process of collecting information must be collaborative and participation of individuals and groups from inside and outside the organization must be encouraged. The organizations, which maintain a policy of secrecy and extreme defense, will find it difficult to gather important information and build confidence among stakeholders. Therefore, the process must be genuine, objective and transparent. This will help in understanding the concerns, priorities and requirements of stakeholders, incorporating their opinions and experiences and safeguarding their interests. A similar process of gathering information must be encouraged within the organizations to involve employees at all levels. All procedures utilized for gathering information further need scanning on a regular basis.

Assessing the vulnerabilities, potential risks and their prevention: The vulnerability of an organization making them crisis prone can often be recognized easily after scanning the existing organizational structure and gathering all relevant information. Once the complete information is collected it needs to be prioritized and an assessment is done to understand the vulnerabilities of organization that are amenable to correction and potential risks which are likely to present as crisis in

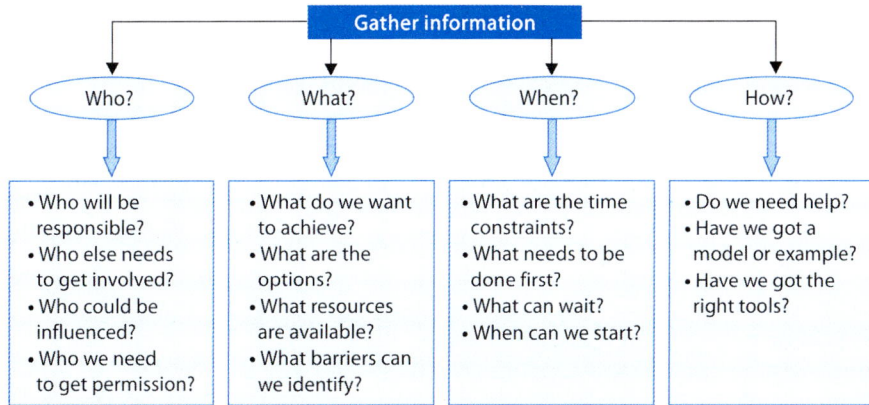

Fig. 10.3: Some of the important questions to be asked in initial stages of crisis management planning

future. At this preventive stage the efforts must be made to recognize the impending crisis and possible actions to correct it before a full-blown crisis precipitates. Such management actions can also be taken from outside the core team and involve:

- Identification of the nature and time course of the action required
- Identification of human resources and ensure their availability for execution of plan
- Allocation of roles and responsibilities to selected staff and their deputies
- Identification of other resources and ensure their availability for execution of plan
- Ensure the continued data collection and documentation
- Time to time scanning of ongoing measures to prevent the precipitation of crisis
- Assess the outcome of management action, with regular reviews and updates.

Define the threshold for declaring a crisis: The identification of a situation amounting to actual or imminent crisis can be highly subjective at times. However, while making a judgment as to the severity of a situation amounting to crisis, certain issues must be considered:

- Concerns of safety and welfare of the patients or public at large
- Immediate and urgent requirement of resources and unusual efforts to limit the damage
- The endpoints of a smoldering crisis if recognized indicate an imminent crisis
- If the problem is in public domain and subject to media attention or the issue is controversial, a quick judgment is required
- Significant external pressure can also influence the decision making.

Once an event or series of events meets the threshold criteria definite authorization procedures must be in place and accordingly authorized person or group must declare the crisis status formally, all those involved must be provided with sufficient information and must be aware of the immediate chain of contact. Further actions will be taken to initiate the crisis management plan.

Establishing Tactical Crisis Management Team

Once the crisis is recognized a targeted approach with the establishment of a tactical crisis management team is required. Teamwork in such situations is always expected to provide better outcomes as compared to when major responsibilities rest upon an individual. The teamwork facilitates the positive outcome by improving cooperation among various departments, accelerated flow of communication and faster decision-making. It is good to ask some of the members of strategic team to be the member of tactical team to maintain the continuity of the process. Besides specialist help can be asked for as the situation may demand. The functions performed by this team can be discussed in two steps:

The First Step

As soon as the crisis is declared or is believed to be imminent, the immediate responsibilities of the team are:
- Define the crisis in terms of its nature, scope and severity
- Estimate the risk involved
- Identify the key executives and authorization procedures
- Enlist the key contacts
- Identify the specialists for support depending upon the nature of crisis
- Identify key stakeholders and ways to communicate with them.

The Second Step

Once the key individuals and groups are recognized the tactical team must organize the individuals in three groups or divisions as per their qualification, experiences and expertise. The three subdivisions of tactical crisis management team look after specific functions in close cooperation with each other. All individuals need to be informed of their roles and responsibilities. As far as possible the specific responsibilities should be assigned to named individuals and precaution must be taken to adequately inform all individuals and groups about the crisis and their roles and responsibilities along with set timelines. The key stakeholders must be assigned specific responsibilities as per requirement and should be adequately informed. Care must be taken while assigning responsibilities to cover the holidays, change over times, busy and peak periods.

Management Division

The management section of tactical management team occupies the chief command post with a designated leader and deputy and directly communicates with the Chief Executives or the Board. The team will get input from the strategic planning team and will take the process further. The important responsibilities of the management division include:

- Taking decision as to the state of crisis, if not declared already. The team must ensure adequate communication regarding current status of crisis and information about the crisis, its context and background to all concerned individuals, groups and authorities. The responsibility must be taken to communicate updates on recent information obtained and response guidelines
- Use pre-established procedures to communicate, mobilize and activate the entire tactical management team, experts and other resources
- All the data, evidences and opinions to be processed and examined
- Look into the legal implications of the situation and accordingly advice the management for any action to be taken or not to taken
- Collect feedback and reports on the impact of implementation of plan. Formulate messages accordingly and communicate appropriately to target audience
- Cooperate and coordinate with other subdivisions
- Manage the budget requirements
- Communicate efficiently about the ongoing plan and its impact to top executives to ensure continued support.

Operational Division

The operational division looks into the technical details of the plan and consists of technical experts from various fields such as drug safety specialist, epidemiologist, pharmacist, clinician, persons with experience in regulatory affairs, etc. In general the operational team must work in cooperation and consultation with other divisions to look after the following activities (Table 10.1):

- To manage, understand and execute the technical aspects of the plan
- To manage, understand and execute the scientific aspects of the plan
- Chart out the requirements accordingly and convey the details to other divisions
- To gather information continuously and offer technical solutions as per requirements
- To develop and implement improved techniques for better outcomes
- To identify for more resource persons and experts for support
- To provide updates to the management team on a regular basis.

Communication Division

The communication division acts as a lifeline for the other two divisions and is the most

Table 10.1: The crisis management plan

Strategic crisis planning team	Tactical crisis management team		
	Management	**Operational**	**Communication**
• Scan existing structure • Gather information • Assess vulnerabilities, risks • Preventive measures • Define threshold to declare crisis	• Define exact status of crisis • Mobilize and activate team • Review data • Assess legal implications • Collect feedback and modify plans • Manage budget • Communicate internally and with stakeholders	• Look into scientific and technical details • Gather info for more improvement • Identify specialist for support • Communicate with other department	• Identify and prepare spokesperson to communicate with press • Activate and maintain hotline • Collect feedback • Communicate with other teams

difficult and sensitive area to handle. All activities of this division must be handled with utmost care by professionals trained in communication skills. A bad implementation by this division can actually create an emergency situation while at times good communication can take care of situations which are likely to become a full blown crisis. The functions of communication division largely involve:

- Well-prepared and well-rehearsed spokesperson from the division is responsible to communicate with external contacts and media
- Activate and maintain the hotlines to answer the queries from outside either immediately of after consultation with other team members
- Maintain adequate flow of information to all stakeholders
- Collect the feedback and other relevant information and convey it to the management division.

ADDITIONAL ACTIVITIES THAT FAVOR "CRISIS PREPARED" ORGANIZATIONAL STRUCTURES

Crisis planning is a dynamic process and preparedness of the organization at times of no crisis is of immense help during the periods of crisis. As stated earlier it is important to encourage a work culture, which has the acceptance for the unexpected events and is capable of reacting efficiently in emergency situations. Following additional activities are essential to further support the crisis management system:

- Create a document of organizational profile giving details of core activities, number of staff, office locations, years in existence, product details and annual productivity figures. This document can be used to provide information to people and groups outside the organization
- A document of simple organization chart showing names, contact details and responsibilities of key persons and their deputies.
- A document showing details of management of previously experienced crisis situations.
- The established crisis management plan must be published with relevant information and should be available to concerned stakeholders. This will help in building confidence and will contribute to organizations credibility and integrity
- Theoretical training and education along with practical rehearsals by running a

simulation of existing management plans on a regular basis
- Continued in-service training of staff to maintain the awareness and abilities to respond during crisis.
- Review of the ongoing crisis management preparation at a regular basis under supervision of a designated individual or group and take remedial measures if required.
- Addition of new techniques and processes with close monitoring and regulat reviews.
- Find the deficiencies in the chain of plan implementation by using real life experiences in the aftermath of real crisis.

CRISIS PREVENTION PRINCIPLES

There are no regulations or guidelines mandating specific company organization for crisis prevention and management. FDA and EMA regulations describe what the organizations should do at the time of crisis or disaster but there is not much information on how to prevent the crisis. However, the general principle of all regulations is focused on detecting and preventing risks and hence indirectly preventing occurrence of a safety crisis. Some of the principles that an organization can follow to prevent occurrence of crisis are as follows:
- Establish and clearly define a Code of Conduct and Compliance
- Establish clear definition and process of fraud and misconduct
- Establish a robust, comprehensive and consistent quality control system with detailed instructions at all levels of activities
- Establish an independent quality assurance system to audit compliance with established standards
- Establish a Safety Governance Model to ensure consistent decision making involving all stakeholders and in line with the organizations' mission and vision.

CONCLUSION

Crisis management in pharmacovigilance is a dynamic process. The most important characteristic of crisis in pharmacovigilance is shortage of time. A rapid action is needed because of a possible serious hazards for patients, imminent threat of regulatory action o and mass media pressure. In this situation, there is urgent need for analysis of all available data, consultations with the experts from various areas, internal discussions within the company, information to various parties and other activities. This situation is normally handled by a task force with an expertise in pharmacovigilance. Besides, preparedness of an organization during no crisis situation has huge impact on the final outcome during real crisis. Only a cooperative organizational effort with support from all external stakeholders during the periods of real crisis can limit the damages. A critical post-crisis review is equally important to strengthen the crisis management in future.

BIBLIOGRAPHY

1. Basic characteristics of a corporate crisis (2003). http://www.bioe2e.org/slides/Bio E2E_Aug_6_03_handout_basic-characteristics.pdf
2. Clair JA, Dufresne RL. Phoenix rising. Positive consequences arising from organizational crisis. In: Giacalone RA, Jurkiewicz CL, Dunn C (Eds). Positive psychology in business ethics and corporate responsibility. Greewich, Conn.: IAP Publishing, 2005;143-64.
3. Crisis management plan for JMD personnel staff. http://www.usdoj.gov/jmd/ps/epm/tab10.pdf
4. Crisis Management and Recovery (CMR) Manual. CQ University Australia. http://facultysite.cqu.edu.au/FCWViewer/view.do?page=4618.
5. Alghabban A. Dictionary of pharmacovigilance. Pharmaceutical Press 2004.
6. Elsubbaugh S, Fildes R, Rose MB. Preparation for crisis management: a proposed model and empirical evidence. Journal of Contingencies and Crisis Management, 2004;12(3):112-27.

7. Glen Trest, Guernsey CH. Effective crisis management, Today's Facility Manager. 2003; http://www.todaysfacilitymanager.com/tfm_03_02_news2.asp.
8. Jaques T. Issue management and crisis management: An integrated, non-linear, relational construct. Public Relation Review. 2007;33(2)147-57.
9. Mitroff II. Why some companies emerge stronger and better from a crisis. New York: Amacom, 2005.
10. Pauchant TC, II Mitroff. Transforming the crisis-prone organization. preventing individual, organizational, and environmental tragedies. San Francisco, CA: Jossey-Bass Publishers, 1992.
11. Sztompka P. The global crisis and the reflexiveness of the social system. In: Edward A (Ed). The global crisis: sociological analyses and responses. Tiryakian Brill Archives. 1984;45-58.
12. Stakeholders in a business crisis. Institute of crisis management, 2008; http://www.crisisexperts.com/stakeholders_main.htm
13. Simola S. Concept of care in organizational crisis prevention. Journal of Business Ethics. 2005;62: 341-53.
14. Talbot JCC, Nilsson BS. Br J Clin Pharmacol 1998;45(5):427–431.
15. The european agency for evaluation of medicinal product, 2004; EMEA/CVMP/159/04.
16. Wang WT. Belardo S. Strategic integration: a knowledge management approach to crisis management. Proceedings of the 38th Hawaii International Conference on System Sciences, 2005.

11
WHO Pharmacovigilance Programme for Global Drug Monitoring

Sushma Srivastava, SK Gupta

Pharmacovigilance is necessary for each and every person who is affected by any form of medical intervention, irrespective of the caste creed or nationality. Medicines have contributed tremendously towards the wellness of human beings, but the world is also facing its darker side in the form of adverse events or adverse drug reactions (ADRs). These are responsible for mild to severe health hazards, disability and sometimes even death to mankind, which can be prevented if a strong pharmacovigilance programme is developed.

The occurrence of adverse drug reactions differs between countries and even in the regions within the country, due to various reasons such as the production of drugs, its distribution and use, pharmaceutical quality and excipients of locally manufactured pharmaceutical products, genetics, diet, traditions of people, use of alternate medicines, etc. The need for the pharmacovigilance system was felt after the thalidomide tragedy. Drug disasters having a high media profile resulted in major changes in drug safety issues, which included the involvement of regulatory systems and the adoption of better epidemiological techniques associated with improvements in information technology. In order to detect the ADRs, not notified during the clinical trials, a pilot pharmacovigilance project was started in 1968 with ten participating countries that had a national pharmacovigilance system (Australia, Canada, Czechoslovakia, Federal Republic of Germany, Ireland, Netherlands, New Zealand, Sweden, United Kingdom, and USA, later joined by Denmark and Norway). World Health Organization (WHO) Programme on International Drug Monitoring was based on the declaration of World Health Assembly to start a project on the feasibility of an international system of monitoring adverse reactions to drugs and was established at WHO headquarters in Geneva, Switzerland. This was later moved to a WHO Collaborating Centre situated in Uppsala, Sweden in 1978 as a part of an agreement between WHO and the Government of Sweden. The operational responsibility was taken up by Sweden while the responsibility of policy matters was retained by the WHO headquarters, Geneva. This WHO Collaborating Centre is now known as the Uppsala Monitoring Centre (UMC). The programme has a networking of National Pharmacovigilance Centres, WHO headquarters, Geneva and Uppsala Monitoring Centre, Sweden.

More than 150 countries have become a member of the WHO Programme for International Drug Monitoring. Presently, 29 countries have applied for membership and are considered as associate members as the technical compatibility of their case reports with the WHO reporting format is being reviewed (Boxes 11.1 and 11.2).[1]

Box 11.1: Full member countries

Afghanistan (2016)
Andorra (2008)
Angola (2013)
Argentina (1994)
Armenia (2001)
Australia (1968)
Austria (1991)
Bangladesh (2014)
Barbados (2008)
Belarus (2006)
Belgium (1977)
Benin (2011)
Bhutan (2014)
Bolivia (2013)
Botswana (2009)
Brazil (2001)
Brunei Darussalam (2005)
Bulgaria (1975)
Burkina Faso (2010)
Cambodia (2012)
Cameroon (2010)
Canada (1968)
Cabo Verde (2012)
Chile (1996)
China (1998)
Colombia (2004)
Dem Rep of Congo (2010)
Costa Rica (1991)
Côte d'Ivoire (2010)
Croatia (1992)
Cuba (1994)
Cyprus (2000)
Czech Republic (1992)
Denmark (1971)
Ecuador (2017)
Egypt (2001)
El Salvador (2017)
Eritrea (2012)
Estonia (1998)
Ethiopia (2008)
Fiji (1999)
Finland (1974)
France (1986)

Germany (1968)
Ghana (2001)
Greece (1990)
Guatemala (2002)
Guinea (2013)
Hungary (1990)
Iceland (1990)
India (1998)
Indonesia (1990)
Islamic Republic of Iran (1998)
Iraq (2010)
Ireland (1968)
Israel (1973)
Italy (1975)
Jamaica (2012)
Japan (1972)
Jordan (2002)
Kazakhstan (2008)
Kenya (2010)
Republic of Korea (1992)
Kyrgyzstan (2003)
Lao People's Democratic Republic (2015)
Latvia (2002)
Liberia (2013)
Lithuania (2005)
Former Yugoslav Republic of Macedonia (2000)
Madagascar (2009)
Malaysia (1990)
Maldives (2016)
Mali (2011)
Malta (2004)
Mauritius (2014)
Mexico (1999)
Republic of Moldova (2003)
Montenegro (2009)
Morocco (1992)
Mozambique (2005)
Namibia (2008)
Nepal (2006)
Netherlands (1968)
New Zealand (1968)
Niger (2012)

Nigeria (2004)
Norway (1971)
Oman (1995)
Panama (2016)
Peru (2002)
Philippines (1995)
Poland (1972)
Portugal (1993)
Romania (1976)
Russian Federation (1998)
Rwanda (2013)
Saudi Arabia (2009)
Senegal (2009)
Serbia (2000)
Sierra Leone (2008)
Singapore (1993)
Slovakia (1993)
Slovenia (2010)
South Africa (1992)
Spain (1984)
Sri Lanka (2000)
Sudan (2008)
Suriname (2007)
Swaziland (2015)
Sweden (1968)
Switzerland (1991)
United Republic of Tanzania (1993)
Thailand (1984)
Togo (2007)
Tunisia (1993)
Turkey (1987)
Uganda (2007)
Ukraine (2002)
United Arab Emirates (2013)
United Kingdom (1968)
Uruguay (2001)
U.S.A. (1968)
Uzbekistan (2006)
Venezuela (1995)
Vietnam (1999)
Zambia (2010)
Zimbabwe (1998)

Box 11.2: Associate member countries

Associate members (29)

Albania	Dominica	Pakistan
Algeria	Gambia	Papua New Guinea
Anguilla	Georgia	Paraguay
Antigua and Barbuda	Grenada	Qatar
Azerbaijan	Guinea-Bissau	Saint Kitts and Nevis
Bahrain	Haiti	Saint Lucia
Bosnia and Herzegovina	Malawi	Saint Vincent and the Grenadines
British Virgin Islands	Mongolia	Syrian Arab Republic
Burundi	Montserrat	Tajikistan
Chad		Zanzibar

ROLE OF WHO PROGRAMME FOR INTERNATIONAL DRUG MONITORING

New Adverse Reaction Signals: Identification and Analysis

Each member country has a National Centre supported by the competent health authority. The centre collects the adverse event report for an individual patient known as Individual Case Safety Reports (ICSRs) from the health professionals or from the various peripheral/regional/zonal centres.[2] These reports are send to the National Centre through VigiFlow, the software owned by WHO-UMC (Sweden). The reports are then processed and analyzed for new adverse reaction signals and sent to UMC for inclusion in the database and also the reports are returned to the professionals on a national basis. These ICSRs are submitted electronically to WHO in a standard ICH E2B compatible format[3,4] and checked for technical correctness and then it is included in the database on a weekly basis. Bayesian Confidence Propagation Neural Network (BCPNN), a data mining approach developed in 1998 is being used at the UMC to support the clinical analysis made by a panel of reviewers.

Reference Source

The WHO database is used as a reference source. Upon receiving a first report of any unfamiliar reaction, the National Centre searches for any other similar reaction elsewhere in the world through the WHO database for signal strengthening. Online search facilities and customized services are available to the national centres for latest information regarding reporting situation.

Information Exchange

Information is exchanged and discussion is stimulated between representatives of National Centres, participating in WHO international drug monitoring programme, through an e-mail information exchange system known as Vigimed, a unique IT drug safety tool. It is a restricted list, open only to individuals connected to the National Centre for Pharmacovigilance or to the drug regulatory authority in participating countries and also in associate countries, managed by the Uppsala Monitoring Centre.[5] A password is needed for the access.

The website of WHO Programme http://www.who-umc.org was started in 1996 which helps in an effective communication between the national centres and UMC. Internet-based seminars and training courses are also being introduced on this site.

Publications

The programme publishes several periodicals, including the 'WHO Pharmaceutical Newsletter' and Uppsala Reports. An adverse reaction Newsletter was provided to the national centres since 1982 to 1999 containing reviews of National Adverse Reaction Bulletins and news of drug-related problems being studied worldwide supplemented with the figures from the WHO register. Later on, this information was incorporated into the WHO Pharmaceutical Newsletter and widely distributed to all member countries of WHO. 'Uppsala Reports' is the UMC's regular news bulletin for everyone concerned with the issues of Pharmacovigilance being published since April 1996. The report is freely available and provides the news about pharmacovigilance, WHO programme, its members and services.[6] Uppsala Reports celebrated 20 years of publication with a visual and editorial makeover in 2016. The content includes current affairs in pharmacovigilance and related fields, and news from UMC and member countries of the WHO PIDM.[7]

UMC plays an important role of a Communication Centre. It provides information on drug safety to regulatory bodies, pharmaceutical industry, researchers, etc.

Several guidelines and books in the areas of pharmacovigilance and risk management are also published.[8,9]

Supply of Tools for Management of Clinical Information

A standardized adverse reaction terminology (WHO-ART) and a comprehensive index of reported drugs (WHO Drug Dictionary or WHO-DD) have been developed by this programme with the purpose of aiding data input and analysis. By linking the recorded case safety data to the corresponding classification, the data can be aggregated and analyzed at different levels of precision. WHO-ART is a terminology used by both regulatory agencies and drug manufacturers. The terminology is flexible and even after so many years can be still improved. Both the tools have importance in monitoring system. They are used in pre-marketing safety area and postmarketing studies. The terminology is made in English and translated in French, German, Portuguese and Spanish. The paper print version is also available for purchase. The International Programme on Chemical Safety has adopted WHO-ART for describing poisoning incidents.

National Centres can use either WHO-ART or MedDRA (Medical Dictionary for Regulatory Activities) terms when reporting to the WHO database. MedDRA is an adverse event classification dictionary endorsed by the International Conference on Harmonization of Technical Requirements for Registration of Pharmaceuticals for Human Use (ICH). It is used in the US, European Union, and Japan. Its use is currently mandated in Europe and Japan for safety reporting. Both terminologies allow for groupings and aggregation of data on different levels, from broad system-organ classes to individual signs and symptoms. Since the database system is not restricted to the use of one medical terminology only, the UMC took a decision to run WHO-ART and MedDRA in parallel so that those who wish can continue using WHO-ART, whereas MedDRA reports need not to be recoded.[4]

All medicinal products referred in ICSRs sent to the WHO database are coded as per WHO Drug Dictionary (WHO-DD) classification by the UMC staff. Drugs reported as 'suspected' of having caused the adverse reaction, and those reported as 'concomitant' or 'interacting' are included. It also includes newly registered drugs put up on the FDA and EMEA websites. The UMC significantly increases the number of products through a collaboration with IMS Health which loads all product data in their system into the WHO-DD.[6] The WHO-DD also includes herbal medicinal products with a unique ATC (Anatomical–Therapeutic–Chemical) based new classification system that links to internationally accepted botanical names and synonyms in view of the increased use of herbals and traditional medicines globally and hence the increased need for safety monitoring of these products. Two extended version of the dictionary have been created WHO Drug Dictionary Enhanced (WHO-DDE) and WHO Herbal Dictionary (WHO-HD). New drugs are added every quarter. WHO-HD is released two times in a year—1st March and 1st September. The WHO Herbal Dictionary (WHO-HD) is the first international dictionary of herbal products, used for identifying the names of herbal products, their active ingredients and therapeutic use, in the course of their drug safety surveillance. It translates a drug name to useful information for coding and analysis of drug safety data—both pre- and post-marketing.[10]

The WHO Drug Dictionary Browser was launched in 2006 that enables direct access to all the features in the Dictionary and is available over the internet. It supplements the current system, which may not have the search capabilities to fully utilize the functionality offered in the browser. Straightforward and more complicated searches are both simplified using Drug Dictionary Browser. It helps to:

- Find 'same name' drugs with different ingredients, listed with a code added to the name in the dictionary B-2 format. The Browser then helps to code the correct entry.
- Search on the active ingredients of concomitant drugs for generic and trade names.
- Code clinical data or case reports
- Understand the active ingredients of the product looked up
- Understand what the ATC codes mean and differentiate between products that have several codes in the interactive tree in the ATC hierarchy.[7]

As of 1st of June 2015 the WHO Drug Dictionary enhanced contains:
- 342,980 unique names
- 2,458,286 different medicinal products and trade names, including, for example, form and strength information
- 13,395 different ingredients mentioned in these products
- Entries from over 133 countries.[11]

From the year 2016 UMC has decided to combine all WHO Drug dictionaries into one dictionary named WHO Drug Global and by releasing the dictionary twice a year, in March and September.[12] It is a combination of WHO Drug Enhanced and WHO Drug Herbal dictionary. Additionally, WHO Drug Global includes Chinese drug names (with Latin characters).

Providing Training and Consultancy Support

World Health Organization is continuously promoting education and communication in pharmacovigilance. Two two-week Pharmacovigilance training programme in AE and AR monitoring are held every year in May at Uppsala, Sweden and the Asia Pacific course, in January-February at Mysuru, India, in collaboration with JSS University for 30 health professionals. The participants are trained in topics vital for effective pharmacovigilance, including sessions to strengthen the performance of members of the WHO Programme, such as pharmacovigilance best practice and tools, signal detection, regulatory aspects and reporting culture.[13]

Several meetings are held locally or at regional level worldwide. WHO participates in these meetings, particularly if held in developing countries, to provide support and technical guidance.

Training Programmes for Pharmacovigilance is being carried out in various countries.

Computer Software for Case Report Management (VigiFlow)

A validated case management system for pharmacovigilance centres and companies has been developed known as VigiFlow.

Uppsala Monitoring Centre made this software available for pharmacovigilance centres in need of a modern system for management of adverse reaction reports. The UMC along with, Swissmedic (IKS), a Swiss medicines agency worked since 2001 to improve ADR reporting and feedback in the age of the internet. A technique for improved communication between reporting and prescribing physicians and a pharmacovigilance centre was made possible because of the internet. When the Swiss national centre needed to upgrade their systems, instead of building something completely new, the UMC worked with them to develop a parallel ADR database with the WHO database. This software 'VigiFlow' (formerly VigiBase Online) has been made available from the UMC for pharmacovigilance centres in need of a modern system for management of adverse reaction reports (there is a charge depending on country size and GDP), and hopefully it would be suitable for others using drug information databases. No local installations and no licenses of database systems and servers are required as this system accesses VigiBase over the internet. Reports can be entered and assessed via a secure internet connection by the doctor reporting an ADR. The report is then accessed by assessors from a regional or national centre. ICSR data can be shared and exchanged (both import and export) in a ICH E2B harmonized format with external stakeholders, e.g. pharmaceutical companies and public health programmes, and with the VigiBase, a WHO global database of individual case safety reports.

The process of developing and maintaining VigiFlow had been validated: version 3.0 of this sophisticated case report management system was successfully released on 28th February 2006, complying with G × P requirements. The validation process is described in Uppsala Reports 32.[14] Till now VigiFlow has seen many upgradations and now version 5.3 is available.

The number of individual case safety reports (ICSRs) in VigiBase June 2014 in the database was 9 million however only a year later it reached over 11 million[11] and in 2016 it was above 13 million (Fig. 11.1).[4]

Vigi portfolio of tools and services[4]
- *VigiBase:* The WHO global ICSRs database. VigiBase includes data on conventional medicines, traditional medicines (herbals), as well as biological medicines, including vaccines.
- *VigiLyze:* A powerful search and analysis tool that provides WHO PIDM members access to more than 13 million ICSRs in VigiBase, submitted by over 100 countries.
- *VigiAccess:* Giving public access to VigiBase through a user interface that allows search and retrival of statistical data on safety issues reported to the WHO PIDM.
- *VigiFlow:* A web-based ICSR management system designed for use by national centres in the WHO PIDM.
- *VigiFlow eReporting:* A web-based module for VigiFlow that allows national centres to capture ICSRs directly from patients and healthcare professionals.

Annual Meetings for Representatives of National Centres

Annually a meeting is organized by WHO and one of the participating countries, representatives of the national centres are invited to attend the meeting for discussing the technical issues in relation to the improvement of the global drug monitoring in general and concerning individual drug safety problems. These meetings have high attendance rates and are important forums for establishing and maintenance of personal relationships and good communication (Box 11.3).

Methodological Research

World Health Organization programme also conducts methodological research for

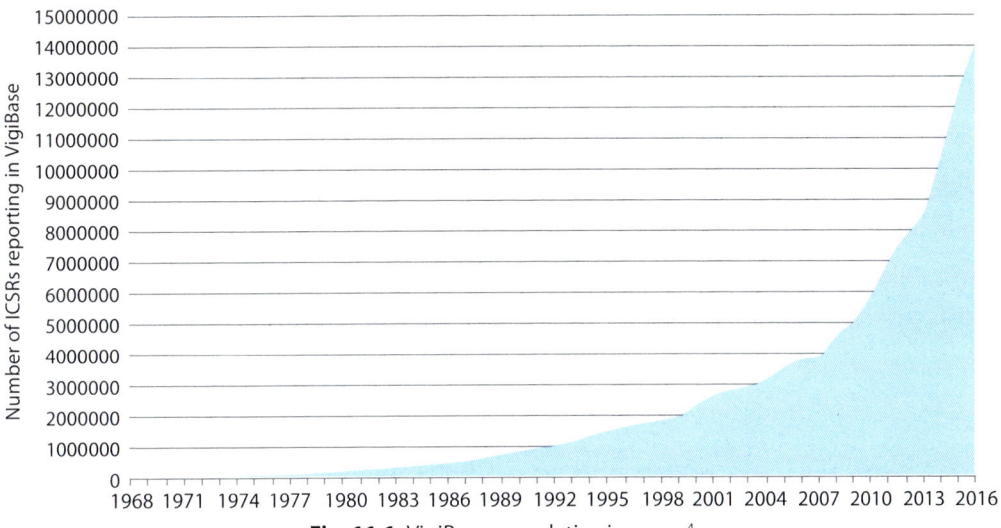

Fig. 11.1: VigiBase cumulative increase[4]

Source: https://www.who-umc.org/media/3081/umc-annual-report-final-version_small.pdf

Box 11.3: Year and venue of the annual meetings of the WHO programme for international drug monitoring

1978 Uppsala, Sweden	1988 Uppsala, Sweden	1998 Tokyo, Japan	2008 Uppsala, Sweden
1979 Geneva, Switzerland	1989 Geneva, Switzerland	1999 Ankara, Turkey	2009 Rabat, Morocco
1980 London, UK	1990 Geneva, Switzerland	2000 Tunis, Tunisia	2010 Accra, Ghana
1981 Uppsala, Sweden	1991 Barcelona, Spain	2001 Dunedin, New Zealand	2011 Dubrovnik, Croatia
1982 Ancona, Italy	1992 Ottawa, Canada	2002 Amsterdam, Netherlands	2012 Brasilia, Brazil
1983 Brussels, Belgium	1993 Geneva, Switzerland	2003 New Delhi, India	2013 Rome, Italy
1984 Washington, DC, USA	1994 Berlin, Germany	2004 Dublin, Ireland	2014 Tianjin, China
1985 Dubrovnik, Yugoslavia	1995 Bangkok, Thailand	2005 Geneva, Switzerland	2015 New Delhi, India
1986 Paris, France	1996 Lisbon, Portugal	2006 Lige, Belgium	2016 Muscat, Oman
1987 Canberra, Australia	1997 Geneva, Switzerland	2007 Buenos Aires, Argentina	2017 Kampala, Uganda

developing pharmacovigilance as a science. Efforts are being made to improve methods for monitoring of traditional medicines and to do methodological research in ADR signal analysis, focused on using international drug utilization data and Bayesian neural network methodology.

Due to the rapid expansion of the use of herbal medicines across the world the safety of herbal medicines has become a major concern to both national health authorities and the general public. To strengthen national capacity in monitoring the safety of herbal medicines and in analyzing the causes of adverse events, and to share safety information at national, regional and global levels WHO has published guidelines on safety monitoring of herbal medicines in pharmacovigilance systems.

GLOBAL PHARMACOVIGILANCE

Uppsala Monitoring Centre (UMC) in close collaboration with WHO and other collaborating centres continues to support countries to develop their pharmacovigilance systems and tries that UMC services adapt to their needs. UMC through its training and education is reaching for a wide audience and aims to work closely with WHO colleagues, public health programmes, academic institutions, and donor organizations to support sustainable, high quality pharmacovigilance systems and practices for all populations. Developing a strategic partnership with regulators, donor organizations, and other influential stakeholders is important for ensuring the continued growth of pharmacovigilance in the world.

JOINING THE WHO PROGRAMME FOR INTERNATIONAL DRUG MONITORING

The WHO Programme for International Drug Monitoring offers an opportunity to WHO member states to collaborate in pharmacovigilance. Countries willing to join should fulfill certain requirements in view of the sensitive nature of the data collected in the programme.

The basic requirements to join the programme include:

1. *General acquaintance with the methodology of spontaneous monitoring:* The country willing to join the programme should have a national programme for the collection of ICSRs in place. The programme should be appropriately funded for maintaining the continuity and be equipped with staff and technical facilities. The staff achieves essential competence to interpret the information received from spontaneous adverse reaction monitoring systems by operating the programme. It is not necessary to cover the whole country or all areas of the health care system by the national system.
2. *National Centre for Drug Monitoring:* It should be designated and recognized by the Ministry of Health (or equivalent). WHO drug monitoring programme includes only member states having a national centre authorized by the competent national health authority. The national centre is mostly part of the national drug regulatory authority, but can also be affiliated to a university institution, a hospital or can work in collaboration with a drug or poison information centre. A central technical advisory committee may be constituted which has the expertise to evaluate the reports and give their suggestions.
3. *Technical competence to fulfill reporting requirements to WHO:* Any national centre has to show its technical competence by way of submitting data in the required format as per the guidelines of UMC prior to its admission in the programme. The ICSRs submitted by the willing country to WHO database can be reviewed as per the policy of WHO and should be freely available for analysis.

Procedure for Joining

A. The country willing to join the programme should write a formal application to WHO headquarters, Geneva through its health authority identifying the institution and the person representing the country. The applicant country is considered as an Associate Member Country from the time its formal membership application is received. Associate members countries get most of the benefits provided to full member countries.
B. The applicant country has to submit a minimum of 20 ICSRs collected in the national pharmacovigilance programme as a sample to the UMC, according to UMC's instructions along with the application or even before submitting the formal application. These sample reports are analyzed by the UMC staff for their technical compatibility. If any deviation is observed then the centre is informed,

however, in case of compatability the WHO headquarter is informed about the National Centre. The WHO headquarter then confirms to the applicant country about its admittance to the programme. Various steps are taken to facilitate the collaboration with UMC.[15]

REFERENCES

1. https://www.who-umc.org/global-pharmacovigilance/who-programme/
2. WHO. International Drug Monitoring: The role of national centres. WHO Technical Series No. 498. 1972.
3. Klepper MJ, Edwards B. Individual case safety reports--how to determine the onset date of an adverse reaction: a survey. Drug Saf. 2011;34(4):299-305.
4. Lindquist M. VigiBase, the WHO Global ICSR Database System: Basic Facts. Drug Information Journal. 2008;42:409-19.
5. Guidelines for Members of the Vigimed Mailing List. Vigimed guide 2007. (last updated 17.4.07)
6. Uppsala Reports 1, April 1996. Available at https://www.who-umc.org/media/2546/ur1-scanned.pdf. Accessed on 2.9.17.
7. https://www.who-umc.org/media/3081/umc-annual-report-final-version_small.pdf
8. Dialogue in pharmacovigilance — more effective communication. Uppsala, Sweden, Uppsala Monitoring Centre, 2002.
9. Effective communications in pharmacovigilance containing The Erice Declaration on communicating medicine safety information. Uppsala, Sweden, Uppsala Monitoring Centre, 1998
10. Uppsala Reports 40, January 2008. Available at: https://www.who-umc.org/media/2632/ur40_med-res.pdf. Accessed on 2.9.2017
11. Uppsala Reports 70. July 2015. Available at: https://www.who-umc.org/media/1699/ 29603.pdf Accessed on 2.9.2017.
12. https://www.who-umc.org/whodrug/whodrug-portfolio/whodrug-global/
13. https://www.who-umc.org/education-training/education-training/asia-pacific-pharmacovigilance-training-course/
14. Uppsala Reports 32, January 2006. Available at www.who-umc.org/Safer-use-of-medicines/uppsala-reports/uppsala-reports-archive/. Accessed on 2.9.2017.
15. http://www.who.int/medicines/areas/quality_safety/safety_efficacy/Joining_the_WHO_Programme.pdf?ua=1

Pharmacovigilance of Herbal Drugs

Rajani Mathur, SK Gupta

INTRODUCTION: WHAT ARE HERBAL MEDICINES?

World Health Organization (WHO) defines Herbal Medicines as a broad term that includes herbs, herbal materials, herbal preparations and finished herbal products (WHO/EDM/TRM/ 2000.1). The term includes herbs including crude plant material such as leaves, flowers, fruit, seed, stems, wood, bark, roots, rhizomes or other plant parts, which may be entire, fragmented or powdered and processed by local procedures and used as established traditionally. The traditional use of herbal medicines has long historical basis, on the basis of which they are widely acknowledged to be safe and effective. Their therapeutic activity encompasses successful prevention, diagnosis and treatment of physical and mental illnesses; improvement of symptoms of illnesses; as well as beneficial alteration or regulation of the physical and mental status of the body.

In 1993, Eisenberg and his colleagues reported that 34% of adults in the United States use at least one type of unconventional form of health care including, herbal products, acupuncture, acupressure, manual or spiritual therapies, yoga, etc. WHO estimates that about 80% or even 90% (BBC NEWS) of population in developing countries rely on traditional medicines, at least for primary health care. Plant derivatives form a predominant part of these approaches (WHO policy perspectives on medicines, 2002). The popularity of herbal products can be further estimated in terms of the trade they generate. The international trade for medicinal plants was US $12.5 billion in 1994 and US $30 billion in 2000, with annual growth rate averaging at 7%. The herbal supplement market had an even higher annual average growth rate of 25% between 1990 and 1997 (Medicinal Plants, International Trade Forum, 2004). In India, the turn over for medicinal plants was approximated to be about ₹5.5 billion/years (Exporting Indian Healthcare, 2002).

Despite the growing popularity of herbal products, they contributed only 7.2% to the trade. In contrast, in other nations, such as Asia, Japan and South Korea the herbal products contribute as much as 35-55% of the total trade. In these nations, traditional medicines are treated with same respect as modern pharmaceuticals and are also included in the national health scheme (Ameh et al. 2010).

The herbal medicines and products with a herbal medicine base are prescribed by physicians across the globe as adjuvant or adjuncts with modern drugs and are dispensed or supplied primarily by pharmacists. Thus, to derive the complete benefit of herbal medicines, the regulations regarding their manufacturing, testing and sale, need to be established by respective governments.

A report of a global survey on national policy on traditional medicine and regulation of herbal medicines indicated that about 50 countries including China, Japan, and Germany already have their national policy and laws on regulations of traditional medicines (Parveen et al, 2015).

In Europe, herbal medicines are registered under two directives, either 'well-established use' or 'traditional herbal medicinal products' both of which have significant requirements for quality (GMP) and safety. Food supplements do not have the same legal requirements for quality control.

In the US, prior to 1994, these products were marketed as foods or drugs, depending on their intended use and whether any health claims were made. In 1994, the Congress passed the Dietary Supplement Health and Education Act (DSHEA) to protect access by consumers to safe dietary supplements (PL No. 103-417). It is understood that the quality of dietary supplements can vary although GMP requirements are issued by the FDA in 2007, and their pharmacovigilance reporting is not compulsory for manufacturers. Thus, all herbs, botanicals, vitamins and minerals that are identified as dietary supplements and regulated under DSHEA have been eliminated from medical ambit (Bass & Raubicheck, 2000; Mills, 2003).

More importantly, under the Food and Drug Regulations, the sale of any natural health product or combination of substances or a traditional medicine is required to be pursuant to a prescription other than when it is sold in accordance with section C.01.043 of the Regulations (Legislation Revision and Consolidation Act, Canada 2009).

In India, the Mashelkar committee on pharma industry has recommended formulation of a national policy to bring herbal and over the counter (OTC) medicines under one umbrella to maintain standards of safety and efficacy (Panel suggests national policy on herbal medicines, 2000).

Recently, Canada has revised Regulations that apply to (a) the sale of natural health products; (b) the manufacturing, packaging, labeling and importation for sale of natural health products; (c) the distribution of natural health products; and (d) the storage of natural health products (Legislation Revision and Consolidation Act, Canada 2009).

Pelargonium (*Pelargonium sidoides* DC and *P. reniforme* Curtis) is reported to have immune modulating properties and antibacterial activity, and Pelargonium extracts have been used for the treatment of respiratory tract and gastrointestinal infections. In the early 1980s in Germany, Umckaloabo® (ISO Arzneimittel), an ethanolic extract of the roots of *P. sidoides* and *P. reniforme*, it was introduced with the claim "no adverse effects". However, till date, the Uppsala Monitoring Centre has received over 34 case reports of allergic hypersensitivity reactions, suspected to be associated with the use of Pelargonium extract (Hugo et al, 2007).

Some of the salient features that are documented in the Regulations are (Legislation Revision and Consolidation Act, Canada 2009):

1. Valid license is essential for the sale of natural health products.
2. It is now required to provide proper name, common name, quantity per dosage unit, potency, source material, and manufacturing process, use, safety and efficacy, etc. about each ingredient of natural product in the application for the license.
3. No false or misleading statement in the application should be made that, in any way, harms the health of the user.
4. Product license can be amended regarding its safety and efficacy, after completing due formalities.
5. There is now provision for licensing authorities to request safety data from licensee and compliance for the same within 15 working days.

6. The product license can be suspended and cancelled, in case of any failure to comply with the regulations.
7. Most importantly, a case report for each serious adverse reaction to the natural health product has to be reported within 15 days by the licensee.
8. Further, an annual summary report containing a concise and critical analysis of all adverse reactions to the natural health product that have possibly occurred, has to be submitted.
9. There is now provision for recall of product, if recommended by licensing authorities, on the basis of the pharmacovigilance report.

The regulations also provide for clinical trials of a natural health product involving human subjects to investigate, discover or verify its clinical, pharmacological or pharmacodynamic effects, to identify any adverse events that are related to its use, to study its absorption, distribution, metabolism, excretion or safety and efficacy. The trials have to be in compliance with Good Clinical Practices (Clinical Trials Involving Human Subjects, 2017).

The various aspects of the standardization of herbal products includes: (i) plant part to be used, (ii) cultivation and harvesting conditions, (iii) species identification, (iv) method of extraction along with the grade and percentage of solvents used, (vi) use of whole extract or specific fraction, (vii) chemical standardization of the product, (viii) bioavailability of the formulation, and (ix) dose, duration, indications, contraindications, adverse effects of the formulation (Kinsel and Straus, 2003).

HERBAL MEDICINES: ARE THEY REALLY SAFE?

Plants have been the primary source of food and medicine for people of every culture throughout the world. Conventionally, the traditional systems of medicine enjoy mass appeal and unshakable faith and have been labeled as 'effective and safe'. However, this mindset is being revised as increasingly reports regarding adverse effects due to herbal medicines are now being generated (Svedlund et al, 2017).

The most common reports of suspected toxicity and adverse events that have been reported with herbal drugs can be classified as (i) side effects (usually predictable), (ii) reactions occurring as a result of overdose, overduration, tolerance, dependence-addiction, (iii) hypersensitivity, allergic and idiosyncratic reactions, (iv) mid-term and long-term toxic effects including liver, renal, cardiac and neurotoxicity also genotoxicity and teratogenicity (Debbie et al, 2012).

Unlike conventional drugs, herbal products are not regulated for purity and potency. Thus, impurities, undeclared adulteration, mineral contamination, batch-to-batch variation, are some of the constant threats in their usage and can also justify many of the reports on their toxic effects (Kinsel & Straus, 2003; Ernst, 2002). The adverse effects and toxicities of herbal drugs pose a significant challenge to health care system and practitioners of traditional medicine need to be more aware of the problems of toxicity. Some of these agents have also been shown to interfere with diagnosis and treatment of modern medicine. Thus, "herbal drugs are safe" is a misnomer and adverse drug reactions (ADRs) with herbal drugs are a reality. The intensity of ADR cannot be marginalized, as they can even prove to be fatal (Abbot et al, 1996; De Smet, 1995). There is common belief that long use of a medicine, based on tradition, assures both its efficacy and safety. Majority of the traditional medicines are now manufactured for global use and they have moved beyond the traditional and cultural framework for which they were originally intended. Consequently, safety of traditional medicines is a serious issue of contention.

Case report: Two patients taking phenytoin 300 mg/day, who had well-controlled seizures who presented with sudden loss of seizure control. A close history taking revealed that they had started taking "Shankhapushpi". Single-dose administration of the drugs did not lead to any change in phenytoin levels but decreased its anti-epileptic effect (Kshirsagar et al, 1992).

The WHO database elaborates that there are presently 16,154 suspected herbal case reports (http://www.who-umc.org). The most commonly reported reactions are:

Pruritus	829
Rash	751
Urticaria	751
Rash erythematous	733
Nausea	682
Vomiting	561
Diarrhea	546
Headache	501
Abdominal pain	497
Fever	460

The most commonly reported critical terms for adverse drug reactions on herbal drugs are:

Hypertension	396
Hepatitis	261
Face edema	243
Death	226
Angiodema	209
Convulsions	195
Chest pain	191
Thrombocytopenia	178
Purpura	150
Dermatitis	129

Recently in an International Symposium on Pharmacovigilance of Herbal Medicines, held in London, on March 28, 2006, the global experience of the WHO Drug Monitoring Programme was elaborated by Dr Ralph Edwards. A total number of 3.6 million ADR were reported of which, 41,439 were listed as due to herbal drug. It was highlighted that in the last twelve years, the number of suspected herbal ADRs has more than tripled. Lack of an internationally standardized classification has been implicated as a major cause for these ADRs (http://ecam.oxfordjournals.org/cgi/reprint/nem022v1.pdf).

The Uppsala Monitoring Centre (UMC) takes ADR reports from over 100 countries around the world. Up to the end of June 2004, the UMC had received more than 11,500 reports of ADRs in which products with one or more herbal ingredients were suspected to be the cause of the reaction. Updated data in 2010 showed, that over 21,000 reports of total 4 million reports were those originating from herbal or natural products (UMC, 2011). At Uppsala, these reports are incorporated in a single database with review of suspected signals carried out by experts in relevant fields.

CHALLENGES RELATING TO THE SAFETY MONITORING OF HERBAL DRUGS

The issue of adverse effects or toxicities that may be associated with herbal drugs is challenging and numerous factors have been identified.

- Ambiguity over nomenclature, variability in content due to diverse climatic conditions, subjective interpretation of traditional descriptions all contribute towards errors in preparation of medicinal plant based products.
- The quality control of the crude plant materials is the most important and challenging. The major difficulty in this is the batch-to-batch variations in the medicinal herb. The reasons are several folds and include ecotype pharmacological variation, soil condition, status of nutrition, seasonal changes and climatic conditions.

Because of the lack of quality control, the amount of the active principle can vary between batches and manufacturers (Marrone, 1999). With regard to Ayurvedic system of medicine, the Charaka Samhita has given guidelines on the quality and purity of medicines and has mentioned that all herbs should be stored in houses that are windless, and guarded against fire, water, moisture, smoke, dust, mice and quadrupeds (Sharma and Dash, 1999).

- Identification and use of medicinal plants in various preparations depending on their natural habitat.

Case report: Two botanical varieties of betel leaf (Piper betle Linn) had two different actions; the Mysuru variety lowered the activity of intestinal enzymes, whereas the Ambadi variety stimulated the enzyme activity (Prabhu et al, 1995).

- Lack of inclusion of herbal materials and preparations in a national/regional pharmacopeia/quality standards/ monographs/formularies keeping in view local availability of plants.
- Many cases of deliberate and naïve adulteration of herbal medicines have come into force. In a screening study conducted at AIIMS, New Delhi, it was highlighted that of the 150 samples screened, over 26% of the samples had been tested positive for presence of corticosteroids (Gupta et al, 2000).

Case report: Pain relief preparation 'Vedana Nigraha Ras' which translates as 'pain relieving tonic', presuming it to be an Ayurvedic medicine based on its name, was taken by a student to relieve pain. Close examination of the bottle label revealed that it actually contained 530 mg of aspirin and 100 mg of paracetamol (Kshirsagar, 1993).

- Liberal use of heavy metals in formulations described in ancient literature also account for some of the adverse events. For example, of the total 6,000 medicines listed in the Ayurvedic texts, at least 35–40% contains heavy metals and about 20–25% of formulations contain more than one heavy metal (Nayak, 2001). Systematic procedures for the preparation of herbo-mineral formulations have been described along with their indications and contraindications. The doses of metals used in practice are based on recommendations given in the ancient Ayurvedic text. However, this is not a guarantee of safety as it is very challenging for trained healthcare provider to prepare, dispense and monitor herbo-mineral formulations. Adverse events with some of the commonly used metals are tabulated (Table 12.1).

Case report: An analysis of 18 samples for lead and 6 for mercury revealed that all samples contained metals in excess of the permissible limits. Patients usually present with anemia and basophilic stippling of the red cells, when peripheral blood smears are analyzed.

Table 12.1: Metals present in herbo-mineral formulations and associated adverse events (Gogtay et al, 2002)

Metal	Adverse event	Max. recommended dose (mg)
Gold	Weakness, urticarial rash, death	15–30
Silver	Weakness, urticarial rash	30–60
Copper	Burning, anorexia, giddiness, hepatitis, tremors, renal dysfunction	8–30
Iron	Erectile dysfunction, cardiac disease, coma, liver injury, renal failure	30–240
Lead	Anemia, dermatological conditions, paraplegia	12–5

- Variety of healthcare professionals serves as qualified provider of herbal medicines. As many herbal medicines are non-prescription medicines, healthcare providers in this category are classically not physicians.
- Lack of proper knowledge on herbal medicines amongst the providers and consumers.
- Wide prevalence of self-medication amongst users of herbal medicines.
- Limited pharmacological data on the therapeutic and safety profile.
- Inadequate and lenient implementation of regulations regarding quality standards for their manufacture, packaging, sale and use.
- Weak national quality assurance measures for labeling, licensing schemes for manufacturing, importing and marketing of herbal products.
- Disparities in regulation of herbal medicines between countries have serious implications for international access to and distribution of such products. For instance, in one country a herbal product may be obtainable only on prescription and from an authorized pharmacy, whereas, in another country it may be obtainable from health food shop, or even, by mail order or internet.
- Unpredictable herb-herb interactions, herb-drug interactions and herb-food interactions are major contributors of adverse reactions. Herbal medicines can cause alter results from laboratory tests and create. Confusion in arriving at a proper diagnosis.
- Majority of people who use herbal medicines do not inform their physicians about their use that can lead to unexpected results of laboratory tests (Dasgupta, 2003). Few examples that may be cited in this regard are:
  - *Ginkgo biloba* has a few side effects. But if combined with warfarin, its antiplatelet activity may cause overcoagulation.
  - Increased effect of antiplatelet and anti-coagulants (warfarin, aspirin, heparin, NSAIDs, clopidogrel, eptifibatide, tirofiban, ticlopidine, dipyridamole, and COX-2 inhibitors), if taken together with *Salvia miltiorrhiza*, *Allium sativum* may lead to bleeding episode (Hu et al, 2005).
  - Decreased plasma concentration of Simvastatin was observed after co-administration with St John's Wort (Hu et al, 2005).
  - Failure of oral contraceptives with Hypericum and breakthrough bleeding (Hu et al, 2005).

MECHANISMS UNDERLYING ADR DUE TO HERBAL DRUGS

Herbal medicines often contain multiple active substances, and the bioactivation of herbal constituents appears to be a critical factor that accounts for the toxicity of some herbs (Fig. 12.1). Broadly defined, the resultant reactive metabolites irreversibly inhibit various CYPs, bind covalently to DNA and proteins leading to organ toxicity and even carcinogenicity (Zhou et al, 2004).

1. *Aristolochic acid nephropathy:* Aristolochic acids (AAs) are nitrophenanthrene carboxylic acids from Aristolochia spp. The consumption of herbs containing AAs have been associated with severe nephropathy which is characterized by renal fibrosis and development of urothelial cancer (Zhu, 2002).
2. *Ginkgo biloba induced thrombocytopenia:* The UMC database contains 11 case reports from two countries (France and Germany) describing thrombocytopenia in suspected connection with oral products containing ingredients derived from *Ginkgo biloba*. In four cases of thrombocytopenia, patients were reported to have recovered; and in

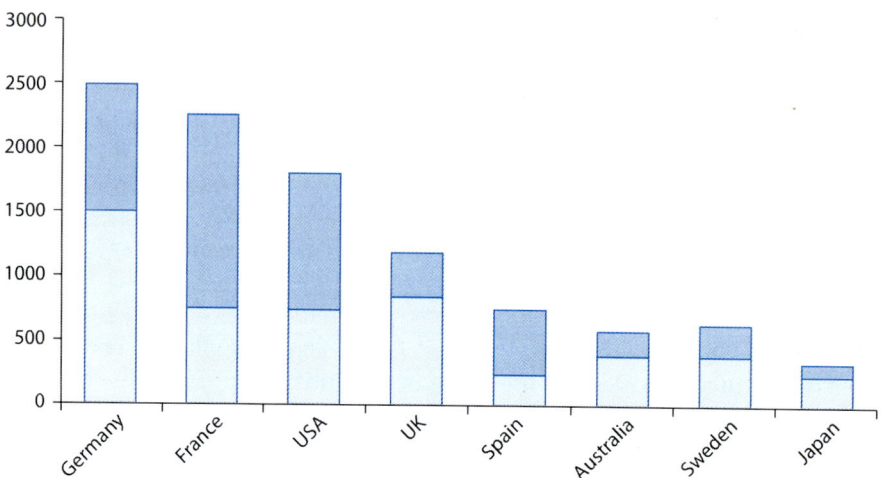

Fig. 12.1: Herbal reports in the WHO database from drugs containing at least one herbal (red or only herbals (blue)
Source: Viewpoint, Part 2.

the remainder, the outcome was either "not yet recovered" or "unknown". In case where the preparation was administered intravenously (*Ginkgo biloba* extract, 175 mg), thrombocytopenia was accompanied by circulatory failure, fever, hypotension, leukocytosis and rigors, after nine days of administration. In the literature, several patients have been described with hemorrhages attributed to the use of products containing *Ginkgo biloba* extract, presumably as a result of impaired platelet aggregation and increased bleeding time (Skogh, 1998; Matthews, 1998; Vale, 1998). In a recent review, fifteen case reports describing a temporal association between usage of *Ginkgo* and bleeding event has been reported (Bent et al, 2005). Most cases involved serious medical conditions, including 8 episodes of intracranial bleeding. Bleeding times were measured in 3 reports and were found to be elevated when patients were taking *Ginkgo*. An assessment of the case reports suggests a possible causal association between *Ginkgo* usage and bleeding events. Patients using *Ginkgo*, particularly those with known bleeding risks, should be counseled about a possible increase in bleeding risk (Bent et al, 2005).

3. *Pulegone toxicity:* Pulegone is a monoterpene ketone present in essential oils from mint species *Mentha pulegium*, and has been used to induce menstruation and abortion. However, high doses of the oil have been associated with hepatic failure, CNS toxicity, gastritis, renal and pulmonary toxicity and death (Anderson et al, 1996).

4. *Germander hepatotoxicity:* Germander (*Teucrium chamaedrys*), a diterpenoid-containing herbal medicine, has been traditionally used for its choleretic and antiseptic effects. Recently, it has been marketed as tea in slimming diets, but numerous cases of hepatotoxicity have been reported with its consumption (Ben Yahia et al, 1993). It has been prohibited in France after confirmation in rechallenge test.

5. *Capsaicin induced inhibition of CYP 450s:* Capsaicin is a major pungent phenolic constituent present in a variety of capsicum fruits. It undergoes bioactivation by *CYP2E1* to reactive species, which are

capable of binding covalently to the active site of CYP2E1 as well as DNA (Surh and Lee, 1995). The interaction with target cell DNA is a double-edged sword as it is responsible for detoxification on one hand but can also trigger mutagenicity and malignant transformation, on the other hand.

6. *Organosulfur compounds induced CYP inhibition:* Organosulfur compounds are the major active components of garlic and have been implicated with hypolipidemic, antiplatelet, immune-enhancing and anticancer activities. A single oral dose of diallyl sulfone inactivated *CYP2E1* dependent activities in liver microsomes (Lin et al, 1996).

7. *Grapefruit juice induced herb-drug interactions:* Grapefruit juice has been found to significantly increase oral bioavailability of some drugs like felodipine, terfenadine, saquinavir, cyclosporine, midazolam, triazolam and verapamil (Bailey et al, 2000). The inhibition of *CYP3A4* activity with no change of *CYP3A4* mRNA and P-glycoprotein is the underlying mechanism (Bailey, 1998).

PHARMACOVIGILANCE OF HERBAL MEDICINES: DEFINITIONS, GOALS AND NEED

As with any system of medicines, pharmacovigilance or safety monitoring of herbal medicines implies detection of any adverse events relating to use of the medicines, assessment and communication of the risks and benefits of medicines and most importantly, educating and informing the patients/consumers. It can be understood as an amalgamation of three complementary actions: preventing adverse events on herbal medicines; when they occur, making them visible, and mitigating their effects. The WHO International Drug Monitoring Programme defines pharmacovigilance as the science of collecting, monitoring, researching, assessing and evaluating information from healthcare providers and patients on the adverse effects of medicines, biological products, herbal medicines and traditional medicines, with a view to identifying new information about hazards, and to preventing harm to patients. Infrequent adverse drug reactions will not be recognized without the existence of a formal system of reporting negative experience. Physicians who have patients taking any particular medicinal plant have to document negative experiences, in order to gather enough scientific information about the adverse effects of the herb. Adverse drug reaction reports are a critical source of herbal drug safety information.

At the outset, an active pharmacovigilance programme requires:
- Increased ability to learn from adverse events occurred, through better reporting systems of adverse events on herbal medicines, skillful technical investigations of incidents and responsible sharing of data
- Greater capacity to anticipate adverse events and probe systemic weaknesses that might lead to an adverse event
- Identifying existing knowledge resources, within and outside the health sector
- Improvements in healthcare delivery system itself, so that structures are reconfigured, incentives are realigned, and safety and quality are placed at the core of the system.

The aim of the pharmacovigilance programme includes:
- Early detection of hitherto unknown adverse reactions and interactions
- Detection of increases in frequency of known adverse reactions
- Identification of risk factors and possible mechanisms underlying adverse reactions
- Estimation of quantitative aspects of benefit/risk and analysis and dissemination of information needed to improve medicines prescribing/dispensing/provision and regulation.

In the WHO International Drug Monitoring Programme that was conducted in September 1991 a consensus on the guidelines for safety monitoring of herbal medicines were drawn. The following objectives were defined:
- To define safety monitoring/pharmacovigilance system of herbal medicines
- To support, strengthen and effectively carry out safety monitoring and pharmacovigilance of herbal medicines
- To provide technical guidance on principle to monitor the safety of herbal medicines and to incorporate herbal medicines into the existing national drug safety monitoring/pharmacovigilance system
- To promote and coordinate international data sharing on pharmacovigilance of herbal medicines.

The need of a sound pharmacovigilance programme can be understood, by the various issues it is meant to address, namely:
- Formulation of drug regulations
- Creating data base
- Classifying and coding the traditional medicines in internationally accepted format of WHO's herbal ATC (Anatomical-Therapeutic-Chemical) classification. The renewed interest in the western world for plants used in traditional medicine, and the rapidly growing interest in developing countries to start research programmes in this area have, unfortunately, not emphasized the great importance of taxonomic botany and documentation for such research. There is a need to adopt the most commonly used binomial names (including their binomial synonyms) for medicinal plants, to eliminate the confusion created by the common names. *Artemisia absinthium* L., for example, contains an active narcotic derivative, which can cause central nervous system disorders and generalized mental deterioration. This herb has at least 11 different common names (Wormwood, Absinthium, Absinth, Absinthe, Madderwort, Wermuth, Mugwort, Mingwort, Warmot, Magenkraut and Herba absinthii), 7 of which bear no resemblance to its botanical name. Because mainly common names are used, *Heliotropium europaeum* (heliotrope), containing pyrrolidine alkaloids, potent hepatoxins, is often confused with *Valeriana officinalis* (garden heliotrope), containing valepotriates, which act as a sedative and muscle relaxant in laboratory animals. The UMC group is collaborating with the Department of Botany, Uppsala University and the Royal Botanical Gardens at Kew in the UK, and with several other international experts to actively address the problem (http://www.who-umc.org)
- Define and code the adverse reaction terms to be used in the pharmacovigilance programme
- Addition of new recognized reporters to the system
- Establishing mutual referencing mechanism of regulatory and quality information on herbal medicines among national pharmacovigilance centres and national drug regulatory authorities
- Strengthening effective global safety information feedback and sharing system on herbal medicines, among national health authorities as well as healthcare professionals and consumers
- Educating the prescribers and consumers
- Creating an environment of openness.

ADVERSE EVENT REPORTING

To explain simply, adverse event reporting is a careful description of relevant clinical feature as a consequence of drug use that ultimately contributes to the growth in understanding about the safety of the herbal medicine that is essential for prescribing physicians and patients to properly weigh anticipated risks and benefits in their therapeutic choices.

The main players that are involved in the system are qualified healthcare professionals, patients, consumers, drug information centres and drug regulatory authorities. The source of information regarding adverse event could either be clinical trial or spontaneous reporting (voluntary, unsolicited communications from healthcare team or consumer), poison information centres, postmarketing surveillance by the industry, intensive hospital monitoring and prescription monitoring.

Assessment of safety of herbal product that has been traditionally used, is based on the guiding principle that in case no harm is demonstrated, there is no specific restrictive regulatory action that should be undertaken. However, if any new evidence to the contrary arises, a revised risk-benefit assessment is demanded. Although, long-term use without any evidence of risk may indicate that a medicine is harmless, it is not always certain how far one can rely solely on long-term usage to provide assurance of innocuity in the light of concern expressed in recent years over the long-term hazards of some herbal medicines (WHO/EDM/TRM/2000.1).

The source of a report is an important factor for the evaluator and determines the feasibility of follow-up. Council for International Organizations of Medical Sciences (CIOMS) Working Group V recommends that as a thumb rule emphasis should be laid on the quality of the report and not on the nature of the source. Thus more important than who made the report is the care and thoroughness with which it is prepared, documented, received, recorded, followed-up, clarified and analyzed. A single report can qualify as a signal and several reports compiled together as a case series becomes a stronger signal.

Thus, a complete report contains the following important information:

- *Title:*
  - It has to be consistent with the content of the report
- *Patient details:*
  - It is essential to provide the age group and sex of the patient
  - In addition, relevant information regarding his weight, height, race, ethnicity, obstetrical status, body mass index and occupation may also be provided
  - The current health status of the patient or the disease or symptoms for which he was being treated with the suspect drug, including the duration of illness, its severity
  - Baseline laboratory findings.
- *Drug:*
  - The suspected drug may be identified by its generic or proprietary name. Herbal products have to be described by Latin binomial of herbal ingredients, plant part used and type of preparation. For herbal extracts it is highly desirable that the type and concentration of the solvent used for extraction be delineated
  - The approximate dosage, duration of therapy, route of administration, and if relevant the adherence of the patient to the regime
  - As assessment of potential contribution of any concomitant therapy is very crucial as it highlights any drug-drug interaction.
- *Adverse event:*
  - A comprehensive description of adverse event and its severity, onset date, duration, and specific treatment meted for its management, if any.
- *Discussion:*
  - Keeping in view the previous reports from literature on relevant topic, along with supporting evidence from dechallenge and rechallenge, diagnostic procedures performed, biological plausibilities and their explanations constitute the discussion portion of the report
  - The report may be rounded off with remarks from regulatory authorities or from principal investigator of the clinical trial, as the case may be.

The assessment of the data has to be done by a multidisciplinary committee constituted by traditional practitioner, general practitioner, clinical pharmacologist, toxicologist, pharmacist, pathologist, phytochemist, etc. In collaboration with botanists, phytochemists and pharmacologists, the Uppsala Monitoring Centre has established a project with the aim of attaining global standardization for herbal medicines and solve the associated problems. Together the data can be objectively assessed and answer two important queries, i.e. (1) 'Can the drug cause the reaction?' and 'Has the drug caused the reaction?' The first question is the basis for signal detection and signal strengthening, while the second pertains to case-causality assessment.

ADVERSE EVENT REPORTING: THE UK LEAD

In the UK at present, the Committee on Safety of Medicines/Medicines and Healthcare products Regulatory Agency's (CSM/MHRA) 'yellow card' scheme for ADR reporting is the main method of monitoring the safety of herbal medicines. The herbal sector in the UK has initiated various spontaneous reporting schemes, based on the Yellow Card scheme, but targeted mainly at herbal-medicine practitioners. It is important that these schemes have a link with the CSM/MHRA so that potential signals are not missed. Several other tools used in pharmacovigilance of conventional medicines, such as prescription-event monitoring, and the use of computerized health-record databases, currently are of no use for evaluating the safety of herbal medicines (Barnes, 2003). The Royal Pharmaceutical Society hosted an international conference entitled "Pharmacovigilance of herbal medicines— current state and future directions" at the Royal College of Obstetrics and Gynaecology London from 26 to 28 April, 2006, wherein Ally Broughton, of the National Institute of Medical Herbalists, reported that a modified Yellow Card scheme had been implemented by the NIMH in 1994 as part of a formal pharmacovigilance reporting system for herbal medicines prescribed by herbal practitioners. A total of 42 yellow card reports have been submitted since the initiation of the scheme (http://www.pjonline.com/Editorial/20060506/forum/forum_herbalmedicines.html).

Despite recent initiatives to stimulate reporting of suspected ADRs associated with herbal medicines, such as extending the scheme to unlicensed herbal products, and including community pharmacists as recognized reporters, numbers of herbal ADR reports received by the CSM/MHRA remain relatively low. Under-reporting, an inevitable and important limitation of spontaneous reporting schemes, is likely to be significant for herbal medicines, since users typically do not seek professional advice about their use of such products, or report if they experience adverse effects (Barnes, 2003).

Other bodies that are actively contributing in documenting ADRs due to herbal medicines include the European Manufacturers Associates (EMA Inc.) and the European Scientific Cooperative on Phytotherapy (ESCOP). Proposed European Union legislation for traditional herbal medicinal products will require manufacturers of products registered under new national schemes to comply with regulatory provisions on pharmacovigilance. In the long-term, other improvements in safety monitoring of herbal medicines may include modifications to existing methodology, patient reporting and greater consideration of pharmacogenetics and pharmacogenomics in optimizing the safety of herbal medicines (Barnes, 2003).

On similar lines the Italian Herb Surveillance Programme of National Institute of Health, the German Producers of Anthroposophic Medicines, the Australian Adverse Drug Reactions Unit, Chinese Drug Regulatory Authorities have also taken up the initiative to report ADRs arising out of herbal medicines. However, a major pitfall that needs to be addressed is the modus operandi for communication between the different systems of data collection (http://ecam.oxfordjournals.org/cgi/reprint/nem022v1.pdf).

TRADITIONAL CHINESE MEDICINES: BOON OR BANE?

Traditional Chinese medicine (TCM) including Chinese materia medica (CMM), is an integral part of Chinese civilization, and is one of the major systems of medical practice today. CMM, with about 1000 kinds of traditional drugs, is comprised of materials derived from plant (>80%), animal and mineral origin. Less than 1% of the CMM used are considered to be toxic. In Chinese history, safety of CMM was accumulated in clinical experience. In Shennong Herbs (Shen-Nong Ben-Cao-Jing, 1st century BC–1st century AD), the drugs were divided into three classes: superior (strengthening), intermediate (effective against diseases with the species' toxicity dependent on dosage) and inferior (toxic and for short-term use) drugs. In Huangdi Inter Medicine (Huang-Di-Nei-Jing), the toxic drugs were divided into four classes: non-toxic, slightly toxic, toxic and very toxic drugs. Traditionally, 18 incompatible medicinal herbs' and 19 mutual restraining medicinal herbs' existed. These were the sum of clinical experience for drug interaction and coadministration of herbs. According to the concepts of TCM, severe side effects may result when two incompatible or mutually restraining drugs are used in coadministration. Recently, reports regarding ADR from TCM have gained much publicity and public concern and have had an enormous effect on the CMM market in the world. Few classical cases may be cited in this regard:

- The induction of renal toxicity was reported for TCM preparations containing *Aristolochia debilis* and *Aristolochia fangchi* containing aristolochic acid.
- Kamisyoyo-san, a TCM for the treatment of seborrheic dermatitis has been reported to induce pneumonitis. Adult respiratory distress syndrome (ARDS) leading to severe hypoxemia was induced and required mechanical ventilation, as an intervention (Shiota, 1996).
- Gynura root has been used extensively in Chinese folk medicine and plays a role in promoting microcirculation and relieving pain and curing injury. Oral ingestion of the roots was associated with the adverse event of hepatic veno-occlusive disease (HVOD), characterized by hyperbilirubinemia, painful hepatomegaly and weight gain due to fluid retention (Dai et al, 2007).
- Unpublished data presented by Dr. Tony Booker, Register of Chinese Herbal Medicine, UK presented at the Symposium of Pharmacovigilance of herbal medicine, that out of a total of 1,265 patients taking Chinese herbs for different diseases, 107 patients (8.5%) developed raised levels of the liver enzyme ALT.

MEASURES TO IMPROVE THE PHARMACOVIGILANCE OF HERBAL MEDICINES

The contemporary practice of Complementary and Alternative Medicine (CAM) with special reference to use of herbal medicines, is vastly different from what was envisaged and practiced in ancient times. In urban settings, the healthcare provider, patient, symptoms, plants, formulations, etc. have undergone a sea-change, thereby making safety and pharmacovigilance a burning issue (Gogtay et al, 2002). Some of the vital steps that need to be taken in order to establish safety and efficacy of these interventions can be enumerated as below:

- Conduct randomized, controlled clinical trial (RCT): RCT remains the gold standard for establishing the safety and efficacy of any intervention. It can easily identify

type A adverse events. However, some stumbling blocks that remain are- use of placebo, blinding, appropriate standard, evaluation paradigms, etc.
- Training of practitioner in recognizing and reporting adverse events
- Introduction of package inserts for herbal medicines
- Public education
- Incorporation of safety monitoring of herbal medicines as part of routine safety monitoring
- Stringent regulations regarding quality and purity.

CONCLUSION

An effective pharmacovigilance programme will go a long way in addressing the gaping lacunae with herbal medicines, i.e. a national regulatory and quality assurance system and rational use of herbal medicines. At present herbal medicines fall in an ambiguous zone with regard to safety, quality and efficacy regulations. Currently, less than 70 countries regulate herbal medicines and few countries have systems in place for the regulation of traditional health practitioners. The herbal medicines urgently need to be incorporated into the regulatory framework and treated at par with other products such as medicines, dietary supplements and food, intended for human use. Ultimately, this exercise will promote safe, therapeutically sound and informed usage of herbal medicines.

New systematic approaches for monitoring the safety of plant-derived medicinal products are being developed. A number of national pharmacovigilance centres are now monitoring the safety of traditional medicines. For that to succeed, the collaboration and support of consumers, traditional health practitioners, providers of traditional and herbal medicines and other experts are necessary. More attention needs to be given to research and to training of healthcare providers and consumers in this area.

A national policy and regulation for herbal medicines will go a long way in defining its role in health care delivery, ensuring that the necessary regulatory and legal mechanisms are created for promoting and maintaining good practice, equitable access, authenticity, safety and efficacy.

BIBLIOGRAPHY

1. Abbot NC, Ernst E, White AR. Complementary medicine. Nature. 1996;381:361.
2. Ameh SJ, Obodozie OO, Abubakar MS, Garba M. Current phytotherapy–An inter-regional perspective on policy, research and development of herbal medicine. J Med Plants Res. 2010;4:1508-16.
3. Anderson IB, Mullen WH, Meeker JE, Khojasteh-Bakht SC, Oishi S, Nelson SD, et al. Pennyroyal toxicity: measurement of toxic metabolite levels in two cases and review of literature. Ann Int Med. 1996;124(8):726-34.
4. Bailey DG, Dresser GR, Kreeft JH, Munoz C, Freeman DJ, Bend JR. Grapefruit-felodipine interaction: effect of unprocessed fruit and probable active ingredients. Clin Pharmacol Ther. 2000;68(5):468-77.
5. Bailey DG, Malcolm J, Arnold O, Spence JD. Grapefruit juice drug interactions. Br J Clin Pharmacol. 1998;46(2):101-11.
6. Barnes J. Pharmacovigilance of herbal medicines: A UK Perspective. Drug Saf. 2003; 26(12):829-51.
7. Bass IS, Raubicheck CJ. Marketing dietary supplements. Washington, DC: Food and Drug Law Inst. 2000. http://www.fda.
8. BBC News. Can Herbal Medicine Combat Aids? Wednesday, 15 March, 2006, 13:10 GMT. [Last accessed on 2013 Apr 16]. Available from: http://www.newsvote.bbc.co.uk/mpapps/pagetools/print/newsbbccouk/2/hi/Africa/4793106.stm
9. Bent S, Goldberg H, Padula A, Avins AL. Spontaneous bleeding associated with Ginkgo biloba-A case report and systematic review of the literature. J Gen Intern Med. 2005;20:657-61.
10. Clinical trials involving human subjects. Natural health products regulations. Amendment Modification Sections. 2017;4:71-3.
11. Dai N, Yu YC, Ren TH, Wu JG, Jiang Y, Shen LG, et al. Gynura root induces hepatic veno-

occlusive disease: a case report and review of the literature. World J Gastroenterol. 2007; 13(10):1628-31.
12. Dasgupta A. Review of abnormal laboratory test results and toxic effects due to use of herbal medicines. Am J Clin Pathol. 2003;120(1):127-37.
13. Debbie S, Graemeb L, DuezPierrec, Elizabethd W, Kelvine C. Pharmacovigilance of herbal medicine. J Ethnopharmacol. 2012;140(3):513-8.
14. de Boer HJ, Hagemann U, Bate J, Meyboom RH. Allergic Reactions to Medicines derived from Pelargonium species. Drug Safe. 2007;30(8):677-80.
15. De Smet PAGM. Health risks of herbal remedies. Drug Safety. 1995;3(2):81-93.
16. Eisenberg DM, Kessler RC, Foster C, et al. Unconventional medicine in the United States. Prevalence, costs and patterns of use. N Engl J Med. 1993;328:246-52.
17. Ernst E. Toxic heavy metals and undeclared drugs in Asian herbal medicines. Trends Pharmacol Sci. 2002;23:136-9.
18. Exporting Indian healthcare. In: Publication of Exim Bank, 2002.
19. Gogtay NJ, Bhatt HA, Dalvi SS, Kshirsagar NA. The use and safety of non-allopathic Indian medicines. Drug Saf. 2002;25(14):1005-19.
20. Gupta SK, Kaleekal T, Joshi S. Misuse of corticosteroids in some of the drugs dispensed as preparations from alternative systems of medicine in India. Pharmacoepidemiol Drug Saf. 2000;9:599-602.
21. http://ecam.oxfordjournals.org/cgi/reprint/nem022v1.pdf {accessed on 7.04.08}
22. http://www.pjonline.com/Editorial/20060506/forum/forum_herbalmedicines.html {accssed on 7.04.08}
23. http://www.who-umc.org {accessed on 3.04.08}
24. Hu Z, Yang X, Ho PC, Chan SY, Heng PW, Chan E, et al. Herb-drug interactions: a literature review. Drugs. 2005; 65(9):1239-82.
25. Kinsel JF, Straus SE. Complementary and alternative therapeutics: rigorous research is needed to support claims. Annu Rev Pharmacol Toxicol. 2003;43:463-84.
26. Kshirsagar NA, Dalvi SS, Joshi MV, et al. Phenytoin and ayurvedic preparation-clinically important interaction in epileptic patients. J Assoc Physicians India. 1992;40: 354-55.
27. Kshirsagar NA. Misleading herbal ayurvedic brand name. Lancet. 1993;341:1595-6.
28. Legislation Revision and Consolidation Act, 1 June, 2009. Published by the Minister of Justice at the following address: http://laws-lois.justice.gc.ca
29. Lin MC, Wang EJ, Patten C, Lee MJ, Xiao F, Reuhl KR, et al. Protective effect of diallyl sulfone against acetaminophen-induced hepatotoxicity in mice. J Biochem Toxicol. 1996;11(1):11-20.
30. Marrone CM. Safety issues with herbal products. Ann Pharmacother. 1999;33:1359-62.
31. Matthews Jr MK. Association of Ginkgo biloba with intracerebral hemorrhage. Neurology. 1998;50:1933.
32. Medicinal plants. In: International Trade Forum. Magazine of International Trade Centre (ITC) UNTCAD/WTO. 2004;p11.
33. Mills S. Clinical research in complementary therapies: principles, problems and solutions. In: Lewith GT, Jonas WB, Walach H, (Eds). Elsevier Science: Churchill Livingstone; 2003. pp. 211-27.
34. Nayak B. Ayurmedline. Ayurvedic drug index. Ayurmedline, Bangalore (India), 2001.
35. Panel suggests national policy on herbal medicines. In: Industry Highlights March 2000. pp. 41.
36. Public Law No. 103-417, 108 Stat. 4325 (Dietary Supplement Health and Education Act of 1994).
37. Sharma RK, Dash B. Charaka Samhita. 6th ed. Vanarasi (India). Chaukhamba Sanskrit Studies, 1999.
38. Shiota Y, Wilson JG, Matsumoto H, Munemasa M, Okamura M, Hiyama J, et al. Adult respiratory distress syndrome induced by a Chinese medicine, Kamisyoyo-San. Int Med.1996;35: 494-6.
39. Skogh M. Extracts of Ginkgo biloba and bleeding or hemorrhage. Lancet, 1998;352:1145.
40. Surh YJ, Lee SS. Capsaicin, a double edged sword: toxicity, metabolism and chemopreventive potential. Life Sci. 1995;56(22):1845-55.
41. Svedlund E, Larsson M, Hägerkvist R. Spontaneously reported adverse reactions for herbal medicinal products and natural remedies in Sweden 2007-15: Report from the Medical Products Agency. Drugs Real World Outcomes. 2017;4(2):119-25. doi: 10.1007/s40801-017-0104-y

42. UMC. 2011. <http://www.who-umc.org/graphics/24727.pdf> (accessed 24.10.11.)
43. Vale S. Subarachnoid hemorrhage associated with Ginkgo biloba. Lancet, 1998;352:36.
44. WHO/EDM/TRM/2000.1. General guidelines for methodologies on research and evaluation of traditional medicine.
45. World Health Organization (WHO). Consultation meeting on traditional medicine. Forty-ninth regional committee meeting, Manila, Phillipines, 18 September, 1998. Manila, WHO Regional Office for the Western Pacific, 1998.
46. Zhou S, Koh H-L, Gao Y, Gong Z-y, Lee EJD. Herbal bioactivation: The good, the bad and the ugly. Life Sci. 2004;74:935-68.
47. Zhu YP. Toxicity of the Chinese herb Mu tong (Aristolochia manshuriensis): What history tells us. Adverse Drug Reactions and Toxicology Reviews. 2002;21(4):171-7.
48. Ben Yahia M, Mavier P, Metreau JM, Zafrani ES, Fabre M, Gatineau-Saillant G, et al. Chronic active hepatitis and cirrhosi induced by wild germander 3 cases. Gastroenterol and Clin Biol. 1993;17(12):959-62.

13

Medical Dictionary for Regulatory Activities: An Overview

Sanjeev Miglani, Arun Gupta, Mugdha Chopra

INTRODUCTION

The Medical Dictionary for Regulatory Activities (MedDRA) is a compilation of clinically validated international medical terminology used by regulatory authorities and the Pharmaceutical companies. The terminology is used throughout the entire regulatory process, from premarketing to postmarketing, and for data entry, retrieval, evaluation, and presentation.[1]

MedDRA results from an identified need for specificity in coding and flexibility in data retrieval, which could not be adequately fulfilled by the former dictionaries (e.g. International Classification of Diseases or WHO-Adverse Reactions Terminology). MedDRA has a rich, complex, hierarchical and multiaxial structure, which enables coding of diagnoses, symptoms, signs, adverse drug reactions, medical and social history, therapeutic indications, investigations, surgical and medical procedures. MedDRA does not comprise a drug or device nomenclature and does not contain the covering study design and patient demographics. Codes are dispatched into 5 nested levels: Lowest level term (LLT) <Preferred term (PT) <High level term < High level group term < System organ class (SOC).[2]

OBJECTIVES OF MedDRA

The objectives of MedDRA are to promote accurate and consistent term selection and understanding of the impact of various options of data retrieval on the accuracy and consistency of the output. In the world wide use of MedDRA this consistency will lay the foundation for increased precision and uniformity in medical terminology and in turn facilitate a common understanding of data shared among academic, commercial, and regulatory entities.[3,4]

APPLICATIONS OF MedDRA[1,4]

The ambit of MedDRA extends to the following uses:
- For the review and analysis of safety data
- Consistent retrieval of specific cases or medical conditions from a database is facilitated
- To include adverse drug reaction/adverse events (ADR/AEs) in tables, analyses, and line listings for reports
- Improvement in consistency of comparing and understanding "safety signals" and aggregated clinical data
- Facilitates electronic interchange of clinical safety information
- Product indications, investigations, medical history, and social history data can be captured and presented
- MedDRA helps in clinical safety Pharmacovigilance, e.g. for AEs in clinical trial databases; Investigator's brochures, core safety information, safety summaries, clinical study reports.

REGULATORY STATUS/ HISTORICAL OVERVIEW[1-3]

MedDRA is based upon the Medical Dictionary for Drug Regulatory Affairs (MedDRA), which was created by the UK Medicines Control Agency (MCA) and was modified by a working party of representatives from pharmaceutical companies.

In September 1994, International consensus meeting recommended that MEDDRA version 1 (v1.0), should form the basis of new standard terminology for drug reaction. In October 1994, International conference on Harmonization adopted MEDDRA v 1.0 as the basis of the new standard medical terminology for drug regulation and finally in November 1994 it was finally released.

In 1997, ICH agreed the implementable version (v2.0) and adopted new name: the Medical Dictionary for Regulatory Activities (MedDRA). The use of MedDRA started in FDA's AE database since 1997. MSSO (MedDRA Maintenance and Support Services Organization) was established in 1998.

The MSSO provides and maintains MedDRA. Currently, the Food and Drug Administration (FDA) encourages the use of MedDRA for the coding of adverse events in individual case safety reports. For electronic submissions of individual case safety reports, Japan and Europe have required the use of MedDRA since 2003. FDA proposed to use MedDRA for postmarketing safety reports in 2003. In 2005, European Union demanded that MedDRA should be used in undesirable effects section in SmPC (Summary of product Characteristics). Subsequently, Volume 9A of the Rules Governing Medicinal Products in the European Union also recommended Standardized MedDRA Queries (SMQs) as a tool for signal detection.

The currently used MedDRA version 20.0 was recently released in March 2017.

MedDRA STRUCTURE[5,6]

The MedDRA dictionary contains 5 hierarchial levels of medical terms coding (Fig. 13.1).
1. LLT: Lowest level term
2. PT: Preferred term
3. HLT: High level term
4. HLGT: High level group term
5. SOC: System Organ Class

Lowest level term (LLT): Lowest level term is the term that most accurately reflects the reporter's verbatim. Many terms from other dictionaries are represented at this level (i.e. culturally unique terms). Multiple LLTs can be linked to a single PT. An LLT can have the following relationships with PT (Fig. 13.2):
- Synonymous (similar meaning)
- Lexical variant (dictionary variation)
- Quasi-synonym (resembling meaning)

Preferred term (PT): Each preferred term represents a single medical concept. LLT is matched with the most clinically relevant PT. There is no limit to the number of LLTs that can be associated with a single PT. Every PT also exists as an identical LLT. PTs can be represented in multiple SOCs. Each PT is assigned to one primary SOC; assignments of that PT to other SOCs are considered secondary.

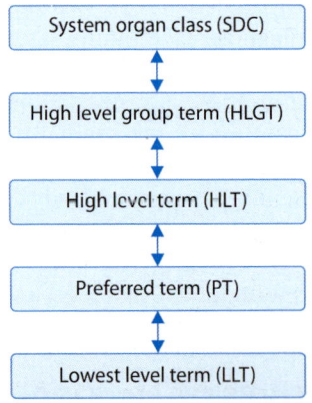

Fig. 13.1: Five levels of medical terms coding

Medical Dictionary for Regulatory Activities: An Overview

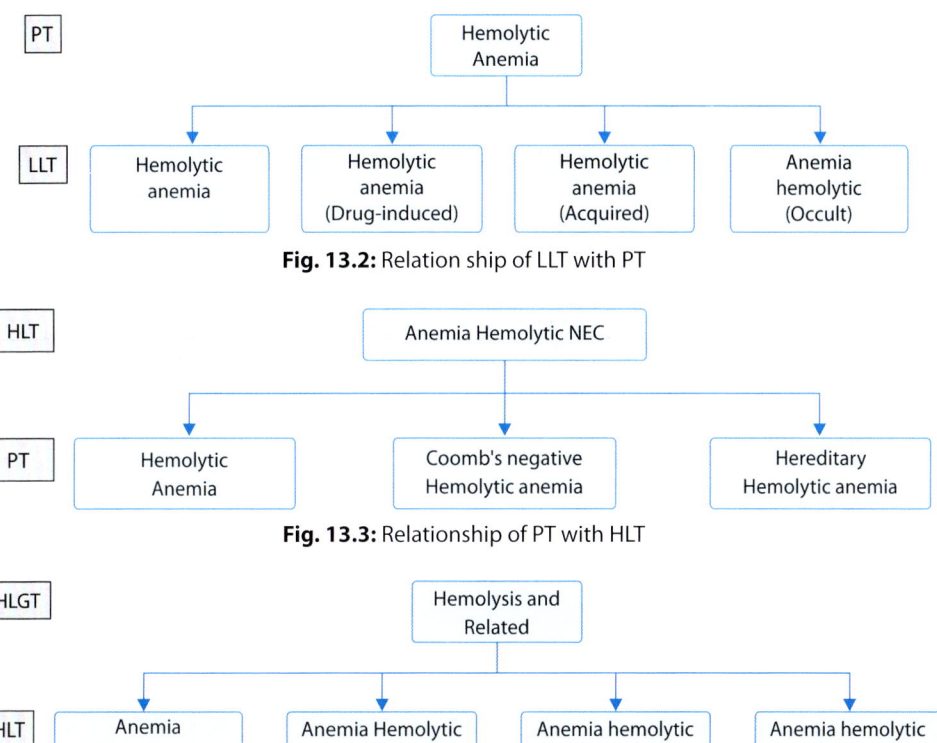

Fig. 13.2: Relation ship of LLT with PT

Fig. 13.3: Relationship of PT with HLT

Fig. 13.4: Relationship of HLT and HLGT

High level term (HLT): It is a more general term used to group closely related PTs. They links PTs related by anatomy, pathology, physiology, etiology, or function (Fig. 13.3). High level terms are linked to at least one SOC via a HLGT. They are solely for data retrieval and presentation purposes.

High level group terms (HLGT): General term grouping of related HLTs. They Link HLTs related by anatomy, pathology, physiology, etiology, or function (Fig. 13.4). They are solely for data retrieval and presentation purposes. There is no limit to the numbers of SOCs to which an HLGT can be linked.

System organ class (SOC): SOCs are the highest level of the hierarchy. SOCs are identified by anatomical or physiological system, etiology (cause) and purpose. SOCs are grouping terms which represent many medical entities from the HLGT level (Fig. 13.5). The SOC is roughly equivalent to "Body System" in other commonly used medical terminologies. Every PT is assigned a primary SOC.

MedDRA system allows terms to be grouped by different points of view (e.g. etiology or manifestation site) for retrieval and presentation. Whereas each LLT is linked to one preferred term (PT), the PT may be linked to several high level terms (HLTs). An HLT may be linked to several High Level Group Terms (HLGTs). Each HLGT may be linked to several SOCs. This implies that each PT may be linked to more than one SOC. One SOC is designated as the primary SOC and other SOCs are called secondary SOCs for a respective PT. The Maintenance and Support Services Organization refers to this property, the representation of a single medical concept

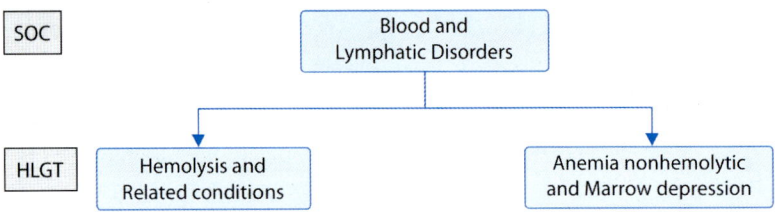

Fig. 13.5: Relationship between HLGT and SOC

in more than one SOC, as multiaxiality. Multiaxiality may start on the HLT, HLGT, or SOC level. Multiaxiality does not apply to 3 of the 26 SOCs: "Investigations," "Surgical and Medical Procedures," and "Social Circumstances."

MedDRA RULES[3,4]

Following general MedDRA rules are recommended to be followed while using MedDRA:

- Some terms are added with NOS (not otherwise specified) or NEC (not elsewhere classified). NOS terms are commonly used terms, which are non-specific; and these are found usually at LLT level only, e.g. Headache NOS. NEC terms are specific terms that do not readily fit into hierarchial classification; and these are only found at HLT and HLGT levels, e.g. respiratory disorders, injuries NOS
- Qualifiers like rare, frequent, severe are usually not used in MedDRA. However, exceptions might be there, e.g. those terms which may give a new meaning to medical term if not used, e.g. severe mental retardation
- Usually abbreviations and acronyms are used up to LLT level only, and these are not incorporated above LLT level. However, there might be few exceptions to this rule, e.g. echocardiography (ECG)
- Natural word order is used at PT and above levels in MedDRA. However, exceptions could be there if reversal allows for similar PT grouping at SOC hierarchies, e.g. pneumonia viral for viral pneumonia.
- Numerical values are usually not used in MedDRA. However, exceptions are there, e.g. 17-α hydroxylase deficiency
- Punctuation marks are usually not used in MedDRA. However, exceptions are there, e.g. Parkinson's disease
- For spellings British English is used from PT and above levels. However, American English may be there at LLT level, e.g. esophagal, estrogen.

CRITERIA FOR TERM SELECTION[3-5,7]

There are usually differences in medical aptitude of different coders, and there could be many more choices to manually code terms in MedDRA. MedDRA users should be aware of the degree of specificity that MedDRA terms may have and the challenges this specificity may pose for appropriate term selection. There might be more than one option for term selection. This is to allow a solution to accommodate different database configurations and historic working practices.

Therefore, to maintain the consistency, the following criteria are recommended to be used for term selection in MedDRA:

- Lowest level term(s) that most accurately reflects the reporter's words should be selected. For term selection, only current LLTs should be used. The use of non-current terms should be restricted to the conversion of historical data
- Medical judgment should be used if an exact match cannot be found, but the medical concept can be adequately represented by an existing term.

Diagnosis

For diagnosis the following parameters should be taken into account:
- If only a single provisional diagnosis, e.g. "suspicion of", "probable", "presumed", "likely", "questionable" is provided, in the absence of additional clinical information, it should be managed just like a confirmed diagnosis. For example, "suspicion of renal failure" is the only information reported, "Renal failure" can be selected
- If both a diagnosis and its characteristic signs and symptoms are provided by the reporter, one can select terms for both, but it is preferable to select a term for only the diagnosis and not for the signs and symptoms. However, terms should also be selected for signs or symptoms that are not generally recognized as part of that diagnosis. For example, if "Bronchial asthma" is reported with dyspnea, cough and wheezing, selecting "bronchial asthma" alone is considered appropriate.
- If both a provisional diagnosis and its characteristic signs and symptoms are provided by the reporter, it is preferable to select terms for both.
- If there are multiple diagnoses or provisional diagnoses without signs and symptoms, terms for each diagnosis or provisional diagnosis can be selected. For example, if a case is reported with the following differential diagnosis: Leptospirosis, typhoid and malaria, then all the three can be selected.
- When an ADR/AE is reported in association with a consequence of an event or a patient outcome, a term for the ADR/AE should be selected and the outcome should be captured in the appropriate field. For example, Death is an outcome and is not usually considered to be an ADR/AE.
- If multiple ADR/AEs are reported in association with a fatal outcome, MedDRA terms for each reported event should be selected. For example, if "septicemia, renal failure, myocardial infarction and patient died" are reported, then "septicemia", "renal failure" and "myocardial infarction" all should be selected and death should be captured as the outcome.

Death

If the only information reported is death, then the most specific death term available should be selected. For example, if a reporter only states that "a patient was found dead", "Found dead" can be selected. If circumstances of the death are provided (e.g. natural, accidental, suicide, homicide), and the term exists, it should be selected.

Hospitalization

Consequences of an event such as hospitalization and disability are not generally considered to be ADR/AEs. For example, if hospitalization is due to diabetic ketoacidosis is reported, then "diabetic ketoacidosis" should be selected. Hospitalization will only serve as seriousness criteria or the consequence of the event. If the only information reported is the outcome term, then the most specific term available should be selected. For example, if a reporter states only that "a patient was hospitalized", "Hospitalization" can be selected.

Suicide

Accurate and consistent term selection for reports of suicide attempts, completed suicides and self-harm is necessary for appropriate data retrieval. It is not acceptable to assume that an overdose is a suicide attempt. Only the appropriate term that describes the overdose can be selected. Similarly, for reports of self-injury that do not mention suicide/suicide attempt, only the appropriate self-injury term should be selected. For example, if the only information received from the reporter is "cutting the wrist", then selecting the term "deliberate self-injury" will be appropriate. In such a case if the reporter mentions that it was a suicide attempt then "attempted suicide" in addition to "deliberate self-injury" should be selected.

Conflicting

When conflicting, ambiguous, or vague information is provided, it can be difficult to select a term that will lead to appropriate data retrieval. In such circumstances, attempts should be made to obtain more specific information. If clarification attempts have failed, the examples below might be helpful. For example, if only hyponatremia is reported and serum sodium is 160 mEq/L, "serum sodium abnormal" can be selected.

Combination term

A combination term in MedDRA is a single medical concept combined with an additional medical term to provide important information on pathophysiology or etiology. A combination term represents an internationally recognized distinct and robust medical concept. When combination terms are reported, medical judgment should be applied.

If encephalopathy is reported in a patient with hepatic disease, then hepatic encephalopathy should be reported. If one term is more specific than the other then the most specific term should be selected, e.g. if dizziness and vertigo are reported then dizziness can be selected.

If splitting provides more appropriate medical information, both the terms should be selected. For example, cardiogenic shock due to myocardial infarction is reported then both the terms "myocardial infarction" and "cardiogenic shock" should be selected.

If the reported term is a combination of an event and a pre-existing condition that has not changed and the combination term does not exist in MedDRA, it is appropriate to select the term for the event. For example, if hemoptysis is reported in a patient with pre-existing mitral stenosis then hemoptysis alone can be selected.

Age and Gender Specific Terms

Some MedDRA terms describe the age group and the event. If available the term with the specific age group and the event should be selected. If dementia in an elderly patient is reported, then senile dementia can be selected. Normally, there are no options for the term "male" and "female" but sometimes these terms are selected for appropriate medical judgment, e.g. male or female orgasmic disorder, male or female pattern baldness.

Body Site Specific Terms

If available the term with both the specific body site and the event should be selected. If polyp in nose is reported nasal polyp can be selected. If a term contains multiple body sites and all link to the same PT, the relevant medical event should have the priority. For example, if a lipoma is found in arm, back, neck, it is appropriate to select the term "lipoma".

MedDRA terms should have both the location and the specific organism/infection. If available the term with both the specific location and the organism can be selected. For example, if gastroenteritis is reported with Shigella then shigella gastroenteritis can be selected.

Pre-existing Medical Conditions

Pre-existing medical conditions that have not changed should generally be classified as medical and/or social history while those that change can be classified as ADR/AEs. If a pre-existing medical condition is modified, the specific MedDRA term should be selected, provided that it exists, e.g. if exacerbation of dyskinesia is reported then "dyskinesia aggravated" can be selected. If progression of a disease ulcerative colitis is reported and there is no appropriate combination term then "ulcerative colitis" and "disease progression" can be selected.

Exposure During Pregnancy and Breastfeeding

MedDRA contains various terms that address exposures to medical products (drug and nondrug) during pregnancy and breastfeeding. To select the most appropriate term(s) to capture the information, first it should be determined if the subject/patient who experienced the event(s) was the mother or the child/fetus. If a pregnant patient experienced adverse event while receiving the study medication, appropriate term for the adverse event and "Drug exposure during pregnancy can be selected". If a child or fetus experience adverse event and was exposed to drug in utero, "maternal drug affecting fetus" can be selected in addition to the appropriate term.

The definition of "congenital" for MedDRA is "any condition present at birth, whether genetically inherited or occurring in utero", e.g if an anomaly of ossicles is reported at birth, congenital anomaly of ossicles can be selected. If the condition is not clearly specified as congenital, e.g. deafness is reported, the term "deafness" can be selected.

Neoplasms

Given the wide variety of neoplasm types, it is not possible to provide specific guidance applicable to all situations.
- The words "cancer" and "carcinoma" are used synonymously
- The word "tumor" is considered neoplastic
- The words "lump" and "mass" are not considered neoplastic.

If a tumor in breast is reported, breast tumor can be selected.

If a cancer growing in ovary is reported, malignant ovarian cancer can be selected.

Surgical and Medical Procedures

The use of the SOC surgical and medical procedures is generally not appropriate for ADR/AEs. The terms in the SOC surgical and medical procedures are not multiaxial in MedDRA. Users should be aware of the impact that use of these terms will have on data retrieval, data analysis, and reporting.

Medication Errors

There are specific medication error terms in MedDRA. Information may be reported describing medication errors with or without clinical consequences. If a medication error results in clinical consequences, term(s) for the medication error and the clinical consequences should be selected. For example, if vomiting due to medication error is reported "vomiting" and medication error can be selected. If medication was given intravenously instead of intramuscular route then the appropriate term to be selected will be "intramuscular formulation administered by the other route" along with the adverse event. Medication errors without clinical consequences are not ARs/AEs. However, it is important to record the occurrence or potential occurrence of a medication error. The term that is closest to the description of medication error reported should be selected.

Drug Interactions

With respect to drug interactions MedDRA does not have specific product names. For examples, if anaphylaxis is reported with the suspected drug interaction then drug interaction and anaphylaxis can be selected.

Device-related Terms

If device-related event reported with clinical consequences is available, a term that reflects both the device-related event and the clinical consequence should be selected. If there is no single MedDRA term reflecting the device-related event and the clinical consequence, both the terms should be selected.

MedDRA VERSIONING[2,4]

This compilation of medical terminology is very dynamic with each recent version representing the best contemporary medical knowledge. To keep pace with the rapidly progressing medical sciences. The six-month update incorporates simple changes and the annual update provides simple plus complex MedDRA changes. Both simple and complex changes impact retrieval and presentation strategies. Organizations should plan and document their strategy for handling MedDRA version updates. When planning or performing data retrieval and presentation, the MedDRA version should be documented.

"**Simple**" **changes** include adding a PT (new medical concept), moving an existing PT from one HLT to another, demoting a PT to the LLT level, adding or removing a link to an existing PT, adding an LLT, moving an existing LLT from one PT to another, promoting an LLT to the PT level, making a current LLT non-current or a non-current LLT current, changing the primary SOC allocation, and changes to SMQs.

"**Complex**" **changes** include adding or changing multiaxial links, adding new grouping terms, merging existing grouping terms, and restructuring a SOC.

STANDARDIZED MedDRA QUERIES (SMQs)[8-10]

To assist medical personnel in locating all the terms related to a specific disease/SOC, SMQs were formulated. Standardized MedDRA Queries (SMQs) are groupings of terms from one or more SOCs that relate to a defined medical condition or area of interest. The terms included could relate to signs, symptoms, diagnoses, syndromes, physical findings, laboratory and other physiologic test data, etc., that are associated with the medical condition or area of interest. SMQs are a joint effort of the Council for International Organizations of Medical Sciences (CIOMS), SMQ Working Group and ICH (MSSO/JMO).

The SMQs are maintained with each release of MedDRA by the MSSO. As of 1-March-2017, 101 level 1 SMQs are in production. Additional SMQs are created as the need arises.

Following are the characteristics of SMQs:
- SMQs are developed from a case definition of a medical condition
- SMQs focus on highly relevant drug safety topics
- SMQs are displayed as a list of PTs, though in some cases all PTs in a HLT, HLGT or SOC may be listed.

SMQs have design concepts such as "narrow" and "broad" sub-searches, hierarchical relationships between related SMQs and/or algorithmic design.

Narrow search provides high specificity where as high sensitivity is offered by the broad search, e.g. the former will identify cases that will highly represent the condition of interest where as latter will identify all the possible cases.

MedDRA AND SMQ IN SIGNAL DETECTION[4,8,9]

Multiaxiality has a significant influence on data retrieval and signal detection. A multiaxiality terminology, in the simplest sense, implies the representation of a concept in more than one SOC. The PT "viral pneumonia" is an example, it is represented primarily in the SOC "Infections and infestation" but also has a secondary link to the SOC "Respiratory, thoracic and mediastinal disorders".

The concept of multiaxiality does not apply to the whole of MedDRA, in fact few PTs have secondary links and this feature is conspicuous by its absence in 3 of the 27 SOCs namely "Investigation", "Surgical and medicinal procedures" and "Social circumstances". Another characteristics of MedDRA that deserves special mention is primary SOC allocation rules as 3 MedDRA SOCs will be primary irrespective of the event. These are "congenital, familial and genetic disorders", "Neoplasms benign, malignant and unspecified (including cysts and polyps)" and "infections and infestations".

Disproportionality studies using proportional method varies across different levels of the terminology. PT level may be best option for indexing a signal but this may not be true in every scenarios. Aggregation of MedDRA according to diagnosis helps in the detection of signals. The novelty of SMQs requires further research to explore their ability to act in this capacity.

The size specificity and multiaxiality are characteristics of MedDRA that impact both the classification and the analysis of data. These characteristics, although potentially helpful, are not always enough. Additional tools such as SMQs are likely to assist in data retrieval and signal detection.

REFERENCES

1. Brown EG, Wood L, Wood S. The medical dictionary for regulatory activities. Drug Safety. 1999;20(2):109-17.
2. Kubler J, Vank R, Beimal S, et al. Adverse event analysis and MedDRA: business as usual or challenge? Drug Information Journal. 2005;39: 63-72.
3. ICH-Endorsed Guide for MedDRA users dated 1-Mar-2017 (MedDRA Term Selection: Point to consider Release 4.13 Based on MedDRA version 20.0).
4. ICH-Endorsed Guide for MedDRA users on Data Output dated 1-Mar-2017 (MedDRA Data Retrieval and presentation: Points to Consider Release 3.13 Based on MedDRA version 20.0).
5. Bousquet C, Lagier G, Louet ALL, et al. Appraisal of the MedDRA and conceptual structure for describing and grouping adverse drug reactions. Drug Safety. 2005;28(1):19-34.
6. Journot V, Tabuteau S, Collin F, et al. About the necessity to manage events coded with MedDRA prior to statistical analysis: Proposal of a strategy with application to a randomized clinical trial, ANRS 099 ALIZE. Contemporary Clinical Trials. 2008;29:95-101.
7. Brown EG. Methods and pitfalls in searching drug safety databases utilizing the Medical Dictionary for Regulatory Activities (MedDRA). Drug Safety. 2003;26(3):145-58.
8. Brown EG. Using MedDRA: implications for risk management. Drug Safety. 2004;27(8):591-602.
9. Mozzicato P. Standardised MedDRA queries. Their role in signal detection. Drug Safety. 2007; 30(7):617-19.
10. Introductory Guide for Standardised MedDRA Queries (SMQs) Version 20.0 -Mar 2017.

14

Pharmacogenetics and Pharmacovigilance

Rajani Mathur

"If it were not for the great variability among individuals, medicine might as well be a science and not an art……"

—Sir William Osler, 1892

ADVERSE DRUG REACTIONS: A CLINICAL PROBLEM

Adverse drug reactions (ADR) remain a major clinical problem. A recent meta-analysis suggested that in the USA alone, ADRs were responsible for >100,000 deaths, making them between the fourth and sixth most common cause of death.[1] ADRs account for 5% of all hospital admissions. ADRs increase the length of stay in hospital by two days at an increased cost of $2500 per patient. They have been reported to affect 10–20% of hospital inpatients and lead to deaths in 0.1% of medical and 0.01% of surgical inpatients. The extent to which ADRs can affect the quality of life of any patient can be a major cause of his noncompliance with the regimen.

WHY ADRs DO NOT AFFECT EVERYBODY EQUALLY?

Perhaps fortunately, ADRs only affect a minority of those taking a particular drug. It is often seen that commonly prescribed drugs, elicit ADR in some, at the same time many remain unaffected. In addition, often, the degree or severity of ADR that will be recorded in susceptible individuals cannot be predicted. The factors that determine susceptibility to ADRs are not clear, though increasingly the pointer is pointing at genetic factors. The role of inheritable variations is not a recent phenomenon and has been well-recognized and recorded since as early as 1950s and 1960s.

A gene can be defined as exhibiting a genetic polymorphism if the variant allele exists in the population at a frequency of at least 1%. Polymorphism can be due to base substitution, deletion or insertion. It could be either in the coding or non- coding region. Polymorphisms are known as non-synonymous or synonymous if they alter amino acid or not, respectively. The polymorphism may be expressed as either an alteration in the function or in the expression level of the protein. Specific populations of some subjects have particular single nucleotide polymorphisms (SNPs) or a set of closely linked SNPs that are also known as haplotypes. The International SNP Map Working Group has recently published a map of 1.42 million SNPs throughout the genome, occurring at an average density of one SNP every 1.9 kilobases. At least 60,000 SNPs are within coding regions and are therefore more likely to be functionally active.

Traditionally, single nucleotide polymorphisms have been associated with some clinically important differences in therapeutic responses to drug therapy. More recently, they have been categorically linked with clinically important differences in ADRs generated as a consequence of the drug regimen. The variations in the genetic constitution of individuals, contribute towards variations in the enzyme system, morphology and physiology of receptors, transporter systems, ion channels, to name a few and this has been sought as an acceptable explanation for the variations in ADRs that are recorded in different individuals.

Broadly categorizing, the ADRs arising due to variability in genetic constitution of an individual are either due to alterations in the pharmacokinetic and/or pharmacodynamic pathways (Flowchart 14.1). Consequently, the ability to identify individuals who are susceptible to ADRs has the potential to reduce the costs, morbidity and mortality associated with any drug regimen.

The problem is being approached with much vigor and several studies have been conducted to establish the role of pharmacogenetic factors with ADRs.[2] Both pre-clinical and clinical evidence (as collected from case controlled or pharmacoepidemiological studies) is available to link the two phenomena. Examples of genes that are known to influence drug responses are provided in several reports.[3] Selected examples where genetic variability is associated with susceptibility to ADRs are given below:

POLYMORPHISM IN GENES ENCODING PHARMACOKINETIC PARAMETERS AND ADRs

Cytochrome P450 Enzyme Family

The family of cytochrome P450 enzyme system is one of the most important enzymes that are involved in the metabolism of a large number of xenobiotics. Consequently, polymorphisms of the genes encoding CYP450s especially *CYP2D6*, have been closely studied for their putative role in generating adverse drug reactions (Table 14.1).

Warfarin, an oral anticoagulant is the drug of choice for the treatment of venous thromboembolism, and prophylaxis against thromboembolism in patients with valvular heart disease and atrial fibrillation.[4] The anticoagulant dose has to be carefully titrated so as to maximize therapeutic benefit against critical risk of hemorrhage. In order to improve the benefit-risk ratio, an accurate prediction of the dosage requirement of warfarin therapy is essential. Further, inter individual variation

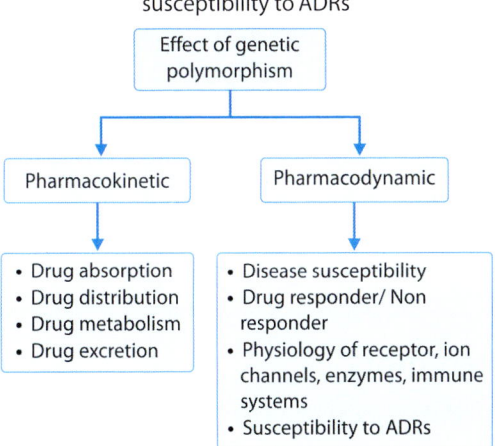

Flowchart 14.1: Genetic variability leading to susceptibility to ADRs

Table 14.1: Selected polymorphisms of *CYP450* enzyme gene and associated ADRs[5]

P450 enzyme	Drug	Adverse Reaction
CYP1A2	Typical antisychotics	Tardive dyskinesia
CYP2C9	Warfarin	Hemorrhage
	Tolbutamide	Hypoglycemia
	Phenytoin	Phenytoin toxicity
CYP2D6	Antiarrhythmics	Arrhythmia
	β-Blockers	Bradycardia
	Tricyclic antidepressant	Confusion

Table 14.2: Gene polymorphisms of phase II metabolizing enzymes and ADRs

Phase II enzyme	Drug	Adverse Reaction
N-acetyltransferase	Sulfonamides, procainamide, isoniazid	Hypersensitivity, SLE
Thiopurine methyltransferase	6-Mercaptopurine	Myelotoxicity
UDP-glucuronosyltransferase	Irinotecan	Diarrhea, myelosuppression

Abbreviations: SLE, systemic lupus erythematosus; UDP, uridine diphosphate.

poses as a challenge and complicates this common clinical problem.

The S-enantiomer of warfarin, which is predominantly responsible for the anti-coagulant effect, is metabolized by CYP2C9. Polymorphisms in the CYP2C9 gene result in two allelic variants. These variant enzymes have been reported to clear warfarin at a slower rate, leading to its accumulation in the body. Hence in such individuals who express the allelic variants, the dose has to be accordingly reduced, so as to avoid the severe ADR of bleeding disorder. Further clinical studies are being conducted to ascertain the need to make genotyping prior to warfarin treatment, a routine practice.[5]

Numerous other ADRs have been associated with *CYP2D6* isoforms and some classical examples include:[6]

- Polymorphisms for *CYP2D6* leading to its absence or reduced activity can lead decreased first pass metabolism and elimination of Metoprolol. This has been explained as the basis of the adverse effect of bradycardia following its therapy, in hypertensive individuals expressing this isoform.
- Reduced metabolism of drugs can lead to its accumulation in the body leading to ADRs. *CYP2D6* poor metabolizers are associated with a higher risk of Perhexilene induced hepatotoxicity and neuropathy can be cited here. It is one of the few drugs that have been withdrawn from the market because of this.

Phase II Metabolizing Enzymes

Polymorphisms in Phase II metabolizing enzymes such as N-acetyltransferase type 2, thiopurine methyltransferase, UDP-glucuronosyl transferase (Table 14.2) has led to the occurrence of ADRs with several drugs.[5]

P-Glycoprotein

Transporter protein P-glycoprotein, or commonly known as P-gp, transmembrane efflux pump that works to extrude drugs and other substrates from cells. P-gp has been isolated in endothelial cells of the gut, kidney, liver and other organs, where it plays a major role in the pharmacokinetics of lipophilic xenobiotics.[7] It is encoded by the ABCB1 gene, which is highly polymorphic and many variant forms of P-gp show significantly reduced transporter function. Because of this, the pharmacokinetics of many drugs can get severely affected and this may contribute to serious ADRs.[8,9] As P-gp transports many drugs including anticancer, statins, digoxin, calcium channel antagonists, angiotensin II receptor antagonist, phenytoin, erythromycin, genetic variation in the function of P-gp increase the risk of adverse outcomes of these drugs.[2]

POLYMORPHISM IN GENES ENCODING PHARMACODYNAMIC PARAMETERS AND ADRs

Drug targets such as receptors, ion channels, enzymes, immune systems are also associated with variations arising due to genetic factors. These variations have been associated with ADRs.

Receptors

Modulation of drug action as a consequence of genetic variations, has been associated with ADRs. For example, drugs acting through dopamine receptors are used as antipsychotic agents. However, serine to glycine substitution in the gene encoding the dopamine D3 receptor has been held responsible for the ADR of tardive dyskinesia following treatment with typical neuroleptic agents. Similarly, unpredictable toxicity of malignant hyperthermia associated with halothane, has also been linked to variations in receptors.

Ion Channels

Various pharmacological agents exert their therapeutic action via modulation of ion channels. Recently, the use of several drugs including terfenadine, cisapride, thioridazine and sertindole has been restricted because of the occurrence of QT- interval prolongation on the electrocardiogram (ECG) and occasionally Torsades de pointes. Mutations in the genes that code for the potassium channel proteins have been reported and held responsible for reduced functioning in transportation of K^+ from the cells, making them susceptible to long QT interval and serious arrhythmias.[10]

PRACTICAL CHALLENGES OF PHARMACOGENOMICS

The human genome is made up of about 3 billion base pairs. An SNP is reported to occur per 300–600 base pairs that totals to about 10 million SNPs per person. The cost of genome SNPscanning can only be reduced or at best limited if:
- Scanning is limited to coding regions only
- Scanning is limited to only non-synonymous SNPs
- Advantage of linkage disequilibrium is taken.

THE WAY FORWARD

There are numerous reports in literature implicating an association between particular polymorphisms in genes and drug response. However, there is paucity of pharma-coepidemiological studies, that consolidate these discrete reports.

Evidence on whether or not selected genetic factor actually represents a risk in the population rests on the findings of such reports. Few studies that have been initiated in this regard provide a lead and way forward.[2]

The Intensive Medicines Monitoring Programme (IMMP) initiated in New Zealand in 1977, aimed to monitor prescriptions of medicines for a period of 4–5 years. ADRs are detected either spontaneously or from answers provided by the prescribing physician in response to the questionnaires that are regular sent to him. As the database includes records of monitored medicines over a known time period, including those patients who have not experienced an adverse event, the incidence of events can be calculated. This allows identification of cases and controls, and easily link genetic variations with increasing susceptibility to the ADRs.

To cite a case in the point, a small pilot nested case-control study was designed to investigate the genetic risk for ADRs. Genetic polymorphisms of transporter proteins P-glycoprotein (P-gp) and cytochrome P450 (CYP) 2C9 can alter their expression at the level of blood-brain barrier. This can lead to significant variations in the substrate (COX-2 inhibitors) concentrations in the brain. An unusual high concentration of the substrate in the brain is held responsible for the visual and psychiatric disturbances experienced by some patients who had been prescribed these drugs. Out of the 37 case and 91 control patients who participated in the study, genotyping of ABCB1 and CYP2C9 was carried out on 15 case and 24 control patients. The results suggested that the selected SNPs may not contribute to the adverse effects associated with the COX-2 inhibitors (Table 14.3).

Traditionally, the approach that has been commonly applied is to conduct studies where,

Table 14.3: Genotype of case and control patients taking COX-2 inhibitors and the ADRs experienced

Event class	Adverse effect	Gene	Case genotype	Control genotype 1 (genotype2)
Celecoxib				
Psychiatric	Depression	ABCB1	C/T	C/T
		CYP2C9	*1*1	*1*1
	Depression	ABCB1	C/T	C/T
		CYP2C	*1*2	*1*1
	Depression	ABCB1	T/T	C/T
		CYP2C	*1*1	*1*1
	Hallucinations	ABCB1	C/C	T/T
		CYP2C9	*1*2	*1*3
	Suicidal ideation	ABCB1	T/T	C/C
Visual		CYP2C9	*1*1	*1*1
	Abnormal vision	ABCB1	T/T	T/T (C/T)
		CYP2C9	*1*2	*1*1 (*1*2)
	Visual field defect	ABCB1	C/T	T/T
		CYP2C9	*1*1	*1*1
Rofecoxib				
Psychiatric	Confusion	ABCB1	C/T	C/T
		CYP2C9	1/1	*1*2
	Depression	ABCB1	T/T	C/T (C/C)
		CYP2C9	*1*3	*1*3 (*1*1)
	Restlessness	ABCB1	C/T	C/T **(T/T)**
		CYP2C9	*1*1	*1*1 (*1*1)
	Low concentration	ABCB1	C/T	C/T
		CYP2C9	*1*1	*1*2
	Delirium	ABCB1	C/C	T/T
		CYP2C9	***1*3**	*1*3
	Anxiety	ABCB1	T/T	C/T
		CYP2C9	*1*1	*1*3
Visual	Blurred vision	ABCB1	C/T	C/T
		CYP2C9	*1*1	*1*1
	Teichopsia	ABCB1	C/C	C/C (C/T)
		CYP2C9	*1*1	*1*1 (*1*2)

Control genotypes 1 and 2 indicate matched controls. A further five controls were genotyped that had been matched to cases that did not consent to genotyping. The genotypes of these control patients were: C/C *1*1; C/T *1*1; C/T *1*2; TT/ *1*1; and T/T *1*3 in only four cases were two matched controls per case able to be obtained for genotyping. Allelic variants that may lead to altered plasma or CNS levels of substrates are show in bold. (*Adapted from:* Clark et al, 2004)

small, selected samples of population, such as those with or without particular variant genes are subjected to short term dosage regimen to determine the link with ADRs. In contrast, it is more helpful to use epidemiological methods to estimate the risk as it allows comparisons to be made between matched populations of patients with the selected ADR (cases) and those without any ADR (controls). A clear indication about a positive or negative link between drug and ADR can be established.

CONCLUSION

Despite mounting evidence that gene polymorphisms can affect the response of therapeutic agents, the clinical practice of prospectively screening the patients for polymorphisms, has not been adopted as a routine practice. Challenges range from financial liabilities, easy access to advanced techniques, quick and reliable results, rigid mindsets, and many more. The promise of pharmacogenetics: "the right drug, right dose for the right patient", can only be achieved in its full glory, once these challenges are met.

REFERENCES

1. Lazarou J, et al. Incidence of adverse drug reactions in hospitalized patients-a meta-analysis of prospective studies. JAm Med Assoc. 1998;279:1200-5.
2. Clark DWJ, Donnelly E, Coulter DM, Roberts RL, Kennedy MA. Linking pharmacovigilance with pharmacogenetics. Drug Saf. 2004;27(15): 1171-84.
3. Tucker G. Pharmacogenetics: expectations and reality. BMJ. 2004;329:4-6.
4. Hart RG, Sherman DG, Easton JD, Cairns JA. Prevention of stroke in patients with nonvalvular atrial fibrillation. Neurology. 1998; 51(3): 674-81.
5. Pirmohamed M, Park BK. Genetic susceptibility to adverse drug reactions. Trends Pharmacol Sci. 2001;22(6):298-305.
6. Meyer UA. Pharmacogenetics and adverse drug reactions. Lancet. 2000;356:1667-71.
7. Seelig A. A general pattern for substrate recognition by P-glycoprotein. Eur J Biochem. 1998;25(1-2):252-61.
8. Kerb R, Aynacioglu AS, Brockmoller J, Schlagenhaufer R, Bauer S, Szekeres T, et al. The predictive value of MDR1, CYP2C9, and CYP2C19 polymorphisms for phaenytoin plasma levels. Pharmacogenomics J. 2001;1(3):204-10.
9. Greiner B, Eichelabaum M, Fritz P, Kreichgauer hp, von Richter O. The role of intestinal P-glycoprotein in the interaction of digoxin and rifampin. J Clin Invest. 1999;104(2):147-53.
10. Guzey C, Spigset O. Genotyping of drug targets: a methods to predict adverse drug reactions? Drug Saf. 2002;25(8):553-60.

15

Pharmacovigilance Regulations in Various Countries

Sushma Srivastava, SK Gupta, Mohit Hans

Sulfanilamide scandal in the US during 1930s and thalidomide tragedy in 1960 made it understood that the drugs can cause adverse events too. Phocomelia, a congenital limb abnormality occurred due to intake of thalidomide during pregnancy for morning sickness, led to serious thinking about drug monitoring all over the world. The methodological researches were initiated. It was found till 1970s that the data collected were not sufficient to assess the frequency of the adverse events. The reporting of the adverse effects (AE) was low and its identification depended upon the knowledge and interpretation of the doctor treating the patient. Several countries started their pharmacovigilance programme and regulations were imposed.

PHARMACOVIGILANCE IN EUROPE

Drug regulation was imposed in Europe in the 1960s after the thalidomide tragedy. Spontaneous adverse drug reactions (ADRs) reporting schemes were developed so that the signals for unexpected hazards can be provided. The medicinal products placed in the market within the European Union (EU) must possess a marketing authorization, excluding some exceptions. This authorization signifies that the product complies with the quality, safety, and efficacy criteria set out in European medicinal product regulatory law. The authorization is granted by the competent authority.[1]

The EU is a political and economic community of 27 member states, located mainly in Europe. The 27 independent sovereign countries which are known as member states are Austria, Belgium, Bulgaria, Cyprus, the Czech Republic, Denmark, Estonia, Finland, France, Germany, Greece, Hungary, Ireland, Italy, Latvia, Lithuania, Luxembourg, Malta, the Netherlands, Poland, Portugal, Romania, Slovakia, Slovenia, Spain, Sweden, and the United Kingdom.[2] Croatia, the former Yugoslav Republic of Macedonia, and Turkey are three official candidate countries; the western Balkan countries of Albania, Bosnia and Herzegovina, Montenegro, and Serbia are officially recognized as potential candidates.[3] Kosovo has been granted similar status.[4]

In the EU, to obtain the market authorization of a drug, ample evidences for the quality, efficacy and safety has to be provided to the authorities even then the EU regulatory authorities give prime importance to pharmacovigilance. The need for continuous monitoring of drugs was felt as the hazard can occur at any time during the life of the product. The spontaneous reporting system was used for the monitoring of adverse drug events, though it has the limitation of under-reporting.

Moreover, a definite number of casualties and frequency of the event cannot be ascertained by this. Apart from the spontaneous reporting other sources of information are also used.

In 1995, European Medicines Evaluation Agency (EMEA) (now known as European Medicines Agency, EMA) and a new regulatory system that included procedures for a centralized authorization and multiple identical authorizations through mutual recognition were established. The EMEA headquarter is in London. The agency intended to protect and promote the health of the people and animals by developing efficient and transparent procedures through a single European marketing authorization, controlling the safety of medicines for humans and animals through the following:[5]

- Pharmacovigilance network
- Fixing safe limits for residues in food-producing animals
- Encouraging research
- Coordination of scientific resources to provide high-quality evaluation of medicinal products
- Providing guidance on research and development programs
- Inspections for ensuring good clinical practice (GCP), good manufacturing practice (GMP) and good laboratory practice (GLP)
- Providing information to users and healthcare professionals.

The Agency, after ten years, implemented all relevant provisions and guidelines of the revised EU pharmaceutical legislation (EC) No 726/2004, in November 2005.[6] In 2005, the Agency besides other initiatives focused on improving pharmacovigilance for safeguarding the quality, safety and efficacy of authorized medicinal products. Pharmacovigilance was introduced in EU Legislation in 1993 through Council Directive 93/39/EEC amending Council Directive 75/319/EEC. However, the first directive on medicines was issued in 1965 (Council directive 65/65/EEC). Medicines legislation of EU is included in a consolidated Directive 2001/83/EC (amended in 2004).[7]

The Council directives harmonize the national legislation of the member states of the EU. The member states have to implement these legal provisions into their national legislation. In most of the states, the pharmacovigilance system is already established. The variation between them occurs due to difference in the health care system.

The pharmacovigilance system in EU is formed with the national pharmacovigilance systems of the member states. It works under the coordination of the EMEA and in cooperation with European Commission. In addition to the member states Norway, Iceland, and Liechtenstein, which are not members but are part of the European Economic Area (EEA) have also been included (EEA Joint Committee, 1999).[1]

The roles and responsibilities for the surveillance of the medicinal products of all the parties are described in Directive 2001/83/EC (amended in 2004) and Council regulation (EEC) No. 2309/93 (replaced by regulation 726/2004) which are described in the guidance documents prepared in 1990s. These guidelines are in accordance with recommendations of International Conference on Harmonization of Technical Requirements for Registration of Pharmaceuticals for Human Use (ICH).[8] These have been revised and compiled.[9] Protection and promotion of human and animal health is the main aim of the EMEA and has the following responsibilities:

- It coordinates the supervision and pharmacovigilance activities of authorized medicinal products in EU
- Provision of access to information on ADRs reported by means of a data processing network that can be accessed by all Member States, EMEA and the Commission (EudraVigilance)
- Maintenance of and variations to the terms of the marketing authorization for centrally authorized products

- Management of referral procedures for nationally authorized products
- Provision of recommendations on measures necessary to ensure safe and effective use of these products.

EMEA published its long-term strategy in 2005[10] for the (i) enhanced safety and support of public and animal health (ii) improvement of Regulatory environment for therapeutic products and (iii) motivation of research and developments in the EU.

The road map had following objectives:
- Top-quality scientific assessment
- Timely access to safe and effective innovative medicines
- Continuous monitoring of medicinal products
- Access to information
- Specific needs for veterinary medicines.

To fulfill these objectives following actions were implemented during 2005:
- Strengthening the quality-assurance system of scientific assessments
- Supporting applicants in the development of new therapeutic approaches and technologies
- Strengthening the Agency's interaction with European industry associations representing the innovative, generic and self-medication industries
- Strengthening interaction with the Agency's stakeholders
- Developing a European Risk Management Strategy (ERMS) for safer medicines
- Addressing antimicrobial resistance: The Committee for Medicinal Products for Veterinary Use (CVMP) made good progress on developing a new strategy on risk management and risk assessment for antimicrobials.

Ensuring adequacy of environmental risk assessment: The CVMP and its Environmental Risk Assessment Working Party (ERAWP) developed guidance to help applicants prepare the environmental risk assessment part of marketing authorization applications. A full environmental risk assessment for all veterinary marketing authorization applications is a new legal requirement.[5]

Rules and regulations governing medicinal products in the European Union are compiled in *EudraLex* which consists of ten volumes. Volume 9 deals with pharmacovigilance. Rules governing medicinal products in the EU are given in the volume 9A "Pharmacovigilance for drugs for human use" which is updated and released in 2008.[11] It was amended to promote international harmonization.

A specific reference to pharmacovigilance in children has been reported. In order to conduct and manage studies involving children, it is underlined the need to consult the new adopted Guideline on Conduct of Pharmacovigilance for Medicines Used by the Pediatric Population,[12] in force from the day of adoption of the EU regulation on medicinal products for pediatric use (26 January 2007). The document also points out the need to report and discuss potential for off-label pediatric use, when the disease or disorder, which is being treated or prevented, is found in the pediatric population.

PROCESS OF REGULATORY PHARMACOVIGILANCE

Regulatory pharmacovigilance depends upon the information gathered or received regarding the clinical effects of marketed medicines in a population. Methods for the collection of ADRs and analyzing them are equally important. The adverse events are evaluated and appropriate actions are taken into consideration such as introducing warnings, contraindications, and information on adverse effects or changes to dose recommendations. Sometimes indications or methods of supply may be restricted. Very rarely a drug is withdrawn from the market for safety reasons. The efficacy of these measures depends upon the

Detection of ADRs

During any stage of the drug development, safety issues can crop up. During the post-authorization period safety issues may arise in initial few years or can arise even after several years in case of long established drugs. The safety issues, which did not arise during the premarketing phase, are tackled promptly. The information regarding that is gathered from multiple sources. The most common way to collect these is spontaneous reports, individual reports from the health practitioners, which they consider as adverse reactions. The term *suspected adverse reaction* might be used in order to avoid the confusion between the adverse event and adverse reaction. Input of data can be achieved from various other sources like screening of international spontaneous reporting database operated by the Uppsala Monitoring Centre (UMC) in Sweden. All member states provide data to UMC. The signal is identified as early as possible and the member states are informed so that the evaluation can be conducted.[1]

Evaluation

Causality, possible mechanisms, frequency and preventability are considered once enough evidence of a hazard is found. To assess these, epidemiological studies may be needed.

Principles relating to post-authorizing studies are given in the guidelines for pharmaceutical companies.[8] New data generated are reviewed and assessed. Risks and benefits of the concerned medicine are discussed and also the possible methods which may facilitate safe use. The opinion of experts in pharmacology and therapeutic areas is taken at the national and international level by involving them in discussions.

Decision-making and Risk Management

The EU competent authority takes regulatory action, justified by scientific evidence and allows the users to make informed decisions and to use medicines safely. In some cases the firm recommendations like contraindications of the drug is given when the benefits and risks are very evident while in other cases less directive advice is needed.

Risk management action varies as per the measures taken for preventing ADR. The adverse effects can be reduced by targeting the drug to the patients who are least likely to be at risk of ADR or by contraindicating in patients prone to risks. Risk of health hazards is mostly related to the dose and duration of the drug. It is a common practice of changing the dosage schedule, keeping in view the safety of the patient, during the post-marketing period.

In case of detecting a new ADR or accumulation of new evidence about a recognized reaction changes in the product information is required that results in variations to market authorizations. Variations in marketing authorization can be proposed either by the competent authorities or the pharmaceutical company. Prior to submission of variation, information is exchanged and discussion occurs between both the parties for speedy execution. The parties when reach to an agreement about the nature and impact of drug safety issue, changes can be implemented voluntarily by the market authorization holder. If the companies do not agree then the regulatory authority exercises its compulsory powers. In case of exceptional urgent public health concerns the authorities act rapidly without a right for appeal by the company, to withdraw the product from the market or to change the product information.

Communication

Handling a safety issue of a marketed product needs a proper communication of the drug-related information to the health professionals and patients. Efforts should be made to communicate the key facts and recommendations explicitly without hiding it with other less important information. The information communicated to the patient should be the same as it is provided to the health professional and the language used should be understandable to him.

The communication period is another important consideration. Information about a new life-threatening ADR should be communicated immediately whereas information about non-serious reaction can be added in the next routine revision of the product information. In the EU immediate measures (within 24 hours) are taken to restrict the use or provide essential additional information on urgent safety grounds.

The Variation Regulations (EC) 541/95 and (EC) 542/95[13,14] were revised by the European Commission. The revision was necessary to provide the same regulatory framework for variations in the Mutual Recognition Procedure (MRP) and the Centralized Procedure and to fulfill the requirements of Directive 2001/83/EC (of 6 November 2001). The new Variations Regulations (Commission Regulation) EC No 1084/2003 for the Mutual Recognition Procedure and EC No 1085/2003 for the centralized procedure are in force since 01 October 2003 for notifications and applications submitted on or after this date.

The drug legislation was under review and Enlargement of European Union was taking place with the involvement of Central and Eastern European Countries. The Pan European Regulatory Forum (PERF) was initiated to involve these countries in medicines regulation and Pharmacovigilance activities. Standards for the conduct of Pharmacovigilance for all the parties involved were developed by Pharmacovigilance Working Party (PhVWP) through an initiative known as good pharmacovigilance practice (GVP). Completion of electronic information network through EudraVigilance was done between all stakeholders. Electronic reporting into the EudraVigilance database became mandatory in November 2005.

The pharmacovigilance legislation was developed on the basis of the observation that adverse drug reactions (ADRs), to a medicine resulted in about 197,000 deaths per year in the EU. The New Directive 2010/84/EU and Regulation (EU) No 1235/2010 were adopted in December 2010, bringing about significant changes in the safety monitoring of medicines across the EU. The new directive and regulation amended Pharmacovigilance laws in the Directive 2001/83/EC and Regulation (EC) No. 726/2004. The New regulation was also accompanied by the Commission Implementing Regulation No 520/2012 of 19 June 2012. In October 2012 this was further amended to Regulation (EU) No 1027/2012 (applicable since 5 June 2013) and Directive 2012/26/EU (applicable since 28 October 2013) for more protection of patient health. Practical measures to facilitate the performance of pharmacovigilance in accordance with the legislation are available in the good pharmacovigilance practice (GVP) guidelines (Annexure 8), which eventually replaced Volume 9A.[11] More information can be obtained from http://www.ema.europa.eu/docs/en_GB/document_library/Regulatory_and_procedural_ guideline/2017/03/WC500224566.pdf.[15,16]

UNITED KINGDOM

Medicines and Healthcare Products Regulatory Agency (MHRA) of United Kingdom (UK) was formed on 1st April 2003 from the merger of the Medicines Control Agency (MCA) and the Medical Devices Agency (MDA) with the objective to safeguard public health by ensuring that the medicines, medical devices and the healthcare products in the UK market are of standard quality and show standard performance efficacy and safety. The safety profile of a medicine at the time of licensing is accompanied with limited data. Its full safety profile can be assessed once it is marketed. The Agency uses various methods of collecting information on medicines. Healthcare professionals and patients are encouraged to report suspected ADRs and there is a legal requirement for companies to report such reactions to their products to MHRA. A register of these suspected adverse reactions is maintained and provides early warnings of potential drug hazards. Defective Medicines Report Centre (DMRC) receives and assesses complaints and reports of actual or suspected defects in medicines. It issues alerts to healthcare professionals and other related parties to inform them when there are any apprehensions about the quality of any medicines. In 2005, 340 defects related to medicines were reported to MHRA and 15 of these products were recalled. The Vigilance and Risk Management of Medicines (VRMM) of the MHRA monitors the safety of all licensed medicines in the United Kingdom. Data regarding adverse reactions are received from various sources, but the main source is Yellow Card Scheme of spontaneous reporting.[17-19]

Good pharmacovigilance practice (GPvP) is the minimum standard for monitoring the safety of medicines on sale to the public in the EU.[20]

HRA inspects marketing authorization holders and their contractors, to ensure they:
- Have an adequate and effective quality system for monitoring the medicines they have licences for
- Maintain a pharmacovigilance system master file
- Document all actions they take
- Have enough competent, appropriately qualified and trained staff to work the system.

Yellow Card Scheme

A system for collecting the adverse drug reaction reports had been developed by several countries after the thalidomide tragedy. In the UK, the Committee on Safety of Drugs was established in 1963, which subsequently became the Committee on Safety of Medicines (CSM) in 1968. In 2005, this became the Commission on Human Medicines (CHM) to spread and publicize the information about the adverse effects of medicines. First time this adverse reaction-reporting scheme was started in 1964 in the UK. Sir Derrick Dunlop, the Chairman of the Committee on Safety of Drugs, wrote to each and every member of the medical community to provide the information regarding any untoward effect of the medicine seen in their patients and provided yellow reporting forms along with his letter. The color of the form had no significance yet the scheme was popularized as Yellow Card Scheme. Till now the scheme is continued with progressive changes. CHM is responsible for the Yellow Card Scheme, which is run on the behalf of CHM by the MHRA. Four regional monitoring centres (RMCs) have been established in 1980s and a fifth centre was launched in 2002. These RMCs were called as Yellow Card Centres. Like all other reporting schemes, this scheme also had some limitations like under-reporting. Initiatives were taken to improve the Scheme by (a) increasing the general reporting base, (b) increasing reporting in specific areas and (c) facilitation of reporting.

The Yellow Card reporting base was widened. Studies were conducted by RMCs on the potential contribution of hospital and community pharmacists to the Yellow Card scheme. It was realized that in comparison to the doctors, hospital pharmacists submitted reports of ADR in greater proportions. This resulted in the extension of the scheme all over the country to include reporting by hospital pharmacists in April 1977. Similar surveys were also carried out by other RMCs. Their findings led to the introduction of nationwide reporting of the community pharmacists in 1999. Gradually, the pharmacists had prescribing powers through patient group directions (PGDs)[21] and by 2004 maximum reports of ADR came through hospital and community pharmacists, making them important contributors to the Yellow Card Scheme (Annexure 2A and B).

During the past few years the role of nurses in patient health care increased. Independent nurse prescribing from the Nurse Prescribers' Formulary for district nurses and health visitors and the Nurse Prescribers' Extended Formulary (NPEF) was introduced. Nurses also were empowered to provide medicines under PGDs and supplementary prescribing was started in 2003. MHRA evaluated the reporting by nurses and found the quality of their reports similar to those of other health professionals. Hence, the scheme was extended to the nurses, midwives, and health visitors in 2002.

Initiatives were taken to improve the reporting of ADRs in the therapeutic areas of special interest such as drugs used in the treatment of HIV/AIDS, ADRs in children, and reactions associated with herbal products including unlicensed remedies.

New drugs for HIV patients became available in the market during 1990s. These drugs had limited safety data at the time of licensing and relatively few ADRs were being reported. Hence HIV Reporting Scheme, which is an extension of the Yellow Card scheme, was started in 1997 by MHRA and CSM in collaboration with Medical Research Council HIV Clinical Trials Centre.

Reporting of ADRs in children for particular diseases under surveillance started in 1986 through the British Paediatric Surveillance Unit's monthly '**orange card**' sent routinely to all consultant pediatricians registered with the Royal College of Paediatrics and Child Health. The EU Regulation on Pediatric Medicines was adopted on 12 December 2006 and came into force on 26 January 2007.

Reports of suspected ADRs to licensed herbal products were collected through **Yellow Card Scheme** till 1996. In 2004, a Directive on traditional herbal medicinal products (Directive 2004/24/EC amending Directive 2001/83/EC) came into force. It required that all the medicinal products being marketed in UK should be registered under the Traditional Herbal Medicines Registration Scheme (THMRS). In order to advice the government on THMRS and on unlicensed herbal remedies supplied under section 12 of the Medicines Act 1968, a new advisory committee on herbal medicines, the Herbal Medicines Advisory Committee (HMAC) was established.

Paper Yellow Card Scheme of Reporting slowly became an inconvenient method of reporting. MHRA launched electronic Yellow Card on MHRA website. Electronic reporting was mandatory for companies under Directive 2004/27/EC from Nov 2005.[22]

Yellow Card Scheme is continuing for over 42 years despite its limitations. It has undergone continual evaluation and development and will continue to carry out its role in UK pharmacovigilance. Reports can be made for:[23]

- Suspected ADRs to all medicines including:
    - Vaccines
    - Blood factors and immunoglobulins
    - Herbal medicines
    - Homeopathic remedies
    - All medical devices available on the UK market
- Defective medicines (those that are not of an acceptable quality)
- Fake or counterfeit medicines or medical devices
- Nicotine-containing electronic cigarettes and refill containers (e-liquids).

Hemovigilance

Hemovigilance as described in The Blood Safety and Quality Regulations 2005 "..... comprises a set of organized surveillance procedures relating to serious adverse or unexpected events or reactions in blood donors or recipients and the epidemiological follow-up of donors. A **serious adverse event** is defined as an unintended occurrence associated with the collection, testing processing, storage and distribution of blood or blood components that might lead to death or life-threatening, disabling or incapacitating conditions for patients or which results in, or prolongs, hospitalization or morbidity. A **serious adverse reaction** is defined as an unintended response in a donor or in a patient associated with the collection or transfusion of blood components that is fatal, life-threatening, disabling or incapacitating, or which results in or prolongs hospitalization or morbidity."[24]

Statutory Instrument 2005 No. 50 relating to blood safety and quality became effective from 8 November 2005. The Regulations set the standards of quality and safety for the collection, testing, processing, storage and distribution of human blood and blood components.

The UK Blood Safety and Quality Regulations 2005 and the EU Blood Safety Directive require that serious adverse events and serious adverse reactions related to blood and blood components are reported to the MHRA, the UK Competent Authority for blood safety.

SABRE

The MHRA's online system for reporting blood safety incidents is **SABRE (Serious Adverse Blood Reactions & Events)**. Blood Establishments, Blood Banks/Hospital Transfusion Teams can register and log in to use the MHRA's secure and confidential online reporting system that allows reporters to electronically submit reports of serious adverse event or serious adverse reaction directly to the MHRA. SABRE has been specifically designed to provide registered reporters by a simple electronic means of submitting haemovigilance reports to the MHRA and to Serious Hazards of Transfusion (SHOT), a professional inquiry service funded by the blood services of England and Wales.

From 8 November 2005, hospital blood banks have been required to confirm compliance with the requirements of the Regulations by submitting an annual Compliance Report to the MHRA.

MHRA works closely with the EMA, and is a trusted source of expertise throughout Europe. It also collaborates with US-FDA and UK Government agencies concerned with healthcare, including the National Patient Safety Agency (NPSA) and the National Institute for Health and Clinical Excellence (NICE).

Recent Regulations

Pharmacovigilance is mainly governed by EU legislation which was updated in 2010 and transcribed into UK law and began being implemented from July 2012.[25] MHRA, the regulator responsible for monitoring pharmacovigilance, is contributing significantly in both the centralized and decentralized regulatory procedures, and maintains its programmes for implementing EU legislation.

The role of MHRA in regulating medical devices and in vitro diagnostic (IVD) devices remains same. It oversees the essential work of the five UK Notified Bodies,[26] which in unison are responsible for evaluating the majority of devices currently found in the EU market. Implementation of proposed new Regulations for Medical Devices and IVDs By MHRA is in process. MHRA maintains its role in vigilance, market surveillance and taking direct action to protect patients and public health, and it continues to coordinate with other Competent Authorities, across Europe and internationally, in these and other areas.[27]

More information regarding post Brexit regulations is available on https://www.

gov.uk/government/news/medicines-and-healthcare-products-regulatory-agency-statement-on-the-outcome-of-the-eu-referendum. Following are the sources for more information on legislations and guidance:
- UK Human Medicines Regulations, Statutory Instrument 2012 No. 1916, Part 11
- Directive 2001/83/EC as amended
- Regulation (EU) No. 726/2004 as amended
- Commission Implementing Regulation (EU) No. 520/2012.
- Good pharmacovigilance practice modules
- Volume 9A of The Rules Governing Medicinal Products in the European Union, September 2008.

FRANCE

The French Pharmacovigilance System was established in 1973. It is a combination of mandatory reporting and intensive hospital surveillance. A national centre was established in 1973 by the French Medical Association and the French Pharmaceutical Manufacturers Association. Six pharmacovigilance centres were also established in the same year and their number grew with the addition of more centres. In mid seventies these centres were recognized officially and a unit was established at Ministry of Health to coordinate the activities. A network of 15 centres existed in 1979, this was expanded and had 29 centres in 1984. In 1984 ADR reporting was made mandatory for prescribers and Marketing Authorization Holders (MAHs). In 1985 online inputs were made possible, data was easily accessed from all the centres. Since 1994 the Pharmacovigilance Unit started working under French Medicines Agency now known as French Agency for the Safety of Health Products (AFSSAPS). Good pharmacovigilance practices were developed and communicated to each and every prescriber in the country. European legislation was imposed for which following two decrees were enforced for extending the mandatory reporting of ADRs to Pharmacists and defining the current general organization of the French pharmacovigilance system.[28]
- The decree of March 1995 on general principles and
- The decree of May 1995 especially related to blood products.

The French system now has a network of [31] regional pharmacovigilance centres (CRPV) under supervision of Pharmacovigilance Unit of AFSSAPS. AFSSAPS stands for Agence Française de Sécurité Sanitaire des Produits de Santé, the French agency responsible for ensuring the effectiveness, quality and proper use of all healthcare products intended for human use. About 10,000 ADR cases are received, assessed and recorded by the regional centres per year, the industry also reports about the similar number of cases to the Drug Agency. A technical committee and a National Commission of Pharmacovigilance centralizes at the AFSSAPS and assesses all data in order to provide consensual advise to the relevant authorities on necessary measures, to prevent or reduce a drug-related adverse effect. Regional Centres work as Drug Information Centres and receive more than 23,000 inquiries per year.[29-30] These centres are decentralized yet coordinated through a national network.[31] An algorithm index is used to assess the relationship between drugs and adverse effects. The adverse reactions alert system is produced by the compilation and analysis of the cases entered in a data bank and by the analysis of queries from general practitioners. The duties of the centres are also to provide information, analyze data and to improve the safe use of drugs.

Many laws and decrees driven by European legislation are implemented in the pharma sector. They are summarized into two laws (called "Codes"):[32]
- The Public Health Code (Code de la Santé Publique, CSP) and

- The Social Security Code (Code de la Sécurité Sociale, CSS).

The French Agency for the Medical Safety of Health Products (AFSSAPS) was created by law on 1 July 1998. It has been effective since 9 March 1999 under the authority of the Ministry of Health. The AFSSAPS scrutinizes the information sent to it by the company/organization distributing the medicinal product and the Regional Pharmacovigilance Centres and ensures correct use of the medicinal product by taking all required actions. The AFSSAPS informs the company or organization distributing the medicinal product of any serious adverse reaction declared or notified to it.[33]

Normally market authorization is obtained under the European Commission (Commission Européenne, EC) Directive 2004/27 in 210 days. A simplified procedure exists for generics by proving the bioequivalence of the pharmaceutical with the original product. Before market authorization is granted, it is possible to put pharmaceuticals on the market with a fast track procedure called a temporary utilization authorization (*Autorisation temporaire d'utilisation*, ATU).[32] Provisions defined in the decree relative to the pharmacovigilance of medicinal products No. 95-278 of 13th March 1995 apply for medicinal products subject to a temporary authorization for use (Art. R.5144.3). A certain number of definitions and recommendations will be amended in this decree to take into account the new directive 2000/38/EC of 5th June 2000.[34]

The pharmacovigilance of plasma-derived medicinal products is subject to the general regulations concerning medicinal products but also to specific rules stipulated by decree No. 95-566 of 6th May 1995.

Order of 28 April 2005 on good pharmacovigilance practices[35] is in pursuance of Articles R. 5121-150 to R. 5121-180 of the Public Health Code, as last amended by Decree No. 2004-99 of 29 January 2004 on pharmacovigilance (Official Journal of 31 January 2004) and Decree No. 2004-802 of 29 July 2004 concerning Parts IV and V (Regulatory provisions) of the Public Health Code and amending certain provisions of that Code (Official Journal of 8 August 2004).

Good pharmacovigilance practices recommend the responsibilities of health professionals, health authorities, and pharmaceutical companies. They are to be taken into account when introducing a quality assurance system in association with the guidelines published by the Commission of the European Communities in Volume 9 'Pharmacovigilance of medicinal products for human and veterinary use' of the "Rules governing medicinal products in the European Community.[36]

France has a new regulator agency known as the National Security Agency for Medicines and Health Products (*Agence nationale de sécurité du médicament et des produits de santé*, ANSM). ANSM replaced the previous agency AFSSAPS which was involved in a controversy related to the diabetes drug mediator and poly Implant Prothése (PIP) breast implant.[37-38] On December 29, 2011, Law No. 2011-2012 was adopted by the French Parliament, on reinforcing drug safety with the goal to restore public trust in the drug regulatory system. As per the new Law, the rules governing disclosure of conflicts of interest with pharmaceutical companies by directors and experts, involved in the drug approval process at the competent regulatory agencies, became more stringent.

ANSM, responsible for assessing the benefits and risks associated with the use of health products, has been given the power to impose administrative sanctions and plays a central role in the new pharmacovigilance system. The law transposed into French law Directive 2010/84/EU in 2010 and amended Directive 2001/83/EC with regard to Pharmacovigilance. Among several measures, the mandatory reporting of adverse drug reactions by health professionals or enterprises exploiting a drug was introduced, failing which a maximum penalty of three years of imprisonment and a fine of €45,000 would be imposed. New pharmacovigilance legislation in France became effective from July 2012 and had significant implications for applicants and holders of EU marketing authorizations.

BRAZIL

Brazil is one of the main countries in Latin America. It has become a favorite destination for the clinical trials and drug development programmes as it has lots of qualified investigators, treatment-naïve patients and an established regulatory system. The Brazilian regulatory process sticks strictly to International Conference on Harmonization (ICH), good clinical practice (GCP) and regional regulations. National Health Surveillance Agency, Agência Nacional de Vigilância Sanitária (ANVISA) is the regulatory agency that is equivalent to the FDA in US. It was established by Law 9.782, on January 26, 1999. It is an independently administered, financially-autonomous regulatory agency, with security of tenure for its directors during the period of their mandates. The Agency is managed by a Collegiate Board of Directors, comprised of five members.[39]

The Agency is associated with the Ministry of Health, under a Management Contract. The agency promotes the protection of the health of the population by implementing sanitary control over production and marketing of products and services subject to sanitary surveillance in addition to coordination of the National Sanitary Surveillance System (SNVS), the National Programme of Blood and Blood Products, and the National Programme of Prevention and Control of Hospital Infections; monitoring of drug prices and prices of medical devices; attributions pertaining to regulation, control and inspection of smoking products; technical support in granting of patents by the National Institute of Industrial Property. ANVISA controls ports, airports and borders and coordinates with the Brazilian Ministry of Foreign Affairs and Foreign institutions over issues related to international aspects of sanitary surveillance.[40]

In the year 2001, Decree no. 696, of the Ministry of Health, created the Brazilian National Drug Monitoring Centre, placed in the Pharmacovigilance Unit, which allowed the insertion of Brazil as the 62nd country in the International Drug Monitoring Programme of the World Health Organization (WHO), coordinated by the Uppsala Monitoring Centre, in Sweden, a WHO collaborative centre.

In October 2005, pharmacovigilance unit was inserted into the Centre for Surveillance of Adverse Events and Quality Deviations, which attributions include proposing, planning, coordinating and establishing the national subsystem of health surveillance for postmarketing products used in humans for diagnosis or therapy, including medicines.

The National System of Pharmacovigilance in Brazil has faced since its creation a strong difficulty among health professionals, including pharmacists: the lack of tradition in reporting adverse events.

Pharmacovigilance practices were required for marketing authorization holders from 2009. Though, the regulatory advancements in pharmacovigilance in Brazil are comparable to international practices, but there is a need of regulations for biosimilars and veterinary medicines. The healthcare professionals need to be encouraged for reporting technical complaints and quality deviations, for the improvement and control of postmarketing drug quality. The strategies need to be developed for the decentralization of pharmacovigilance actions in the whole country.[41]

INDIA

In India the import, manufacture, sale and distribution of drugs is regulated under Drugs and Cosmetics Act 1940 and Drugs and Cosmetic Rules 1945 which have been amended from time to time. Central Government through Central Drugs Standard Control Organization (CDSCO), headed by Drug Controller General of India (DCGI), regulates pharmacovigilance system, new drugs/clinical trials approval, licensing of special products, legislation and imports, etc. The drug regulatory authorities of India initiated the setting up of the pharmacovigilance centres in the country in 1986. In 1997, India joined the Adverse Drug Reaction Monitoring Programme of WHO. The National pharmacovigilance centre was started at Department of Pharmacology, AIIMS, New Delhi. Besides two, WHO special centres were also initiated in KEM Hospital, Mumbai and JLN Hospital, Aligarh Muslim University, Aligarh. The prime role of these centres was to monitor and collect information of ADRs to marketed drugs in India and report them to the DCGI who is the drug regulatory authority of India. The safety monitoring of drugs was slowed down due to various factors such as large rural population, poor spontaneous reporting, lack of awareness among the physicians and patients, use of traditional medicines, fast development of new molecules and inadequate postmarketing surveillance. In 2005, the WHO-sponsored and World Bank-funded National Pharmacovigilance Programme for India was established.[42]

The National Pharmacovigilance Programme (NPP) was established in January 2005 under National Pharmacovigilance Advisory Committee based in the CDSCO, New Delhi under the guidance of DGHS, Ministry of Health and Family Welfare, Government of India. Two zonal centres were started: (i) the South-West zonal centre, located in the Department of Clinical Pharmacology, Seth GS Medical College and KEM Hospital, Mumbai and (ii) the North-East zonal centre located in the Department of Pharmacology, AIIMS, New Delhi. These centres gather information from all over the country and send it to the NPAC and to the UMC in Sweden. Five regional centres and 24 peripheral centres were also established in different parts of the country with an objective to promote a reporting culture and to involve a large number of healthcare professionals in the systems in information dissemination and to make efforts in making the programme to be a benchmark for global drug monitoring. Measures were undertaken by the regulatory authorities to promote safety monitoring. Department of Indian System of Medicine was created by the Government of India which had a role in standardization, improving the availability and quality of raw materials, research, creating awareness among the physicians and patients and involving them in the national health care. GMP guidelines were released for non-allopathic systems of medicine. The Regulatory Authority for India has introduced and implemented the Schedule Y, which describes the requirement and guidelines on clinical trials for import and manufacture of new drug. Any company having a marketing license should have proper pharmacovigilance system as specified in Schedule Y. All adverse reaction reports and the information about the benefit-risk analysis of a product should be communicated to DCGI.[43]

The guidance for the legislative requirements of pharmacovigilance in India is given in Schedule Y of the Drugs and Cosmetics Act 1945. The Schedule Y deals with regulations relating to pre-clinical and clinical studies for development of a new drug as well as clinical trial requirements for import, manufacture, and obtaining marketing approval for a new drug in India. Schedule Y was thoroughly reviewed and was amended in January 2005. It indicates the liability of DCGI to ensure adequate compliance of pharmacovigilance obligations of the pharmaceutical companies. In the amended Schedule Y, an attempt has been made to better define the responsibilities of pharmaceutical companies for their marketed products as well as relating to the reporting of adverse events from clinical trials. The section entitled postmarketing surveillance includes the requirement for submission of periodic safety update reports (PSURs), PSUR cycle, template for PSUR, and the timelines and conditions for expedited reporting.[43]

Bill No. LVII of 2007, The Drugs and Cosmetics (Amendment) bill, 200744 was produced in Rajya Sabha to amend the Drugs and Cosmetics Act, 1940. The Drugs and Cosmetics Act, 1940 (the Act) is a consumer protection legislation, mainly concerned with the standards and quality of drugs and regulates the import, manufacture, sale and distribution of drugs and cosmetics. An expert committee was constituted in January 2003 under the Chairmanship of Dr RA Mashelker, DG CSIR to undertake a comprehensive examination of drug regulatory issues, together with the problem of spurious drugs and to suggest measures to improve the drug administration in the country.

The Committee recommended setting up of a Central Drugs Authority reporting directly to the Ministry of Health and Family Welfare and a system of centralized licensing. The Central Government considered the recommendations of the Committee and proposes to make amendments in the Act, in order to facilitate setting up of a Central Drugs Authority and introduction of Centralized licensing for manufacture of drugs in pursuance of the said recommendations. The Drugs and Cosmetics (Amendment) Bill, 2007, *inter alia*, provides for:

- Substitution of the "Drugs Technical Advisory Board" as well as the "Drugs Technical Advisory Board for Ayurvedic, Siddha and Unani Drugs" by the "Central Drugs Authority"
- Insertion of a new Chapter IA with a view to providing the constitution of the Central Drugs Authority and other connected or incidental matters
- Insertion of a new Chapter IB in the Act, providing for grant of permission for clinical trials, punishment for conducting clinical trial without permission, trial of offences, etc.
- Expansion of the compositions of the Drugs Consultative Committees.

Certain consequential changes in the Act were also proposed to make it in Consonance with proposal for setting up of the Central Drugs Authority.[44]

Pharmacovigilance Program of India

Pharmacovigilance Programme of India (PvPI) became functional from 14th July 2010, with AIIMS, New Delhi as the National Coordination Centre (NCC). The monitoring of the ADRs all over India was done with the help of 22 ADR Monitoring Centres (AMCs) including AIIMS, New Delhi. Afterwards the NCC was shifted to Indian Pharmacopoeia Commission (IPC) on 15th April 2011, Ghaziabad. The main aim was to generate an independent data on the safety of drugs to match the global drug safety monitoring standards. The PvPI works with the mission to safeguard the health of the Indian population by ensuring that the benefit of use of medicine outweighs the risks associated with its use.[45] The PvPI has succeeded in establishing 250 adverse drug monitoring centres all over India. The ADRs are reported through ADR forms which are in english for healthcare professionals and in 10 vernacular languages for consumers (Annexures 1A and B). The information received in the form of Individual Case Safety Reports (ICSRs) through them and HCPs, pharmacists and other non-HCPs (Medical Colleges & Hospitals, Medical/Central/Autonomous Institutes or Corporate Hospitals not enrolled under PvPI) is collated and analyzed by the PvPI and the inferences are used to recommend informed regulatory interventions. Concurrently, it informs the healthcare professionals and the consumers about the risks associated with the medicines. The PvPI is also targeting towards the detection of substandard medicines; prescribing, dispensing and administration errors to achieve better patient safety. Simultaneously, the PvPI is trying to address other challenges like counterfeit drugs, antimicrobial resistance, and surveillance during mass vaccinations and other national programs. The following are the objectives of the program:[46]

- To create a nationwide system for patient safety reporting
- To identify and analyze new signals from the reported cases
- To analyze the benefit-risk ratio of marketed medications
- To generate evidence-based information on safety of medicines
- To support regulatory agencies in the decision-making process on the use of medications
- To communicate the safety information on the use of medicines to various stakeholders to minimize the risk
- To emerge as a national centre of excellence for pharmacovigilance activities
- To collaborate with other national centres for the exchange of information and data management
- To provide training and consultancy support to other national pharmacovigilance centres across globe
- To promote rational use of medicine.

CHINA

The Ministry of Health of the People's Republic of China was established on November 21, 1949. It is a member of the State Council with a mandate in health. The drug administration law was enforced in 1984 and was amended in 2001. The State Food and Drug Administration (SFDA) was founded in 2003 on the basis of the State Drug Administration (SDA) as per the restructuring plan of the State Council that was approved by the First Plenary Session of the 10th National People's Congress and "the State Council Notice on Government Structuring" (No.8.2003.). The SFDA is directly under the State Council, which is responsible for comprehensive supervision on the safety management of food, health food and cosmetics and is the national regulatory authority of drug and medical device.[47,48]

Several technical institutes are affiliated with SFDA such as National Institute for the Control of Pharmaceuticals and Biological Products, State Pharmacopoeia Commission, Drug Evaluation Centre, Drug Reevaluation Centre, Drug Certification Centre and National Committee on the Assessment of Protected TCM Products. Centre for Drug Reevaluation is functioning as the National Centre for ADR Monitoring since 1989.

A National Centre for Adverse Drug Reaction (ADR) Monitoring was established in 1989 in China, which was affiliated to Ministry of Health. The centre joined SFDA in 1999. Out of the 31 provinces the branch centres were established in only 12 states, however the numbers increased to 31 in 2005. In 1998, China became a member of the WHO's Programme for International Drug Monitoring. During March 2004, the final Regulations on Adverse Drug Reaction Reporting and Monitoring were announced.[49]

Drug administration Law of the People's Republic of China was revised and came into effect since December 1, 2001. Regulation for implementation of Law of the People's Republic of China came into force from September 15, 2002. Regulation for the distribution and vaccination of vaccines came into effect since June 1st, 2005.[48]

As per the procedure the pharmaceutical industries and healthcare professionals should report ADR events quarterly, but new, uncommon, serious or 'group' ADRs are required to be reported within a shorter time period. Reports are sent to local centres, which then analyze and transmit them to the national ADR Centre operated by China's State Food and Drug Administration (SFDA). The national authority then further studies, publishes formal warning announcements or prohibits use of a product.[49]

Article 71 of Drug Administration Law of the People's of China states, 'The national government shall implement a monitoring system of ADRs. Drug manufacturing enterprises, operation enterprises and medical institutions shall frequently inspect the quality, efficacy and medical effects of the drugs. Any serious adverse reactions shall be duly reported to the local drug administration department and the health administration department of the people's government of the province, autonomous region or municipal city. Relevant regulations shall be promulgated by SDA together with MOH'.

'For a drug that is confirmed to have serious drug reactions, SDA or the drug administration departments of the provinces, autonomous regions and municipal cities may adopt emergency measures to stop the manufacture, sale and use of the drug, and organize relevant experts to evaluate within five days. The administrative decision shall be according to relevant laws, and made within fifteen days from the delivery of evaluators' determination.[50]

Measures for the administration on report and monitoring of the side effects of pharmaceuticals (2004) were adopted by the Ministry of Health of the People's Republic of China and the State Food and Drug Administration.[50] http//www.lehmanlaw.com/resource-centre/laws-and-regulations/pharma/regulation-for-monitoring-adverse-srug-reactions 1999.html). As per the Article 7 of Chapter 2 the Food and Drug Administrations of the provinces, autonomous regions, and municipalities directly under the Central Government shall be responsible for the administration in monitoring the side effect of pharmaceuticals within their own administrative districts and perform their duties mentioned in the article. Details regarding reporting of side effects are mentioned in Chapter 3. The report of new or serious side effect of pharmaceuticals should be made to the monitoring centre within 15 days from the date they are found by the personnel responsible for reporting the side effect of the pharmaceuticals. Individuals can also directly report any new or serious side effect caused by the pharmaceutical to the local monitoring centre or food and drug administrations of the provinces, autonomous regions and municipalities under the central government. The monitoring centres analyze the reports and sent them and the appraisal opinions to the SFDA (Annexure 9). SFDA on the basis of these, takes measures like suspending the production, sales and use, etc. It circulates notices on the report and monitoring of pharmaceuticals side effect of the state time to time. Punishment is imposed if the circumstance is serious enough and cause serious consequences.[51] In 2013, the State Food and Drug Administration (SFDA), has been renamed as China Food and Drug Administration (CFDA). The adverse events following immunization (AFEI) are reported to Chinese Centres for Disease Control and Prevention (CDC), and medical device reports are reported to CFDA by standardized report forms.

China has an online spontaneous reporting system known as China Adverse Drug Reaction Monitoring System (CADRMS), which connects the four-level pharmacovigilance network (national, provincial, municipal and county) By 2013, CADRMS had received over 6.6 million ADR case reports. After integrating and analyzing pharmacovigilance data, the National Centre for ADR Monitoring (NCADRM) publishes medication safety information by releasing ADR bulletins, National ADR Annual Reports and International Pharmacovigilance Newsletters. The NCADRM also routinely provides CADRMS data feedback to manufacturers.

The CFDA implemented risk management through several approaches, including arranging 'manufacturer communication meetings', modification of medication package inserts, and restriction, suspension or withdrawal of marketing authorizations. Seamless information exchange with overseas regulatory authorities and organizations remains an area for improvement. Further development of the China pharmacovigilance system in terms of signal generation, post-marketing pharmacoepidemiology research and education is also needed.[52-55]

Regulations for Traditional Chinese Medicine

Traditional Chinese medicine (TCM) products are in existence for more than 4000 years. The use of TCM products has increased globally, hence these are also regulated as drugs in China. Chinese ADR monitoring is useful in its reporting of ADRs related with TCM.[47] The constitution of People's Republic of China insisted for the development of modern and traditional medicines simultaneously. The TCM developed continuously and they are considered as medicinal medicines in China. The marketing requires a quality dossier, safety and efficacy evaluation and special labeling. New drugs are examined and approved by the Drug Administration Law, which was enacted in 1984. The articles 3, 5, 6, 11, 15, 21, 22, 29, 31 of Drug Administration Law of the People's of China govern the issues related to the TCM.[48]

JAPAN

A trilateral partnership between the regulatory authorities of Japan, the USA, and the European Union (EU) led to the establishment of the International Conference on Harmonization of Technical Requirements for Registration of Pharmaceuticals for Human Use (ICH) in 1990. Since its inception ICH has been standardizing regulations on drugs in cooperation with the main trade organizations of the pharmaceutical industry. The pharmaceutical industry of Japan that has gradually expanded over the years is facing challenges related to compliance with internationally standardized regulations.

Ministry of Health, Labor and Welfare (MHLW) is in charge of pharmaceutical regulatory affairs in Japan and works together with Pharmaceuticals and Medical Devices Agency (PMDA) which was established in April 1, 2004. MHLW was established in 2001 by the union of Ministry of Health & Welfare (MHW) and Ministry of Labor. MHW has reorganized and combined the departments for Drug Safety Measures and General Medical Practices in order to establish a new Pharmaceutical and Medical Safety Bureau (PMSB). PMSB, formerly the Pharmaceutical Affairs Bureau (PAB), is responsible for the main duties and functions of the ministry which include: (1) the efficacy/safety of prescription and over-the-counter drugs, cosmetics and medical devices; (2) adequate blood supply; (3) regulation of poisonous and deleterious substances; and (4) promotion measures against narcotics.

Various laws and regulations have been imposed for the pharmaceutical administration in Japan. One of these is Pharmaceutical Affairs Law (PAL), which assures the quality, efficacy, and safety of drugs, cosmetics, and medical devises through regulations. Besides it promotes R&D of drugs and medical devices essential for health care.

Initially in 1889 the Regulations on Handling and Sales of Medicines were enacted. Later on in 1943 the Pharmaceutical Law was passed which underwent several revisions in 1948 and 1960 (Law no. 145). In 2002, the Pharmaceutical Law was revised (Law no. 96, July 31, 2002) based on demands for augmentation of safety assurance in keeping with the age of biotechnology and genomics, augmentation of post marketing surveillance policies, revision of the approval and licensing system.[56] After the revision of PAL in 2002, reporting of ADR has become a legal duty of doctors, dentists, pharmacists and other health professionals. In 1997 the duty of the drug companies to send the ADR reports to the regulatory body was clearly specified in PAL (Article 77-4-2) and ICH-E2A guideline. Electronic submission of safety reports with E2B/M2 format was made mandatory in 2003. The amendment of PAL in 2002 is characterized by (i) the enhancement of post marketing safety measures (ii) introduction of new regulations for safety of biological products and (iii) introduction of a marketing authorization holder (MAH) license and (iv) establishment of Pharmaceutical and Medical Device Agency (PMDA).

A system of re-examination and re-evaluation of marketed drugs has been adopted in Japan in 1971. All new drugs are re-examined after a stipulated time, and if no major problem is indicated then are only marketed. In April 1997 basic plan of the postmarketing studies was required to be submitted during the approval of the new products and the results of the study were required to be included in the periodic safety update report (PSUR) (notification no. 32 of the PMSB). In 2001 regulation on Early-Phase Postmarketing vigilance was introduced which is unique to Japan. These regulations are given in good postmarketing surveillance practice (GPMSP) along with the regulations on ADR reports and risk communication. In 2004 GPMSP was divided into two ministerial ordinances of 'good parmacovigilance practice (GVP) and Good Postmarketing Study Practice (GPSP) for the regulations of the ADR reports and risk communication and of the investigational studies respectively.

According to GVP before April 2005 a drug company has to submit the domestic report of moderate unexpected reaction within 30 calendar days form the first receipt of the report and also the domestic reports of the expected serious reactions should also be submitted within the same time period. But after 2005 a domestic report of expected serious reaction should be reported within 15 calendar days. All expected serious reactions are required to be reported within 15 calendar days during the EPPV and during the first 2 years after the approval of a new chemical entity.

The drug companies in Japan had the legal duty to carry out the Drug Use Investigations (DUIs), i.e. patients treated with newly launched products should be registered by the prescribers to monitor and report any suspected ADR. The spontaneous reporting system (SRS) was improved during the last decade changing the role of DUIs. In 2004, the GPMSP was amended and only for special cases DUI was carried out. In 2004 an agreement was reached between Japan, USA and EU for the guideline of pharmacovigilance planning (PVP), also known as E2E guideline, in the ICH. The ICH harmonized guideline has been included into Japanese regulation rule in 2005 as per the notice of MHLW. In Japan, the Pharmaceutical and Medical Device Agency (PMDA), established by the Ministry of Health, Labour and Welfare in 2004, offered free access to part of its database, i.e. the Japanese Adverse Drug Event Report (JADER), in April 2012.[57,58]

AUSTRALIA

Therapeutic Goods Administration (TGA) is the regulatory agency of australia for registration and marketing of all therapeutic products. Australian guideline for pharmacovigilance responsibilities of sponsors of registered medicines regulated by drug safety and evaluation branch' was prepared in July 2003 which was amended on 31 May 2005. This guideline is specifically for the reporting of adverse reactions to registered medicines regulated by the Drug Safety and Evaluation Branch (DSEB) of the TGA. It established a pharmacovigilance system for the collection and evaluation of information relevant to the benefit to risk balance of registered medicinal products. The TGA monitors the safety profile of the products available in Australia and takes appropriate action where necessary.

Any ADR expected or unexpected should be reported to adverse drug reaction unit. This has a preferred format for reporting the ADRs. The format is printed on a small 'Blue Card' which can be downloaded from the TGA website or can be obtained upon request from the adverse drug reaction unit (Annexure 10).

ADRs can be reported by telephone by using the consumer Adverse Medicine Events Line: Ph 1300 134 237.[59] This service is provided by the Mater Hospital, Brisbane for the general public who suspect that they have experienced an adverse drug event. This service forwards reports of suspected adverse reactions to the Adverse Drug Reactions Advisory Committee (ADRAC). ADRs can be reported online using TGA online services, i.e. Australian Adverse Drug Reaction Reporting System.

The guidance for the pharmacovigilance responsibilities of sponsors of medicines is included on the Australian Register of Therapeutic Goods (ARTG) and regulated by the TGA. It gives the mandatory reporting requirements and offers recommendations on pharmacovigilance best practice.[60] The Therapeutic Goods Administration (TGA) receives adverse event reports associated with medicines and medical devices from members of the public, general practitioners, nurses, other health professionals and the therapeutic goods industry.

Two types of Database of Adverse Event Notifications (DAEN) are there which provide information about adverse events.[61]

1. **DAEN-medicines** gives information about adverse events of **medicines and vaccines** used in Australia.
2. **DAEN-medical devices** provides information about adverse events related to **medical devices** used in Australia.

The revised pharmacovigilance document came into effect on 10 November 2012 with the Therapeutic Goods Amendment Regulation 2012 [No. 3].

Australian legislation in full text is available on the website of Federal Register of Legislation.[62]

CANADA

Health Canada is the regulatory authority of Canada. The Health Products and Food Branch (HPFB) of Health Canada monitor the safety, efficacy and quality of all health products available for sale in Canada. Within HPFB, postmarket surveillance activities are the responsibility of the Marketed Health Products Directorate (MHPD).

MHPD in collaboration with other HPFB directorates carries out postmarket surveillance. It reviews health-product safety data, conducts risk assessments and evaluates their therapeutic efficacy. MHPD communicates the new product safety information to the public and the health care community and can take measures to remove a product from the market. Adverse reactions to drugs are collected and assessed by MHPD in coordination with Canadian Adverse Drug Reaction Monitoring Programme (CADRMP). Once a drug is licensed for use or marketed, the MHPD no longer has sufficient resources to routinely determine the chances that a particular drug has caused a reported adverse effect. The postmarket surveillance system depends mainly on voluntary reporting by health professionals and consumers, although reporting by health professionals may become mandatory in the near future. These voluntary reports are submitted either to the drug manufacturer or directly to CADRMP now known as Canada Vigilance Program. It maintains a computerized database of filed reports known as the Canadian Adverse Drug Reaction Information System (CADRIS). Manufacturers are required to submit reports of serious reactions within 15 days of receiving them. Health Canada advises manufacturers that a report of harm, suspected to be caused by a drug can be reported if the minimum reporting criteria are met and the report is considered relevant by a medical professional in the industry. The Canada Vigilance Programme is Health Canada's postmarket surveillance programme that collects and assesses reports of suspected adverse reactions to health products marketed in Canada. Postmarket surveillance helps Health Canada in monitoring the safety profile of health products once marketed and ensures that the benefits of the products are more than the risks. *A Draft Guidance Document for Industry, Reporting Adverse Reactions to Marketed Health Products* has been prepared which is intended to replace and supersede the 1996 *Guidelines for the Canadian Pharmaceutical Industry on Reporting Adverse Reactions to Marketed Drugs (Vaccines Excluded)* and its 2001 revision.[63]

The Canada Vigilance Programme is collecting reports of suspected adverse reactions since 1965. Adverse reaction reports are submitted by health professionals and consumers on a voluntary basis either directly to Health Canada or via Market Authorization Holders. The following health products marketed in Canada are collected by the program: prescription and non-prescription medications, biologics (including fractionated blood products, as well as therapeutic and diagnostic vaccines), natural health products and radiopharmaceuticals. The information collected by the programme can be accessed through the Canada Vigilance Online Database. Information related to vaccines used for immunization has been included in the database since January 1, 2011 and information concerning human blood and blood components has been included in the database since September 1, 2015.[64]

The Canada Vigilance Programme is supported by seven Canada Vigilance Regional Offices who provide a regional point-of-contact for health professionals and consumers. Reports are collected by the regional offices before being forwarded to the Canada Vigilance National Office for further analysis.

Health professionals and consumers can report suspected adverse reactions online, by phone or by submitting the Canada Vigilance Reporting Form by fax or mail (Annexures 11A to C).

It is mandatory to report any serious adverse reaction to Health Canada by the drug manufacturers. Reporting can also be done by the health professionals and patients. In case of serious adverse reaction MHPD takes appropriate action. MHPD also brings out a quarterly daily, *The Canadian Adverse Reaction Newsletter,* which raises safety issues. The regulations and guidelines for the advertising of marketed health products in Canada have been developed by MHPD. Health care is a shared responsibility and depends on the input and collaboration of consumers, industry and health professionals both within Canada and abroad, to ensure the continued postmarket safety, efficacy and quality of drugs and other marketed health products.[64-67]

UNITED STATES OF AMERICA

The US Food and Drug Administration is a scientific, regulatory, and public health agency. Most food products (other than meat and poultry), human and animal drugs, therapeutic agents of biological origin, medical devices, radiation-emitting products for consumer, medical, and occupational use, cosmetics, and animal feed come under its jurisdiction. The agency was established in 1862 in the US Department of Agriculture as the Division of Chemistry and after July 1901 became the Bureau of Chemistry. The Federal Food and Drugs Act were passed in 1906 and the agency had regulatory functions along with scientific role. The Bureau of Chemistry's name changed to the Food, Drug, and Insecticide Administration in July 1927 and its nonregulatory research work was transferred elsewhere in the department. In July 1930 the present name was given. FDA was under the Department of Agriculture until June 1940. In April 1953, the agency again was transferred, to the Department of Health, Education, and Welfare (HEW). Fifteen years later FDA became part of the Public Health Service within HEW, and in May 1980 the education function was removed from HEW to create the Department of Health and Human Services, FDA's current home.

Legal requirement for the development, approval and marketing of drugs are contained in Federal Food, Drug and Cosmetic Act (FDCA). In order to know the legal standards for Pharmacovigilance in the United States a pharma company has to go through the laws, regulations and guidance documents. FDA has prepared some guidance documents for the industry. The law governing the pharmacovigilance requirements in the US for the drugs is section 505 of the FDCA (21 USC §355). FDA is authorized to regulate investigational drugs under Section 505(i). Biological products are treated as drugs during the investigational stage and are regulated accordingly (21 CFR § 312.2(a); § 601.21). Section 505(k) of the FDCA (21 USC § 355(k) is the basis in law for pharmacovigilance.

In Code of Federal Regulations, Title 21 deals with Food and drugs.[68] Section 314 of subchapter D and Chapter 1 deals with the issues related to the applications for FDA approval to market a new drug. Current regulations for postmarketing reporting of adverse drug experiences are described in Sec. 314.80 of CFR 21.

Sec. 314.80 Postmarketing reporting of adverse drug experiences
Title 21: Food and Drugs
Chapter I: Food And Drug Administration Department of Health And Human Services
Subchapter D: Drugs For Human Use
Part 314 : Applications For FDA Approval To Market A New Drug

Subpart B—Applications
Sec. 314.80 Postmarketing reporting of adverse drug experiences.
a. *Definitions:* The following definitions of terms apply to this section:
   Adverse drug experience: Any adverse event associated with the use of a drug in humans, whether or not considered drug related, including the following: An adverse event occurring in the course of the use of a drug product in professional practice; an adverse event occurring from drug overdose whether accidental or intentional; an adverse event occurring from drug abuse; an adverse event occurring from drug withdrawal; and any failure of expected pharmacological action.
   Individual case safety report (ICSR). A description of an adverse drug experience related to an individual patient or subject.
   ICSR attachments: Documents related to the adverse drug experience described in an ICSR, such as medical records, hospital discharge summaries, or other documentation.
   Disability: A substantial disruption of a person's ability to conduct normal life functions.
   Life-threatening adverse drug experience: Any adverse drug experience that places the patient, in the view of the initial reporter, at *immediate* risk of death from the adverse drug experience as it occurred, i.e. it does not include an adverse drug experience that, had it occurred in a more severe form, might have caused death.
   Serious adverse drug experience: Any adverse drug experience occurring at any dose that results in any of the following outcomes: Death, a life-threatening adverse drug experience, inpatient hospitalization or prolongation of existing hospitalization, a persistent or significant disability/incapacity, or a congenital anomaly/birth defect. Important medical events that may not result in death, be life-threatening,

Contd...

Contd...

or require hospitalization may be considered a serious adverse drug experience when, based upon appropriate medical judgment, they may jeopardize the patient or subject and may require medical or surgical intervention to prevent one of the outcomes listed in this definition. Examples of such medical events include allergic bronchospasm requiring intensive treatment in an emergency room or at home, blood dyscrasias or convulsions that do not result in inpatient hospitalization, or the development of drug dependency or drug abuse.

Unexpected adverse drug experience: Any adverse drug experience that is not listed in the current labeling for the drug product. This includes events that may be symptomatically and pathophysiologically related to an event listed in the labeling, but differ from the event because of greater severity or specificity. For example, under this definition, hepatic necrosis would be unexpected (by virtue of greater severity) if the labeling only referred to elevated hepatic enzymes or hepatitis. Similarly, cerebral thromboembolism and cerebral vasculitis would be unexpected (by virtue of greater specificity) if the labeling only listed cerebral vascular accidents. "Unexpected," as used in this definition, refers to an adverse drug experience that has not been previously observed (*i.e.* included in the labeling) rather than from the perspective of such experience not being anticipated from the pharmacological properties of the pharmaceutical product.

b. *Review of adverse drug experiences:* Each applicant having an approved application under 314.50 or, in the case of a 505(b)(2) application, an effective approved application, must promptly review all adverse drug experience information obtained or otherwise received by the applicant from any source, foreign or domestic, including information derived from commercial marketing experience, postmarketing clinical investigations, postmarketing epidemiological/surveillance studies, reports in the scientific literature, and unpublished scientific papers. Applicants are not required to resubmit to FDA adverse drug experience reports forwarded to the applicant by FDA; however, applicants must submit all follow-up information on such reports to FDA. Any person subject to the reporting requirements under paragraph (c) of this section must also develop written procedures for the surveillance, receipt, evaluation, and reporting of postmarketing adverse drug experiences to FDA.

c. *Reporting requirements.* The applicant must submit to FDA adverse drug experience information as described in this section. Except as provided in paragraph (g)(2) of this section, these reports must be submitted to the Agency in electronic format as described in paragraph (g)(1) of this section.

   1. i. *Postmarketing 15-day "Alert reports":* The applicant must report each adverse drug experience that is both serious and unexpected, whether foreign or domestic, as soon as possible but no later than 15 calendar days from initial receipt of the information by the applicant.

   ii. *Postmarketing 15-day "Alert reports"—follow up:* The applicant must promptly investigate all adverse drug experiences that are the subject of these postmarketing 15-day Alert reports and must submit follow-up reports within 15 calendar days of receipt of new information or as requested by FDA. If additional information is not obtainable, records should be maintained of the unsuccessful steps taken to seek additional information.

   iii. *Submission of reports:* The requirements of paragraphs (c)(1)(i) and (c)(1)(ii) of this section, concerning the submission of postmarketing 15-day Alert reports, also apply to any person other than the applicant whose name appears on the label of an approved drug product as a manufacturer, packer, or distributor (nonapplicant). To avoid unnecessary duplication in the submission to FDA of reports required by paragraphs (c)(1)(i) and (c)(1)(ii) of this section, obligations of a nonapplicant may be met by submission of all reports of serious adverse drug experiences to the applicant. If a nonapplicant elects to submit adverse drug experience reports to the applicant rather than to FDA, the nonapplicant must submit, by any appropriate means, each report to the applicant within 5 calendar days of initial receipt of the information by the nonapplicant, and the applicant must then comply with the requirements of this section. Under this circumstance, the nonapplicant must maintain a record of this action which must include:

Contd...

Contd...
- A copy of each adverse drug experience report;
- The date the report was received by the nonapplicant;
- The date the report was submitted to the applicant; and
- The name and address of the applicant.

2. *Periodic adverse drug experience reports:* (i) The applicant must report each adverse drug experience not reported under paragraph (c)(1)(i) of this section at quarterly intervals, for 3 years from the date of approval of the application, and then at annual intervals. The applicant must submit each quarterly report within 30 days of the close of the quarter (the first quarter beginning on the date of approval of the application) and each annual report within 60 days of the anniversary date of approval of the application. Upon written notice, FDA may extend or reestablish the requirement that an applicant submit quarterly reports, or require that the applicant submit reports under this section at different times than those stated. For example, the agency may re-establish a quarterly reporting requirement following the approval of a major supplement. Follow-up information to adverse drug experiences submitted in a periodic report may be submitted in the next periodic report.
    ii. Each periodic report is required to contain:
    - *Descriptive information:* (1) A narrative summary and analysis of the information in the report; (2) An analysis of the 15-day Alert reports submitted during the reporting interval (all 15-day Alert reports being appropriately referenced by the applicant's patient identification code, adverse reaction term(s), and date of submission to FDA); (3) A history of actions taken since the last report because of adverse drug experiences (for example, labeling changes or studies initiated); and (4) An index consisting of a line listing of the applicant's patient identification code, and adverse reaction term(s) for all ICSRs submitted under paragraph (c)(2)(ii)(B) of this section.
    - *ICSRs for serious, expected, and nonserious adverse drug experiences:* An ICSR for each adverse drug experience not reported under paragraph (c)(1)(i) of this section (all serious, expected and nonserious adverse drug experiences). All such ICSRs must be submitted to FDA (either individually or in one or more batches) within the timeframe specified in paragraph (c)(2)(i) of this section. ICSRs must only be submitted to FDA once.
    iii. Periodic reporting, except for information regarding 15-day Alert reports, does not apply to adverse drug experience information obtained from postmarketing studies (whether or not conducted under an investigational new drug application), from reports in the scientific literature, and from foreign marketing experience.
d. *Scientific literature:* A 15-day Alert report based on information in the scientific literature must be accompanied by a copy of the published article. The 15-day reporting requirements in paragraph (c)(1)(i) of this section (*i.e.* serious, unexpected adverse drug experiences) apply only to reports found in scientific and medical journals either as case reports or as the result of a formal clinical trial.
e. *Postmarketing studies:* An applicant is not required to submit a 15-day Alert report under paragraph (c) of this section for an adverse drug experience obtained from a postmarketing study (whether or not conducted under an investigational new drug application) unless the applicant concludes that there is a reasonable possibility that the drug caused the adverse experience.
f. *Information reported on ICSRs:* ICSRs include the following information:
    1. *Patient information.*
        i. Patient identification code;
        ii. Patient age at the time of adverse drug experience, or date of birth;
        iii. Patient gender; and
        iv. Patient weight.
    2. *Adverse drug experience.*
        i. Outcome attributed to adverse drug experience;

Contd...

Contd...

  ii. Date of adverse drug experience;
  iii. Date of ICSR submission;
  iv. Description of adverse drug experience (including a concise medical narrative);
  v. Adverse drug experience term(s);
  vi. Description of relevant tests, including dates and laboratory data; and
  vii. Other relevant patient history, including pre-existing medical conditions.
 3. *Suspect medical product(s).*
  i. Name;
  ii. Dose, frequency, and route of administration used;
  iii. Therapy dates;
  iv. Diagnosis for use (indication);
  v. Whether the product is a prescription or nonprescription product;
  vi. Whether the product is a combination product as defined in 3.2(e) of this chapter;
  vii. Whether adverse drug experience abated after drug use stopped or dose reduced;
  viii. Whether adverse drug experience reappeared after reintroduction of drug;
  ix. Lot number;
  x. Expiration date;
  xi. National Drug Code (NDC) number; and
  xii. Concomitant medical products and therapy dates.
 4. *Initial reporter information.*
  i. Name, address, and telephone number;
  ii. Whether the initial reporter is a health care professional; and
  iii. Occupation, if a health care professional.
 5. *Applicant information.*
  i. Applicant name and contact office address;
  ii. Telephone number;
  iii. Report source, such as spontaneous, literature, or study;
  iv. Date the report was received by applicant;
  v. Application number and type;
  vi. Whether the ICSR is a 15-day "Alert report";
  vii. Whether the ICSR is an initial report or follow-up report; and
  viii. Unique case identification number, which must be the same in the initial report and any subsequent follow-up report(s).

g. *Electronic format for submissions:*
(1) Safety report submissions, including ICSRs, ICSR attachments, and the descriptive information in periodic reports, must be in an electronic format that FDA can process, review, and archive. FDA will issue guidance on how to provide the electronic submission (e.g. method of transmission, media, file formats, preparation and organization of files).
(2) An applicant or nonapplicant may request, in writing, a temporary waiver of the requirements in paragraph (g)(1) of this section. These waivers will be granted on a limited basis for good cause shown. FDA will issue guidance on requesting a waiver of the requirements in paragraph (g)(1) of this section.

h. *Multiple reports:* An applicant should not include in reports under this section any adverse drug experiences that occurred in clinical trials if they were previously submitted as part of the approved application. If a report applies to a drug for which an applicant holds more than one approved application, the applicant should submit the report to the application that was first approved. If a report refers to more than one drug marketed by an applicant, the applicant should submit the report to the application for the drug listed first in the report.

Contd...

Contd...

i. *Patient privacy:* An applicant should not include in reports under this section the names and addresses of individual patients; instead, the applicant should assign a unique code for identification of the patient. The applicant should include the name of the reporter from whom the information was received as part of the initial reporter information, even when the reporter is the patient. The names of patients, health care professionals, hospitals, and geographical identifiers in adverse drug experience reports are not releasable to the public under FDA's public information regulations in part 20 of this chapter.

j. *Record-keeping:* The applicant must maintain for a period of 10 years records of all adverse drug experiences known to the applicant, including raw data and any correspondence relating to adverse drug experiences.

k. *Withdrawal of approval:* If an applicant fails to establish and maintain records and make reports required under this section, FDA may withdraw approval of the application and, thus, prohibit continued marketing of the drug product that is the subject of the application.

l. *Disclaimer:* A report or information submitted by an applicant under this section (and any release by FDA of that report or information) does not necessarily reflect a conclusion by the applicant or FDA that the report or information constitutes an admission that the drug caused or contributed to an adverse effect. An applicant need not admit, and may deny, that the report or information submitted under this section constitutes an admission that the drug caused or contributed to an adverse effect. For purposes of this provision, the term "applicant" also includes any person reporting under paragraph (c)(1)(iii) of this section.

[50 FR 7493, Feb. 22, 1985; 50 FR 14212, Apr. 11, 1985, as amended at 50 FR 21238, May 23, 1985; 51 FR 24481, July 3, 1986; 52 FR 37936, Oct. 13, 1987; 55 FR 11580, Mar. 29, 1990; 57 FR 17983, Apr. 28, 1992; 62 FR 34168, June 25, 1997; 62 FR 52251, Oct. 7, 1997; 63 FR 14611, Mar. 26, 1998; 67 FR 9586, Mar. 4, 2002; 69 FR 13473, Mar. 23, 2004; 74 FR 13113, Mar. 26, 2009; 79 FR 33088, June 10, 2014]

The FDA keeps on reviewing the benefits and risks of marketed drugs, throughout the life of the drug, mainly on the basis of ADR reports. Health professionals or consumers sent the ADR report to FDA or the drug manufacturer directly, and it is mandatory for the drug manufacturers to submit all received ADR reports (Annexures 3A to C) to FDA as per 21 CFR 314.80. FDA has a computerized repository to store these reports since 1969 and with time it has undergone several changes and improvement. In 1997 the FDA redesigned the database, which is referred as Adverse Event Reporting System (AERS), FDA shifted from using coding symbols for Thesaurus of Adverse Reaction Terms (COSTART) to Medical Dictionary for Regulatory Activities (MedDRA) coding technologies. MedDRA is based upon the Medical Dictionary for Drug Regulatory Affairs (MedDRA), created by the UK Medicines Control Agency (MCA). FDA started to use MedDRA in its database since 1997.

FDA has a provision for establishing a system for analyzing the ADR reports and submitting them to FDA. The regulatory requirements for ADR reporting of any marketed or investigational product is same and is of international standards. FDA published a proposed regulation in March 2003 that amended pre and postmarketing reporting regulations. Till 2005 no action was taken in this regard and the existing regulations prevailed.

Data from AERS was moved to FAERS for the launch of FAERS on September 10, 2012. Adverse Event Reporting System (AERS) is now known as FDA Adverse Event Reporting System (FAERS) and it supports the FDA's postmarketing safety surveillance programme for all marketed drug and therapeutic biologic products. It contains adverse event reports FDA has received from manufacturers as required by regulation along with reports received directly from consumers and healthcare professionals. Adverse events and medication errors are coded to terms in the terminology.[69]

The adverse events following vaccination reports are reported to the Vaccine Adverse Event Reporting System (VAERS) US; whereas, reports of adverse events involving medical devices are included in Manufacturer and User Facility Device Experience (MAUDE) Database. The Medical Device Reporting (MDR) regulation (21 CFR 803) contains mandatory requirements for manufacturers, importers, and device user facilities to report certain device-related adverse events and product problems to the FDA.[70]

Food and Drug Administration Amendments Act (FDAAA), 2007[71]

In September 2007 to expand the FDA's post-market surveillance powers, in accordance with the reauthorization of the Prescription Drug User Fee Act (PDUFA), the US Government passed new laws relating to the drug safety. This legislation, entitled 'the FDA Amendments Act (FDAAA) included provisions in the areas of:[72]
- Additional encouragement of specialized pediatric medical device development
- The creation of Reagan-Udall foundation to modernize product development, accelerate innovation, and enhance product safety
- Food safety provisions
- Advisory committee provisions
- Clinical trial registries
- Provisions intended to enhance drug safety.

FDAAA reauthorized *Prescription Drug User Fee Act (PDUFA) and Medical Device User Fee and Modernization Act (MDUFMA)* to help fund reviews of new drugs and to make significant improvements in the medical device review programme respectively.

FDAAA reauthorized other laws, including the Best Pharmaceuticals for Children Act (BPCA) and the Pediatric Research Equity Act (PREA). Both of these were designed to encourage more research into, and more development of, treatments for children.

FDAAA also included drug safety provisions which addressed safety-related labeling changes, risk evaluation and mitigations strategies, post-approval clinical trials and observational studies, and active postmarket risk identification and analysis.[71-73]

A comparison of pharmacovigilance regulations in various countries using 18 parameters have been given in Table 15.1.[74]

Table 15.1: Comparison of pharmacovigilance regulations of various countries					
Sl. No.	Components	United States	United Kingdom	India	Canada
1.	Regulatory Authority	FDA	MHRA	CDSCO	Health Canada
2.	Pharmacovigilance Responsible Body (Centre for Regulatory Pharmacovigilance)	CDER & CBER	CHM	NCC PvPI, IPC	Marketed Health Products, Directorate of the Health Products and Food Branch
3.	Guidelines	21CFR 314.80; 314.98, Guidance for Industry GVP and pharmacoepidemiologic Assessment	Article 106 of Directive 2001/20/EC, Directive 2001/83/EC & Article 26 of Regulation (EC) No.726/2004	Schedule Y of Drug and Cosmetics Rules, 1945	GVP Guidelines (GUI-0102)

Contd...

Contd...

Sl. No.	Components	United States	United Kingdom	India	Canada
4.	Process for reporting	Through MedWatch Form and Online through FAERS	Through yellow card form or via online reporting through yellow card portal, or via email	Paper ADR reporting Form, through Mobile app, or via email	Canada Vigilance Programme (MedEffect Canada) either online, by fax/mail or through telephone at Canada Vigilance Regional Office
5.	Pharmacovigilance system master file	Not mentioned	Maintained by European Union for each member countries	Not mentioned	Not mentioned
6.	Pharmacovigilance inspection	Via PADE inspections	Via Risk assessment strategy	Not mentioned	GVP inspection programme Inspection Strategy for GVP for drugs (POL-0041)
7.	Pharmacovigilance audit	Via Post approval audit inspections	In accordance to EU Good pharmacovigilance practice guidelines	Not mentioned	In accordance with the GVP guidelines (GUI-0102)
8.	Risk management system	Given in risk management Guidance under Guidance for industry GVP and pharmacoepidemiologic assessment	Follows risk management plan as per EMA guidance	Mentioned in Guidance Document for spontaneous adverse drug reaction reporting	Mentioned in guidance document—Submission of risk management plans and follow-up commitments
9.	Serious adverse drug reactions reporting time period	Within 15 calendar days of occurrence	Within 15 calendar days reporting by QPPV	Within 24 hours of occurrence	Within 15 calendar days of occurrence of ADR
10.	Database	FAERS database	Yellow Card database	WHO ICSR database (VigiBase)	Canada vigilance adverse reaction online database
11.	Types of different ADR reporting form	Three: 1. Form 3500 2. Form 3500A 3. Form 3500B	MHRA Yellow Card adverse drug reaction Reporting Form	Two: 1. Suspected ADR reporting form for Healthcare personnel 2. Medicines side effect reporting form for Consumers	Two: 1. Form for suspected adverse drug reaction to marketed products by industry 2. Form for suspected adverse drug

Contd...

Contd...

Sl. No.	Components	United States	United Kingdom	India	Canada
					reaction reporting by consumers
12.	PSUR submission	To CDER for drug products and CBER for biological products	To PSUR repository	To DCGI and PvPI	To submission and information policy division Therapeutic Products Directorate Health Canada
13.	Data lock point for PSUR	70/90 days	6 months after the commission date	30 days of the last reporting period	70/90 days
14.	Safety communication	Solicited communication via FDA website release	Communicated via MHRA website and press release	Communicated via CDSCO press release and also PvPI newsletters	Communicated via Health Canada website
15.	Risk minimization measures	Done through risk MAP guidelines	Not mentioned	Not mentioned	Guidance Document—submission of risk management plans and rollow-up commitments
16.	Toll-free/Helpline Number	Yes 1-800-332-1088	Yes 0808-100-3352	Yes 1800-180-3024	Yes 1-866-337-7705
17.	Connection with UMC	Yes, FAERS data is communicated to WHO UMC	Yes, Yellow Card reports are reported to UMC after causality assessment	Yes, The ICSRs are directly reported to UMC database via VigiFlow	Yes, via MedEffect programme

Abbreviations: FDA, food and drug administration; MHRA, medicines and healthcare products regulatory agency; CDSCO, central drugs standard control organization; CDER, centre for drug evaluation and research; CBER, centre for biologics evaluation and research; NCC, national coordination centre; PvPI, pharmacovigilance programme of India; IPC, Indian pharmacopoeia commission; CHM, commission of human medicines; GVP, good pharmacovigilance practice; FAERS, FDA adverse event reporting system; PADE, postmarketing adverse drug experience; EU, European union; EMA, European Medicines Agency, QPP, qualified personnel for pharmacovigilance; ADR, adverse drug reaction; ICSR, Individual case safety reports; PSUR, periodic safety update report; DCGI, Drug Controller general of India; UMC, uppsala monitoring centre

REFERENCES

1. Bahri P, Tsintis P 2007 Pharmacovigilance, Ed Mann Edwards Arora Deepa. Pharmacovigilance obligations of the pharmaceutical companies in India. Indian J Pharmacol. 2008;40(7):13-6.
2. European Countries. Europa (web portal). Retrieved on 2007-09-05.
3. European Commission-Enlargement- Candidate and Potential Candidate Countries. Europa (web portal). Retrieved on 2007-06-26.
4. EU/Kosovo Factsheet. European Union - Delegation of the European Commission to the United States. Retrieved on 2007-03-27.
5. Annual report 2005 EMEA/MB/63019/2006
6. OJ L 136, 30.04.2004, p. 1.
7. Directive 2001/83/EC
8. Recommendations of International Conference on Harmonization of Technical Requirements for Registration of Pharmaceuticals for Human Use (ICH).
9. European Commission, 2006.

10. European Medicines Agency Road Map to 2010.
11. Eudralex- Volume 9A of The Rules Governing Medicinal Products in the European Union–Guidelines on Pharmacovigilance for Medicinal Products for Human Use.
12. EMEA/CHMP/PhVWP/235910/2005- rev.1
13. Commission Regulation (EC) No 541/95 of 10 March 1995 (as amended in 1998), concerning the examination of variations to the terms of a marketing authorization granted by a competent authority of a Member State.
14. Commission Regulation (EC) No 542/95 of 10 March 1995 (as amended in 1998), concerning the examination of variations to the terms of a marketing authorization falling within scope of Council Regulation (EEC) No 2309/93.
15. http://www.gmp-compliance.org/gmp-news/important-changes-at-emea. Accessed on Sept 2017.
16. OJ L 159, 20.6.2012, p5
17. Davis S, et al. Pharmacovigilance, 2nd edition. Eds Ronald D Mann and Elizabeth B Andrews 2007, John Wiley & Sons
18. http://www.mhra.gov.uk/ Safetyinformation/index.htm
19. MHRA-Medicines and medical devices regulations 2007: what you need to know
20. https://www.gov.uk/guidance/good-pharmacovigilance-practice-gpvp: accessed on 24.9.17
21. Health Service Circular 2000/026
22. Directive 2004/27/EC. Accessed on Sept 2017.
23. https://www.gov.uk/guidance/the-yellow-card-scheme-guidance-for-healthcare-professionals. Accessed on Sept 2017.
24. http://www.mhra.gov.uk/Safetyinformation/Howwemonitorthesafetyofproducts/Blood/index.htm. Accessed on Sept 2017.
25. http://www.pmlive.com/blogs/digital_intelligence/archive/2013/february/new_guidance_on_dataprotection_in_pharmacovigilance_for_uk_pharma_463520. Accessed on Sept 2017.
26. https://www.gov.uk/government/publications/medical-devices-uk-notified-bodies/uk-notified-bodies-for-medical-devices. Accessed on Sept 2017.
27. https://s3.amazonaws.com/thegovernmentsays-files/content/147/1470161.html
28. Moore N, Kreft-Jais C, Dhanani A. Spontaneous reporting –France. In: Mann RD, Andrews EB (Eds). Pharmacovigilance 2nd edition. John Wiley & Sons. 2007;217-226.21.
29. Welsch M, Alt M, Richard MH, Imbs JL. The French pharmacovigilance system: structure and missions. Presse Med. 2000;29(2):102-6.
30. Bégaud B, Chaslerie A, Haramburu F. Organization and results of drug vigilance in France. Rev Epidemiol Sante Publique. 1994;42(5):416-23.
31. Royer RJ. Pharmacovigilance. The French system. Drug Saf. 1990; 5(Suppl 1):137-40.
32. Pharmaceutical Pricing and Reimbursement Information, FRANCE, October 2007, Commissioned by European Commission, Health and Consumer Protection Directorate-General and Austrian Ministry of Health, Family and Youth.
33. Article R.5144-8 of the French Public Health Code
34. Bélorgey C. Temporary Authorisations for Use (ATU), Agence Francaise De Securite Sanitaire Des Produits De Sante, Division For The Evaluation Of Medicinal And Biological Products, June 2001.
35. Journal officiel de la République française, Lois et Décrets, 26 May 2005, No. 121, pp. 9087-9102, Text No. 14, NOR: SANP0521624A
36. http://www.legifrance.gouv.fr/WAspad/UnTexteDeJorf?numjo=SANP0521624A. Accessed on Sept 2017.
37. http://www.pmlive.com/pharma_news/new_french_regulatory_agency_ansm_afssaps_402076. accessed on Sept 2017
38. Lochouarn M. France launches new drug regulatory agency. Lancet. 2012;379(9832): p2136,
39. http//:www.anvisa.gov.br/legis/law_9782.htm
40. http://www.anvisa.gov.br/eng/index.htm. Accessed on Sept 2017.
41. De Carvalho PM, Varallo FR, Dagli-Hernandez C (2016) Brazilian Regulation in Pharmacovigilance: A Review. Pharmaceut Reg Affairs 5:164. doi:10.4172/2167-7689.1000164
42. Biswas P, Biswas AK. Setting standards for proactive pharmacovigilance in India. Indian J Pharmacol. 2007;39:124-8.
43. Arora D. Pharmacovigilance obligations of the pharmaceutical companies in India. Indian J Pharmacol. 2008; 40 (7): 13-16.

44. Bill No. LVII of 2007, The Drugs and Cosmetics (Amendment) bill, 2007 to be produced in Rajya Sabha June 2007)
45. http://www.ipc.gov.in/PvPI1/pv_about.html. Accessed on Sept 2017.
46. Dhamija P, Kara S, Sharma PK, et al. Indian College of Physicians (ICP) position Statement on Pharmacovigilance. J Assoc Physicians India. 2017; 65: 63-66.
47. http://eng.sfda.gov.cn/cmsweb/webportal/W43879538/index.html)
48. Chen X. An Overview of SFDA and Current Drug Administration in China State Food and Drug Administration, September 6 2005, (http//www.bpfk.gov.my-chinachenxy.ppt.url).
49. Zhou, Yibing, Miller, Victor, Hogan, Matthew, Callahan Larry. 2006. An Overview of Adverse Drug Reaction Monitoring in China. International Journal of Pharmaceutical Medicine. 2006;20(2):79-85(7).
50. Drug Administration Law of China 2001. Available at http://www.lehmanlaw.com/resource-centre/laws-and-regulations/pharma/the-drug-administration-law-of-the-peoples-republic-of-china-2001.html. Accessed on Sept 2017.
51. Measures for the administration on report and monitoring of the side effects of pharmaceuticals 2004.
52. http://eng.sfda.gov.cn/WS03/CL0757/172239.html. Accessed on Sept 2017.
53. Zhang L, Wong LYL, He Y, et al. Drug Saf 2014;37:765. https://doi.org/10.1007/s40264-014-0222-3.
54. Chan K, Zhang H, Lin ZX. An overview on adverse drug reactions to traditional Chinese medicines Br J Clin Pharmacol. 2015;80(4):834-43. Published online 2015 May 19. doi: 10.1111/bcp.12598
55. Hou Y, Li X, Wu G, Ye X. National ADR Monitoring System in China. Drug Saf. 2016;39(11):1043-51.
56. Pharmaceutical Administration and Regulation in Japan, 2007.
57. Fujiwara M, Kawasaki Y, Yamada H. A Pharmacovigilance Approach for Post-Marketing in Japan Using the Japanese Adverse Drug Event Report (JADER) Database and Association Analysis. PLoS One. 2016; 11(4): e0154425. Published online 2016 Apr 27. doi: 10.1371/journal.pone.0154425
58. https://www.jstage.jst.go.jp/article/jjpe/19/1/19_14/_pdf
59. https://www.adea.com.au/wp-content/uploads/2013/08/How_to_report_Problems_with_medicine.pdf
60. https://www.tga.gov.au/book/export/html/763772 (accessed on Sept 2017)
61. https://www.tga.gov.au/database-adverse-event-notifications-daen
62. https://www.legislation.gov.au/
63. https://www.canada.ca/en/health-canada/services/drugs-health-products/reports-publications/medeffect-canada/guidance-document-industry-reporting-adverse-reactions-marketed-health-products-health-canada-2011.html. Accessed on Sept 2017.
64. https://www.canada.ca/en/health-canada/services/drugs-health-products/medeffect-canada/adverse-reaction-database.html (accessed on Sept 2017)
65. Health Canada: Your Health & Safety - Our Priority Health Products and Food Branch 02/2006 Post-market Surveillance(http://www.hc-sc.gc.ca/ahc-asc/alt_formats/hpfb-dgpsa/pdf/3kitfiche/factsheet_fiches- info _07 -eng.pdf)
66. http://www.hc-sc.gc.ca/dhp-mps/medeff/vigilance-eng.php. Accessed on Sept 2017.
67. https://www.canada.ca/en/health-canada/services/drugs-health-products.html. Accessed on Sept 2017.
68. CFR 21, Volume 5, Revised as of April 1, 2017. (Accessed on Sept 2017)
69. https://www.fda.gov/Drugs/GuidanceComplianceRegulatoryInformation/Surveillance/AdverseDrugEffects/default.htm (Accessed on Sept 2017).
70. https://www.fda.gov/MedicalDevices/Safety/ReportaProblem/default.htm(accessed on September 2017
71. https://www.fda.gov/ForConsumers/ConsumerUpdates/ucm061229.htm (accessed on Sept 2017)
72. Food and Drug Administration Amendments Act of 2007 (https://www.fda.gov/Regulatory-Information/LawsEnforcedbyFDA/Significant Amendments to the FDC Act/Food and Drug Administration Amendments Act of 2007/default.htm).
73. Gerald J. Update on Post-marketing Drug Safety Activities at the US FDA. UR40 January 2008 (www.who-umc.org) page 10.
74. Hans M, Gupta SK. Unpublished Report (2016).

16
Pharmacoepidemiology and Pharmacovigilance

SK Gupta, Mohit Hans, Sushma Srivastava

INTRODUCTION

Pharmacoepidemiology involves the application of the epidemiological methods in order to study the clinical use of drugs in populations. Therefore, pharmacoepidemiology can be defined as the study of the use and effects/side-effects of drugs in large numbers of people with the purpose of supporting the rational and cost-effective use of drugs in the population thereby improving health outcomes.

Pharmacoepidemiology may be either drug-oriented, emphasizing the safety and effectiveness of the individual drug or groups of drugs, or utilization-oriented which aims to improve the quality of drug therapy through educational intervention. Drug utilization research can also be divided into descriptive and analytical studies. The emphasis of the descriptive studies has been to describe patterns of drug utilization and to identify problems deserving more detailed studies.

Analytical studies try to relate or link the data on drug utilization to the figures on morbidity, the outcome of treatment and quality of care with the ultimate goal of assessing whether the drug therapy is rational or not. Sophisticated utilization-oriented pharmacoepidemiology on the other side focuses on the drug (e.g. dose-effect and concentration-effect relationships), the prescriber (e.g. quality indices of the prescription), or the patient (e.g. selection of drug and dose, and comparisons of kidney function, drug metabolic phenotype/genotype, age, etc.).

Since, the description of the extent, nature and determinants of drug exposure is explained through dug utilization research, therefore, it becomes an essential part of the pharmacoepidemiology. The distinction between these two terms has been less sharp over the time, therefore they are sometimes used interchangeably. However, while drug utilization studies often employ various sources of information that focus on drugs (e.g. aggregate data from wholesale and prescription registers), the term epidemiology implies to defined populations in which drug use can be expressed in terms of incidence and prevalence. Together, drug utilization research and pharmacoepidemiology may provide insights into the following aspects of drug use and drug prescribing.

The initial focus of pharmacoepidemiology was on the safety of individual drug products, i.e. pharmacosurveillance, but now it also includes studies of their beneficial effects as well. The driving force behind this development was a growing awareness that the health outcomes of drug use in the rigorous setting of randomized clinical trials are not necessarily the same as the health outcomes of drug use in real world scenario. Since, the randomized controlled trials needed to obtain the market authorization for new drugs, involve limited numbers of carefully selected patients, who are treated and followed-up for a relatively short time in strictly controlled conditions. As a result, a clear indication of the effect of the drug on health outcomes of the large population in real world scenario cannot be assessed under everyday circumstances.

Pharmacoepidemiological studies often make the useful contributions to the knowledge about efficacy and safety, because, unlike clinical trials, they assess drug effects in larger, heterogeneous populations of patients over longer periods. Drug utilization research also provide insights into the efficiency of drug use, i.e. whether a certain drug therapy provides value for money and the results of such research can be used to help to set priorities for the rational allocation of health care budgets.

Since, the clinicians apply the knowledge of the benefits and risks of pharmaceuticals to individual and population-based patient care, therefore, practice of pharmacotherapy presents numerous challenges to their practice. Understanding about the efficacy and safety of drugs arises from well-controlled studies or the randomized controlled trials (RCTs) conducted during the drug development and approval process. However, many additional risks and benefits are identified after the drug approval process, i.e. when the drug is utilized by the masses. A potential gap in the knowledge of risk and benefits of the pharmacotherapy is due to the pre-approval studies as they involve limited sample size, short study follow-ups, limited characteristics of patient studied and differences in the setting from the real-world scenario. Benefits and risk founded during post-approval follow-up may range from minor to clinically important effects. A close monitoring of the medicinal product must also be followed up closely after the drug is marketed as this information adds value to the clinical practice. The term effectiveness is generally used whether or not the drug achieves its desired effect in the real world in contrast to its therapeutic effect in the randomized controlled trials.

Drug effectiveness studies are generally conducted using observational study designs. Although, RCTs also play an important role in determining a drug's effectiveness, it is widely accepted that results from an RCT offers the best evidence that the investigational drug will perform under ideal conditions or the real-world conditions, and it is likely that the "well-controlled" design of RCTs will continue to be required for new drug applications to the Food and Drug Administration (FDA).

Reports of the adequate and well-controlled investigations form a primary basis for determining the substantial evidence in support of the claims of the effectiveness of new drug. Thus, pharmacoepidemiology provides precious information about the clinical and economic outcomes of the drug or a device or biologics particularly after they are marketed.

Methodology developed in general epidemiology can benefit pharmacoepidemiology and can be further developed for application uniquely to pharmacoepidemiology. Some areas that are altogether unique to pharmacoepidemiology include pharmacovigilance. Pharmacovigilance is a continual monitoring process or activity for recognizing the unwanted effects and other safety-related aspects of drugs that are already on the market. Practically pharmacovigilance involves spontaneous reporting systems which allow health care professionals and others to report adverse drug reactions to a central agency which then combine reports to produce a more informative safety profile for the drug product based on one or a few reports from one or a few health care professionals.

In situations where it is either infeasible or unethical to assign patients randomly to active treatment or placebo epidemiologic study designs are an essential aspect of evaluating drug safety and effectiveness.

Although the randomized, controlled, blinded trial is the standard against which other designs are measured, it is often unsuitable in terms of safety aspect within the domain of pharmacoepidemiology.

METHODOLOGIES IN PHARMACOEPIDEMIOLOGIC STUDIES

A number of study designs and methods are used to generate data on the uses and risks of new and older drugs (Flowchart 16.1). Study designs used in pharmacoepidemiology are classified into two categories, i.e. experimental and observational. In experimental studies individuals are usually randomized to the exposure of the drug under investigation and then follow-up of individuals to detect the effects of exposure (Table 16.1).

While observational epidemiologic study designs, such as case-control, cohort, and cross-sectional studies, are used extensively. Large automated databases, meta-analyses, RCTs, and hybrid designs, such as nested case-control studies, also play an important role in pharmacoepidemiology.

Typically in an epidemiologic study, a randomization plan is not required to determine who will receive a particular drug exposure. Rather, associations between exposure(s) and disease(s) under study are determined through the use of observational study designs and statistical analyses. Observational methods are used in most situations because they limit the use of experimentation due to ethics and cost factors.

Case Reports

Case reports, also referred to as spontaneous case reports or passive surveillance, is an unsolicited communication by a healthcare professionals or consumers to a company, regulatory authority or other organization (e.g. World Health Organization, or regional centres) describe a single patient who was exposed to a medicinal product and experienced a particular adverse drug reaction and this information has not been obtained from a study or any organized data collection. The FDA receives approximately 400,000 reports of suspected adverse events annually. Well-documented case reports can be viewed as a safety signal of ADR related any drug-

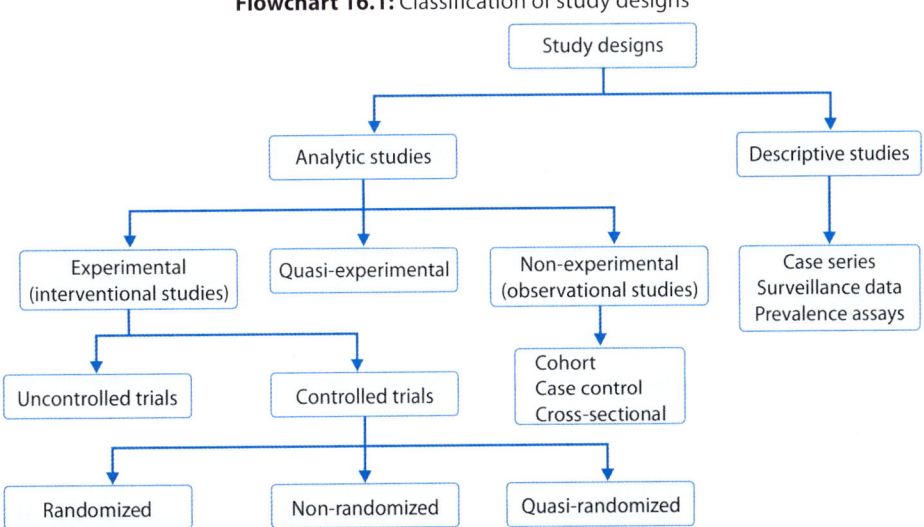

Flowchart 16.1: Classification of study designs

Table 16.1: Summary of the pharmacoepidemiological study designs

Study design	Characteristics	Advantages	Disadvantages
Case reports and case series	Detailed description of case(s) without a control group	• Fast • Inexpensive • First publication of the case	• Selection bias • Limited potential for establishing causal effects
Cross-sectional study	Exposure and outcomes measured at a same time and compared with subjects who may or may not have outcome	• Fast • Inexpensive • Description of the prevalence of disease	• Selection bias • Survival bias • Limited potential for establishing causal effects
Case-control study	Cases are compared with controls	• Relatively inexpensive • Efficient method • Suitable for studying rare outcomes and multiple exposures	• Selection bias • Control group selection can be difficult • Some potential in establishment of causal effect
Cohort study	Cohort of individuals free from outcome is followed and compared based on the exposure	• High generalizability • Suitable for studying multiple or rare exposures and multiple outcomes	• Selection bias • Can be expensive • Long period • Some potential in establishment of causal effect
Randomized controlled trials	Allocation of the study subject to either treatment or placebo group in randomized manner	• Suitable for studying more than one intervention • Establishment of the causal effect	• Very expensive • Longer duration • Not for studying rare events • Selection bias

drug interaction, alerting to the possibility of a rare adverse event not previously detected in premarketing studies. A signal is defined as a possible relationship between an adverse event and a drug and the relationship being unknown or incompletely documented previously. The results or the consequences drawn from the spontaneous reports are taken into account by the prescribers and the regulators for the purpose of prescribing. A valuable information on at-risk groups, risk factors, and clinical characteristics of known serious adverse drug reactions can be obtained from the spontaneous reports. Spontaneous reporting systems can be easily found at local, regional or national levels. The various reporting systems include:
- US FDA MedWatch
- UK Yellow Card
- WHO International system
- National Pharmacovigilance System: India

Case Series

Case series are a collection of patients who represents a single exposure. Their clinical outcomes are evaluated and described. They play an important role in communicating previously unidentified risk and benefits of the drugs. These are beneficial in quantifying the incidence of an adverse reaction, particularly for a newly approved drug. Case series basically serve as the markers that the incidence of the concerned adverse effect does not occur in the population that is larger than that studies prior to drug's marketing. It is very uncommon to make a causation statement based on the case series report. Since, the major disadvantage of the case series study is that it lacks a control study group, therefore, a conclusion cannot be inferred for a situation which requires comparison with the control group.

Case-control Studies

A case-control study involves a group of cases (people who have the disease of interest) and controls (people who do not). The exposure histories of the cases and the controls are determined to establish the extent of association between exposure(s) of interest and disease. Case-control studies compare patients with a specific disease with a control group composed of similar people but without the disease. In these studies cases of disease or events are identified and controls or the patients without the disease are then selected from the source population that give rise to the cases. The selection of the controls must be such that the prevalence among controls should represent the prevalence among the source population. The exposure status among two groups is compared using the odd ratio, which gives the estimate of the relative risk of disease in the two groups. Case control studies attempt to identify the risk factors for a disease by examining differences in antecedent exposure variables between cases and controls. Under specific conditions the case control studies can provide the absolute incidence rate of the adverse event. If all the cases of interest are captured in an area and the fraction of the controls from the source population is known, then an incidence rate can be calculated. This study design has been widely used to estimate the safety of the pharmaceuticals.

Cohort Studies

In cohort studies, group of individuals or the cohorts are identified and characterized and then followed over time to determine the incidence of some predetermined outcome or outcomes. Basically, a cohort study involves a group of individuals or persons without the disease of interest at the onset of the study, monitoring the exposure status of each individual and then follow the cohort over time to determine the development of the disease in exposed and non-exposed individuals. A comparison of the incidence of one or more outcomes among those individuals who received a drug or some other exposure of interest with the incidence of the event(s) for acomparison group can be done with the cohort study design. A controlled cohort study having one cohort characterized by exposure to the drug being evaluated and a second cohort untreated or treated with an alternative drug is more suitable than an uncontrolled cohort study which do not involve any control group. A cohort study can either be done prospectively or retrospectively. A retrospective cohort design is useful when comparing exposed cohorts to the non-exposed cohort which can be identified from a time point in the past from the existing large databases and followed from that time to the present with regard to the incidence of the given outcome. Since, the exposure is assessed before the outcome occurs therefore, a prospective cohort study can provide strong evidence of associations between the drugs and the diseases.

Experimental Study Designs

The experimental study designs include the RCTs which are the gold standard for the evaluation of the therapy or the intervention. A major advantage of the RCT is that they can provide an evidence of the causal relationship because they exclude the selection bias and selection by prognosis, i.e. confounding by indication. A controlled trial is a prospective study design which involves two or more treatments groups and controls who may be treated with an active drug or a placebo or both. It is characterized by a random and unbiased allocation of the active substance or placebo to the treatment and the control groups. A more stringent form of an RCT involves a double blinded technique where the patient and the physician both do not know about which treatment is being allocated to which group.

PHARMACOEPIDEMIOLOGY IN DRUG DEVELOPMENT

Epidemiological data and methods are utilized during each and every phase or aspect of the drug development lifecycle. However, the extent of involvement is dependent on the knowledge base and interactions between factors that are specific to the molecule. Many factors are responsible for affecting both the exposure and response to drug therapy which ultimately means that the core of drug development has always been the randomized controlled trial, preferably double blinded. These randomized, blinded designs restrict the involvement of known and unknown confounding factors, both those affecting the physician's decision to prescribe and those affecting patient response, to ensure that different treatment groups are as similar as possible at baseline, so that the impact (both benefits and risks) of the new treatment can be adequately assessed.

These randomized studies are often too expensive to conduct because they are very resource intensive, often too short to identify long-term treatment effects. Furthermore, the studies are usually designed to establish efficacy and therefore they do not provide sufficient information regarding the safety outcomes.

Once the drug is marketed and prescribed within the general population the epidemiology data can provide estimate of the size of the target population along with its geographic distribution, quantify and describe demographic and clinical characteristics, and help in determining the potential public health impact of a target treatment.

Once the drug is in phase II or III clinical trials a more robust and clear understanding of the target population is required in order to establish the efficacy and safety hence, the epidemiology study design, i.e. observational study design (cohort, case-control, cross-sectional) is needed to generate potential information to specific queries regarding the population. Proper estimates of the total number of individuals currently impacted as well as future estimates by utilizing current and projected prevalence and incidence rates can be obtained through the population epidemiology of a disease.

The epidemiological data is very useful in pre-approval drug development phases as it is used to generate potential information regarding the target population. This helps in the identification of the potential target population which can be included in the clinical trial and on the other hand to identify those groups of population, which require further follow-up post-authorization. Pharmacoepidemiological studies can also be used to identify any causal relationship between the drug treatment and the major comorbidities of the disease under study.

The pharmacoepidemiology principles can provide a broad overview of population epidemiology, treated natural history and burden of disease in the lifecycle of drug development.

In population epidemiology, the pharmacoepidemiology can provide an overview of the condition for which the product is being developed, including the incidence rate, i.e. the rate of new cases in a population within a specified time frame, prevalence rate, i.e. the number of existing cases stratified by geography, patient demographics in a population within a specified time frame, clinical characteristics, trends over time and recommendations relating to studies needed to address data gaps.

In case of the treated natural history, pharmacoepidemiology provides an overview of clinical course of the condition for which the product is being developed. It focuses on detailing disease progression, defining a patient profile, quantifying rates of common comorbidities, treatments and treatment practices, disease outcome rates (e.g. morbidity, mortality, survival) and rates of potential drug-related adverse events. This provides information in understanding the types of adverse events associated with the indication and its common therapies and to quantify the frequency (i.e. risk) of these adverse events within the general population and to estimate the potential benefit of the product under development.

For the burden of disease, the pharmacoepidemiology provides an overview focusing on the negative disease-related impact for the individual suffering and their social network, as well as the incurred direct and indirect costs in the real-world setting.

So, it can be concluded that pharmacoepidemiologic studies can help in optimizing the therapeutic response to a drug during the post-approval phase. These studies can provide valuable information regarding the relationship between medicinal products and the adverse events and beneficial outcomes. Provision of evidence-based medicine can be assisted through the information generated by epidemiological studies as they provide with the important insights regarding the safety, pattern of drug utilization and effectiveness.

BIBLIOGRAPHY

1. Stergachis A, Hazlet TK, Boudreau D. Pharmacoepidemiology. Foundation Issues Section 1. The McGraw-Hill Companies, Inc. 2008;pp.46-55.
2. Wise L. Risks and benefits of (pharmaco) epidemiology. Therapeutic advances in drug safety. 2011;2(3):95-102.
3. Manack A, Turkel CC, Kaplowitz H. Role of epidemiological data within the drug development lifecycle: a chronic migraine case study. INTECH Open Access Publisher; 2012.

Hospitalization due to Adverse Drug Reactions and its Economic Burden

SK Gupta, Mohit Hans, Sushma Srivastava

INTRODUCTION

Adverse drug reactions (ADRs) have become a global problem and a major concern of patient safety and clinical practice. Today most of the patients are treated with multiple drugs or in simple terms. The concept of polypharmacy have led to an increase in the number of ADRs that are inevitable. Understanding the healthcare burden of ADRs as well as the relevant types and drugs involved represents an important gap in our knowledge.

The World Health Organization (WHO) defines an ADR as "a response to a drug which is noxious and unintended, and which occurs at doses normally used in man for the prophylaxis, diagnosis, or therapy of disease, or for the modification of physiological function".[1] In general practice, medication-related adverse events (AEs) represent an important cause of morbidity and are thought to cause 10% to 30% of all hospital admissions.[2] These AEs are defined as "any untoward medical occurrences that may present during treatment with a pharmaceutical product but which does not necessarily have a causal relationship with this treatment".[3] Among these AEs, ADRs represent a major burden, significantly contributing to morbidity, mortality, and health care costs.[4,5] A severe ADR is one which is life-threatening, causing permanent damage or requiring intensive care whereas moderate ADRs require hospital admission, a change in therapy, or some specific treatment. In a meta-analysis of prospective studies, 1,00,000 deaths per year could be attributed to ADRs in the USA, which marks the seriousness and extent of the problem. ADRs were reported to be the fourth to sixth leading cause of death in the United States and serious adverse drug reactions contributed to 6.7% of total hospitalization.[6]

A major limitation in ADR research is that we lack reliable data on the true prevalence and burden of ADRs. This relates to the fact that information about ADRs is captured traditionally through voluntary reporting systems, which on a large scale under report the true number of ADRs,[7] and do not capture information about the number of patients at risk thus making an impossible assessment of the relative frequencies of different ADRs. It was reported that Singapore has one of the highest per capita rates of spontaneous ADR reporting in the world.[8] An inability in the calculation of the true prevalence of ADRs can be contributed to under-reporting, incomplete information and reporting bias.[7] Furthermore, a Swedish study reported that 3.1% of deaths in the general population (including subjects who died in and outside hospitals) were attributed to ADRs itself.[9] In order to relate an ADR to a medication, it has been reported to encompass certain (definite), probable and possible probabilities into the total number of ADRs.[10]

Some of the risk factors contributing to drug related hospitalizations included increased use of medicines, the existence of multiple inter current disease states and polypharmacy. A high incidence of hospitalization was reported with geriatric population. This can be attributed to pharmacological and pathological changes leading to alteration in pharmacodynamic and pharmacokinetic parameters of drug absorption, distribution, metabolism and excretion in elderly patients. Certain classes of drugs such as antiplatelets, antineoplastics, anticoagulants, diuretics, immunosuppressive, antidiabetics and antibiotics were reported to have a high profile of drug-related problems. In many reported studies on geriatrics, majority of hospitalized patients presented with chief complaints of weakness due to dehydration, electrolyte imbalance; bleeding, gastrointestinal disturbances, anemia, hypoglycemia, secondary infections, etc. Therefore, it has been reported that problems associated with the use of medications have contributed to a major portion of the health expenses in most of the countries.[11]

A study conducted by Gallagher et al.[12] in UK to ascertain the occurrence of ADRs causing hospital attendance in children reported an incidence of 2.9% over the 1-year period. In another study conducted earlier by Gallagher et al.[13] the estimated incidence of hospital admissions was 4%. Langerova et al. reported that 2.2% of pediatric hospital admissions were caused by ADRs.[10] A systematic review by Smyth et al. (2012)[14] reported a range of 0.4% to 10.3% incidence rate of ADRs causing hospital admissions, with a pooled estimate of 2.9%. Another study performed by Posthumus et al.[15] reported a 6.9% of ADR-related acute admissions in children.

Various studies have reported that drug-related problems (DRP) leading to hospitalizations on an average have accounted for 8.36%, thus DRP admissions need high attention. According to the literature on drug related hospital admissions, around 5–10% of hospital admissions were due to drug-related problems out of which 50% of them were avoidable.[11]

In one of the study conducted by Jamuna Rani and Priyam (2014)[16] regarding analysis of adverse drug reaction related hospital admissions from various departments of a tertiary care hospitals it was reported that 33 admissions were due to ADR. However, the ADR related hospitalization was lower as compared to studies reported with western population. Jamuna Rani and Priyam (2013)[17] conducted a retrospective analysis of hospitalization caused by ADRs in a tertiary care hospital in south India. Out of 23 cases of hospital admission, 10 were males and 13 were females. An elderly age group comprised of 30.4%, most implicated drugs causing ADRs were antibiotics followed by NSAIDs and the remaining adverse reactions were due to antiepileptic and hormonal drugs.

Seasonal influenza epidemics continue to have a substantial economic and public health burden in the United States. On an average, it is estimated that over 200,000 people are hospitalized each year due to respiratory and circulatory complications associated with the seasonal influenza. Young-Xu et al. performed an analysis of the annual burden of seasonal influenza in the US Veterans Affairs population. In the five-year study period from 2010 to 2014, they estimated the influenza attributed outcomes with a statistical regression model using observed emergency department (ED) visits, hospitalizations and deaths from the Veterans Health Administration of the Department of Veterans Affairs (VA) electronic medical records and respiratory viral surveillance data from the Centres for Disease Control and Prevention (CDC). It was reported that over the five-year observation period, the number of patients rose from 5,294,641 in 2010 to 5,754,615 in 2014. The reported average cost over the five-year duration for 10,674 VA ED visits was $6.2 million, 2,538 VA hospitalizations was $41.7 million and 5,522 all-cause deaths with monetary losses was $1.1 billion. Combined cost estimated was $1.2 billion contributing to the total annual influenza-attributed societal burden.[18]

In Europe, ADRs cause a considerable amount of morbidity and mortality. It has been reported that approximately 5% of all hospital admissions were due to ADRs and that 5% of hospitalized patients experienced an ADR during their hospital stay and ADRs cause 197,000 deaths annually throughout the European Union (EU).[19] These estimates lead to a major reform in the European regulatory system for pharmacovigilance which was implemented in July 2012.

A review of observational studies published since 1 January 2000 estimating the epidemiology of ADRs in hospital settings was performed in a European country by Bouvy et al.[20] They identified 47 published studies since 1 January 2000, whether prospective or retrospective observational, reporting the ADR occurrence rate among the European population. In total, 32 studies, performed in 12 different countries (France, UK, Germany, Italy, Switzerland, Greece, Spain, Romania, Slovenia, Austria, Netherlands, and Norway), reported the percentage of patients admitted to the hospital due to an ADR. Twenty-two studies, performed in nine different countries (Germany, France, Netherlands, Switzerland, UK, Norway, Italy, Romania, and Spain), reported the percentage of patients experiencing an ADR during hospitalization, five studies reported ADRs which occurred in various outpatient settings in three different countries while one study reported ADRs as a cause of in hospital deaths in a Finnish hospital. It was reported that on an average, the ADR occurrence rate at hospital admission was 3.6% of all hospitalizations (median; mean 4.6%) in 22 published studies that reported the rate of occurrence of ADRs in unselected patient populations. Furthermore, the ADR occurrence rate during hospitalization was 10.1% of all the patients (median; mean 17.0%). The review reported that, in Europe, approximately 3.6% of all hospital admissions were caused by ADRs, and up to 10% of patients in European hospitals develop an ADR during their stay. Furthermore, the percentage of hospitalizations leading in a fatal ADR is likely to be lower than 0.5%.

A retrospective study reported by Wu et al, assessed the incidence and economic burden of ADR among elderly patients in Ontario emergency department (ED). They collected data of the ADR related ED visits. The incidence and costs of ADR-related ED visits and subsequent hospital admissions were reported for all adults aged 66 years and above for the period April 2003–March 2008. All costs in EDs and inpatient medical care are paid by provincial single-payer insurance programmes in Canada. It was reported that approximately 0.75% of total annual ED visits were found to be ADR-related which included adults aged 66 years and above and among these patients 21.6% were hospitalized. In 2007, the cost of ADR-related visits was reported to be $333 per ED visit and $7528 per hospitalization for a total annual cost of $13.6 million in Ontario, or an estimated $35.7 million in Canada. Severe ADRs were associated with sex, age, comorbid disease burden, multiple drugs, multiple pharmacies, newly prescribed drugs, recent ED visit, recent hospitalization and long-term care (LTC) residence.[20]

There are certain conditions, for good outpatient care, which can potentially prevent the need for hospitalization or for which early intervention can prevent complications or more severe disease. These are recognized as the Prevention Quality Indicators (PQIs) which can be combined with hospital inpatient discharge data to identify quality of care for "ambulatory care sensitive conditions." These PQIs are population based and adjusted for covariates. Even though these indicators are hospital inpatient data based, they provide an insight into the community health care system or services outside the hospital setting. For example, patients with diabetes may be hospitalized for complications originating due to diabetes if their condition is not adequately monitored or if they do not receive the proper education needed for appropriate self-management.

The PQIs can be used as a "screening tool" to help mark the potential health care quality problem areas which needs further investigation; provide a quick check on primary care access or outpatient services in a community by utilizing the patient data from a typical hospital discharge abstract; and, can help public health agencies, State data organizations, health care systems, and other organizations interested in improving health care quality in their communities.

With a high-quality, community-based primary care, hospitalization for such illnesses can be avoided. Although other factors not under the direct control of the health care system, such as poor environmental conditions or lack of patient adherence to recommended treatments, can result in hospitalization, the PQIs provide a suitable starting point for assessing the quality of health services in the community. Since, the PQIs are calculated using the available hospital administrative data, they are an easy-to-use and inexpensive screening tool. They can also be used to provide a window into the community—to identify unmet community health care needs, to monitor how well the complications from a number of common conditions are avoided in an outpatient setting, and in comparison, of performance of local health care systems across communities.[21]

ECONOMIC BURDEN OF ADRs

The impact and management of ADRs is complex and in the USA, may cost up to 30.1 billion dollars annually. ADRs may increase costs due to increased hospitalization, prolongation of hospital stay and additional clinical investigations in more serious cases.

Talking of the cost incurred due to ADRs during 90s, several studies have been published that analyzed the cost and economic burden due to adverse drug reactions. In addition, ADRs may trigger a cascade of prescriptions when some new medications are being prescribed for conditions that are a consequence of another medication, which is often regarded an unrecognized ADR. Examples include: the use of antipsychotics in patients with Parkinson's disease treated with dopaminergic drugs or the use of anticholinergic for the purpose of urinary retention in Alzheimer's disease patients treated with cholinesterase inhibitors.[22] This will lead an increase in the costs of pharmacotherapy as well as compounding a further risk to different ADRs.

Out of incident ADRs resulting in hospitalization, the cost per preventable ADR was reported to be higher than for non-preventable ADRs.[23] Another study in an inpatient setting reported the cost to be $US 2262 per ADR.[24] The costs of ADRs incurred in an inpatient setting varied within different hospital wards, costing up to $US 13,994 in a non-intensive care unit, but $US 19,685 in an intensive care unit.[25] Addition, reported drug surveillance studies have been able to identify the following ADRs which pose the greatest economic burden in hospital setting: fever, bleeding, diarrhea and cardiac arrhythmia, in decreasing order.[24] NSAIDs, antibacterial agents, anticoagulant agents and antineoplastic agents have been a major cause of ADR-related costs.[26]

Both the extended duration of hospitalization as well as the outpatient care as a result of ADRs constitute the major source of financial burden.[27] The main costs of ADRs in a hospital are constituted by wages, disposable goods and medications.[28] Besides from the direct financial costs, there are also several indirect costs for patients and their care givers which are incurred by ADRs, such as missed days from work and/or morbidity such as anxiety due to the ADR episode.[29]

In most of the economic and business decision making processes whether private or public, the term 'cost' is always considered with variation in its counterparts from benefit (in cost-benefit analysis, CBA), to effectiveness (in cost-effectiveness analysis, CEA), and especially in healthcare fields, to quality-adjusted life years (QALYs) or latent utility (in cost-utility analysis, CUA). Costs are most commonly measured in monetary terms for a direct comparison among available alternative options.

Cost of illness (COI), known as the burden of disease (BOD), is a definition that includes various aspects of the disease which cause a great impact on the health outcomes in a country, specific regions, communities, and even individuals. The COI category ranges from the epidemiology of the disease to its effect on longevity and morbidity along with the downfall in health status and quality of life (QoL), and financial aspects including direct and indirect expenses as a result of premature death, disability or injury due to corresponding disease and/or its comorbidities.

In order to formulate and prioritize health care policies and interventions and to achieve a proper allocation of health care resources in line with the budget constraints an accurate knowledge of the COI is important so as to achieve policy efficiency.

The basic goal of a COI study is to evaluate or assess the economic burden caused by illness on the society as a whole. As clearly stated in Jefferson et al. (2002), "the aim of COI studies is descriptive: to itemize, value, and sum the costs of a particular problem with the aim of giving an idea of its economic burden." So, in order to conduct a COI study, researchers are required to recognize, identify, list, measure and value the costs which a disease and its comorbidities will generate.[30]

A prospective study conducted by Patel et al. (2007) over a period of 6 weeks in a tertiary referral centre among the adult patients reported that ADRs accounted for 3.84% of the patients presented to the emergency department. Out of these, 141 were admitted and thus 53.21% of the total patients reporting to the emergency department were hospitalized with an average cost of USD 150 per patient contributing to the significant economic burden.[31]

In prospect of carrying out COI studies, an underlying assumption should be kept in mind that the economic aspect of COI represents the 'potential benefits of a health care intervention' if it had completely eradicated the illness. In this direction, the COI studies generally include some amount of 'health loss' and tries to measure the resource costs incurred in treating the related condition. The BOD studies specifically measure the 'burden' of years of life (YLL) that have been lost because of the premature death, and the years lost due to disability or morbidity (YLD). These two categories together encompass a cost called as total DALY (disability-adjusted life years), which combines the health care costs and the 'lost economic or societal contribution' resulting from premature death or disability.

A systematic review was reported by Clabaugh et al. 2008 who, examined the methods used by researchers in developing COI studies. The aim of the review was to categorize the approaches that the published literature used in terms of perspective, scope, components of care analyzed in the literature, datasets, and valuation approaches used for direct cost. It reported conclusions regarding the adequacy of current COI research methods and makes recommendations on improving them. It was concluded that analyzing the cost of illness presented useful opportunities and a link for communication with the public and policymakers on the relative importance of specific diseases and injuries. The research indicated that COI studies employ varied approaches and many articles have methodological limitations. Without the well-accepted standards in order to guide researchers in their execution of these studies, policymakers and the general public must be cautious of the methods applied in their calculation and subsequent results.[32]

TYPES OF COST

The COI studies traditionally divide costs into three categories, i.e. direct, indirect, and intangible costs. Because of the seldom quantification of the intangible costs in COI studies due to the measurement difficulties and related controversies, the main focus will be on the first two cost categories.

Direct Cost

The direct costs consist of healthcare costs and non-healthcare costs since it is being incurred by the health system, society, family and individual patient. The former is defined as the medical care expenditures for diagnosis, treatment, and rehabilitation, while the latter is associated with the consumption of non-healthcare resources like transportation, household expenditures, relocating, property losses, and informal cares of any kinds. The estimated direct cost associated with chronic diseases are higher than those of acute diseases or communicable diseases on terms and condition that the effective and efficacious treatments and prevention methods were adopted.

Indirect Cost

In comparison to the accounting and business disciplines where the 'indirect' cost is indicative of the supporting and overhead activities that need to be shared among the users, the term 'indirect' in COI studies basically refers to productivity losses due to morbidity and mortality, beard by the individual, family, society, or the employer. In general, the indirect cost is a part of the social welfare losses attributed to diseases, while the remaining welfare losses are associated by the losses in healthy time resulting from pain, suffering and grief caused by diseases. Three method can be applied in order to calculate the indirect cost which include: Human capital method, friction cost method and willingness to pay method.[30]

In 2015, US health care spending increased to 5.8% to reach $3.2 trillion, or $9,990 per person. As a result of in the Affordable Care Act the coverage expansion that began in 2014, continued to have an impact on the growth of health care spending in 2015. Additionally, it was reported that the major drivers for a faster growth in total health care spending in 2015 was, stronger growth in expenses for private health insurance, hospital care, physician and clinical services, and the continued strong growth in Medicaid and retail prescription drug spending. The overall share of the US economy committed to health care spending was 17.8% in 2015, up from 17.4% in 2014.[33]

A global systematic review was conducted (Seuring et al. 2015) in order to review the global incidence of cost of type 2 diabetes. An extensive search was carried out in order to assess the studies reporting the economic burden of type 2 diabetes published from 2001 to 2014. It was reported that direct costs were generally higher than indirect costs. Direct costs reported to be ranging from $242 for a study on out-of-pocket expenditures in Mexico to $11,917 for a study on the cost of diabetes in the US, while indirect costs ranged from $45 for Pakistan to $16,914 for the Bahamas. In low and middle income countries in contrast to high income countries—a substantial part of the cost burden was attributed to patients via out-of-pocket treatment costs. It was reported that regression analysis revealed that direct diabetes costs are closely and positively associated with a country's gross domestic product (GDP) per capita, and that the USA stood out as having particularly high costs, even after controlling for GDP per capita.[34]

COST OF ADRs

The estimation of the direct and indirect costs resulting from ADRs is difficult as description of the endpoint of most adverse reactions is very limited. Identification and measurement of the costs of those cases where ADRs are probable causes of death or lead to hospitalization is possible. It is also possible to get some information about the severity of the effects and make cost estimations from the description of the nature of adverse reactions. However, it is not possible to recognize, for example, the medical expenditures or number of days lost from work due to all kinds of ADRs.

A systematic review assessing the cost of ADRs induced hospitalization was reported with an aim to systematically review the economic cost of ADR induces hospitalizations. Based on the included 12 studies in the review it was reported that the incidence of ADR admissions ranged from 0.60% to 7.0% with the median length of hospital stay ranging from 3 to 8.7 days. Direct medical cost was evaluated in all studies while indirect cost was calculated in only 2 studies. It was reported that cost per case of ADR induced hospitalization ranged between US$ 180 to 7,038 in 2013.[35]

There is no reliable estimate of the social direct or indirect cost of the ADRs, however, if we could manage to establish the causal link between drug consumption, ADRs, and the cost incurred to manage ADR-related illness using the necessary epidemiological information then it can be used as a reliable estimate of the cost. Estimating cost can also be beneficial in other ways as well like comparing the cost of different interventions and to study changes over a specific period of time. These estimations can also provide some idea of alterations in healthcare policies in order to improve the balance between cost and benefits. The COI studies are considered to be an important and inevitable technique in health and medical sciences. It helps the policy and decision makers to correctly implement and allocate different resources through estimation and comparison of the economic burden of disease to the society.

In general, the COI studies are the descriptive studies which can provide information in order to support the political process as well as the managerial functions of a various tiers of health care providers and organizations. To carry out a successful COI study, the study should be designed in such an innovative way that it can eventually identify the different subjects who bear the costs and explain the possibility that the results of COI can vary across different study designs.

REFERENCES

1. http://www.adr-database.com/What%20are%20ADRs.html
2. Royal S, Smeaton L, Avery AJ, Hurwitz B, Sheikh A. Interventions in primary care to reduce medication related adverse events and hospital admissions: systematic review and meta-analysis. Qual Saf Health Care. 2006;15(1):23-31.
3. Nebeker JR, Barach P, Samore MH. Clarifying adverse drug events: a clinician's guide to terminology, documentation, and reporting. Ann Intern Med. 2004;140(10):795-801.
4. Onder G, van der Cammen TJ, Petrovic M, Somers A, Rajkumar C. Strategies to reduce the risk of iatrogenic illness in complex older adults. Age Ageing. 2013;42(3):284-91.
5. Onder G, Pedone C, Landi F, et al. Adverse drug reactions as cause of hospital admissions: results from the Italian Group of Pharmacoepidemiology in the Elderly (GIFA). J Am Geriatr Soc. 2002;50(12):1962-8.
6. Lazarou J, Pomeranz BH, Corey PN. Incidence of adverse drug reactions in hospitalized patients: a meta-analysis of prospective studies. JAMA. 1998;279(15):1200-5.
7. Wise L, Parkinson J, Raine J, Breckenridge A. New approaches to drug safety: a pharmacovigilance tool kit. Nat Rev Drug Discov. 2009; 8: 779-82.
8. Viklund A, Biriell C. VigiBase scales new heights. Uppsala Reports. 2015;70:5.

9. Wester K, Jonsson AK, Spigset O, Druid H, Hagg S. Incidence of fatal adverse drug reactions: a population based study. Br J Clin Pharmacol. 2008;65(4):573-9.
10. Langerova P, Vrtal J, Urbanek K. Adverse drug reactions causing hospital admissions in childhood: A prospective, observational, single-center study. Basic Clin Pharmacol Toxicol. 2008;102:408-11.
11. Nivya K, Kiran VS, Ragoo N, Jayaprakash B, Sekhar MS. Systemic review on drug related hospital admissions–A pubmed based search. Saudi Pharmaceutical Journal. 2015;23(1):1-8.
12. Gallagher RM, Mason JR, Bird KA, Kirkham JJ, Peak M, Williamson PR, et al. Adverse drug reactions causing admission to a pediatric hospital. PLoS One. 2012;7:e50127.
13. Gallagher RM, Bird KA, Mason JR, Peak M, Williamson PR, Nunn AJ, et al. Adverse drug reactions causing admission to a pediatric hospital: A pilot study. J Clin Pharm Ther. 2011;36:194-9.
14. Smyth RM, Gargon E, Kirkham J, Cresswell L, Golder S, Smyth R, et al. Adverse drug reactions in children – A systematic review. PLoS One. 2012;7:e24061.
15. Posthumus AA, Alingh CC, Zwaan CC, VanGrootheest KK, Hanff LL, Witjes BB, et al. Adverse drug reaction-related admissions in pediatrics, a prospective single-center study. BMJ Open. 2012;2:E000934.
16. Jamunarani R, Priya M. Analysis of Adverse Drug Reaction related hospital admissions and common challenges encountered in ADR reporting in a tertiary care teaching hospital. Asian J Pharm Clin Res. 2014;7(Suppl 1):141-3.
17. Rani J, Priya M. Hospitalization caused by adverse drug reactions(ADRs) in a tertiary care hospital in south India: aretrospective study. NJBMS. 2013;3(3):227-30.
18. Young-Xu Y, van Aalst R, Russo E, Lee JKH, Chit A. The Annual Burden of Seasonal Influenza in the US Veterans Affairs Population. PLoS ONE. 2017;12(1): e0169344.
19. European Commission. Proposal for a regulation amending, as regards pharmacovigilance of medicinal products for human use. Regulation (EC) No 726/2004. Impact assessment. 2008. Available at: http://ec.europa.eu/health/files/pharmacos/pharmpack_12_2008/pharmacovigilance-ia-vol1_en.pdf. Accessed 10 Jan 2017.
20. Wu C, Bell CM, Wodchis WP. Incidence and economic burden of adverse drug reactions among elderly patients in Ontario Emergency Departments. Drug Safety. 2012;35(9):769-81.
21. http://www.qualityindicators.ahrq.gov/modules/pqi_overview.aspx
22. Kalisch LM, Caughey GE, Roughead RE, Gilbert AL. The prescribing cascade. Aust Prescr. 2011;34:162-6.
23. Bates DW, Spell N, Cullen DJ, Burdick E, Laird N, Petersen LA, et al. The costs of adverse drug events in hospitalized patients. Adverse Drug Events Prevention Study Group. JAMA. 1997;277:307-11.
24. Classen DC, Pestotnik SL, Evans RS, Lloyd JF, Burke JP. Adverse drug events in hospitalized patients. Excess length of stay, extra costs, and attributable mortality. JAMA. 1997;277:301-6.
25. Cullen DJ, Sweitzer BJ, Bates DW, Burdick E, Edmondson A, Leape LL. Preventable adverse drug events in hospitalized patients: a comparative study of intensive care and general care units. Crit Care Med. 1997;25:1289-97.
26. White TJ, Arakelian A, Rho JP. Counting the costs of drug-related adverse events. Pharmacoeconomics. 1999;15:445-58.
27. Field TS, Gilman BH, Subramanian S, Fuller JC, Bates DW, Gurwitz JH. The costs associated with adverse drug events among older adults in the ambulatory setting. Med Care. 2005;43:1171-6.
28. Wasserfallen J, Livio F, Buclin T, Tillet L, Yersin B, Biollaz J. Rate, type, and cost of adverse drug reactions in emergency department admissions. Eur J Intern Med. 2001;12:442-7.
29. Wu WK, Pantaleo N. Evaluation of outpatient adverse drug reactions leading to hospitalization. Am J Health Syst Pharm. 2003;60:253-9.
30. Jo C. Cost-of-illness studies: concepts, scopes, and methods. Clinical and molecular hepatology. 2014;20(4):327-37.
31. Patel KJ, Kedia MS, Bajpai D, Mehta SS, Kshirsagar NA, Gogtay NJ. Evaluation of the prevalence and economic burden of adverse drug reactions presenting to the medical emergency department of a tertiary referral centre: a prospective study. BMC Clinical Pharmacology. 2007;7(1):1-5.

32. Clabaugh G, Ward MM. Cost of Illness Studies in the United States: a systematic review of methodologies used for direct cost. Value in Health. 2008;11(1):13-21.
33. National Health Expenditure 2015 highlights available from https://www.cms.gov/Research-Statistics-Data-and-Systems/Statistics-Trends-and-Reports/NationalHealthExpendData/downloads/highlights.pdf
34. Seuring T, Archangelidi O, Suhrcke M. The economic costs of type 2 diabetes: a global systematic review. Pharmacoeconomics. 2015;33(8):811-31.
35. Siltharm C, Thavorncharoensap M. Cost of adverse drug reactions (ADRs) induced hospitalization: a systematic review. Mahidol Univ J Pharm Sci. 2013;40:40-9.

18
Vigilance Systems for Medical Devices

SK Gupta, Sushma Srivastava, Mohit Hans

INTRODUCTION

Medical devices are the crucial components of health care system, especially the patient care which may include uncomplicated devices employed during medical examinations, such as tongue depressors and thermometers, or sophisticated life-saving implants like heart valves and coronary stents. They play an increasingly vital role in health care delivery globally.[1]

Typically, the purpose of a medical device is not attained through any pharmacological, immunological or metabolic means. Medical equipment excludes implantable, disposable or single-use medical devices. Medical equipment is used for the specific purposes of diagnosis and treatment of disease or rehabilitation following disease or injury and it can be used either alone or in combination with any accessory, consumable or another piece of medical equipment.[2]

Medical devices contribute to the achievement of the highest standards of health of individuals. Without them common medical procedures like from bandaging a sprained ankle, to diagnosing HIV/AIDS, implanting an artificial hip or any surgical intervention—would not be have been so easy. Medical devices are used in many diverse settings: for example, by lay persons at home; by paramedical staff and clinicians in remote clinics; by opticians and dentists; or by healthcare professionals in advanced medical facilities; for prevention and screening, and in palliative care. Such health technologies are widely used in diagnosing an illness, monitoring treatments, assisting disabled persons, or intervening and treating illnesses, both acute and chronic. There are an estimated 5 million different kinds of medical devices in the world market, segregated into more than 22,000 generic devices groups.[3]

World Health Organization (WHO) defines a medical device as an article, instrument, apparatus or machine that is used in the prevention, diagnosis or treatment of illness or disease, or for detecting, measuring, restoring, correcting or modifying the structure or function of the body for any health purpose.[2]

US Food and Drugs Administration (USFDA) defines a medical device under section 201(h) of the Federal Food, Drug & Cosmetic (FD&C) Act as "an instrument, apparatus, implement, machine, contrivance, implant, in vitro reagent, or other similar or related article, including a component part, or accessory which is:
- Recognized in the Official National Formulary, or the United States Pharmacopoeia, or any supplement to them
- Intended for use in the diagnosis of disease or other conditions, or in the cure,

mitigation, treatment, or prevention of disease, in man or other animals
- Intended to affect the structure or any function of the body of man or other animals, and which does not achieve its primary intended purposes through chemical action within or on the body of man or other animals and which is not dependent upon being metabolized for the achievement of any of its primary intended purposes."[4]

Medicines and Healthcare Products Regulatory Agency (MHRA) as per its Medical Devices Directive (Directive 93/42/EEC) defines a medical device as any instrument, apparatus, appliance, software, material or other article, whether used alone or in combination, including the software intended by its manufacturer to be used specifically for diagnostic and/or therapeutic purposes and necessary for its proper application, intended by the manufacturer to be used for human beings for the purpose of:
- Diagnosis, prevention, monitoring, treatment or alleviation of disease
- Diagnosis, monitoring, treatment, alleviation of or compensation for an injury or handicap
- Investigation, replacement or modification of the anatomy or of a physiological process
- Control of conception.

It does not achieve its principal intended action in or on the human body by pharmacological, immunological or metabolic means, but which may be assisted in its function by such means.[5]

As per Central Drug Standard Control Organization (CDSCO), a medical device means:
- Any instrument, apparatus, appliance, implant, material or another article, whether used alone or in combination, including the software, intended by its manufacturer to be used especially for human beings or animals for one or more of the specific purposes of:
  - Diagnosis, prevention, monitoring, treatment or alleviation of any disease or disorder
  - Diagnosis, monitoring, treatment, alleviation or assistance for, any injury or disability
  - Investigation, replacement or modification or support of the anatomy or of a physiological process
  - Supporting or sustaining life
  - Disinfection of medical devices
  - Control of conception

  It does not achieve the primary intended action in or on the human body or animals by any pharmacological or immunological or metabolic means, but which may be assisted in its intended function by such means, and covered under sub-clause (iv) of clause (b) of section 3of the Drugs and Cosmetics Act,1940 (23 of 1940);
- An accessory to such an instrument, apparatus, appliance, material or other article
- Substances covered under sub-clause (i) of clause (b) of section 3 of the Drugs and Cosmetics Act, 1940 (23 of 1940) used for in vitro diagnosis which is a reagent, calibrator, control material, kit, instrument, apparatus, equipment or system, specimen receptacle, whether used alone or in combination with any other reagent, calibrator, control material, kit, instrument, apparatus, equipment or system, that is intended by its manufacturer to be used *in vitro* for examination of any specimen, including any blood or tissue donation, derived from the human body, solely or principally for the purpose of providing information:
  - Concerning a physiological or pathological state or a congenital abnormality
  - To determine the safety and compatibility of any blood or tissue donation with a potential recipient thereof

- To monitor therapeutic measures.
- Substances in the nature of medical devices covered by sub-clause (ii) of clause (b) of section 3 of the Drugs and Cosmetics Act, 1940 (23 of 1940).[6]

According to the Department of Health, Therapeutic Goods Administration, Australia the Therapeutic Goods Act 1989 defines a medical device as:

- Any instrument, apparatus, appliance, material or other article (whether used alone or in combination, and including the software necessary for its proper application) intended, by the person under whose name it is or is to be supplied, to be used for human beings for the purpose of one or more of the following:
  - Diagnosis, prevention, monitoring, treatment or alleviation of disease
  - Diagnosis, monitoring, treatment, alleviation of or compensation for an injury or handicap
  - Investigation, replacement or modification of the anatomy or of a physiological process
  - Control of conception

and that does not achieve its principal intended action in or on the human body by pharmacological, immunological or metabolic means, but that may be assisted in its function by such means

- An accessory to such an instrument, apparatus, appliance, material or other article.[7]

The Global Harmonization Task Force (GHTF) has proposed the following harmonized definition for medical devices. Medical device means any instrument, apparatus, implement, machine, appliance, implant, in vitro reagent or calibrator, software, material or other similar or related article, intended by the manufacturer to be used, alone or in combination, for human beings for one or more of the specific purposes of:

- Diagnosis, prevention, monitoring, treatment or alleviation of disease
- Diagnosis, monitoring, treatment, alleviation of or compensation for an injury
- Investigation, replacement, modification, or support of the anatomy or of a physiological process
- Supporting or sustaining life
- Control of conception
- Disinfection of medical devices
- Providing information for medical purposes by means of in vitro examination of specimens derived from the human body

and which does not achieve its primary intended action in or on the human body by pharmacological, immunological or metabolic means, but which may be assisted in its function by such means.[1]

Table 18.1: Salient features of medical device regulations of US, EU, Japan, Australia and Canada[1]

	United States	European Union (EU)	Japan	Australia	Canada
Regulation of medical device	The Federal Food, Drug and Cosmetic Act	Medical Device Directive (MDD)			
Pre- and postmarket supervision of medical devices	Centre for Device and Radiological Health (CDRH), within FDA	Regulatory control enacted by NB which are autonomous private enterprise and have the authority to grant CE mark	Pharmaceutical, Medical Device Agency (PMDA)	The Therapeutic Goods Administration (TGA)	Therapeutic Products Division (TPD) of Health Canada
Risk classification	Three tiered system: Class I Class II Class III	Four class scheme: Class I (Is and Im) Class IIa Class IIb Class III	General medical device (class I) Controlled medical devices (class II) Specially controlled medical devices (class III and IV)	Class I, Class I-supplied sterile, Class I- incorporating a measuring device, class IIa, class IIb, class III and active implantable medical devices (AIMD)	Four-tier classification [Class I is at lower risk and class IV pose the highest risk]
Approval system	Class I- general controls Class II: 510(k) process Class III: PMA process	Manufacturers need to exhibit CE marking on their products in order to ensure devices are safe and it for use	Class I needs device notification Class II needs a device certificate Class III and IV need a device approval	Both the device and manufacture process adhere to the requirement of the therapeutic good legislation	Class I device: Only post marketing monitoring Class II: Safety, efficacy, quality and the post market control Class III and IV: Premarket safety and efficacy assessment

Table 18.2: Comparison of vigilance systems of US, UK, Australia, and India[8]

Parameters	FDA	TGA (Australia)	MHRA	CDSCO (India)
Definition of medical device	Includes all instruments, appliances, materials, machines, in vitro diagnostic agents, implants, software, accessories, and disinfectants	Excludes tampons and hospital, household, and commercial-grade disinfectants	Excludes materials used for disinfection of medical devices	10-device category regulated as a drug
Medical device classification	3 classes: class I, class II, and class III	5 classes: class I, classes II a and II b, class III, and class AIMD	4 classes: Class I, class IIa, class IIb, and class III	No defined classes for devices
Basis of classification	• Level of control • Medical specialties	Classification rules	Classification rules	NA

Postmarketing surveillance activities	• Medical device tracking
	• MDR
	• MDR event files, records, and written procedures
	• Complaint handling
	• Recall procedure and seizures
		• Adverse event reporting
		• Vigilance exchange programme
		• Enforcement activities
		• Distribution records
		• Audits
			• Adverse event reporting
			• FSCA and field safety notices
			• Investigations
			• Enforcement
			• Postmarket clinical follow-up
			• Records
				• Adverse event reporting
				• For importers
				  ○ Complaint handling
				  ○ Adverse event reporting
				  ○ Procedure for distribution of records
				  ○ Procedure for recall

Medical device tracking	Have established tracking system since 1993	IMDTS developed recently for tracking of patients with implantable medical devices	AITS developed to investigate the failure modes of the device by assessment of user reports	In labeling provisions, the lot number/batch number for a device is mandatory for easy traceability
Who needs to report AE	Manufacturers, importers, user facilities, users, distributors, and health professionals	Manufacturers, sponsors, users, health professionals, and TGA	Manufacturers, users, health professionals, authorized representatives, and MHRA	Manufacturers only
Criteria for reporting	• Death or serious injury • Device malfunctions • User error • Injury/illness requiring medical intervention	• Event has occurred • Medical device's association with the event • Event led/might lead to death/serious injury	• Event has occurred • Medical device's association with the event • Event led/might lead to death/serious injury	• Event has occurred • Medical device's association with the event • Event led/might lead to death/serious injury

Contd...

Contd...

Parameters	FDA	TGA (Australia)	MHRA	CDSCO (India)
Not-reportable incidents/events	Manufacturers can apply for RAE, e.g. • Erroneous information • When another manufacturer makes the device	• User-detected deficiencies • Root cause of the adverse event is due to the patients' pre-existing condition • Exceeded service life of device • Likelihood of adverse event is acceptable after risk assessment • Side effects clearly identified in the manufacturer's labeling and documented in device master record	• User-detected deficiencies • Root cause of the adverse event is due to the patients' pre-existing condition • Exceeded service life of device • Likelihood of adverse event is acceptable after risk assessment • Side effects clearly identified in the manufacturer's labeling and documented in device master record	• User-detected deficiencies • Root cause of the adverse event is due to the patients' pre-existing condition • Exceeded service life of device • Likelihood of adverse event is acceptable after risk assessment • Side effects clearly identified in the manufacturer's labeling and documented in device master record
Reporting time frame	• Manufacture: Death, serious injury, and malfunctions—30 calendar days, and events requiring immediate remedial action—5 working days • User facility: Death and serious injury—10 working days • Distributors and importers: Death, serious injury, and malfunction to manufacturer—10 working days	• Death/serious deterioration—10 calendar days • Reportable near adverse event—30 calendar days • Serious public health threat requiring remedial action—48 hours	• Serious public threat—2 calendar days • Death/serious deterioration—10 elapsed calendar days • Other incidents—30 elapsed calendar days • After receiving user reports from MHRA, reporting 3 working days	• Unanticipated death or serious injury within 14 days • All other reportable events not later than 30 elapsed calendar days
Types of report	• 30-day reports • 5-day reports • Baseline reporting • Supplemental reporting • Annual reports	• Adverse event report for each incident or medical device • Annual report	• Initial reporting of adverse events • Final reports • Periodic summary reporting • Trend reporting	• Initial reporting • Trend reporting • Final reporting

Contd...

Contd...

Parameters	FDA	TGA (Australia)	MHRA	CDSCO (India)
Applicable forms	• Form 3500 – online • Form 3500A for manufacturers, importers, and distributors • Form 3419 • Form 3417 • Form 3381	• Form MDIR01 • Form UDIR01 – online	• Manufacturer's incident report form • Online reporting for manufacturers by MORE	Adverse event reporting form
Vigilance exchange	NA	With overseas regulatory agencies	Exchange information for similar incidents and for FSCA within and outside	Not defined
Vigilance exchange form	NA	No	Yes	NA
Records	• AE records • Evaluation records • Records for follow-up and inspection • Investigation protocol • Copies of test, laboratory reports, and service records	• Distribution records • Records for products manufactured • Records of problem report, its evaluation, and appropriate action taken	• AE records • Evaluation records • Customer/user complaint record • Records for products manufactured • Records of distributors • CAPA records	A mandatory specification for importers only
Recall/FSCA	Manufacturers need to initiate recall	Sponsors need to initiate a recall	Manufacturers need to initiate a recall	A mandatory specification for importers only
Recall communication	• Telephone calls, telegrams, and mailgrams • First class letters approved by FDA • General public warning • Public warning through specialized news media	• Recall letters approved within 48 hours of recall agreement • Paid advertisements to consumer/retail level approved by TGA	• FSN approved by MHRA as per specified format within 48 hours of FSCA agreement • In case of urgency, through telephone, fax, or by a visit	–

Abbreviations: AE, adverse event; AIMD, active implantable medical device; AITS, Adverse Incident Tracking System; CAPA, corrective and preventive actions; CDSCO, Central Drug Standard Control Organization; FDA, Food and Drug Administration; FSCA, field safety corrective actions; FSN, field safety notice; IMDTS, Implantable Medical Device Tracking Subcommittee; MDR, medical device reporting; MHRA, Medicines and Healthcare products Regulatory Agency; RAE, remedial action exemption; TGA, Therapeutic Goods and Administration.

Table 18.3: Comparison of the Device Adverse Reporting Systems in GHTF five members[9]

Purpose

Europe	USA	Canada	Australia	Japan
The purpose of the vigilance system is to improve the protection of health and safety of patients, users and others by reducing the likelihood of the same type of adverse incident being repeated in different places at different times. This is to be achieved by the evaluation of reported incidents and, where appropriate, dissemination of information which could be used to prevent such repetitions, or to alleviate the consequences of such incidents. The vigilance system is intended to allow data to be correlated between Competent Authorities and manufacturers and so facilitate corrective action earlier than would be the case if data were collected and action taken on a State by State basis	The purpose of the Medical Device Reporting Regulation is to ensure that manufacturers, (including those foreign), and importers promptly inform FDA of all serious injuries, deaths or malfunctions associated with marketed devices. User facilities report deaths and serious injuries. As the principal US public health agency responsible for ensuring that devices are safe and effective, FDA needs such information to evaluate the risk associated with a device in order to take whatever action is necessary to reduce or eliminate the public's exposure to this risk	The purpose of Mandatory Problem Reporting is to reduce the likelihood of recurrence of serious adverse incidents related to medical devices by evaluation of reported incidents and, where appropriate, dissemination of information which could be used to prevent repetitions or to alleviate the consequences of such incidents	The purpose of the Incident Reporting and Investigation Scheme is to support the Post-market monitoring processes under the Therapeutic Goods Act. Only a small, select group of high-risk, registered devices are evaluated by the TGA prior to being approved for sale on the market, the majority of products being listed on the Australian Register of Therapeutic Goods without evaluation. Postmarket monitoring is considered an important process to evaluate on-going quality, safety and efficacy of therapeutic devices available in the market	The purpose is to ensure that safety and effectiveness have been carefully evaluated before approval time, and expected adverse events and contraindications must be described on the labeling. Before the approval stage, the number of patients is restricted and only narrow ranged group of patients is involved in clinical trial. After approval, the device is used for a wide range of patients, and there is the possibility of unexpected adverse events which cannot be foreseen when the device is being approved. Therefore, any adverse events must be tracked to ensure safety for marketed device

Applicability

Europe	USA	Canada	Australia	Japan
These guidelines cover the activities of: • The Commission • Competent authorities • Notified bodies	The Medical Device Reporting regulation establishes requirements for: • Manufacturers • Importers • User facilities	The Medical Devices Regulations cover the activities of: • Medical Device Bureau • Bureau of Compliance and Enforcement	The Therapeutic Goods Act cover the activities of: • The Therapeutic Goods Administration • Manufacturers • Sponsors (manufacturers and importers)	These guidelines cover the activities of: • MHW (Ministry of Health & Welfare) • Medical facility (voluntary)

Contd...

Contd...

Europe	USA	Canada	Australia	Japan
• Manufacturers (including their authorized representatives and persons responsible for placing on the market, see Article 14 of the MDD) • Users and others concerned with the continuing safety of medical devices	Health professionals (physicians, physician assistants, pharmacists, nurses) and other consumers are encouraged to voluntarily report serious adverse events and product problems	• Manufacturers • Distributors	• Postmarket reporting of adverse events is mandatory for device sponsors when they become aware of a serious injury or death involving a device • A device sponsor is generally the legal entity which manufactures or imports a therapeutic device • Postmarket reporting of adverse events is voluntary, but strongly encouraged, of healthcare institutions or practitioners	• Manufacturer/Importer/Domestic agent for foreign manufacturer

Reporting Timing

Europe	USA	Canada	Australia	Japan
Mandatory reporting				

The report should be made as soon as possible. The time given below is the maximum elapsed time for determining the relevant facts and making an initial report. The time runs from the manufacturer first being informed of the incident, to the relevant Competent Authority receiving the notification from the manufacturer.
Incidents: 10 days
Near incidents: 30 days
	Adverse event report: The time from the date the manufacturer or user facility became aware of information that reasonably suggests that a device has or may have caused or contributed to the event to the date of the report.
	• Manufacturer
	  • Death, serious injury, reportable malfunctions: to FDA within 30 calendar days
	• User facility
	  • Death: to FDA and manufacturer within 10 working days
		Manufacturers and importers must report within the following time period the device related adverse events to the Bureau of Compliance and Enforcement.
		Incident: 10 days
		Near incident: 30 days
			Reporting times are not specified, but are predicated on the phrase "…as soon as possible after the sponsor becomes aware…"	Medical device manufacturers, importers and domestic agents for foreign manufacturers report within the following time period to the Safety Division of MHW after they become aware of an event:
				• Unlabeled serious incidents or near incidents—15 days
				• Labeled serious incidents or near incidents—30 days
				• Unlabeled medium level incidents or near incidence—30 days

Contd...

Contd...

Europe	USA	Canada	Australia	Japan

Mandatory reporting	Serious injury: To manufacturer within 10 working days. (Such reports shall be submitted to FDA if the device manufacturer is not known)
	• Distributor
	  • Death, serious injury, and malfunctions: To manufacturer within 10 working days
	  • Death, serious injury to FDA within 10 working days
	Manufacturer 5-Day Report: The time runs (in working days) from the manufacturer became aware that a reportable MDR event necessitated remedial action to prevent an unreasonable risk of substantial harm to the public health to the date of the report; or becoming aware of a reportable event for which FDA has made a written request for the submission of a 5-day report. When such a request is made, the manufacturer shall submit, without further requests, a 5-day report of all subsequent events of the same nature that involve substantially similar devices for the time period specified in the written request.
	Manufacturer Baseline Report: to be submitted for a device when the device model is first reported and to be updated annually on the anniversary month of the initial submission (Pending Guidance)
				• Serious incidents by infectious diseases that could be caused by using medical devices—15 days

Reporting Criteria	Europe	USA	Canada	Australia	Japan
Death/Serious injury	Death or serious deterioration in state of health: • Life-threatening illness or injury • Permanent impairment of a body function • Permanent impairment to a body structure	Death, or serious injury, which means an injury or illness that: • Is life-threatening • Results in permanent damage to a body structure • Results in permanent impairment of a body function (Permanent means irreversible, but not trivial, impairment or damage to a body structure or function)	Death or serious deterioration in state of health: • Life-threatening • Permanent damage to a body structure • Permanent impairment to a body function	Death or serious injury, is not specifically defined, but is taken to be: • Life-threatening • Resulting in permanent damage to a body structure • Resulting in permanent impairment of a body function.	Death or Serious injury means an injury or illness that: • Is life-threatening • Results in permanent damage to a body structure • Results in permanent impairment of a body function
Conditional serious injury	A condition necessitating medical or surgical intervention to prevent permanent impairment of a body function or permanent impairment of a body structure	An injury or illness that necessitates medical or surgical intervention to preclude permanent damage to a body structure or permanent impairment of a body function	Condition which necessitates medical or surgical intervention to prevent: • Permanent damage to a body structure • Permanent impairment to a body function	Conditional serious injury is not specifically defined, but is taken to be: • An injury requiring clinical intervention to prevent serious injury	Condition which necessitates medical or surgical intervention to prevent: • Permanent damage to a body structure • Permanent impairment to a body function
Malfunction	All reportable adverse events require there to have been a malfunction or deterioration in the characteristics and/or performance of a device which led to or might have led to death or a serious deterioration in health. Where	Device malfunction (or failure to meet performance specifications or otherwise perform as intended) such that the device or a similar device would be likely to cause a death or serious injury if the malfunction was to recur.	Malfunction or deterioration in the characteristics and/or performance of a device which might have led to death or serious deterioration in health: • Incident occurred and	Malfunction is not specifically defined, but is taken to be: • A failure of the device to perform as expected which has the potential to compromise patient or operator safety	Failure, malfunction, improper/inadequate design, manufacturing problem and improper/inadequate labeling which has led or may lead to death or damage if malfunctions re-occurs

Contd...

Contd...

Malfunction	
no serious injury/death occurred, it is sufficient that if the event occurred again in might lead to death/serious deterioration in health and is known as a near incident	• Performance specifications include all claims made in the labeling for the device • Intended use may be shown by labeling claims; advertising matter; oral or written statements A malfunction is considered likely to cause or contribute to a death or serious injury if: • The chance of it causing such an event is not remote or minute • It affects the device in a catastrophic manner that may lead to a death or serious injury • The manufacturer takes or would be required to take action to prevent a hazard to health as a result of the malfunction • A malfunction of the same type has actually caused or contributed to a death or serious injury in the past two years	• Is such that if it occurred again, it might lead to death or serious deterioration in health

User error	
User errors are generally outside of the adverse reporting system except when: • Examination of the device or labeling (inaccuracies in the instruction leaflet or instruction for use include omissions and deficiencies) indicated some factors which could lead to an incident involving death	• Use error (errors induced by poor design, poor labeling, poor instruction, etc. which could lead to an incident involving death or serious injury)	• Examination of the device or labeling (inaccuracies in the instruction leaflet or instruction for use include omissions and deficiencies) indicated some factors which could lead to an incident involving death or	User error is not specifically defined, but is taken to be: • A situation where patient or operator injury, or near injury, is caused by incorrect use, i.e. not following instructions or labeling when these are assessed as adequate for a "normal" or "reasonable" user	• Recall provisions address inadequate labeling which could lead to an incident involving death or serious injury. There are no such definite provisions in adverse incident reporting

Contd...

Contd...

User Error			
or serious deterioration in health	"Off label" use when either the device is not specified for the application or specifically contraindicated within the instructions for use or labeling	serious deterioration in health	Research literature which indicates the following items: • Serious effect to human health • Great change of the trend of adverse events • No effectiveness

Literature analysis			
No such guideline exists and the EU Vigilance guideline states "These guidelines make no recommendations on the structure of the systems by which manufacturers gather information concerning the use of devices in the post production phase". However, the directive indicates that "The manufacturer must undertake to institute and keep up to date a systematic procedure to review experience gained from device in the post production phase"	Reporting is required when the manufacturer becomes aware of a reportable incident regardless of its source such as literature reports	The Regulations do not specify how the manufacturer or importer becomes aware of reportable incidents, but simply that they must report them within certain time limits based on when they become "aware"	The Therapeutic Goods Act does not specify how a sponsor becomes aware of reportable events, but conditions imposed under the Act require that "Where the goods are distributed overseas as well as in Australia, product recall or any similar regulatory action taken in relation to the goods outside Australia which has or may have relevance to the quality safety or efficacy of the goods distributed in Australia must be notified. immediately the action or information is known to the sponsor"

Remedial action			
Not applicable	5-Day Manufacturer Report means a report submitted upon: • Becoming aware that a reportable event or events, necessitates remedial action to prevent an unreasonable risk of substantial harm to public health; or	Not applicable	Not applicable

Contd...

Contd...

	Remedial Action	Voluntary reports
	• Becoming aware of a reportable event for which FDA has made a written request for the submission of a 5-day report. When such a request is made, the manufacturer shall submit, without further requests, a 5-day report for all subsequent events of the same nature that involve substantially similar devices for the time period specified in the written request	
Voluntary reports		
Voluntary reports may be submitted at any time and may be other than death, serious injury or malfunction as defined	Voluntary reports may be submitted at any time and may be other than death, serious injury or malfunction as defined	Voluntary reports may be submitted at any time and may be other than death or serious injury or malfunction as defined. Reports of incidents (including those involving death or serious deterioration in health) from those other than manufacturers and importers (for example, hospitals, coroners, the public, etc.) are also considered voluntary reports	Voluntary reports may be submitted at any time and may be other than death or serious injury	Voluntary reports may be submitted at any time and may be other than death, serious injury or malfunction as defined

Vigilance Systems for Medical Devices

Applicable Forms

Europe	USA	Canada	Australia	Japan
• Initial Incident Report • Final Incident Report	• Mandatory adverse event report (MedWatch Form 3500A) for manufacturers, user facilities and importers • Voluntary adverse event report (MedWatch Form 3500) for health professionals and others • Baseline report for manufacturers (Form 3417) • Annual user facility report (Form 3419)	• A proforma incident reporting form (Medical Devices Problem Reporting Form; 1 July 1998) is available and preferred, but is not considered mandatory, providing that all information that would be required in the form is submitted	• A proforma incident reporting form is available but is not considered mandatory	• Initial and final reports as identified in form number 3-2

Not Reportable Incidents/Events

Europe	USA	Canada	Australia	Japan
• Single fault conditions for which the manufacturer has made provisions • Normal aging of the device* predicted in the information supplied with the device • Mishandling or user error* • Expected side effects* Risk was foreseeable and clinically acceptable in view of potential patient benefit • Outcome of the incident was adversely affected by a pre-existing condition of the patient • Events occurred outside of the European Union	• Adverse events for which there is information that would cause a person who is qualified to make a medical judgment (e.g. a physician, nurse, risk manager or biomedical engineer) to reach a reasonable conclusion that a device did not cause or contribute to a death or serious injury or that a malfunction would not be likely to cause or contribute to a death or serious injury if it were to recur • FDA may grant exemptions, variances or alternatives from, or to, any or all of the reporting requirements	• The Regulations have no provision for "Not Reportable Events". This topic may be covered in future guidance documents • Events occurred outside of Canada	• The Therapeutic Goods Act has no provision for "not reportable events" but these will be conferred in future guidance documents • Events occurred outside of Australia	• There are no definite provisions for "Not Reportable Events" except for mishandling or user error. Reporting is not required when an incident has obviously been caused by user's mishandling or error resulting from inadequate knowledge or techniques

* If provisions are made in labeling information

MEDICAL DEVICE REGULATIONS AND NEED FOR HARMONIZATION

Earlier there was rare existence of medical device regulations in most of the countries worldwide and there were limited regulatory controls in order to prohibit the use of low quality devices. Hence, there was a compulsion to draft regulatory policies for medical devices in order to assess their quality, safety and efficacy. Fortunately, since the early 1980s, there was an exceptional change in the regulatory paradigm for medical devices.[1,10]

Regulations are primarily concerned with enabling patient access to high quality, safe and effective medical devices, and restricting access to those products that are unsafe or have limited clinical use. When regulations are appropriately implemented they ensure benefit of the public health and the safety of patients, health care workers and the community. In this direction, the assisting member states of the WHO, through regulatory guidance, training, coordination and promotion of international best practices has set-up this as a priority for the Diagnostic Imaging and Medical Devices (DIM) team.

WHO has a mandate, as outlined in the World Health Assembly (WHA) Resolution 60.29 "to encourage member states to draw up national or regional guidelines for good manufacturing and regulatory practices, to establish surveillance systems and other measures to ensure the quality, safety and efficacy of medical devices and, where appropriate, to participate in international harmonization". Furthermore, WHO's Strategic Objective 11 states that it is necessary for WHO: "to ensure improved access, quality and use of medical products and technologies".

The 67th World Health Assembly (WHA) approved the resolution 20 named: "Regulatory system strengthening for medical products. It stated the importance of the regulations of medical devices as one of the medical products, for better outcome of the public health and to increase the access to safe, effective and quality medical products; and acknowledged the need for supporting the area of medical devices.

Some important notes in the WHA67.20 resolution reference to medical devices are the following:

- It URGES Member States: to strengthen national regulatory systems, to engage in global, regional and sub-regional networks of national regulatory authorities, and to promote international cooperation, as appropriate
- It REQUESTS the Director-General WHO: to prioritize support for establishing and strengthening regional and sub-regional networks of regulatory authorities, as appropriate, including strengthening areas of regulation of health products that are the least developed, such as regulation of medical devices, including diagnostics; and to support the building-up of effective national and regional regulatory bodies and networks. To report in five years to the WHA on the implementation.[11]

Policies, strategies, and action plans for health technologies, specifically for medical devices, are required in any national health plan. In accordance with the context of a robust health system they ensure access to safe, effective, and high-quality medical devices that prevent, diagnose, and treat disease and injury, and assist patients in their rehabilitation. As per the WHO guidance document on Development of medical device policies, it is necessary to create awareness of the importance of developing and implementing health technology policies—comprising of the regulatory, health technology management, and health technology assessment components in the context of the national health plan. It emphasizes on the role of medical devices in global health care and the prioritization of needs within Member States and discusses the key components of an effective policy, the organizational systems necessary for implementation of the policy, and the methodology for measuring progress.[12]

Now due to the availability of varying regulations of the countries or region on medical devices, there is a need to harmonize regulations in order to overcome regulatory hurdles and expedite access to high quality, safe and efficacious medical devices.

The idea of regulatory harmonization can improve the efficiency of national economies and their ability to adapt to change and to remain competitive. Firms can become more efficient, innovative, and competitive through harmonization sharpening the competitive pressures which provides powerful incentives. These reforms will boost the productivity of entire industries and often bring sharp and swift price reductions and will in turn leads to improvements in the quality and range of products and services, to the benefit of consumers and user industries.

After the era of liberalization followed by globalization, international boundaries are no longer an obstacle and the whole world is termed as a Global Village. In addition, concentrating little on changes in the world economy then it can be found that there is a slower growth in USA, EU, and Japan while the growth is robust in developing countries with sustained and rapid growth in China and India continuing their higher growth potential. Developing economies have a desire to ensure safety and performance of products brought to their markets. The pricing pressure is gradually increasing due to competitive pressure. There is an impromptu need for a better operating model because traditional methods of business, technology, and competition are blurring; the definition of customer is changing; regulatory scrutiny is increasing; because of continuous regulatory pressure on governments and industry with scarcity of resources both human and financial; international market is big and getting bigger; and demographic trends are driving fundamental changes in the global economy.[1,13]

Regulatory systems for medical devices are less developed than those for other health products such as medicinal products or vaccines. According to the 2013 WHO Baseline Country Survey on Medical Devices, only 69% of 175 responding countries had a national authority responsible for implementing and enforcing medical device regulations (Fig. 18.1).

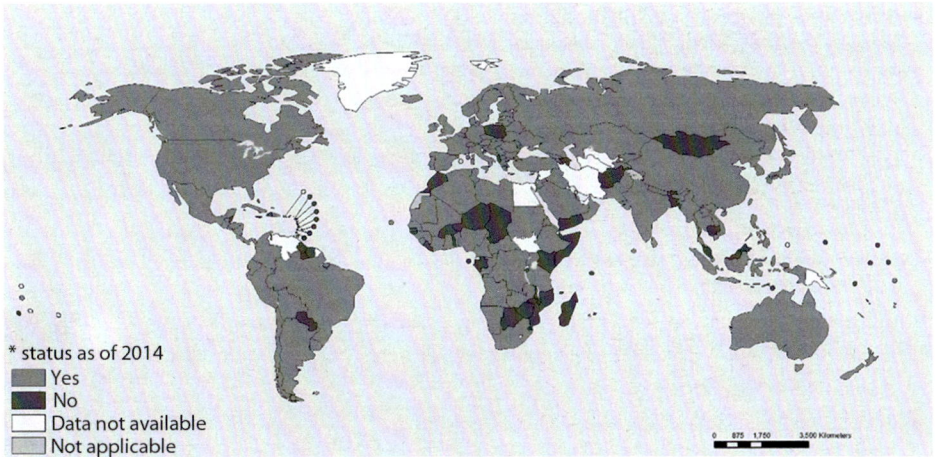

Fig. 18.1: Global distribution of National Regulatory Agency for Medical Devices, WHO 2014.

Many of those governments that have drafted regulations have made little progress in implementing them. WHO has a clear role and mandate in building regulatory capacity through training and harmonization and is committed to this important work, with the support of all stakeholders.[14]

Elements of effective national health policies, strategies, and plans
National health policies, strategies, and plans must articulate in a comprehensive, balanced, and coherent fashion:[12]

- Vision, values, goals, targets, and intersectoral policy alignment
- A robust *situation analysis*, covering:
  - Assessment of social determinants of health and health needs, including current and projected disease burdens and health challenges
  - Assessment of expectations, including current and projected demand for services as well as social expectations
  - Assessment of health system performance and of performance gaps in responding to needs and expectations
  - Assessment of the capacity of the health sector to respond to current and to anticipate future challenges
  - Assessment of health system resources (human, physical, financial, informational) and of resource gaps in responding to needs and expectations
  - Assessment of stakeholder positions (including, where appropriate, of external partners)
- The possible scenarios and policy directions for:
  - Improving health equity
  - Making services people-centred so as to respond to priority needs and expectations
  - Protecting and promoting the health of communities and public health
  - Building the capacity to deal with crisis and future challenges
- A comprehensive strategy to respond to the challenges and implement the policy directions
- The implications of these policy directions for:
  - Service delivery (service networks as well as programmes, actions aimed at individuals as well as public health actions aimed at populations)
  - Health workforce; medical products and technologies, and infrastructure
  - Information
  - Health financing, and
  - Governance of the health sector
- Their implications for working with other sectors:
  - Their resource implications and the associated costs
  - The investment strategy and a strategy for mobilizing the funds required
  - The leadership and governance arrangements for implementing the strategy in terms of:
    - Role of various institutions and stakeholders
    - Monitoring performance, measuring outcomes, organizing research and adapting the strategy to changing circumstances
    - Regulatory and legal frameworks to ensure sustain ability;
    - Working with other sectors to ensure health is taken into consideration in all policies;
    - Dealing with the donor community in countries where donor funding is an important contributor to financing the health sector.

How these content components are sequenced and partitioned among policy, strategy and planning documents, and where the emphasis is put, depends to quite some extent on the specific country-context.

MEDICAL DEVICE REGULATIONS

The initiation of the postmarket surveillance of medical devices was in the United States with the enforcement of the Food and Drug Administration Modernization Act 1970 under Section 522 for class II and class III devices. In 1989, the Therapeutic Goods Act was introduced in Australia which provided the legal basis for uniform national controls over goods used in the prevention, diagnosis, curing, or alleviation of a disease, ailment, defect, or injury. In June 1993, the vigilance requirement for medical devices for member states and manufacturers was published as Council Directive 90/385/EEC and 93/42/EEC, followed by incorporation of amendments of revision 5 of MEDDEV guidance 2.12–1 [1] in 2007 by the European Union. In order to achieve uniformity between the national medical device regulatory systems and to increase the access to safe, effective, and clinically beneficial medical technologies, the Global Harmonization Task Force (GHTF) was conceived in 1992 by five members: European Union, United States, Australia, Japan, and Canada wherein the vigilance of devices was among the study groups.[8]

India

The Central Drug Standards Control Organization (CDSCO) which is a part of the Ministry of Health and Family Welfare is currently regulating the medical devices in India. In 2006, Medical Devices Regulation Bill (MDRB) was introduced with an aim to enforce and strengthen laws related to medical devices and institute the Medical Device Regulatory Authority of India (MDRA). The motive of the bill was to create and sustain a national system of controls for the quality, safety and accessibility of medical devices in India. Currently, actions related to medical devices are governed by the Drugs and Cosmetics Act, 1940 and Rules, 1945. Most recently in August, 2013, the Drugs and Cosmetics (Amendment) Bill, 2013 was introduced. Among the other things, this bill also includes a separate chapter for regulatory measures for import, manufacture, sale, distribution and export of medical devices in India. For the purpose of import of medical devices in India, the procedure for registration and import license as prescribed under the Drugs and Cosmetics Rules shall be followed. Imported medical devices that have already obtained approval in the United States (by the FDA) or the European Union (by CE Marking) are allowed on the Indian market-without undergoing separate conformity assessment procedures however it applies to those devices that are notified in the list.[1]

United States

In the United States, the Federal Food Drug and Cosmetic Act regulates the medical device. The marketing application must be submitted to the Food and Drug Administration (FDA) and approval must be received before marketing the medical device in the United States. The Centre for Devices and Radiological Health (CDRH) within FDA is primarily accountable for pre-and postmarket supervision of medical devices in the United States. A risk-based classification for medical devices has been adopted in the United States wherein the devices are classified according to the risk associated with the use of the device. Devices are classified into a 3-tiered system (Class I-lowest risk; Class II-intermediate risk; Class III highest risk).

Class I Devices

This class comprise of devices that do not lead to a likely preposterous hazard of patient ailment or injury. These low-risk devices are regulated with general controls, which are well-accepted norms related to labeling, manufacturing, postmarket surveillance, and

Flowchart 18.1: Simplified overview of the regulatory process in India[15]

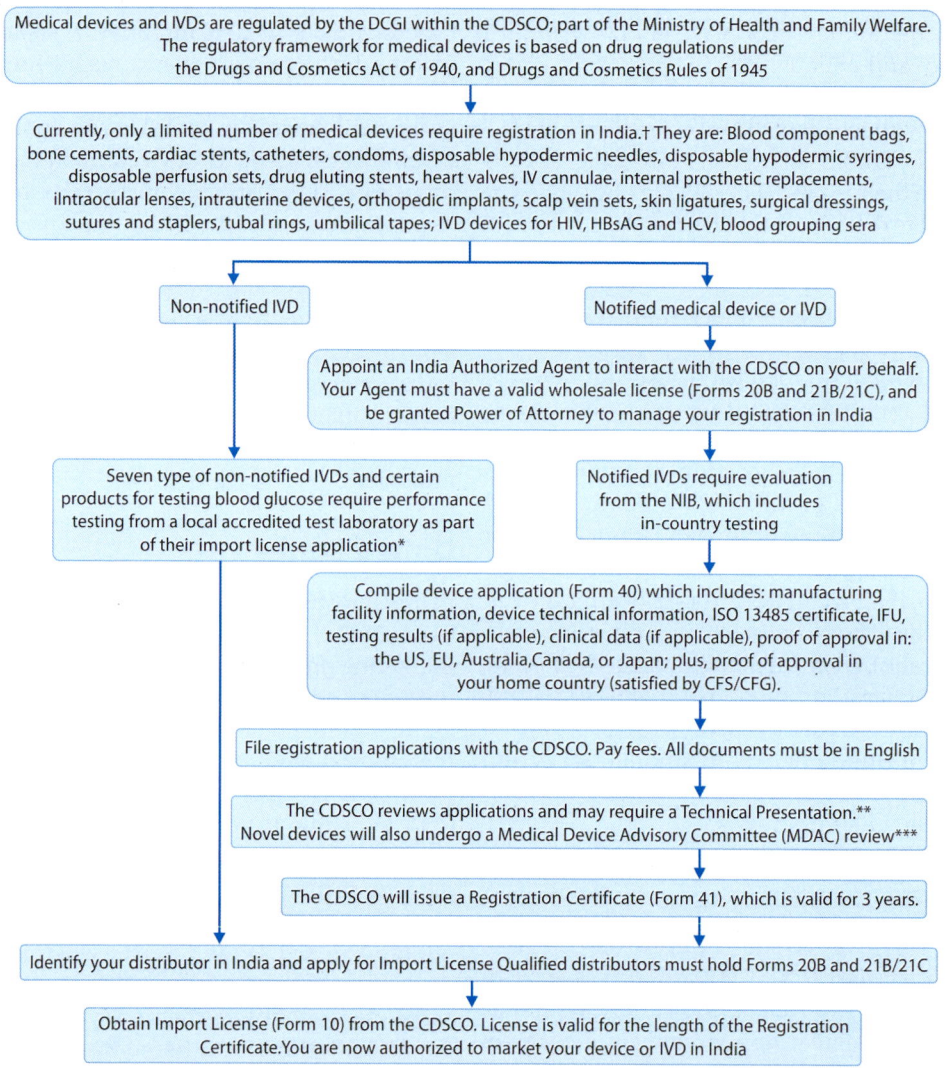

Abbreviations: DCGI, Drug Controller General of India; CDSCO, central drug standard control organization; IV, intravenous; HIV, human immunodeficiency virus; HBsAG, hepatitis B surface antigen; HCV, hepatitis C virus; IVD, in vitro diagnostic device; NIB, National Institute of Biological

† Please note some products, e.g. dental implants, do not appear on the official list, however, they do require registration. All IVDs require an Import License before they may be brought to market. Medical devices which do not require registration have no restrictions and may be imported directly. Please contact us for details.

* The seven types of non-notified IVDs requiring performance testing are: malaria, dengue, chikungunya, syphilis, typhoid, tuberculosis, and cancer markers. Blood glucose test strips and fully automated analyzer based glucose reagents will require performance testing from NIB, similar to Notified IVDs.

** Approximately 75% of applications will require a formal Technical Presentation with the CDSCO in India. The technical presentation is an in-person discussion about the product, any predicates on the market, market research, etc. A representative from the manufacturer (such as an engineer) is expected to attend this meeting along with the India Authorized Agent.

*** Devices novel to the Indian market (new material or intended use, etc.) may require clinical studies conducted in India before a Registration Certificate will be granted, or possibly a restricted approval, with the requirement to actively collect and submit post-market data. The MDAC meeting will include local surgeons and experts, who will weigh in on the acceptability of the existing clinical data.

reporting. Devices are assigned class I status when there is a credible surety that general controls alone will be sufficient to assure safety and effectiveness. Moreover, counter measures such as seizure, recall prerogative, etc. have been granted to the FDA. Formal FDA scrutiny is not intended for most class I devices before their market launch. The FDA does not evaluate these products separately nor is there a requirement that safety and effectiveness of the individual product be confirmed before launch. Some examples of products in class I category are handheld surgical instruments, tongue depressors and crutches, etc.

Class II Devices

Class II devices are those higher-risk devices for which only general controls are insufficient to establish safety and effectiveness, and for which, there are sufficient data to substantiate special controls. Because these devices pose a greater risk of harm compared to class I devices and hence they are scrutinized by added regulation of special controls, which may be confirmed by the FDA. Also, the majority of class II devices need FDA clearance of a premarket notification 510(k) process before the device is launched. In the 510(k) process, the medical device manufacturer must submit data to demonstrate that the new device is comparable to a legally marketed device. Even though this can generally be corroborated based on the bench and animal testing alone, very few 510(k) applications need to submit clinical data. Generally, this class of device includes high technology products such as cardiac monitors, tampons, infusion pumps, surgical drapes and oxygen masks.

Class III Devices

The class III devices are those which are either life-sustaining/supporting or of considerable importance in supporting impairment of human health. Examples of class III devices are pacemakers, heart valves, coronary stents, etc. Since, they are judged to pose the highest potential risk of illness or injury, hence, general and special controls alone are insufficient to establish safety and effectiveness. Therefore, most class III devices need premarket approval (PMA) from FDA before they can be launched.

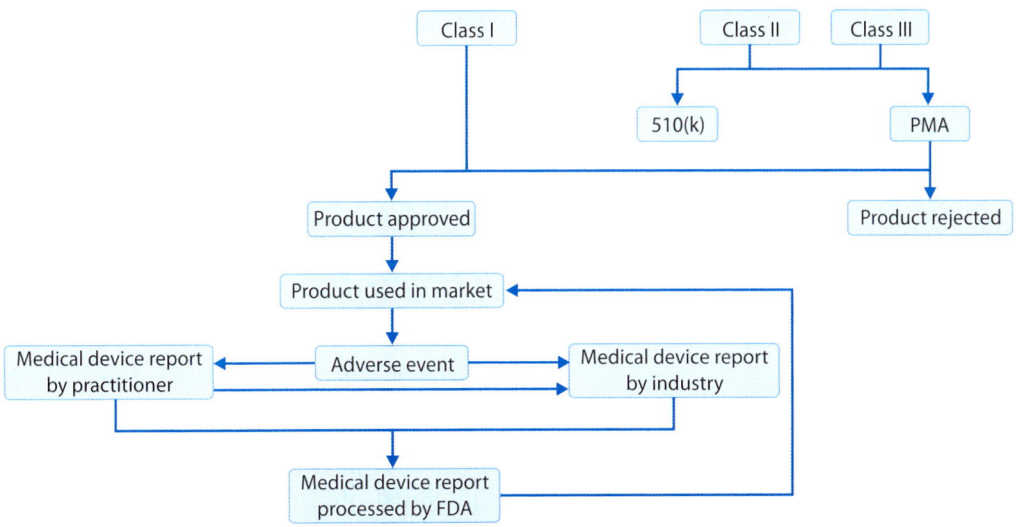

Flowchart 18.2: Medical device regulation and reporting pathway in US[16]
Abbreviations: PMA, postmarket approval; FDA, Food and Drug Administration

Postmarket Approval Process

To assess the safety and efficacy for all class III devices a postmarket approval (PMA) review process is followed. This is the most rigorous regulatory procedures for medical devices. The PMA process requires clinical study to demonstrate the safety and effectiveness prior to marketing approval because class III devices are either life sustaining/supporting or of considerable importance in averting impairment of human health. Due to the high level of risk associated with Class III devices, FDA has determined that general and special controls alone are insufficient to assure the safety and effectiveness of class III devices. Therefore, these devices require a PMA application under section 515 of the FD&C Act in order to obtain marketing clearance. It is the most stringent type of device marketing application required by FDA. The applicant must receive FDA approval of its PMA application prior to marketing the device. In order to get a postmarket approval, the application is based on a determination by FDA that the PMA contains sufficient valid scientific evidence to assure that the device is safe and effective for its intended use(s). An approved PMA is, in effect, a private license granting the applicant (or owner) permission to market the device. FDA regulations provide 180 days to review the PMA and make a determination. The regulation governing premarket approval is stated in Title 21 Code of Federal Regulations (CFR) Part 814, Premarket Approval. A class III device that fails to meet PMA requirements is considered to be adulterated under section 501(f) of the FD&C Act and cannot be marketed.

Premarket Notification 510(K) Process

A 510(k) process is a premarket submission made to the FDA in order to establish that the device to be marketed is safe and effective. Most class II devices need pre-market entry notification (termed 510k). It is basically a regulatory review process which is less rigorous compared to the PMA process. The 510k submission must demonstrate that the new device is comparable to an already marketed device in the United States. It is the duty of the sponsor to ascertain a suitable device to which they need to demonstrate that their new device is comparable. Before marketing clearance, the manufacturer must also ensure that the device is adequately labeled in accordance with FDA's labeling requirements. Most device applications receiving marketing clearance under the 510(k) process are on the basis of preclinical testing only. Sometimes when there are apprehensions regarding safety and effectiveness, the FDA can demand clinical data for 510(k) clearance.[1]

Canada

The medical device is classified based on the Canadian Risk-Based Classification System (RBCS), under the aegis of the Therapeutic Products Division (TPD) of Health Canada. Health Canada has adopted a four-tier classification system for medical devices based on their risk to the human body. Devices posing the lowest risk to the human body have been classified under Class I and Class IV poses the highest risk. The scrutiny increases with the risk of the device since Health Canada employs a risk-based process for the regulation of medical devices. Class I devices are reckoned to be lower risk device and postmarket monitoring is adjudged to be enough. Class II devices are licensed and are subject to the safety and efficacy needs of the regulations. In addition, manufacturers must acquire a valid Quality Systems certification, along with the post market controls. The higher risk devices of Class III and IV have the added obligations and must fulfil the regulatory prerequisites of a premarket safety and efficacy assessment.[1]

Japan

In Japan, the analysis, assessment and suggestions on decisions regarding the medical devices are taken by the Pharmaceuticals Medical Devices Agency (PMDA), a regulatory agency founded in 2004, which is further suggested to the Ministry of Health, Labor and Welfare (MHLW) as PMDA has no jurisdiction to take eventual decisions. The whole medical device regulatory scheme, in addition to the national health protection system, public health, medical facilities and labor and welfare matters are seen by the MHLW which is a powerful central ministry amalgamating political authorization and accountability. A new law was passed in the year 2005 in harmonization with the international stipulations. The law is known as the New Pharmaceutical Affairs Law (PAL). There is some difference as compared to the international stipulations as the additional requirements are needed for manufacturing and building spaces. So, a manufacturer has to work in accordance with the market authorization holder (MAH) process and the former is only accountable for production while the latter holds the responsibility of launching the product to market. In Japan, medical devices are classified into General Medical devices (Class I), Controlled Medical Devices (Class II) and Specially Controlled Medical Devices (Class III and IV). A manufacturer must also get a device notification, device certificate or device approval based on the class of device. Medical devices in class I need a device notification, medical devices in class II need a device certificate and medical devices class III and IV need a device approval. Clinical trials are not required for class I, in principle not necessary for class II, sometimes necessary for class III and in principle compulsory for class IV. In Japan, it is compulsory to follow good pharmacovigilance practice (GVP).[1]

Table 18.2: MHRA classification of general medical devices[8]

Class of device	Risk level	Requirements	Example
Class I	Low risk	Premarket notification	Dressings
Class IIa	Low–medium risk	Certification by notified body	X-ray film
Class IIb	Medium–high-risk	Certification by notified body	Blood bags, contact lens care products
Class II	High-risk	Certification by notified body	Bone cement, cardiac stents

MEDICAL DEVICE MARKET: FOCUSING *BRICS*

These leading emerging economies represent a total medical market of US$ 26.8 billion. But how might the impact of the economic downturn affect them? Where do commercial opportunities exist for medical device companies now, and what are the future prospects?

With an enormous population of 30 billion people and with significant unmet medical needs, there are considerable challenges and opportunities of the *BRIC* markets. The economic downturn has affected these markets varyingly; for example, the Brazilian import market may be affected by disadvantageous US$ exchange rates, but China is affected more by a weak economy in the USA, in its major market significant growth rates are impressive, but the low starting point—along with a range of other operational issues—means companies must be targeted in the opportunities they pursue.

There are wide regional differences in the expenditure levels within the *BRIC* countries as compared to the developed countries where health systems have evolved to provide a more uniform level of coverage. All four countries have a relatively wealthy urban population with a greater spending power than their respective national average. These urban populations have grown rapidly, and number hundreds of millions. The challenge for these countries is the extension of this level of wealth to the rest of the population, in order to provide an affordable level of healthcare.

The prevailing economic woes have to be considered over the long-term. Since, this is evolution not revolution and change will be incremental. Short-term opportunities exist in meeting the health demands of the burgeoning middle classes, and future prospects are bright, where steady growth in *BRIC* markets will erode commercial differences with the established markets in North America, Japan and Europe.

Highlights from the Region

Brazil

Brazil has the largest economy and medical device market in Latin America, but per capita medical expenditure is still very low. The highest expenditure is in the large cities, such as Sao Paulo or Rio de Janeiro, but producers are moving into regional markets outside the major state capitals. GDP growth was 3.5% in 2013 and is expected to grow to an average of 4.1% through 2018. With a growing economy, if inflation is kept in check, there will be more money available to spend on healthcare both in the public and private sectors.

Russia

In 2012, the Russian market for medical equipment and supplies was estimated at US$ 5,455.7 million. Despite the rapid growth, especially of imported products, in the 2007-11 period the per capita spending is low by European standards at US$39 per capita. Russian medical device manufacturers are generally small and under-capitalized, and tend to produce obsolete products; they can only compete with Western products in terms of cost. The country has a strong scientific research base with no experience of commercializing new products. Exports are low and centreed on other former USSR markets. In November 2010, the government developed a strategy that will help the medical device industry to attract investment, create new jobs and produce competitive, safe, good quality and affordable products to fulfill the healthcare system's requirements. Currently, the bulk of high-tech medical equipment comes from abroad. If the objectives of the plan are realized, by 2020, the local industry will be able to meet 50% of the local demand for medical devices.

India

The Indian market for medical equipment and supplies ranks among the world's top 20 but, despite strong growth rates, the market remains disproportionately small with per capita spending of US$24. The dominant healthcare provider is the private sector, particularly in urban areas, and as such is the major end-user of medical equipment. High quality, high tech products are sought after, particularly by facilities run by corporate groups such as Apollo Hospitals and Fortis Healthcare. The latest Five Year Plan (2012-17) proposed an ambitious expansion of healthcare services including doubling the level of public health spending to 2.5% of GDP and increasing health insurance coverage from 25 to 75%. Because of the lack of healthcare infrastructure, the government's plans mark an opportunity for private investors, and manufacturers of medical devices, as new facilities are constructed and existing ones are upgraded. Central Drugs Standard Control Organization (CDSCO), Ministry of Health and Family Welfare, Government of India issued Medical Device Rules 2017 vide G.S.R. 78(E) dated 31st January 2017, which will be effective from 1st January 2018.

China

For 2012, Espicom estimates market growth to be in the region of 21.4%; one of the fastest growing markets in the world. High rates of growth are not uncommon in the Asian region, but on the back of a huge market size, China's growth is particularly pronounced. Annual data till December 2012 reported that imports have grown very strongly during the period, rising by 20.8% to reach US$10,329 million. All product categories posted strong growth during the period, with orthopedic and prosthetic products leading the way with a rise of 51.4% over the previous year. All other categories achieved at least 15% growth during the period. The prospects for medical device spending is huge; the government has committed heavily in the construction of thousands of hospitals, healthcare centres, clinics and this will inevitably lead to spending on capital goods, most notably medical devices, equipment and furniture at an unprecedented rate in a relatively short space of time. In addition, there is a continuous encouragement by the government for the development of the private sector in order to cater for the growing needs of China's middle classes and restrictions on foreign investors operating hospitals have also been lifted.

South Africa

South Africa has a particularly low provision of doctors at less than one doctor (0.7) per thousand population. In 2008, of the total 34,687 doctors or medical practitioners registered with the Health Professions Council of South Africa (HPCSA), only 30.7%, or 10,653, were working in the public sector with the majority working in the private sector. This means the provision rate for doctors in the public sector is just 0.2 per thousand population. The long-term growth prospects of the South African medical device market will be strongly influenced by the ANC government's policies in regards to the new National Health Insurance (NHI) scheme, the promotion of public-private partnerships to develop and upgrade hospitals, the serious shortage of healthcare personnel and an urgent need to effectively address the AIDS crisis in the country. The government has committed itself to increasing the level of healthcare spending and has launched a 14-year programme to implement universal healthcare coverage. A key driver of growth can be the public-private partnerships to develop hospitals in South Africa but this could be tempered slightly, by a depreciating rate against the US dollar and the general state of the South African economy. The medium-term prospects for the medical device industry look encouraging; based on current trends, the market, of which over 90% is supplied by imports, is expected to grow at a CAGR of 8.7% from 2012-2017. Imports reached a new record high of US$1,178.9 million in 2011, rising by 20.3% over the previous year and expanding at a CAGR of 8.1% during the 2007-2011 period. Imports fell in 2009 following poor economic conditions but bounced back with two consecutive years of growth.[17]

REFERENCES

1. Gupta SK. Medical device regulations: a Current perspective. Journal of Young Pharmacists. 2016;8(1):6-11.
2. http://www.who.int/medical_devices/definitions/en/.
3. WHO global model regulatory framework for medical devices including IVD medical devices. Available at http://www.who.int/medicines/areas/quality_safety/quality_ assurance/ModelregulatoryFramework_MedDev_QAS16-664Rev2.pdf?ua=1

4. Medical device definition available at http://www.fda.gov/MedicalDevices/DeviceRegulationandGuidance/Overview/ClassifyYourDevice/ucm051512.htm.
5. Definition of medical devices from Medical Devices Directive (Directive 93/42/EEC) available at https://www.gov.uk/guidance/decide-if-your-product-is-a-medicine-or-a-medical-device.
6. Definition of medical device from medical device rules, 2016 assessed at http://www.cdsco.nic.in/writereaddata/Draft_Medical%20Devices%20Rules%202016.pdf.
7. Definition available at https://www.tga.gov.au/what-medical-device.
8. Gupta P, Janodia MD, Jagadish PC, Udupa N. Medical device vigilance systems: India, US, UK, and Australia. Medical Devices (Auckland, NZ). 2010;3:67-79.
9. Comparison of the Device Adverse Reporting Systems in USA, Europe, Canada, Australia & Japan. Final document of the global harmonization task force. Available at http://www3.hbmsp.sipa.gov.tw/itri/tw/images/download/zy/GHTF/Guidance_1-5.pdf.
10. Brolin S. Global Regulatory Requirements for Medical Devices. 2008. Available from: URL: http://mdh.divaportal.org/smash/get/diva2:121327/FULLTEXT01.Pdf
11. Quality and safety regulations for medical devices available at http://www.who.int/medical_devices/safety/en/.
12. WHO guidance document on Development of medical device policies. Available at http://apps.who.int/iris/bitstream/10665/44600/1/9789241501637_eng.pdf.
13. Saini KS, Kaushik A, Anil B, Rambabu S. Harmonized medical device regulation: need, challenges, and risks of not harmonizing the regulation in Asia. Journal of Young Pharmacists. 2010;2(1):101-6.
14. Global statistics and map available at http://www.who.int/medical_devices/safety/en/.
15. Regulatory process overview of India available at www.Emergogroup.com/india.
16. Teow N, Siegel SJ. FDA Regulation of Medical Devices and Medical Device Reporting. Pharmaceut Reg Affairs 2013;2(2):110.
17. BRICS medical device market report available at http://www.reportlinker.com/p01201769-summary/BRICS-Medical-Device-Market-Reports.html.

19

Data Management in Pharmacovigilance

Kamal Akhtar, Manoj Sharma

INTRODUCTION

Pharmacovigilance is a term that has originated from two separate terms:
Pharmakon (Greek) = Medical substance
Vigilia (Latin) = To keep watch

Pharmacovigilance (PV) is defined as the science and activities relating to the detection, assessment, understanding and prevention of adverse effects or any other drug-related problem.[1]

It includes premarketing (clinical development) as well as postmarketing (surveillance) stages of analyzing the safety of the drug. The various aspects of drug safety that can captured during the different stages of drug development can be seen in Figure 19.1.

The objectives of pharmacovigilance are:
- To detect the side effects of the drug that were unknown
- To evaluate the benefits against risks
- To identify the information that could be useful for consumers
- To overcome the risks to make the drug safe for use
- To monitor the drug during consumption for trends.

ROLE OF SOFTWARE/COMPUTER-BASED SYSTEMS

Pharmacovigilance requires collection and assimilation of data from all sources including but not limiting to spontaneous reports,

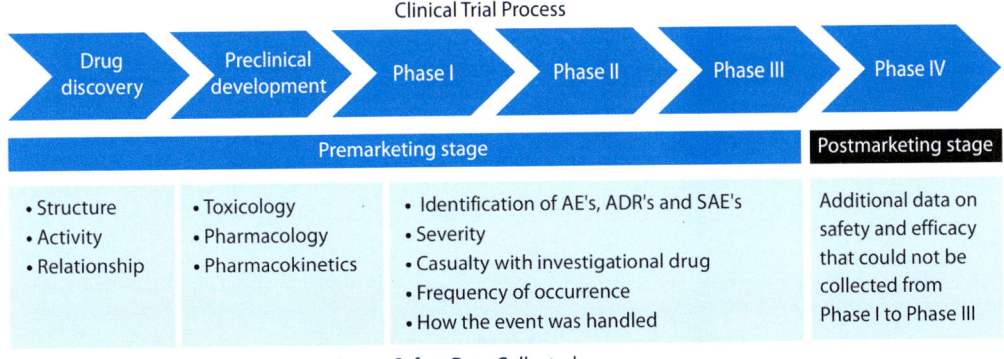

Fig. 19.1: Safety data collected during the various phases of drug development

literature reports, media reports, clinical trials and other sources. The data collected requires the processing of data, i.e. data entry, data reconciliation from the source documents, data review, and finally data analysis. The handling of data in a paper based format involves a plethora of challenges especially at the time when huge data is received by the MAH.

With the advent of softwares and computer-based systems the work load and administrative burdens can be reduced. In case of pharmacovigilance activities where data is generated from clinical trial source, the software helps investigators to easily create the protocol, track the participants enrollment and their progress. It not only tracks the financial activity associated in a clinical trial but also facilitates the better communication between team members. For administrators it helps to maintain trials and financial activity related to multiple departments, investigators and participants, facilitate compliance and support institution-specific processes.

Softwares are broadly divided into different domains.[2]
1. Clinical trial management system.
2. Clinical data management (CDM).
3. Softwares for pharmacovigilance.

Clinical Trial Management System

Clinical trial management system (CTMS) is involved in management and recruitment of subjects, investigator management of investigator at the study site and CRO site. This software system maintains and manages planning, performing and reporting functions. It is used at the sites where clinical research is conducted such as research hospitals, physician practices, academic medical centres and cancer centres and pharmaceutical and biotechnology industries. For example, the softwares for CTMS include: Open clinica: Realtime CTMS: Allergo CTMS and others.

Clinical Data Management

Clinical data management (CDM) is the process of collection, cleaning, and management of subject data in compliance with regulatory standards. The primary objective of CDM processes is to provide high-quality data by keeping the number of errors and missing data as low as possible and gather maximum data for analysis. To meet this objective, best practices are adopted to ensure that data are complete, reliable, and processed correctly. This has been facilitated by the use of software applications that maintain an audit trail and provide easy identification and resolution of data discrepancies. Sophisticated innovations have enabled CDM to handle large trials and ensure the data quality even in complex trials.

Some of the processes involved in CDM include: Case report form (CRF) designing, CRF annotation, data base designing, data entry, data validation, discrepancy management, medical coding, data extraction and data base locking.[2]

Tools for CDM

Many software tools are available for data management, and these are called clinical data management systems (CDMS). In multicentric trials, a CDMS has become essential to handle the huge amount of data. Most of the CDMS used in pharmaceutical companies are commercial, but a few open source tools are available as well. Commonly used CDM tools are ORACLE CLINICAL, CLINTRIAL, MACRO, RAVE, and eClinical Suite. In terms of functionality, these software tools are more or less similar and there is no significant advantage of one system over the other. These software tools are expensive and need sophisticated Information Technology infrastructure to function. Additionally, some multinational pharmaceutical giants use custom-made CDMS tools to suit their operational needs and procedures. Among the open source tools, the most prominent ones are OpenClinica, openCDMS, TrialDB, and PhOSCo. These CDM software are available free of cost and are as good as their commercial counterparts in terms of functionality. These open source software can be downloaded from their respective websites.[2]

In regulatory submission studies, maintaining an audit trail of data management activities is of paramount importance. These CDM tools ensure the audit trail and help in the management of discrepancies. According to the roles and responsibilities (explained later), multiple user IDs can be created with access limitation to data entry, medical coding, database designing, or quality check. This ensures that each user can access only the respective functionalities allotted to that user ID and cannot make any other change in the database. For responsibilities where changes are permitted to be made in the data, the software will record the change made, the user ID that made the change and the time and date of change, for audit purposes (audit trail). During a regulatory audit, the auditors can verify the discrepancy management process; the changes made and can confirm that no unauthorized or false changes were made.

In clinical data management process, the adverse events received are coded using Medical dictionary for coding of events. The coding classifies the medical terms on the CRF to standard dictionary terms so as to avoid unnecessary duplication and to maintain the uniformity in the process. It helps in proper coding of medical terminologies related to the trial. Various medical dictionaries are used which are available online, commonly, Medical Dictionary for Regulatory Activities (MedDRA) is used for the coding of adverse events as well as other illnesses. WHO-DDE (World Health Organization Drug Dictionary Enhanced)—coding the medications. WHO-ART (World Health Organization-Adverse Reactions Terminoogy). WHO-HD—World Health Organization Herbal Dictionary and concomitant medications (CM).[3]

Softwares for Pharmacovigilance

The softwares used in the management of individual case safety reports are known as safety databases. These databases are used by the personnel working in the drug safety department to perform the following functions:
- Data entry
- Review of the ICSR
- Medical review
- Generation of report in the reporting format viz. Council for International Organization of Medical Sciences Form (CIOMS I), Standard Generalized Markup Language (SGML), Form 3500A, etc.

The safety data base is also used for signal detection in adverse drug reactions.

Commonly used Safety Databases (Softwares for Pharmacovigilance)

- **Aris G:** It's the world's leading pharmacovigilance and clinical safety system. It manages adverse event reporting and adverse reaction requirements not just for drugs but also for vaccines, biologics and devices. It is flexible and fully scalable that is it can be used by both small companies in the early stages of clinical Trials for reporting severe adverse events and large organizations with worldwide pharmacovigilance operations.
- **ARGUS:** It provides comprehensive foundation for case management and reporting also helps to manage the data from multiple sources, meet strict global compliance guidelines and have access to flexible drug safety databases.

- **Oracle AERS:** Provides single global solution in managing worldwide safety information. It involves reporting and analysis of serious adverse events for all medicinal products including drugs, medical devices, vaccines, biologics, gene therapies.

HAROM (Human Adverse Reaction Online Monitoring System): One of it's kind is the world's most comprehensive real-time source of individual case safety reports (ICSRs) management. It is used to maintain continually updated information of ICSRs in more than 150 countries. It provides a single source to carry out an easy processing and reporting of ICSRs for legal pharmacovigilance obligation globally. HAROM has been designed to fasten the process of Case Processing in Pharmacovigilance which helps Pharmaceutical and Clinical Research Organizations to manage ICSRs data from multiple sources, meeting strict global compliance guidelines, and access with ease.[5]

Tools for Postmarketing Surveillance

VigiFlow: It helps in the collection and analysis of individual case safety reports.

VigiLyze: This facilitates the analysis of VigiBase data. It is a powerful search and analysis tool that provides access to Global, regional or National view of an ADR and Monitor international patient safety data.

VigiBase: Gives the information about safety profile of drugs and competitive products and optimize the queries.

PaniFlow: Helps to monitor ADR following administration of drugs and vaccines against influenza virus during the pandemic.[6]

METHODS OF SAFETY DATA ANALYSIS

There are essentially two methods of analysis of safety data:

1. **Paper-based method:** This method involves the comparison of data stored in the database against primary medical records. The analysis obtained is audited by a second party which follows the same procedure. The drawback of this method is that the analysis is not reproducible (subsequent analysis cannot query this analysis for results) and there is no real-time auditing of the data.
2. **Computer-based methods:** The traditional computer-based methods were similar to paper-based methods as they consisted of discrete and ad hoc processes. They consist of COTS (commercial off the shelf) software. The software has the ability to analyze safety data using various methods. The drawbacks of these methods are that no real time auditing is possible, analysis is not reproducible and the analysis process is non-systematic and not well-integrated. The most common computer-based methods are:
   - *Indexing and hyperlinking*: The tools that use this method can analyze the safety data as they have the ability to search for terms within an electronic document/e-CRF through full-text indexing, hyperlinking, and built in navigational modules. Examples of some of these tools are Adobe Acrobat, Microsoft Word and Excel.
   - *Importation:* The tools that use this method can analyze safety data as they have the ability to import tabulations of the Case Report Forms using a method known as the ECRT (Electronic Case Report Tabulation). Examples of some of these tools are SAS, Microsoft Access and JMP.

Until the year 1968 the FDA collected and analyzed safety data using traditional methods of pen and paper. It was in 1968 that the FDA developed a computerized repository where adverse drug reactions could be voluntarily reported by consumers during postmarketing surveillance. However, even then the analysis was still done manually until the 1980s.

In 1990s there was an IT boom. Personal computers were common and softwares were developed to computationally analyze the adverse drug reactions. However, these softwares were standalone and were lacking common standards, interoperatibility and integration to provide true systematic computational analysis of safety data.

As a result of the lack of reproducibility and real time auditing, negative results may be suppressed in the analysis and safety issues may remain hidden. Thus, there is a requirement that all the postmarketing safety data should be readily accessible to take an effective, informed decision during post-marketing surveillance.

FDA started out in the effort to implement standardized interoperable systems and databases to collect both premarketing and postmarketing safety data for systematic analysis and decision making. The effort has shown huge benefits in the collection and assessment of safety data.

Today there are several issues in pharmacovigilance that need to be addressed. Some of them are as follows:
1. Many ADR's mimic the disease and vice versa—Can you truly determine whether it is an ADR or the symptom of the disease itself?
2. Absence of standards for collection, transformation and presentation of Safety data.
Lack of integrated systems to systematically access premarketing and postmarketing data and absence of standard tools for conducting the analysis.

INFORMATICS IN PHARMACOVIGILANCE— A NEW PARADIGM

There is a need to shift to advanced methods of safety data management and pharmacovigilance using integrated systems to achieve integration, reproducibility and real time auditing capability. Partial computer based approaches mimic paper based methods as they are ad hoc in nature. These need to be replaced with a fully computerized informatics approach.

"Informatics is the science of storing, manipulating, analyzing and visualizing information with the help of computer systems."

The informatics approach considers safety data collection, transformation and analysis as a single re-usable, reproducible system that can be audited in real time. This may sound simpler than it is really is because for the implementation of an informatics approach for the analysis of safety data several requirements must be met.

The following are some of the requirements that must be met by a system as well as by the data that is used for analysis:
1. Data standards and interoperable systems
2. High quality safety data
3. Re-structuring capabilities
4. Data analysis
5. Reproducibility
6. Maintenance

Let us discuss each of these:

Data Standards and Interoperable Systems

Every computer systems used in data analysis requires the data to adhere to some standards. The data standards may consist of:
- Naming convention of the data file
- Standard elements of the data file
- Standardized names of each data element
- Standardized definition for each data element.

The importance of the above standards is that their implementation allows for data from one system to be used in the other and vice versa thus making the systems interoperable. If the data does not adhere to these standards then it may be recognized by one system but its format might not be understood by another. Another benefit of laying these standards is that it allows for the creation of standardized data analysis systems/tools that function on the data adhering to a common standard. These tools can then be used by all safety analysts to perform pharmacovigilance consistently around the globe.

This can be explained with an example: Suppose we have adverse event data in the oracle clinical database and the total number of adverse events = "n".

Now let us take any adverse event say "Coronary Thrombosis". If while entering this event into the Oracle Clinical database we used the <TAB> key or the <ENTER> key, this event would contain white-spaces and would be stored as:
- Coronary
- Thrombosis

The term should actually have been stored as "Coronary Thrombosis" but the white-spaces have led two the term being thrown across two columns. In this above case when the data goes to the analysis system for example SAS, it will take "Coronary" and "Thrombosis" as two different records as they fall in a different column.

This will cause the total number of adverse events in the analysis to be (n + 1). Apart from this each of the terms will not be coded correctly by the medical dictionary. Thus, white-spaces have resulted in irregularity in the interpretation and analysis of safety data. Had there been a standard governing the usage of white-spaces within any AE term, the errors would have occurred.

High Quality Safety Data

We may establish standards as well as have interoperable systems, but for them to function efficiently we require the data to be of high quality. To ensure the data is of good quality some of the following aspects should be kept in mind while collecting safety data.

Patient Identification

Single unique IDs should be used consistently across the database and special characters such as spaces and hyphens should be avoided.

Some of the common issues are the presence of hyphens, commas and additional zeroes in patient IDs. Also there are instances when it may be seen that the same patient in a study has different IDs in different tables. Following data table depicts how the addition of zeroes changes the identification of the patient in the data table as compared to the narrative table.

Unique patient identifier in data tables	Unique patient identifier in narrative table
1023507	Patient 01-023-507 is a 50-year-old Indian male, etc.
2076309	Patient 02-076-309 is a 42-years-old Hispanic female, etc.

Categorical Variables

These include questions such as race and gender which should have well-defined responses used consistently across the database. One of the common issues include gender being accepted as either "M", "Male" or "male" and sometimes even being coded to "1" and "2". Due to this, the question Gender may be answered differently at various sites. Some investigators would write "1" for male and others would write "Male". This creates issues during analysis. Thus, only one method should be used to capture predefined responses. The best method is to have a discrete value group (DVG) defined for such variables to maintain consistency.

Formatting Dates

The dates should be accepted in a standard format. It may be dd-mm-yy or mm-dd-yy or any other. However, the internationally accepted format today in which dates are captured for multinational studies is dd-mmm-yyyy for example 01-JAN-2008.

One of the common issues could be for example if the Date of birth is collected as 21-FEB-1982 and Visit date is collected as 10-01-2008. We cannot make out if visit date is the 10th of January or the 1st of October. Thus, all dates should be collected and managed in common format.

Coding of Adverse Events

The terms for drug names, medical history, concomitant medications and adverse events as reported by the investigator are called verbatim terms. These may not be standard medical terms and thus need to be consistently coded as per standard medical dictionaries such as MedDRA (Medical Dictionary for Regulatory Activities) and the WHO Drug and their conventions.

One of the common issues encountered is if two verbatim terms are reported, which essentially mean the same but have different case (either using all lower case, all upper case or a combination). The coding dictionary counts these are two different terms and will code them accordingly.

Drug Name Errors

Sometimes multiple names may exist for the same medication. It is essential to utilize a standard name as per a medical dictionary such as WHO Drug.

One of the common issues are for example, two names are recorded for concomitant medications which essentially are the same compound because they have not been coded correctly. In one of the NDA received by the FDA it was found that for 150 unique medications 900 different names were provided in the submission. Another NDA recorded 34,000 drug names for 2000 unique concomitant medications because the investigators at different sites were using different names.

Numerical Data Errors

The attributes for every question should be well-defined (whether it is numeric, character, data-time variable or alphanumeric). Also the coding should be taken into account.

Some of the common issues that may be encountered if the attributes are not well-defined include things such as a question is entered as a character in one study and numeric in the other such as. For example, Dose is measured as "80 mg" in one study (both character and numeric variable), while in another it is measured as "80" (numeric variable). Such inconsistency may create problems in the analysis of the data.

Missing Information

For both premarketing and postmarketing data lots of information may be missing because the patient may have left the trial in the middle due to several reasons.

Thus, common issues may be encountered for example, all adverse events may not be reported by the patient voluntarily or the patient may withdraw before reporting them at all. Also Tight-windows for AE reporting are not possible for drugs that have greater half-life.

Another issue may be that the external data such as laboratory reports, biopsy, hospital records, etc. may not have been received in time and are thus excluded from the final database.

Restructuring Capabilities

It is necessary for both the data as well as the database to have the capability to be restructured as per requirements. This helps achieve several objectives. In premarketing the data may be pooled from different sites to create a larger database of clinical data which makes the data statistically significant. In postmarketing the data may be pooled from different countries where adverse drug reactions are reported or may even be collected from different resources such as patients, doctors and drug companies so that maximum safety information about the drug can be gathered.

The ability of the data to be restructured allows it to be pooled together for deciphering safety information such as drug toxicity for a specific sub-group. The larger the data pool the easier is the data mining—a process that allows for searching of meaningful information from a large quantity of given data. Data mining of safety data allows for the creation of relationships between drug-drug, drug-disease and drug-demography associations.

Despite of seeming a lucrative option of safety information gathering there are several issues in pooling data together. Some of them are:
- Combining data may obscure meaningful information. For example, combining the term "tumor" and "brain tumor" may result in misinterpretation of the type of tumor.
- Different coding dictionaries are used in different countries and they may create coding inconsistencies. Thus, combining the data would be an issue as we have two terms meaning the same disease/drug because they have been coded as two different terms.
- The effects of drug vary with the heterogeneity of the population. Thus pooling data in multicentric trial might be a problem.

Not only the data needs to be restructured but also the database needs to be reconfigured if they have been maintained over a long period of time. Also after any change made to the database it needs to be validated again.

An example of this is the Oracle AERS database used by the FDA which stores the adverse events reported during any study. Initially (1968-1997), Oracle AERS was mapped to COSTART (Coding Symbols for a Thesaurus of Adverse reaction Terms) which only contained 1200 event codes, but later with the creation of the MedDRA dictionary which contained 15,000 event codes, Oracle AERS was reconfigured and mapped to MedDRA.

The process of restructuring, mapping and validation of any database is a labor intensive process but increases the efficiency of data analysis. Any integrated system should be able to restructure the data and the database in a transparent way.

Data Analysis

The process of data analysis requires the data collected to be cleaned, reconfigured and standardized. However, data collection at different sites occurs using their respective personal standards. Some sites use CRFs, some e-CRFs and some EDC methods. Thus, potentially useful information may not always be translated into the database effectively.

The informatics approach capitalizes on the fact that the data is reported into an integrated system using a consistent collection mechanism and is cleaned and reconfigured prior to data analysis. The key aspects that influence data analysis are:
- *Large size of the database:* Larger database allows for better benefit-risk decision.
- *High-dimension of data:* Clinical data for any patient may be several records of multiple tests, readings, scores, etc. So many variables make the analysis of the data difficult. The systematic analysis of all these variables while keeping focus on the safety parameters still poses problems.
- *Heterogeneous patients:* For premarketing data the clinical information should be obtained from a heterogeneous population so that the drug could be universally marketed. This is accomplished by choosing patients of varied age, gender, race, body weight and risk groups.

However, this same requirement poses the issue that any safety information obtained cannot be generalized for all the patients. The informatics approach overcomes this by performing stratified analysis.
- *Adverse event relationship:* The relationship of an event with a drug is essential to know causality. However, we cannot judge the causality by comparing treatment group against control group as there are several factors such as inconsistent time taken by the drug to show its effect and varied effect of the drug in a heterogeneous population. If we can compare the treatment group to the control group, the decision to continue/discontinue the drug can be easily taken. This is not possible by using data arranged in a tabular format. The Informatics approach allows for such information to be depicted graphically which can highlight the difference and lead to easy inference of the safety information.
- *Effect of concomitant medications:* To judge the safety profile of the drug, its interaction with concomitant medications being taken must be clear because the concomitant medication may be having an additive or antagonistic effect on the investigational drug. Also certain foods and supplements being taken may cause interference and result in adverse events.
So how do we know that the effect is due to the investigational drug, concomitant medication or the food and supplement? This is still a question that needs to be addressed.
- *Effect of pre-existing disease:* If a subject is already suffering from another disease and he is given the investigational drug, it may affect the underlying condition or may even induce another adverse reaction. Thus, the effect of the drug is confounded with the existing disease. So, we need to make sure that did the drug cause the AE or was it the interference of the drug with the underlying disease? This affects data analysis.
- *Volume of data for analysis:* Finally, the volume of data plays an important role in analysis. Large amount of data is generated from premarketing and postmarketing stages that needs to be analyzed. Take for example, the Oracle AERS database of the FDA which contains 2.5 million records collected since 1968. FDA receives around 1000 new reports of adverse events each day.

With this huge amount of data it is necessary to follow an informatics approach, so that the right variables (drug exposure data, underlying disease condition, etc.) can be chosen to run analysis so as to get meaningful results.

The informatics approach allows for the use of integrated, standardized software that can be used easily every time a new adverse event is reported and the results can be reproduced and audited in real time.

EMERGING TECHNOLOGIES/ COMPUTER-BASED TOOLS FOR PHARMACOVIGILANCE

Until now there was no specific safety analysis tool was a gold standard which was uniformly accepted or utilized. No tools were available which could analyze all aspects of toxicity of a drug or generalize its effect on any given population. Moreover there are several different standards of collecting, transforming and submitting clinical data today that make safety data analysis more difficult. Between 1990 and 1995, the FDA received submissions for clinical trials in which a total of 500,000 patients were enrolled. Lack of integrated, standardized and interoperable computer-based tools prevented analysis of such vast amount of data.

Ideally the FDA would have liked to integrate the data from all studies received, into a safety dataset for analysis. However since different New Drug Applications (NDA) had different data structure and different variable names this was not possible. In July 2004 the FDA adopted the Submission Data Tabulation Model (SDTM) of the CDISC (Clinical Data Interchange Standards Consortium).

Since a common standards is adopted in which the clinical data needs to be submitted in SDTM format, thus comprehensive software's/tools could be developed that support standard analysis of all NDA's. This has given rise to Emerging Technologies/ Computer Based Tools for assessing safety data.

These advanced computer based methods/software/tools allows for the analysis of large databases to get meaningful information in a systematic way. The practical use of these systems is assisting in the endeavor to achieve a gold standard by identifying both positive and negative signals. This in turn has helped in creating a full proof method for safety data analysis.

Some tools have emerged for analysis of pre-marketing data and some for postmarketing data. Others have the ability to perform both these tasks. The following are some of the emerging tools and their features.

WebSDM™ FOR ANALYSIS OF PREMARKETING SAFETY DATA

Premarketing safety data can be analyzed today using several emerging tools that are compliant with the SDTM standard of the CDISC.

WebSDM™ is one such tool developed by Lincoln Technologies, which is now a part of a company called Phase Forward. This tool is implemented by the FDA to analyze two new drug applications (NDA) in real time.

WebSDM™ ensures that the data submitted to the FDA is compliant with the submission standards of the CDISC and also allows for the automation of analytical processes.

MGPS AND HBLR FOR ANALYSIS OF POSTMARKETING DATA

There are several emerging tools available for the analysis of postmarketing safety data. Multi-Item Gamma Poisson Shrinker (MGPS) and Hierarchical Bayesian Logistic Regression (HBLR) are two such tools.

Multi-item Gamma Poisson Shrinker (MGPS) is a tool used in postmarketing surveillance. It is a statistical algorithm used by the FDA. MGPS can detect signals of higher than expected drug adverse event associations in postmarketing safety databases.

Hierarchical Bayesian Logistic Regression (HBLR) on the other hand in another tool being explored by the FDA. It detects signals generally occurring due to the use of multiple drugs together (polypharmacy). It has the potential to correct the confounding that occurs with the use of concomitant medications, so it can be readily predicted whether the investigational drug is causing an adverse event or not.

Apart from the ones discussed here, there are several other emerging tools, technologies and products in the market, aimed for integrated pharmacovigilance. Some of them are:

1. Aris Global Total Safety Suite: ARISg™, ARISj™, agXchange™, agSignals™ and agComposer™
2. Galt Safety Suite: DrugSafety.com, dsNavigator, dsGateway, dsAnalysis and Informatics Online
3. Insightful Safety™
4. Empirica Suite™
5. Oracle AERS™
6. Argus Insight™, Argus Interchange™ and Argus Perceptive™
7. VigiFlow™: The modern solution for ADR management
8. ClinTrace™

Data Management in Pharmacovigilance

DRUG SAFETY TECHNOLOGY VENDORS

There are several companies/vendors that have come out with Safety Systems specific to pharmacovigilance. Some of these vendors provide standalone products to suit a specific pharmacovigilance function while others have developed a suite of applications for integrated pharmacovigilance, data mining and signal detection. Some of these vendors are:
1. ArisGlobal
2. Galt Associates Inc.
3. Insightful
4. Oracle
5. Phase Forward
6. Relsys Inc.
7. eResearch Technology (eRT)
8. SAIC

The following Vendor Profiles are a description of these vendors, their services, geographical presence and the pharmacovigilance products they have in the market.

VENDOR PROFILE—ARIS GLOBAL

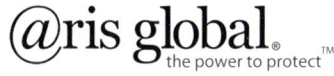

Business profile	ARIS GLOBAL is the leading provider of Pharmacovigilance, Drug Safety Monitoring and Drug Safety Software. It has been providing such solutions for the last 15 years. It also provides software's for Clinical Trials Management and Medical Communications.
Geography	The company has its offices in US, UK, Germany, India and Japan. It has over 100 pharmaceutical and medical devices companies as its customers.
Services	Aris Global provides services ranging from providing software solutions for pharmaceutical companies in the area of trial management and pharmacovigilance to consulting companies in the implementation and validation of this software as well as in preparing project plans.
Products	ARIS GLOBAL Total Safety Suite The suite includes 6 applications that can be independently deployed:

1.	ARISg™	Used for the Collection, Coding, Assessment and Reporting of Adverse Events Data.
2.	ARISj™	ARISg™ supports Japanese language for domestic reporting.
3.	agXchange™	Facilitates electronic exchange of safety data. It is database independent
4.	ARISg for Complaints™	Management of product complaints
5.	agSignals™	Signal detection through benefit-risk assessment
6.	agComposer™	Scheduling and automatic preparation of PSUR's

ARIS GLOBAL TOTAL SAFETY SUITE

The ARIS GLOBAL Total Safety Suite consists of 6 applications that can be independently deployed. The various applications and their functionality span the area of pharmacovigilance, clinical safety and risk management. When deployed together the applications are compliant with ethical standards for clinical trials. The Total safety suite has features for case management, risk assessment, report preparation and submissions of safety data electronically. The various applications that form a part of the suite are described below:

ARISg™

ARISg is one of the leading software for adverse event management and reporting. It is deployed at over 120 life science organizations throughout the globe. This includes 20 of the top 50 biotech pharmaceutical and biotechnology companies. It is compliant with the regulatory requirements for drug safety data reporting. ARISg supports the collection of spontaneous safety reports globally, medical coding of verbatim terms that have been reported and collection of adverse events.

The collaborative framework of the software allows entering the adverse event data logically, while routing specific cases (based on company's methods for handling cases) to relevant personnel for expedited reporting. The software can create AE reports in several different formats such as CIOMS and E2B.

ARISj™

ARISj has functionality similar to ARISg and essentially boasts of its capabilities to support all domestic reporting in Japanese (Kanji) format. It is the only solution that allows for reporting in Japanese and is successfully deployed at many of the leading pharmaceutical companies in Japan. This software enhances collaboration amongst the major ICH regions supporting GCP which include the US, European Union and Japan.

ARISg and ARISj can be installed on a central database so that they utilize the same data entry templates and workflow for centralized management and analysis of the safety data but decentralized reporting in localized format and language.

agXchange™

The regulatory agencies in US and Europe have made it mandatory that safety data be submitted electronically. agXchange enables the submission of safety data in the form of ICSRs and suspected unexpected serious adverse events to the various regulatory agencies electronically.

Since, electronic transmission needs to be secure, the software has encryption protocols integrated within it which make the exchange of safety data secure. Also the system has the ability to send the data individually or in batch mode and also receive the receipt of transmission once the data is uploaded at the destination.

Safety data can be displayed with agXchange before being imported to the production database, thus making it less error prone. The software is database independent and can operate with any safety database.

ARISg for Complaints™

Postmarketing safety data is important to know the grievance that the consumer has about the medicinal product. ARISg for complaints is the software within the global suite which enables the collection, management and assessment of these product complaints received globally on a regular basis.

agSignals™

agSignals is the application within the total suite that provides comprehensive benefit-risk assessment. It was formerly known as SafetyMart. The software is used for the detection of signals and mining of potentially useful information from the available safety data which is utilized for determining the risks involved in the use of the medicinal product and also the potential benefits.

The software has simple to use interface allowing for simple visualization of complex relationships through the use of tables and graphs. The data can be exported to other analysis applications as well. The architecture of agSignals is an optimized database with a front end interface for conducting the analysis and generating reports. The database can be queried for complex relationships in an intuitive manner allowing for extensive epidemiological adverse event analysis.

agComposer™

agComposer supports the preparation and submission of Periodic Safety Database Reports, while also integrating the information form the annual safety reports. The software is database independent and can work effectively with any safety system for the preparation of periodic safety update reports (PSURs).

The software has predefined format and design of a standard PSUR and picks up the data from the safety system to be automatically inserted into the tables of the report hence automating the process.

If another adverse event is reported immediately after the analysis the event cannot be incorporated in the analysis output and the whole analysis needs to be run again as the output is not reproducible in nature.

Reference ranges used, especially for laboratory data may vary from country to country and lab to lab. Thus, it becomes difficult combining two datasets having different ranges.

VENDOR PROFILE – GALT ASSOCIATES INC

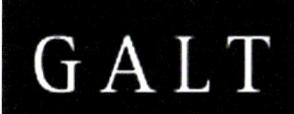

Business profile	Galt Associates, Inc. is a pharmacovigilance support company, specializing in the delivery of web-based compliance and analysis solutions for the pharmaceutical industry. This helps pharmaceutical companies manage drug safety data.
Geography	The company has its offices in several locations around the globe.
Services	Galt builds life science applications utilizing their comprehensive knowledge of the pharmaceutical industry, as well as their extensive research and consulting experience in safety analysis, disease modeling, outcomes research and health economics.
Products	Galt Suite of Life Science Applications The suite includes 5 application modules: DrugSafety.com dsNavigator dsGateway dsAnalysis Informatics-Online

VENDOR PROFILE - INSIGHTFUL

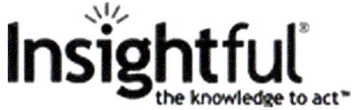

Business profile	Insightful Corporation is a leading provider of scalable data analysis solutions that drive better decisions faster by integrating statistics into business processes. Insightful delivers software and solutions for predictive analytics that have enabled thousands of companies to discern the patterns, trends, and relationships hidden in the data they collect.	
Geography	Headquartered in Seattle, USA, it has offices in France, Switzerland, UK and Hong Kong.	
Services	Insightful is a leading provider of real clinical data solutions through software, training, support and consulting services.	
Products	Insightful safety	
	The suite allows for the analysis of safety data.	
	Insightful safety	Quantify treatment effects on safety endpoints
		Identify safety signals quickly and accurately
		Select the best dose in early-phase trials
		Identify patients with lab and/or AE issues early in all trials
		Uses advanced statistical methods such as Bayesian hierarchical models and machine learning models

VENDOR PROFILE – ORACLE CORP

ORACLE®

Business profile	Oracle Corporation is a leading supplier of software across many industries, with a Pharmaceutical and Life Sciences offering across Discovery, Development, Manufacturing and Marketing. Founded in 1977 the organization now has over 40,000 employees.
Geography	US based but with Global presence.
Services	Oracle provides leading Life Sciences Products such as Oracle Pharmaceutical Applications Suite, and consulting in the implementation and validation of its applications.
Products	Oracle AERS and Oracle TMS
	These are safety data management products of the Oracle Pharmaceutical Applications (OPA) Suite.
	Oracle AERS — Global Collection and Management of Adverse Event Data
	Oracle TMS — Consistent Coding of Drug and Event Terminologies

VENDOR PROFILE – PHASE FORWARD

PHASE•FORWARD

Business profile	Phase Forward was founded in 1997 and has been providing clinical data solutions since its inception. It evolved through organic growth and acquisition acquiring Provenda in March 2001 and Clinsoft in August 2001.		
Geography	It is Headquartered in the US in Massachusetts with other offices in Washington, California, UK, Australia, Japan and France		
Services	Phase Forward provides life science applications for pharmaceutical companies. It also provides services of implementation, validation and integration of these applications. Phase Forwards Lincoln Technologies Safety division provides safety data management tools and services.		
Products	Solutions from Lincoln Safety Group		
	These tools allow for signal detection, strategic pharmacovigilance and adverse event reporting		
	Signal detection	CTSD™	Based of WebSDM, that was created in association with FDA. It enables creating of a SDTM CDISC standard compliant data repository and automated screening for safety issues during premarketing stage. Also allows for graphical analysis and interpretation of safety data.
	Strategic pharmacovigilance	WebVDME™	Detection and quantification of safety signals through advanced data mining against safety databases. It is being used at 7 of top 10 pharmaceutical companies as well as at FDA, NIH and UK's MHRA
		WebVDM™ signal detection module	Tracking and managing signals detected by WebVDME™. Reviewing earlier results, comparing and decision making.
	Adverse event reporting	Empirica™ Trace	Collection, coding, analyzing and reporting adverse events. Electronic submission of safety data and regulatory compliance

Data Management in Pharmacovigilance

VENDOR PROFILE – RELSYS INC.

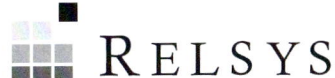

Business profile	Relsys Inc. is the market leader in the area of drug safety and regulatory affairs. It provides software for unparalleled success in the area of drug safety. Relsys Inc. has been in operation since 1987 and has a global presence
Geography	Relsys Inc. is located in North America, Europe, Japan, and India.
Services	Relsys has been providing safety solutions, both products and services, to the global pharmaceutical industry. It offers implementation and support service offerings for its line of products.
Products	Argus safety suite

The suite contains the following safety applications:

Argus Affiliate™	Centralized tracking of events reported through affiliates
Argus Assurance™	Systematic pharmacovigilance by providing preventive QC measures and retrospective QA measures for safety leadership.
Argus Beacon™	Provides key performance indicators to "keep the finger on the pulse" of the trial.
Argus Dossier™	Submission and Management of Periodic Safety Update Reports (PSUR's)
Argus Insight™	Multidimensional analysis of safety data and generating pre-formatted, filterable safety reports. Formerly sold as power reports.
Argus Interchange™	Scheduling and Submission of Safety Reports Electronically.
ArgusJ™	Provides support of domestic Japanese reporting required in Kanji format.
Argus Perceptive™	Intergrated solution of pharmacovigilance and risk management. Formerly called ArgusPV™.

VENDOR PROFILE – ERESEARCH TECHNOLOGIES (ERT)

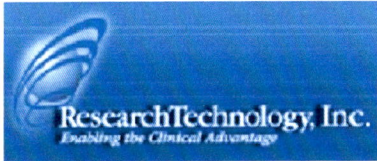

Business profile	eResearchTechnology, Inc. (eRT) is a provider of technology-based products and services for the pharmaceutical industry. It had products used in the area of safety data management.
Geography	eRT has offices located essentially in US and UK.
Services	eResearchTechnology, Inc. (eRT) provides technology and services that enable researchers to collect, interpret and distribute cardiac safety and clinical data accurately and efficiently. eRT has a wide range of products directed towards managing cardiac safety data.
Products	Individual software/web based solutions to manage safety

The following are some applications specifically for pharmacovigilance:

EXPeRT Direct™	Web based tool for cardiac safety data monitoring for reviewing safety data and generating reports.
EXPeRT eClinical Adverse Event Reporting	Real time access to key safety metrics and support proactive decision making.

VENDOR PROFILE – SAIC

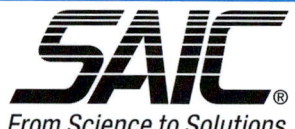

Business profile	SAIC's has approximately 44,000 employees and supports government and commercial customers in all phases for drug development: Discovery, Pre-Clinical and Clinical Development, and Operations & Compliance. SAIC had annual revenues of $8.9 billion for its fiscal year ended January 31, 2008. SAIC is the partner of FDA in technical support and enhancement of its Oracle AERS system
Geography	Headquartered in San Diego, California, it has a global presence.
Services	SAIC is focused on enhancing the cycle times and success rates in clinical development and provides technical products and services in all areas of drug development including but not limited to pharmacovigilance and risk management.
Products	Services in the area of pharmacovigilance and risk management
	The following are some areas of SAIC expertise:
SAIC expertise and offerings	Risk Management Practices and Risk Strategy development.
	Pharmacovigilance system requirement analysis
	Evaluation of COTS safety and signal detection system and gap analysis
	Development of statistical algorithms for signal detection
	Designing data mining, visualization and reporting tools for signal detection
	System integration and enterprise safety portal development

VENDOR PROFILE - SAS

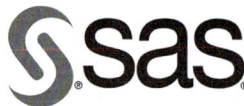

Business Profile	SAS is the leader in business intelligence and analytical software and services for all industries. SAS solutions are used at 44,000 sites in 109 countries—including 96 of the top 100 FORTUNE Global 500® companies. SAS has more than 10,000 employees.
Geography	SAS has 400 offices in more than 50 countries. It has a global presence.
Services	SAS delivers integrated set software for all industries in the area of business intelligence, Risk Intelligence and performance management. It also provides these well-focused solutions specifically for the Life Sciences sector. In the Pharmaceutical sector SAS has developed technology based on the CDISC standards. It is the de facto standard for clinical data analysis and the FDA standard for electronic submissions.
Products	SAS Technology Solutions
	The following are some areas where SAS software ensures pharmacovigilance and signal detection:
SAS technology solutions	Summary analysis and graphical visualization of safety analysis
	Multidimensional analysis of variables for signal detection in specific disease populations
	Predictive Modelling and Data Mining using SAS Miner™
	De Facto standard of submission and reporting to the regulatory authorities.

CASE STUDIES

WedSDM™

WebSDM™ (Web Submissions Data Manager) is an analytical tool provided by Lincoln Technologies. It utilizes the CDISC standards and thus data needs to be converted as per the SDTM (Study Data Tabulation Model) before being loaded into the tool. This software has been implemented by the FDA to analyze two NDA's in real time.

From a sponsors perspective this simultaneous analysis saves time and also ensures that the data submitted to the FDA complies with the CDISC standard while from the perspective of the FDA time is saved as the data received does not need to be standardized and can be directly analyzed by the standard FDA tools.

WebSDM™ has the "Sector Map Graphical Tool" for visual analysis of clinical trial data. It has the ability to highlight unexpected adverse events in treatment versus control group and thus simplifies the interactive analysis of data.

MGPS™

MGPS™ (Multi-item Gamma Poisson Shrinker) is a statistical algorithm used in postmarketing surveillance. It is a tool used by the FDA for pharmacovigilance.

MGPS is used in signal detection of unexpected adverse events and their relationship with drugs in postmarketing safety databases. It uses dispropotionality analysis and Bayesian Shrinkage as the statistical analysis methods.

The software also has the ability to perform "stratification" of the data. When used against the Oracle AERS database it systematically stratifies the data by over 1000 categories. This helps in the signal detection process. It also has "Sector Map" tool for graphical analysis of the data.

MGPS has recently been adopted by the British Medicines and Healthcare Products Regulatory Agency (MHRA) for pharmacovigilance.

HBLR™

HBLR (Hierarchical Bayesian Logistic Regression) is a statistical algorithm used in postmarketing surveillance. This tool is currently being explored by the FDA.

HBLR is used for detection of signals created due to the use of many medications simultaneously (polypharmacy). It removes the confounding creating by concomitant medications. It overcomes two important aspects during signal detection:

- *Signal absorption:* Signal absorption is a phenomenon whereby an "innocent bystander" drug is falsely signalled as being associated with an adverse event thus creating "false positive" signal
- *Signal masking:* Signal masking is a phenomenon when a weak signal for a drug causing an adverse event is not detected because of the presence strong signals from other drugs. This is usually because of similarity of two drugs in a database.

Oracle AERS™

Oracle AERS (Adverse Event Reporting System) is a safety management system and a product of Oracle Corporation. The software forms a part of a large suite of clinical applications called the Oracle Pharmaceutical Applications (OPA) suite.

Oracle AERS has been implemented by the FDA. It can be used for both premarketing as well as postmarketing management of safety data and allows for consistent coding of reported terms for drug names and events using standard medical dictionaries such as MedDRA. The "data query" functionality of the software helps answer complex questions about risk-benefit.

AERS allows for reporting of events using standardized reports adhering to various formats such as CIOMS and E2B.

SAS™

SAS (Statistical Analysis System) is essentially an analysis tool. It is used by the Life Science Industry as well as FDA.

The FDA used SAS for scientific intelligence in many departments such as CDER, CDRH and CBER. In the area of pharmacovigilance SAS is used in different phases such as:
- Summary analysis and visualization of adverse event reports
- Longitudinal analysis of data regarding adverse events.
- Analysis of multiple variables to determine patterns and signals in specific populations.

SAS is moving from being an analysis system for "detection" to a system for "prediction" of safety concerns in the area of pharmacovigilance.

VigiFlow™

VigiFlow™ is the modern solution for ADR management. It complies with the GxP and E2B standards and focuses more on the management of data than the technology for its analysis.

VigiFlow™ is used at the Uppsala Monitoring Centre (UMC) run by the World Health Organization (WHO) and has the WHO Drug dictionary integrated within it. It is web-based and is designed to be used by multiple users simultaneously.

The software is installed and maintained centrally at the UMC and companies can have secured access to it without the need to go into the technical aspects. All reports submitted by any pharmaceutical company are not accessible to the others and thus confidentiality of the reports is ensured.

DATA MINING AND SIGNAL DETECTION

Data mining is the process of analyzing databases that store a large amount of data (Data warehouses) and picking out relevant information to identify signals or relationships. In Pharmacovigilance data mining uses statistical method for determining if an adverse experience is more likely to occur with one investigational product as compared to all of the other products on the market. Data mining helps in the following:
- Identifying subtle realationships among any number of variables in a large database (drug-drug or drug-event or drug-medical history or drug-gender relationships)
- Identifying potential toxicities of a drug early on
- Analyzing complex relationships
- Generating signals for further evaluation.

A signal is defined by the World Health Organization as:
- "Reported information on a possible causal association between an adverse event and a drug, the relationship being unclear or incompletely documented previously"
- Signal detection is a key objective of pharmacovigilance and helps in the evaluation of benefits and risks. The various sources of signals in pharmacovigilance are:
  - Observation by investigators and patients
  - Case report forms
  - Adverse event report assessment
  - Clinical databases.

The use of cutting edge information technology tools and systems are bringing about automation of signal detection. They can compare the safety profile of a drug against other products in a database using statistical methods.

There are several analysis strategies that may be used for signal detection. The most common ones are:
- **Safety database querying:** This strategy involves systematic querying of clinical safety databases to identify potential association between product and adverse events that may be of regulatory interest. The strength of this identified signal can then be supported by utilizing other methods.
- **Safety database mining:** This strategy involves systematic querying of large database/database warehouses to identify association among two or more safety variables that occur at a frequency which is higher than expected (for example, drug-event relationship, drug-drug interaction). Once such patterns are observed, the strength of the signals can be explored using other signal detection methods.

Irrespective of the strategy being followed for signal detection there are standard techniques that are applied to get meaningful information from the data. These techniques are nothing but statistical methods. Some of the most common techniques applied in signal detection include:
- Multi-Gamma Poisson Shrinker (MGPS) adopted by the FDA
- Bayesian Confidence Propagation Neural Network (BCPNN) Information Component (IC) and Relative Odds Ratio (ROR) adopted by Uppsala Monitoring Centre and World Health Organization
- Proportional Reporting Ratio (PRR) adopted by Medicines Control Agency (MCA) of the EMEA
- Adjusted Residual Score (Adjusted R) is a statistical measure recently introduced by SAS in its signal detection module.

Data mining and signal detection helps detect even those safety issues which have not been expected during the study, thus making pharmacovigilance a more "predictive" approach.

UPPSALA MONITORING CENTER

With the growing safety concerns there has been a focus on pharmacovigilance by the all the regulatory authorities around the globe. The initiative taken by the WHO has led to true internationalization of safety initiatives. In 1968 the WHO collaboration centre was located in Geneva. In 1969, there was an agreement between Sweden and WHO and the centre was moved to Uppsala and came to be known as the Uppsala Monitoring Centre.

WHO-UMC is a non-profit foundation having an international representation. It has over 82 official member countries and 17 associate member countries. The centre holds close to 3.7 million adverse drug reactions (ADRs) reports in its database.

The following are the objectives of the Uppsala Monitoring Centre:
- Exchange of drug safety information on an international level
- Development of new methods and pharmacovigilance tools
- Signal detection and analysis
- Collection and analysis of safety data on a global scale
- Early detection and decision making capability
- Reviewing and updating the WHO Drug dictionary.

The UMC creates and distributes a report called "SIGNALS" which contains an Analysis of adverse drug reactions in the WHO database. This report is written by 40 experts around the world and it is sent to all UMC National Centres and individually accessible by the industry. The recipients are encouraged to comment on the topics presented.

The Uppsala Monitoring Centre uses a web based tool which is a modern solution for ADR management called VigiFlow™.

CONCLUSION

Even with the Food, Drug and Cosmetics Act in place, most of the hospitalizations in the US are still due adverse events of medicines taken. Traditional methods are not enough to ensure safety and thus new pharmacovigilance approaches are needed to be adopted.

The solution to ensure effective pharmacovigilance is the use of new tools that utilize the power of modern computer technology provide innovative means of analyzing drug safety information in a systematic way.

These tools help compare analysis results from one safety database with other independent databases (medical database, health insurance company records, etc.) to identify signals. They are based on standards such as CDISC are thus interoperable, making the process integrated.

Today data mining and signal detection is based on complex algorithms and ensure that important decisions can be taken about the drug safety.

Pharmacovigilance is moving into a new era, where cutting edge technologies and integrated systems make it possible to "predict" unexpected safety issues that otherwise would have been impossible to "detect" hence ensuring that the medicines that are marketed today can be safely consumed.

BIBLIOGRAPHY

1. A pharmacovigilance software solution for adverse events reporting. Pcv Manager. Available at http://www.knowledgenet.in/pharmacovigilance.html.
2. Apoorva BM, Kiran LJ, Kumar S C. Softwares in Pharmacovigilance and Clinical trials. World Journal of Pharmaceutical Research. 2015;4(845)·544-9.
3. ARISg. Available at http://arisglobal.com/total-safety/arisg/. Accessed on 05 July, 2017.
4. http://haromsolutions.com/Pharmacovigilance_software.php. Accessed on 05 July 2017.
5. http://www.who.int/medicines/areas/quality_safety/safety_efficacy/pharmvigi/en/.Accessed on 04 July 2017.
6. Pharmacovigilance. Uppsala Monitoring Centre – Who-umc.org Available at http://www.who-umc.org/.

ANNEXURES

ANNEXURE 1A

ADR form for Health Care Professionals, India

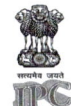

Version-1.2

SUSPECTED ADVERSE DRUG REACTION REPORTING FORM
For VOLUNTARY reporting of Adverse Drug Reactions by Healthcare Professionals

INDIAN PHARMACOPOEIA COMMISSION
(National Coordination Centre-Pharmacovigilance Programme of India)
Ministry of Health & Family Welfare, Government of India
Sector-23, Raj Nagar, Ghaziabad-201002

FOR AMC/NCC USE ONLY
AMC Report No.   :
Worldwide Unique No. :

Report Type ☐ Initial ☐ Follow up

A. PATIENT INFORMATION
1. Patient Initials _____
2. Age at time of Event or Date of Birth _____
3. M ☐   F ☐   Other ☐
4. Weight _____ Kgs

12. Relevant tests/ laboratory data with dates

B. SUSPECTED ADVERSE REACTION
5. Date of reaction started (dd/mm/yyyy)
6. Date of recovery   (dd/mm/yyyy)
7. Describe reaction or problem

13. Relevant medical/ medication history (e.g. allergies, race, pregnancy, smoking, alcohol use, hepatic/renal dysfunction etc.)

14. Seriousness of the reaction: No ☐ if Yes ☐ (please tick anyone)
- ☐ Death (dd/mm/yyyy)   ☐ Congenital-anomaly
- ☐ Life threatening   ☐ Required intervention to Prevent permanent
- ☐ Hospitalization/Prolonged   impairment/damage
- ☐ Disability   ☐ Other (specify)

15. Outcomes
- ☐ Recovered   ☐ Recovering   ☐ Not recovered
- ☐ Fatal   ☐ Recovered with sequelae ☐ Unknown

C. SUSPECTED MEDICATION(S)

S.No	8. Name (Brand/Generic)	Manufacturer (if known)	Batch No. / Lot No.	Exp. Date (If known)	Dose used	Route used	Frequency (OD, BD etc.)	Therapy dates Date started	Therapy dates Date stopped	Indication	Causality Assessment
i											
ii											
iii											
iv											

S.No as per C	9. Action Taken (please tick)						10. Reaction reappeared after reintroduction (please tick)			
	Drug withdrawn	Dose increased	Dose reduced	Dose not changed	Not applicable	Unknown	Yes	No	Effect unknown	Dose (if reintroduced)
i										
ii										
iii										
iv										

11. Concomitant medical product including self-medication and herbal remedies with therapy dates (Exclude those used to treat reaction)

S.No	Name (Brand/Generic)	Dose used	Route used	Frequency (OD, BD, etc.)	Therapy dates Date started	Therapy dates Date stopped	Indication
i							
ii							
iii							

Additional Information:

D. REPORTER DETAILS
16. Name and Professional Address: _____
_____
Pin: _____ E-mail _____
Tel. No. (with STD code) _____
Occupation: _____ Signature: _____

17. Date of this report (dd/mm/yyyy):

Confidentiality: The patient's identity is held in strict confidence and protected to the fullest extent. Programme staff is not expected to and will not disclose the reporter's identity in response to a request from the public. Submission of a report does not constitute an admission that medical personnel or manufacturer or the product caused or contributed to the reaction.

National Coordination Centre
Pharmacovigilance Programme of India
Ministry of Health & Family Welfare,
Government of India
Sector-23, Raj Nagar, Ghaziabad-201002
Tel.: 0120-2783400, 2783401, 2783392
Fax: 0120-2783311
www.ipc.nic.in

Pharmacovigilance Programme of India for Assuring Drug Safety

ADVICE ABOUT REPORTING

A. What to report

- Report serious adverse drug reactions. A reaction is serious when the patient outcome is:
  - Death
  - Life-threatening
  - Hospitalization (initial or prolonged)
  - Disability (significant, persistent or permanent)
  - Congenital anomaly
  - Required intervention to prevent permanent impairment or damage
- Report non-serious, known or unknown, frequent or rare adverse drug reactions due to Medicines, Vaccines and Herbal products.

B. Who can report

- All healthcare professionals (Clinicians, Dentists, Pharmacists and Nurses) can report adverse drug reactions

C. Where to report

- Duly filled Suspected Adverse Drug Reaction Reporting Form can be send to the nearest Adverse Drug Reaction Monitoring Centre (AMC) or directly to the National Coordination Centre (NCC).
- Call on Helpline (Toll Free) 1800 180 3024 to report ADRs.
- Or can directly mail this filled form to pvpi@ipcindia.net or pvpi.ipcindia@gmail.com
- A list of nationwide AMCs is available at:
  http://www.ipc.gov.in, http://www.ipc.gov.in/PvPI/pv_home.html

D. What happens to the submitted information

- Information provided in this form is handled in strict confidence. The causality assessment is carried out at AMCs by using WHO-UMC scale. The analyzed forms are forwarded to the NCC through ADR database. Finally the data is analyzed and forwarded to the Global Pharmacovigilance Database managed by WHO Uppsala Monitoring Centre in Sweden.
- The reports are periodically reviewed by the NCC-PvPI. The information generated on the basis of these reports helps in continuous assessment of the benefit-risk ratio of medicines.
- The information is submitted to the Steering committee of PvPI constituted by the Ministry of Health & Family Welfare. The Committee is entrusted with the responsibility to review the data and suggest any interventions that may be required.

E. Mandatory field for suspected ADR reporting form

- Patient initials, age at onset of reaction, reaction term(s), date of onset of reaction, suspected medication(s) and reporter information.

For ADRs Reporting Call on PvPI Helpline (Toll Free)
1800 180 3024
(9:00 AM to 5:30 PM, Working Days)

ANNEXURE 1B

ADR form for Consumers in Hindi

Version 1.0
संस्करण 1.0

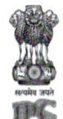

MEDICINES SIDE EFFECT REPORTING FORM (FOR CONSUMERS)
औषधि दुष्प्रभाव सूचना फॉर्म (उपभोक्ताओं के लिए)

Indian Pharmacopoeia Commission, National Coordination Centre- Pharmacovigilance Programme of India, Ministry of Health & Family Welfare, Government of India.
भारतीय भेषज संहिता आयोग, राष्ट्रीय समन्वय केंद्र – भारतीय फार्माकोविजिलेंस कार्यक्रम,
स्वास्थ्य एवं परिवार कल्याण मंत्रालय, भारत सरकार।

1. Patient Details/ रोगी का विवरण

Patient Initials/ रोगी के आद्याक्षर:: ☐   Gender/ लिंग (√): Male/ पुरुष ☐ Female/ स्त्री ☐ Other/ अन्य ☐   Age (Year or Month)/ आयु (वर्ष या माह):

2. Health Information/ स्वास्थ्य संबंधी जानकारी

a. Reason(s) for taking medicine(s)(Disease/Symptoms)/ दवा(दवाएं) लेने का कारण (रोग / लक्षण):

b. Medicines Advised by/ दवाई की सलाह देने वाला (√): Doctor/ डॉक्टर ☐ Pharmacist/ फॉर्मासिस्ट ☐ Friends/Relatives/ मित्र / रिश्तेदार ☐
Self (Past disease experienced/No past disease experienced)/ स्वयं (पूर्व बीमारी का अनुभव / पूर्व बीमारी का कोई अनुभव नहीं) ☐

3. Details of Person Reporting the Side Effect/ दुष्प्रभाव की सूचना देने वाले व्यक्ति का विवरण

Name (Optional)/ नाम (वैकल्पिक):

Address/ पता:

Telephone No/ टेलीफोन नं:   Email/ ईमेल:

4. Details of Medicine Taking/Taken/ ली जा रही है / ली जा चुकी दवाई का विवरण

Name of Medicines/ दवाइयों के नाम	Quantity of Medicines taken (e.g. 250 mg, Two times a day)/ ली गई दवाई की मात्रा (उदाहरण के लिए 250 मिग्रा, एक दिन में दो बार)	Expiry Date of Medicines/ दवा के निष्क्रिय होने की तिथि	Date of Start of Medicines/ दवाइयां आरंभ करने की तिथि	Date of Stop of Medicines/ दवाइयां रोकने की तिथि

Dosage form/खुराक का स्वरूप (√) : Tablet/ गोली (टेबलेट) ☐ Capsule/ कैप्सूल ☐ Injection/ इंजेक्शन ☐ Oral Liquids/ मौखिक तरल ☐ If Others (Please Specify........................)/यदि अन्य (कृपया निर्दिष्ट करें................)

5. About the Side Effect/ दुष्प्रभाव के बारे में

When did the side effect start?/ दुष्प्रभाव की शुरुआत कब हुई थी?   Side Effect is still Continuing (Yes/No)/
When did the side effect stop?/ दुष्प्रभाव कब समाप्त हुआ था?   क्या दुष्प्रभाव जारी हैं (हां / नहीं):

6. How bad was the Side Effect? (Please √ the boxes that Apply)/ दुष्प्रभाव कितने हानिकारक थे? (कृपया जो लागू हो, उस पर √ का निशान लगाएं)

☐ Did not affect daily activities/ दैनिक गतिविधियां प्रभावित नहीं हुई थी   ☐ Affect daily activities/ दैनिक गतिविधियां प्रभावित हुई
☐ Admitted to hospital/ अस्पताल ले जाना पड़ा   ☐ Death/ मृत्यु
☐ Others/ अन्य

7. Describe the Side Effect (What did you do to manage the side effect?)/ दुष्प्रभाव की व्याख्या करें (आपने दुष्प्रभावों से छुटकारा प्राप्त करने के लिए क्या किया?):

This reporting is voluntary, has no legal implication and aims to improve patient safety. Your active participation is valuable. The information provided in this form will be forwarded to ADR Monitoring Centre for follow-up. You are requested to cooperate with the programme officials when they contact you for more details. Please do report even if you do not have all the information.
यह रिपोर्टिंग स्वैच्छिक है, कोई कानूनी निहितार्थ नहीं है और इसका लक्ष्य मरीज की सुरक्षा में सुधार करना है। आपकी सक्रिय भागीदारी मूल्यवान है। इस फॉर्म में दी गई जानकारी की अनुवर्ती कार्रवाई हेतु एडीआर निगरानी केंद्र को भेजा जाएगा। आपसे अनुरोध है कि आप कार्यक्रम के अधिकारियों का सहयोग करें जब वे अधिक जानकारी प्राप्त करने के लिए आपसे संपर्क करें। कृपया पूर्ण जानकारी न होने पर भी सूचित करें।

Please turn the page to read the instructions
निर्देशों को पढ़ने के लिए कृपया पेज पलटें

Send your report by mail or Fax to/ मेल या फैक्स के द्वारा अपनी रिपोर्ट निम्न पते पर भेजें

Pharmacovigilance Programme of India
National Coordination Centre,
Indian Pharmacopoeia Commission,
Ministry of Health & Family Welfare, Govt. of India
Sector-23,Rajnagar,Ghaziabad-201002.Uttar Pradesh
Tel.:0120-2783400, 2783401, 2783392
FAX: 0120-2783311
Email: pvpi.compat@gmail.com
For more information visit us at *www.ipc.gov.in*

Call us on Helpline/ हेल्पलाइन पर हमें फोन करें
1800-180-3024 (Toll Free/
(टोल फ्री))
(9:00 AM to 5:30 PM, weekdays/ प्रातः 9:00 बजे 5:30 बजे तक, प्रत्येक कार्यदिवस पर)

Confidentiality: The patient's identity is held in strict confidence and protected to the fullest extent. Programme staff is not expected to and will not disclose the reporter's identity in response to a request from the public.
गोपनीयताः रोगी की पहचान को पूर्णतः गुप्त और सुरक्षित रखा जाएगा है। कार्यक्रम के स्टाफ से उम्मीद की जाती है कि स्टाफ का कोई भी व्यक्ति सार्वजनिक अनुरोध पर रिपोर्ट देने वाले की पहचान का खुलासा नहीं करेगा।

Instructions to Complete the Reporting Form
सूचना फॉर्म को पूरा करने के लिए निर्देश

Section 1 - Patient Details
- ✓ In patient Initial, write first letter of the name and first letter of the surname (e.g. Pradeep Sharma-PS).
- ✓ Provide personal information (Gender, Age).

Section -2 Health Information
- ✓ Provide reason(s) for taking medicines and medicines advised by (Doctor, Pharmacists, Friends/ Relatives and Self).

Section 3 - Details of Person Reporting the Side Effect
- ✓ Provide the name (optional), address; telephone no. and email are necessary to assess the report.

Section 4 - Details of the Medicines Taking/Taken
- ✓ Give all details about the Medicines (Name of Medicines, Quantity of Medicines taken, Expiry Date, start and stop date of Medicines) that have caused side effect.
- ✓ Please provide Dosage form (Tablets, Capsule, injections, Oral liquid) and if others please specify.

Section 5 - About the Side Effect
- ✓ Provide side effect start and stop dates and also specify whether the side effect is still continuing.

Section 6 - How bad was the Side Effect
- ✓ Please tick marks the appropriate boxes that apply.

Section 7- Describe the Side Effect
- ✓ Please describe the details of side effect and what treatment was taken to manage the side effect.

निर्देश 1 – रोगी का विवरण
- ✓ रोगी के आद्याक्षर में, नाम का पहला अक्षर लिखें और उपनाम का प्रथम अक्षर लिखें (जैसे प्रदीप शर्मा–प्रश)।
- ✓ व्यक्तिगत जानकारी (लिंग, आयु) प्रदान करें।

निर्देश –2 स्वास्थ्य संबंधी जानकारी
- ✓ दवा लेने के कारण और परामर्शदाता का नाम दें (डॉक्टर, फार्मासिस्ट, मित्र/रिश्तेदार और स्वयं)।

निर्देश 3 – दुष्प्रभाव की रिपोर्ट करने वाले व्यक्ति का विवरण दें
- ✓ रिपोर्ट के मूल्यांकन हेतु नाम (वैकल्पिक), पता, टेलीफोन नं और ई–मेल उपलब्ध कराएं।

निर्देश 4 – ली जा रही है / ली जा चुकी दवाइयों का विवरण
- ✓ उन दवाइयों (दवाइयों) का नाम, ली गई दवाइयों, निष्क्रिय होने की तिथि, दवाइयां शुरू करने एवं रोकने की तिथि) का विवरण दें जिनके कारण आपको दुष्प्रभाव हुआ है।
- ✓ खुराक का स्वरूप (गोली (टेबलेट), कैप्सूल, इंजेक्शन, मौखिक तरल (पीने वाली दवा) और यदि कोई अन्य हो तो निर्दिष्ट करें।

निर्देश 5 – दुष्प्रभाव के प्रभाव के बारे में
- ✓ दुष्प्रभाव आरंभ और समाप्त होने की तिथि बताएं और यह भी निर्दिष्ट करें कि क्या दुष्प्रभाव अभी भी जारी हैं।

निर्देश 6 – दुष्प्रभाव कितने हानिकारक थे?
- ✓ कृपया उचित डब्बे पर निशान लगाएं।

निर्देश 7– दुष्प्रभाव की व्याख्या करें
- ✓ कृपया दुष्प्रभाव का विवरण और उस दुष्प्रभाव से छुटकारा पाने के लिए क्या उपचार किया गया, विवेचना करें।

इस फॉर्म को पूरा करने के लिए अपना समय देने हेतु आपका धन्यवाद।

ANNEXURE 2A

MHRA-Yellow-Card-patient-form-to-report-side-effects

Tear along the dotted line

Confidential

✹ Yellow Card

Use blue or black ink. Complete all the lines marked with ✸ and give as much other information as you can

1 About the suspected side effect

✸ **What were the symptoms of the suspected side effect, and how did it happen?** If there isn't enough space here, attach an extra sheet of paper.

_____
_____
_____
_____

How bad was the suspected side effect? Tick the box that best describes how bad the symptoms were.

✸ ☐ Mild ☐ Unpleasant, but did not affect everyday activities ☐ Bad enough to affect everyday activities ☐ Bad enough to see doctor
☐ Bad enough to be admitted to hospital ☐ Caused very serious illness ☐ Caused death ☐ Other _____

When did the side effect start?

How is the person feeling now? Tick the box that best describes whether the person still has symptoms of the suspected side effect.

✸ ☐ Better (no more symptoms) ☐ Getting better ☐ Still has symptoms ☐ More seriously ill ☐ Died ☐ Other

Can you give any more details? For example, did the person take or receive any other treatment for the symptoms? Did they stop taking the medicine as a result of the side effect?

_____
_____
_____
_____

2 About the person who had the suspected side effect

Who had the suspected side effect? **Is the patient pregnant?**

✸ ☐ You ☐ Your child ☐ Someone else ☐ Yes ☐ No ☐ Unknown ☐ N/A

Information about the person Supply as much information as you can, even if you prefer not to give a name.

First name or initials _____ Family name _____ ☐ Male ☐ Female

✸ Age _____ Weight _____ ☐ kg ☐ stones/pounds Height _____ ☐ metres ☐ feet/inches

Any other relevant information? For example, does the patient have any medical conditions or allergies? If the patient is pregnant, please provide date of last menstrual period and as much information as you can about this and any previous pregnancies.

_____
_____

Make sure you have completed all the lines marked ✸ **Please turn over →**

3 About the medicine(s) which might have caused the side effect

Give details of the medicine you suspect of causing the side effect.

* **Name of the medicine** _____ ☐ prescription ☐ bought in pharmacy ☐ bought elsewhere

Dosage (for example, one 250 mg tablet, twice a day) _____ ☐ bought on the internet

What was it taken for? _____

Start date: _____ End date: _____ Did you stop because of side effects? ☐ Yes ☐ No

If you (or the person you're reporting for) were taking any other medicine at the same time (which might have caused an interaction), give details of it. If you need to give details of more than one other medicine, attach an extra sheet of paper.

Name of other medicine _____ ☐ prescription ☐ bought in pharmacy ☐ bought elsewhere

Dosage (for example, one 250 mg tablet, twice a day) _____ ☐ bought on the internet

What was it taken for? _____

Do you think this medicine might also have caused the side effect? ☐ Yes ☐ No ☐ Possibly

Start date: _____ End date: _____ Did you stop because of side effects? ☐ Yes ☐ No

Have you taken any other medicines or herbal remedies (as well as the above) **within the last 3 months?** ☐ Yes ☐ No

4 About your doctor *(optional)*

Would you like a copy of this report to be sent to your doctor?

☐ Yes ☐ No If Yes, give the doctor's name and address.

If you want us to send a copy of this report to any other healthcare professional, attach a separate sheet with their contact details.

If we need more medical information (such as test results), do we have your permission to contact your doctor directly for it?

☐ Yes ☐ No

Doctor's name _____

Address _____

_____

_____ Postcode _____

5 About you — the person making the report

We need contact details — please supply a full postal address, even if you prefer not to give a phone number or email address.

* Title _____ First name or initials _____ Family name _____

* Address _____

* _____ Postcode _____

Telephone number _____ Email address _____

Please sign and date this form

I agree that the Medicines and Healthcare products Regulatory Agency (MHRA) can contact me to discuss the suspected side effect, and to ask for more information that might help understanding of the case.

* Signed _____ Date _____

Please return this form in the envelope provided to: FREEPOST YELLOW CARD. (No other address details are required) © Crown Copyright 2015

ANNEXURE 2B

MHRA Yellow-Card-Healthcare-professional-form-February-2017

In Confidence

REPORT OF SUSPECTED ADVERSE DRUG REACTIONS
COMMISSION ON HUMAN MEDICINES (CHM)
It's easy to report online: mhra.gov.uk/yellowcard or via the app

Yellow Card
Making medicines safer

If you suspect an adverse reaction may be related to one or more drugs/vaccines/complementary remedies, please complete this Yellow Card. See 'Adverse reactions to drugs' section in the British National Formulary (BNF), visit **mhra.gov.uk/yellowcard**, or see the back of this form for guidance. Do not be put off reporting because some details are not known.

PATIENT DETAILS Patient Initials:_____ Sex: M / F Ethnicity:_____ Pregnant? Y / N Weight (kg):_____
Age (at time of reaction):_____ Identification number (e.g. Your Practice or Hospital Ref):_____

SUSPECTED DRUG(S)/VACCINE(S)

Drug/Vaccine (Brand if known)	Batch	Route	Dosage	Date started	Date stopped	Prescribed for

SUSPECTED REACTION(S) Please describe the reaction(s) and any treatment given:
(Please attach additional pages if necessary)

Outcome
Recovered ☐
Recovering ☐
Continuing ☐
Other ☐

Date reaction(s) started:_____ Date reaction(s) stopped: _____
Do you consider the reaction(s) to be serious? Yes / No
If yes, please indicate why the reaction is considered to be serious (please tick all that apply):

☐ Patient died due to reaction   ☐ Involved or prolonged inpatient hospitalisation
☐ Life threatening   ☐ Involved persistent or significant disability or incapacity
☐ Congenital abnormality   ☐ If medically significant, please give details:

Do you consider that the suspected reaction(s) resulted from a medication error? Yes/No

OTHER DRUG(S) (including self-medication and complementary remedies)
Did the patient take any other medicines/vaccines/complementary remedies in the last 3 months prior to the reaction? Yes / No
If yes, please give the following information if known:

Drug/Vaccine (Brand if known)	Batch	Route	Dosage	Date started	Date stopped	Prescribed for

Additional relevant information e.g. medical history, test results, known allergies, rechallenge (if performed), further details about any medication error (e.g. errors in prescription, dosing, dispensing or administration). For reactions relating to use of a medicine during pregnancy please state all other drugs taken during pregnancy, the last menstrual period, information on previous pregnancies, ultrasound scans, any delivery complications, birth defects or developmental concerns.

Please list any medicines obtained from the internet:

REPORTER DETAILS
Name and Professional Address: _____

Postcode:_____ Tel No: _____
Email: _____
Speciality: _____
Signature:_____ Date: _____

CLINICIAN (if not the reporter)
Name and Professional Address: _____

Postcode:_____ Tel No: _____
Email: _____
Speciality: _____
Date: _____

MHRA Interactive information on suspected adverse drug reactions received by the MHRA is available at **mhra.gov.uk/yellowcard** under Drug Analysis Profiles. Stay up-to-date on the latest advice for the safe use of medicines with our monthly bulletin *Drug Safety Update* at **gov.uk/drug-safety-update**

Please attach additional pages if necessary. Send to: FREEPOST YELLOW CARD (no other address details or postage required)

FREEPOST YELLOW CARD

SECOND FOLD HERE

GUIDELINES FOR YELLOW CARD REPORTING: SUSPECTED ADVERSE DRUG REACTIONS

Please use the Yellow Card Scheme to tell us about:

- **All** suspected adverse drug reactions (ADRs) **for new medicines** – identified by a black triangle ▼ symbol
- **All serious*** suspected ADRs in adults and children for established vaccines and medicines, including unlicensed medicines, herbal or homeopathic remedies, and medicines used off-label
- **All medication errors that result in an adverse reaction** (e.g. any reactions from unintentional errors in prescription, dosing, dispensing, or administration). There are no repercussions from reporting any such errors to the Scheme.

*Reactions which are fatal, life-threatening, a congenital abnormality, disabling or incapacitating, result in or prolong hospitalisation, or medically significant are considered serious.

If you are unsure, please report anyway

For more information contact Yellow Card Information Service: Freephone 0800 731 6789 or yellowcard@mhra.gsi.gov.uk

It's easy to report suspected ADRs online: www.mhra.gov.uk/yellowcard or via the **Yellow Card app (ADRs only)**.

You can also report a Yellow Card **online** for suspected problems or incidents relating to medical devices adverse incidents, defective medicines, counterfeit healthcare products, or safety concerns for e-cigarettes or their refill containers (e-liquids).

FIRST FOLD HERE

ANNEXURE 3A

Form FDA- 3500

U.S. Department of Health and Human Services

MedWatch
The FDA Safety Information and Adverse Event Reporting Program

For VOLUNTARY reporting of adverse events, product problems and product use errors

Page 1 of 3

Form Approved: OMB No. 0910-0291, Expires: 9/30/2018
See PRA statement on reverse.

FDA USE ONLY
Triage unit sequence #
FDA Rec. Date

Note: For date prompts of "dd-mmm-yyyy" please use 2-digit day, 3-letter month abbreviation, and 4-digit year; for example, 01-Jul-2015.

A. PATIENT INFORMATION

1. Patient Identifier
2. Age
   - ☐ Year(s) ☐ Month(s)
   - ☐ Week(s) ☐ Days(s)
   - or Date of Birth (e.g., 08 Feb 1925)
   - In Confidence
3. Sex
   - ☐ Female
   - ☐ Male
4. Weight
   - ☐ lb
   - ☐ kg

5.a. Ethnicity (Check single best answer)
- ☐ Hispanic/Latino
- ☐ Not Hispanic/Latino

5.b. Race (Check all that apply)
- ☐ Asian ☐ American Indian or Alaskan Native
- ☐ Black or African American ☐ White
- ☐ Native Hawaiian or Other Pacific Islander

B. ADVERSE EVENT, PRODUCT PROBLEM

1. Check all that apply
   - ☐ Adverse Event ☐ Product Problem (e.g., defects/malfunctions)
   - ☐ Product Use Error ☐ Problem with Different Manufacturer of Same Medicine

2. Outcome Attributed to Adverse Event (Check all that apply)
   - ☐ Death Include date (dd-mmm-yyyy): _ _ - _ _ _ - _ _ _ _
   - ☐ Life-threatening ☐ Disability or Permanent Damage
   - ☐ Hospitalization – initial or prolonged ☐ Congenital Anomaly/Birth Defects
   - ☐ Other Serious (Important Medical Events)
   - ☐ Required Intervention to Prevent Permanent Impairment/Damage (Devices)

3. Date of Event (dd-mmm-yyyy)
4. Date of this Report (dd-mmm-yyyy)

5. Describe Event, Problem or Product Use Error

(Continue on page 3)

6. Relevant Tests/Laboratory Data, Including Dates

(Continue on page 3)

7. Other Relevant History, Including Preexisting Medical Conditions (e.g., allergies, pregnancy, smoking and alcohol use, liver/kidney problems, etc.)

(Continue on page 3)

C. PRODUCT AVAILABILITY

2. Product Available for Evaluation? (Do not send product to FDA)
   - ☐ Yes ☐ No ☐ Returned to Manufacturer on (dd-mmm-yyyy)

D. SUSPECT PRODUCTS

1. Name, Manufacturer/Compounder, Strength (from product label)

#1 – Name and Strength	#1 – NDC # or Unique ID
#1 – Manufacturer/Compounder	#1 – Lot #
#2 – Name and Strength	#2 – NDC # or Unique ID
#2 – Manufacturer/Compounder	#2 – Lot #

---

3. Dose or Amount | Frequency | Route
   #1
   #2

4. Dates of Use (From/To for each) (If unknown, give duration, or best guess) (dd-mmm-yyyy)
   #1
   #2

5. Diagnosis or Reason for Use (indication)
   #1
   #2

6. Is the Product Compounded?
   #1 ☐ Yes ☐ No
   #2 ☐ Yes ☐ No

7. Is the Product Over-the-Counter?
   #1 ☐ Yes ☐ No
   #2 ☐ Yes ☐ No

8. Expiration Date (dd-mmm-yyyy)
   #1 _ _ - _ _ _ - _ _ _ _ #2 _ _ - _ _ _ - _ _ _ _

9. Event Abated After Use Stopped or Dose Reduced?
   #1 ☐ Yes ☐ No ☐ Doesn't apply
   #2 ☐ Yes ☐ No ☐ Doesn't apply

10. Event Reappeared After Reintroduction?
    #1 ☐ Yes ☐ No ☐ Doesn't apply
    #2 ☐ Yes ☐ No ☐ Doesn't apply

E. SUSPECT MEDICAL DEVICE

1. Brand Name
2. Common Device Name | 2b. Procode
3. Manufacturer Name, City and State
4. Model # | Lot #
   Catalog # | Expiration Date (dd-mmm-yyyy)
   Serial # | Unique Identifier (UDI) #
5. Operator of Device
   - ☐ Health Professional
   - ☐ Lay User/Patient
   - ☐ Other

6. If Implanted, Give Date (dd-mmm-yyyy)
7. If Explanted, Give Date (dd-mmm-yyyy)

8. Is this a single-use device that was reprocessed and reused on a patient? ☐ Yes ☐ No

9. If Yes to Item 8, Enter Name and Address of Reprocessor

F. OTHER (CONCOMITANT) MEDICAL PRODUCTS

Product names and therapy dates (Exclude treatment of event)

(Continue on page 3)

G. REPORTER (See confidentiality section on back)

1. Name and Address
   - Last Name: | First Name:
   - Address:
   - City: | State/Province/Region:
   - Country: | ZIP/Postal Code:
   - Phone #: | Email:

2. Health Professional? ☐ Yes ☐ No
3. Occupation
4. Also Reported to:
   - ☐ Manufacturer/Compounder
   - ☐ User Facility
   - ☐ Distributor/Importer

5. If you do NOT want your identity disclosed to the manufacturer, please mark this box: ☐

PLEASE TYPE OR USE BLACK INK

FORM FDA 3500 (10/15) Submission of a report does not constitute an admission that medical personnel or the product caused or contributed to the event.

ADVICE ABOUT VOLUNTARY REPORTING

Detailed instructions available at: http://www.fda.gov/medwatch/report/consumer/instruct.htm

Report adverse events, product problems or product use errors with:
- Medications *(drugs or biologics)*
- Medical devices *(including in-vitro diagnostics)*
- Combination products *(medication & medical devices)*
- Human cells, tissues, and cellular and tissue-based products
- Special nutritional products *(dietary supplements, medical foods, infant formulas)*
- Cosmetics
- Food *(including beverages and ingredients added to foods)*

Report product problems - quality, performance or safety concerns such as:
- Suspected counterfeit product
- Suspected contamination
- Questionable stability
- Defective components
- Poor packaging or labeling
- Therapeutic failures (product didn't work)

Report SERIOUS adverse events. An event is serious when the patient outcome is:
- Death
- Life-threatening
- Hospitalization - initial or prolonged
- Disability or permanent damage
- Congenital anomaly/birth defect
- Required intervention to prevent permanent impairment or damage (devices)
- Other serious (important medical events)

Report even if:
- You're not certain the product caused the event
- You don't have all the details

How to report:
- Just fill in the sections that apply to your report
- Use section D for all products except medical devices
- Attach additional pages if needed
- Use a separate form for each patient
- Report either to FDA or the manufacturer *(or both)*

Other methods of reporting:
- 1-800-FDA-0178 - To FAX report
- 1-800-FDA-1088 - To report by phone
- www.fda.gov/medwatch/report.htm - To report online

If your report involves a serious adverse event with a device and it occurred in a facility outside a doctor's office, that facility may be legally required to report to FDA and/or the manufacturer. Please notify the person in that facility who would handle such reporting.

If your report involves a serious adverse event with a vaccine, call 1-800-822-7967 to report.

Confidentiality: The patient's identity is held in strict confidence by FDA and protected to the fullest extent of the law. The reporter's identity, including the identity of a self-reporter, may be shared with the manufacturer unless requested otherwise.

The information in this box applies only to requirements of the Paperwork Reduction Act of 1995

The burden time for this collection of information has been estimated to average 40 minutes per response, including the time to review instructions, search existing data sources, gather and maintain the data needed, and complete and review the collection of information. Send comments regarding this burden estimate or any other aspect of this collection of information, including suggestions for reducing this burden to:

Department of Health and Human Services
Food and Drug Administration
Office of Chief Information Officer
Paperwork Reduction Act (PRA) Staff
PRAStaff@fda.hhs.gov

Please DO NOT RETURN this form to the PRA Staff e-mail to the left.

OMB statement:
"An agency may not conduct or sponsor, and a person is not required to respond to, a collection of information unless it displays a currently valid OMB control number."

U.S. DEPARTMENT OF HEALTH AND HUMAN SERVICES
Food and Drug Administration

FORM FDA 3500 (10/15) (Back)   Please Use Address Provided Below -- Fold in Thirds, Tape and Mail

---

DEPARTMENT OF
HEALTH & HUMAN SERVICES

Public Health Service
Food and Drug Administration
Rockville, MD 20857

Official Business
Penalty for Private Use $300

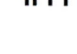

BUSINESS REPLY MAIL
FIRST CLASS MAIL PERMIT NO. 946 ROCKVILLE MD

POSTAGE WILL BE PAID BY FOOD AND DRUG ADMINISTRATION

MEDWATCH
The FDA Safety Information and Adverse Event Reporting Program
Food and Drug Administration
5600 Fishers Lane
Rockville, MD 20852-9787

NO POSTAGE
NECESSARY
IF MAILED
IN THE
UNITED STATES
OR APO/FPO

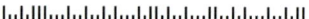

Annexure 3A: Form FDA-3500

U.S. Department of Health and Human Services

MedWatch
The FDA Safety Information and
Adverse Event Reporting Program

FORM FDA 3500 (10/15) *(continued)*

(CONTINUATION PAGE)

For VOLUNTARY reporting of adverse events and product problems

Page 3 of 3

B.5. Describe Event or Problem *(continued)*

B.6. Relevant Tests/Laboratory Data, Including Dates *(continued)*

B.7. Other Relevant History, Including Preexisting Medical Conditions *(e.g., allergies, pregnancy, smoking and alcohol use, hepatic/renal dysfunction, etc.)* *(continued)*

F. Concomitant Medical Products and Therapy Dates *(Exclude treatment of event)* *(continued)*

SPECIMEN COPY

ANNEXURE 3B

Form FDA- 3500A

U.S. Department of Health and Human Services
Food and Drug Administration

MEDWATCH
FORM FDA 3500A (10/15)

For use by user-facilities, importers, distributors and manufacturers for MANDATORY reporting

Page 1 of 3

Form Approved: OMB No. 0910-0291, Expires: 9/30/2018
See PRA statement on reverse.

Mfr Report #

UF/Importer Report #

FDA Use Only

Note: For date prompts of "dd-mmm-yyyy" please use 2-digit day, 3-letter month abbreviation, and 4-digit year; for example, 01-Jul-2015.

A. PATIENT INFORMATION

1. Patient Identifier
   In Confidence
2. Age
   ☐ Year(s) ☐ Month(s)
   ☐ Week(s) ☐ Days(s)
   or Date of Birth (e.g., 08 Feb 1925)
3. Sex
   ☐ Female
   ☐ Male
4. Weight
   ☐ lb
   ☐ kg

5.a. Ethnicity (Check single best answer)
   ☐ Hispanic/Latino
   ☐ Not Hispanic/Latino

5.b. Race (Check all that apply)
   ☐ Asian ☐ American Indian or Alaskan Native
   ☐ Black or African American ☐ White
   ☐ Native Hawaiian or Other Pacific Islander

B. ADVERSE EVENT OR PRODUCT PROBLEM

1. ☐ Adverse Event and/or ☐ Product Problem (e.g., defects/malfunctions)
2. Outcome Attributed to Adverse Event (Check all that apply)
   ☐ Death Include date (dd-mmm-yyyy): _____
   ☐ Life-threatening
   ☐ Hospitalization – initial or prolonged
   ☐ Disability or Permanent Damage
   ☐ Congenital Anomaly/Birth Defects
   ☐ Other Serious (Important Medical Events)
   ☐ Required Intervention to Prevent Permanent Impairment/Damage (Devices)

3. Date of Event (dd-mmm-yyyy)
4. Date of this Report (dd-mmm-yyyy)

5. Describe Event or Problem

(Continue on page 3)

6. Relevant Tests/Laboratory Data, Including Dates

(Continue on page 3)

7. Other Relevant History, Including Preexisting Medical Conditions (e.g., allergies, pregnancy, smoking and alcohol use, liver/kidney problems, etc.)

(Continue on page 3)

C. SUSPECT PRODUCT(S)

1. Name, Manufacturer/Compounder, Strength

#1 – Name and Strength	#1 – NDC # or Unique ID
#1 – Manufacturer/Compounder	#1 – Lot #
#2 – Name and Strength	#2 – NDC # or Unique ID
#2 – Manufacturer/Compounder	#2 – Lot #

2. Concomitant Medical Products and Therapy Dates (Exclude treatment of event)

(Continue on page 3)

Submission of a report does not constitute an admission that medical personnel, user facility, importer, distributor, manufacturer or product caused or contributed to the event.

PLEASE TYPE OR USE BLACK INK

3. Dose | Frequency | Route Used
#1
#2

4. Therapy Dates (If unknown, give duration) from/to (or best estimate) (dd-mmm-yyyy)
#1
#2

5. Diagnosis for Use (Indication)
#1
#2

6. Is the Product Compounded?
#1 ☐ Yes ☐ No
#2 ☐ Yes ☐ No

7. Is the Product Over-the-Counter?
#1 ☐ Yes ☐ No
#2 ☐ Yes ☐ No

8. Expiration Date (dd-mmm-yyyy)
#1 _____ #2 _____

9. Event Abated After Use Stopped or Dose Reduced?
#1 ☐ Yes ☐ No ☐ Doesn't apply
#2 ☐ Yes ☐ No ☐ Doesn't apply

10. Event Reappeared After Reintroduction?
#1 ☐ Yes ☐ No ☐ Doesn't apply
#2 ☐ Yes ☐ No ☐ Doesn't apply

D. SUSPECT MEDICAL DEVICE

1. Brand Name
2. Common Device Name | 2b. Procode
3. Manufacturer Name, City and State

4. Model #	Lot #	5. Operator of Device
Catalog #	Expiration Date (dd-mmm-yyyy)	☐ Health Professional
Serial #	Unique Identifier (UDI) #	☐ Lay User/Patient ☐ Other

6. If Implanted, Give Date (dd-mmm-yyyy)
7. If Explanted, Give Date (dd-mmm-yyyy)

8. Is this a single-use device that was reprocessed and reused on a patient? ☐ Yes ☐ No
9. If Yes to Item 8, Enter Name and Address of Reprocessor

10. Device Available for Evaluation? (Do not send to FDA)
   ☐ Yes ☐ No ☐ Returned to Manufacturer on: _____

11. Concomitant Medical Products and Therapy Dates (Exclude treatment of event)

(Continue on page 3)

E. INITIAL REPORTER

1. Name and Address
   Last Name: | First Name:
   Address:
   City: | State/Province/Region:
   Country: | ZIP/Postal Code:
   Phone #: | Email:

2. Health Professional?
   ☐ Yes ☐ No

3. Occupation (Select from list)

4. Initial Reporter Also Sent Report to FDA
   ☐ Yes ☐ No ☐ Unk

Annexure 3B: Form FDA- 3500A

MedWatch
FORM FDA 3500A (10/15) *(continued)*

Page 2 of 3

F. FOR USE BY USER FACILITY/IMPORTER *(Devices Only)*

1. Check One
   - ☐ User Facility
   - ☐ Importer
2. UF/Importer Report Number
3. User Facility or Importer Name/Address
4. Contact Person
5. Phone Number
6. Date User Facility or Importer Became Aware of Event *(dd-mmm-yyyy)*
7. Type of Report
   - ☐ Initial
   - ☐ Follow-up #
8. Date of This Report *(dd-mmm-yyyy)*
9. Approximate Age of Device
10. Event Problem Codes *(Refer to coding manual)*
    - Patient Code
    - Device Code
11. Report Sent to FDA? *(If Yes, enter date (dd-mmm-yyyy))*
    - ☐ Yes
    - ☐ No
12. Location Where Event Occurred
    - ☐ Hospital
    - ☐ Home
    - ☐ Nursing Home
    - ☐ Outpatient Treatment Facility
    - ☐ Outpatient Diagnostic Facility
    - ☐ Ambulatory Surgical Facility
    - ☐ Other: _____ *(Specify)*
13. Report Sent to Manufacturer? *(If Yes, enter date (dd-mmm-yyyy))*
    - ☐ Yes
    - ☐ No
14. Manufacturer Name/Address

G. ALL MANUFACTURERS

1. Contact Office (and Manufacturing Site for Devices)
   - Name
   - Address
   - Email Address
   - Compounding Outsourcing Facility 503B? ☐ Yes
2. Phone Number
3. Report Source *(Check all that apply)*
   - ☐ Foreign
   - ☐ Study
   - ☐ Literature
   - ☐ Consumer
   - ☐ Health Professional
   - ☐ User Facility
   - ☐ Company Representative
   - ☐ Distributor
   - ☐ Other: _____
4. Date Received by Manufacturer *(dd-mmm-yyyy)*
5. NDA # _____ ANDA # _____ IND # _____ BLA # _____ PMA/510(k) # _____
6. If IND, Give Protocol #
7. Type of Report *(Check all that apply)*
   - ☐ 5-day
   - ☐ 7-day
   - ☐ 10-day
   - ☐ 15-day
   - ☐ 30-day
   - ☐ Periodic
   - ☐ Initial
   - ☐ Follow-up # _____
   - Combination Product ☐ Yes
   - Pre-1938 ☐ Yes
   - OTC ☐ Yes
8. Adverse Event Term(s)
9. Manufacturer Report Number

H. DEVICE MANUFACTURERS ONLY

1. Type of Reportable Event
   - ☐ Death
   - ☐ Serious Injury
   - ☐ Malfunction
2. If Follow-up, What Type?
   - ☐ Correction
   - ☐ Additional Information
   - ☐ Response to FDA Request
   - ☐ Device Evaluation
3. Device Evaluated by Manufacturer?
   - ☐ Not Returned to Manufacturer
   - ☐ Yes ☐ Evaluation Summary Attached
   - ☐ No *(Attach page to explain why not)* or provide code:
4. Device Manufacture Date *(dd-mmm-yyyy)*
5. Labeled for Single Use?
   - ☐ Yes ☐ No
6. Event Problem and Evaluation Codes *(Refer to coding manual)*
   - Patient Code
   - Device Code
   - Method
   - Results
   - Conclusions
7. If Remedial Action Initiated, Check Type
   - ☐ Recall
   - ☐ Repair
   - ☐ Replace
   - ☐ Relabeling
   - ☐ Notification
   - ☐ Inspection
   - ☐ Patient Monitoring
   - ☐ Modification/Adjustment
   - ☐ Other: _____
8. Usage of Device
   - ☐ Initial Use of Device
   - ☐ Reuse
   - ☐ Unknown
9. If action reported to FDA under 21 USC 360i(f), list correction/removal reporting number:
10. ☐ Additional Manufacturer Narrative   and / or   11. ☐ Corrected Data

---

This section applies only to requirements of the Paperwork Reduction Act of 1995.
The public reporting burden for this collection of information has been estimated to average 73 minutes per response, including the time for reviewing instructions, searching existing data sources, gathering and maintaining the data needed, and completing and reviewing the collection of information. Send comments regarding this burden estimate or any other aspect of this collection of information, including suggestions for reducing this burden to:

Department of Health and Human Services
Food and Drug Administration
Office of Chief Information Officer
Paperwork Reduction Act (PRA) Staff
PRAStaff@fda.hhs.gov
Please DO NOT RETURN this form to the above PRA Staff email address.

OMB Statement: "An agency may not conduct or sponsor, and a person is not required to respond to, a collection of information unless it displays a currently valid OMB control number."

MEDWATCH
FORM FDA 3500A (10/15) *(continued)*

(CONTINUATION PAGE)
For use by user-facilities,
importers, distributors, and manufacturers
for MANDATORY reporting
Page 3 of 3

B.5. **Describe Event or Problem** *(continued)*

B.6. **Relevant Tests/Laboratory Data, Including Dates** *(continued)*

B.7. **Other Relevant History, Including Preexisting Medical Conditions** *(e.g., allergies, pregnancy, smoking and alcohol use, hepatic/renal dysfunction, etc.) (continued)*

Concomitant Medical Products and Therapy Dates *(Exclude treatment of event) (For continuation of C.2 and/or D.11; please distinguish)*

Other Remarks

ANNEXURE 3C

Form FDA-3500B

DEPARTMENT OF HEALTH AND HUMAN SERVICES
Food and Drug Administration

Form Approved: OMB No. 0910-0291
Expiration Date: 9/30/2018
(See PRA Statement below)

MedWatch Consumer Voluntary Reporting
(FORM FDA 3500B)

When do I use this form?

- You were hurt or had a bad side effect (including new or worsening symptoms) after taking a drug or using a medical device or product.
- You used a drug, product, or medical device incorrectly which could have or led to unsafe use.
- You noticed a problem with the quality of the drug, product or medical device.
- You had problems with how a drug worked after switching from one maker to another maker.

Don't use this form to report:

- Vaccines – report problems to the Vaccine Adverse Event Reporting System (VAERS).
- Investigational drugs or medical devices (those being studied) – report problems to your doctor or to the contact person listed in the clinical trial.

Will the information I report be kept private?

The FDA recognizes that privacy is an important concern, so you should know:

- We ask only for the name and contact information of the person filling out the form in case we need more information.
- Your name and contact information may be shared with the company that makes the product to help them better understand the problem you are reporting, unless you request otherwise (see Section E).

What types of products should I use this form for?

- Drugs, including prescription or over-the-counter medicines, and biologics, such as human cells and tissues used for transplantation (for example, tendons, ligaments, and bone) and gene therapies

- Medical devices, including any health-related kit, test, tool, or piece of equipment (such as breast implants, pacemakers, diabetes glucose-test kits, hearing aids, breast pumps, and many others)
- Nutrition products including vitamins and minerals, herbal remedies, infant formulas, medical foods, such as those labeled for people with a specific disease or condition
- Cosmetics such as moisturizers, makeup, shampoos and conditioners, face and body washes, deodorants, nail care products, hair dyes and relaxers, and tattoos
- Foods (including beverages and ingredients added to foods)

Are there specific instructions for filling out the form?

- Fill in as much information as possible and send in the report even if you do not have all the information.
- You can fill out this form yourself or have someone fill it out for you. If you need help, you may want to talk with your health professional.
- Feel free to include or attach an image of the product. Please do not send the products to the FDA.

How will I know the FDA has received my form?

- You will receive a reply from the FDA after we receive your report. We will personally contact you only if we need additional information.
- Your report will become part of a database so that it can be reviewed and compared to other reports by an FDA safety evaluator who will determine what steps to take.

How can I contact the FDA if I have questions?

Toll-free line: 1-800-332-1088
www.fda.gov/reportinghelp
To report online: www.fda.gov/medwatch/report.htm

The information below applies only to requirements of the Paperwork Reduction Act of 1995.

The burden time for this collection of information is estimated to average 30 minutes per response, including the time to review instructions, search existing data sources, gather and maintain the data needed and complete and review the collection of information. Send comments regarding this burden estimate or any other aspect of this information collection, including suggestions for reducing this burden to the address to the right:

OMB Statement: "An agency may not conduct or sponsor, and a person is not required to respond to, a collection of information unless it displays a currently valid OMB number."

Department of Health and Human Services
Food and Drug Administration
Office of Chief Information Officer
Paperwork Reduction Act (PRA) Staff
PRAStaff@fda.hhs.gov

DO NOT SEND YOUR COMPLETED FORM TO THIS PRA STAFF ADDRESS.

FORM FDA 3500B (10/15)   **MedWatch** Consumer Voluntary Reporting   General Information Page
EF

DEPARTMENT OF HEALTH AND HUMAN SERVICES
Food and Drug Administration

Form Approved: OMB No. 0910-0291
Expiration Date: 9/30/2018
(See PRA Statement on preceding general information page)

MedWatch Consumer Voluntary Reporting
(FORM FDA 3500B)

Note: For date prompts of "dd-mmm-yyyy" please use 2-digit day, 3-letter month abbreviation, and 4-digit year; for example, 01-Jul-2015.

Section A – About the Problem

What kind of problem was it? *(Check all that apply)*

☐ Were hurt or had a bad side effect *(including new or worsening symptoms)*
☐ Used a product incorrectly which could have or led to a problem
☐ Noticed a problem with the quality of the product
☐ Had problems after switching from one product maker to another maker

Did any of the following happen? *(Check all that apply)*

☐ Hospitalization – admitted or stayed longer
☐ Required help to prevent permanent harm *(for medical devices only)*
☐ Disability or health problem
☐ Birth defect
☐ Life-threatening
☐ Death *(include date)(dd-mmm-yyyy):* __ __ - __ __ __ - __ __ __ __
☐ Other serious/important medical incident *(Please describe below)*

Date the problem occurred *(dd-mmm-yyyy)*
__ __ - __ __ __ - __ __ __ __

Tell us what happened and how it happened. *(Include as many details as possible)*

[Continuation Page]

List any relevant tests or laboratory data if you know them. *(Include dates)*

[Continuation Page]

For a problem with a product, including
- prescription or over-the-counter medicine
- biologics, such as human cells and tissues used for transplantation (for example, tendons, ligaments, and bone) and gene therapies
- nutrition products, such as vitamins and minerals, herbal remedies, infant formulas, and medical foods
- cosmetics or make-up products
- foods (including beverages and ingredients added to foods)

➡ **Go to Section B**

For a problem with a medical device, including
- any health-related test, tool, or piece of equipment
- health-related kits, such as glucose monitoring kits or blood pressure cuffs
- implants, such as breast implants, pacemakers, or catheters
- other consumer health products, such as contact lenses, hearing aids, and breast pumps

➡ **Go to Section C (Skip Section B)**

For more information, visit http://www.fda.gov/MedWatch

Submission of a report does not constitute an admission that medical personnel or the product caused or contributed to the event.

FORM FDA 3500B (10/15)   **MedWatch** Consumer Voluntary Reporting   Page 1 of 3
EF

Annexure 3C: Form FDA- 3500B

Section B – About the Products

Name of the product as it appears on the box, bottle, or package *(Include as many names as you see)*

Name of the company that makes (or compounds) the product

Is the Product Compounded? *(Your health professional may be able to help you identify whether the drug was compounded.)*	☐ Yes ☐ No	Is the Product Over-the-Counter?	☐ Yes ☐ No

Expiration date *(dd-mmm-yyyy)* __ __ - __ __ __ - __ __ __ __ **Lot number** **NDC number**

Strength *(for example, 250 mg per 500 mL or 1 g)*	Quantity *(for example, 2 pills, 2 puffs, or 1 teaspoon, etc.)*	Frequency *(for example, twice daily or at bedtime)*	How was it taken or used *(for example, by mouth, injection, or on the skin)?*

Date the person first started taking or using the product *(dd-mmm-yyyy):* __ __ - __ __ __ - __ __ __ __

Date the person stopped taking or using the product *(dd-mmm-yyyy):* __ __ - __ __ __ - __ __ __ __

Why was the person using the product? *(such as, what condition was it supposed to treat)*

Did the problem stop after the person reduced the dose or stopped taking or using the product? ☐ Yes ☐ No

Did the problem return if the person started taking or using the product again? ☐ Yes ☐ No ☐ Didn't restart

Do you still have the product in case we need to evaluate it? *(Do not send the product to FDA. We will contact you directly if we need it.)* ☐ Yes ☐ No

➡ **Go to Section D (Skip Section C)**

Section C – About the Medical Device

Name of medical device

Name of the company that makes the medical device

Other identifying information *(The model, catalog, lot, serial, or UDI number, and the expiration date, if you can locate them)*

Was someone operating the medical device when the problem occurred? ☐ Yes ☐ No	If yes, who was using it? ☐ The person who had the problem ☐ A health professional *(such as a doctor, nurse, or aide)* ☐ Someone else *(Please explain who)*

For implanted medical devices ONLY *(such as pacemakers, breast implants, etc.)*

Date the implant was put in *(dd-mmm-yyyy)* __ __ - __ __ __ - __ __ __ __   **Date the implant was taken out** *(If relevant) (dd-mmm-yyyy)* __ __ - __ __ __ - __ __ __ __

➡ **Go to Section D**

For more information, visit http://www.fda.gov/MedWatch

Submission of a report does not constitute an admission that medical personnel or the product caused or contributed to the event.

Section D – About the Person Who Had the Problem

Person's Initials	Sex ☐ Female ☐ Male	Age *(specify unit of time for age)* ☐ Year(s)　☐ Month(s) ☐ Week(s)　☐ Day(s)	Date of Birth *(dd-mmm-yyyy)* __ __ - __ __ __ - __ __ __ __	Weight *(Specify lbs or kg)* ☐ lb　☐ kg
Race/ Ethnicity	Ethnicity *(Choose only one)* ☐ Hispanic/Latino ☐ Not Hispanic/Latino	Race *(Choose all that apply)* ☐ American Indian or Alaskan Native ☐ Native Hawaiian or Other Pacific Islander	☐ Asian ☐ White	☐ Black or African American

List known medical conditions. *(Such as diabetes, high blood pressure, cancer, heart disease, or others)*

Please list all allergies *(such as to drugs, foods, pollen or others)*

List any other important information about the person *(such as smoking, pregnancy, alcohol use, etc.)*

List all current prescription medications and medical devices being used.

[Continuation Page]

List all over-the-counter medications and any vitamins, minerals, supplements, and herbal remedies being used.

[Continuation Page]

➡ **Go to Section E**

Section E – About the Person Filling Out This Form

We will contact you only if we need additional information.

Last name	First name
Number/Street	City and State/Province
Country	ZIP or Postal code
Telephone number	Email address	Today's date *(dd-mmm-yyyy)*

Did you report this problem to the company that makes the product (the manufacturer/compounder)?　☐ Yes　☐ No

If you do NOT want your identity disclosed to the manufacturer, place an 'X' in this box:　☐

Send This Report by Mail or Fax

Keep the product in case the FDA wants to contact you for more information. Please do not send products to the FDA. Mail or fax the form to: MedWatch, Food and Drug Administration, 5600 Fishers Lane, Rockville, MD 20852; FAX: 800-332-0178 (toll-free).

Thank you for helping us protect the public health.

For more information, visit http://www.fda.gov/MedWatch	Submission of a report does not constitute an admission that medical personnel or the product caused or contributed to the event.

FORM FDA 3500B (10/15)　　**MedWatch** Consumer Voluntary Reporting

Annexure 3C: Form FDA- 3500B

Continued Entries
CONTINUED ENTRY FOR: Tell us what happened and how it happened. *(Include as many details as possible)*
CONTINUED ENTRY FOR: List any relevant tests or laboratory data if you know them. *(Include dates)*
CONTINUED ENTRY FOR: List all current prescription medications and medical devices being used.
CONTINUED ENTRY FOR: List all over-the-counter medications and any vitamins, minerals, and herbal remedies being used.

FORM FDA 3500B (10/15)   **MedWatch** – Consumer Voluntary Reporting   Continuation Page

General Instructions for Completing the MedWatch Form FDA 3500

For use by health professionals and consumers for VOLUNTARY reporting of adverse events, product use errors and product quality problems with:
- drugs
- biologics, (including blood components, blood derivatives, allergenics, human cells, tissues, and cellular and tissue-based products (HCT/Ps)
- medical devices (including *in vitro* diagnostics)
- combination products (e.g. durg-device, biologic-device)
- special nutritional products (dietary supplements, infant formulas, medical foods)
- cosmetics

Adverse events involving vaccines should be reported to the Vaccine Adverse Event Reporting System (VAERS), http://vaers.hhs.gov/pdf/vaers_form.pdf. Adverse events involving investigation (study) drugs **such as those relating to investigational New Drug (IND) application** should be reported as required in the study protocol and sent to the address and contact person listed in the study protocol. They should generally not be submitted to FDA MedWatch as voluntary reports.

Note for consumers: If possible, please take the 3500 form to your health professional (e.g. doctor or pharmacist) so that information based on your medical record that can help in the evaluation of your report will be provided. If, for whatever reason, you do not wish to have your health professional fill out the form, you are welcome to do so yourself.

GENERAL INSTRUCTIONS
- Please make sure that all entries are either typed, printed in a font no smaller than 8 point, or written using black ink
- Please complete all sections that apply to your report
- Dates should be entered as mm/dd/yyyy (e.g., June 3, 2005 = 06/03/2005). If exact dates are unknown, please provide the best estimate (see B3)
- For narrative entries, if the fields do not provide adequate space, attach additional pages as needed
- If attaching additional pages, please do the following:
  - Identify all attached pages as Page_____ of _____
  - Indicate the appropriate section and block number next to the narrative continuation
  - Include the phrase continued at the end of each field that has additional information continued onto another page
- **Section D,** Suspect product(s), should be used to report on special nutritional products and cosmetics as well as drugs or biologics, including human cells, tissues, and cellular and tissue-based products (HCT/Ps)
- If your report involves a serious adverse event with a device and it occurred in a facility other than a doctor's office, that facility may be legally required to report to FDA and/or manufacturer. Please notify the person in that facility who would handle such reporting.

QUESTIONS AND VOLUNTARY REPORTING?
Call MedWatch at 800-FDA-1088 or 301-796-1935

Annexure 3C: Form FDA- 3500B

SECTION A: PATIENT INFORMATION

Complete a separate form for each patient, unless the report involves a medical device where multiple patients were adversely affected through the use of the same device. In that case, please indicate the number of patients in block B5 (Describe event or problem) and complete Section A and blocks B2, B5, B6, B7 and F for each patient. Enter the corresponding patient identifier in block A1 for each patient involved in the event.

Parent-child/fetus report(s) are those cases in which either a fetus/breastfeeding infant or the mother, or both, have an adverse event that is possibly associated with a product administered to the mother during pregnancy. Several general principles are used for filing these reports:

- If there has been no event affecting the child/fetus, report only on the parent
- For those cases describing fetal death, miscarriage or abortion, report the parent as the patient in the report
- When only the child/fetus has an adverse reaction/event (other than fetal death, miscarriage or abortion), the information provided in section A applies to the child/fetus. However, the information in Section D would apply to the parent who was the source of exposure to the product.
- When a newborn baby is found to have a birth defect/congenital anomaly that the initial report considers possibly associated with a product administered to the mother during pregnancy, the patient is the newborn baby
- If both the parent and the child/fetus have adverse events, separate reports should be submitted for each patient.

A1: Patient Identifier

Please provide the patient's initials or some other type of identifier that will allow you, the reporter, to readily locate the case if you are contacted for more information. Do not use the patient's name or social security number.

The patient's identity is held in strict confidence by FDA and protected to the fullest extent of the law. The FDA will not disclose the reporter's identity in response to a request from the public, pursuant to the Freedom of Information Act.

If no patient was involved (such as may be the case with a product problem), enter none.

A2: Age at Time of Event or Date of Birth

Provide the most precise information available. Enter the patient's birth date, if known, or the patient's age at the time of event onset. For age, indicate time units used (e.g. years, months, days).

- If the patient is 3 years or older, use years (e.g. 4 years)
- If the patient is less than 3 years old, use months (e.g. 24 months)
- If the patient is less than 1 month old, use days (e.g. 5 days)
- Provide the best estimate if exact age is unknown.

A3: Sex

Enter the patient's gender. If the adverse event is a congenital anomaly/birth defect, report the sex of the child.

A4: Weight

Indicate whether the weight is in pounds (lb) or kilograms (kg). Make a best estimate if exact weight is unknown.

SECTION B: ADVERSE EVENT, PRODUCT PROBLEM, PRODUCT USE ERROR

B1: Adverse Event, Product Problem, Product Use Error, or Problem with Different Manufacturer of Same Medicine

Choose the appropriate box(es). If a product problem may have caused or contributed to the adverse event, check the both boxes.

Adverse event: Any incident where the use of a medication (drug or biologic, including HCT/P), at any dose, medical device (including *in vitro diagnostics*) or a special nutritional product (e.g. dietary supplement, infant formula or medical food) is suspected to have resulted in an adverse outcome in a patient.

To report, it is not necessary to be certain of a cause/effect relationship between the adverse event and the use of the medical product(s) in question. Suspicion of an association is sufficient reason to report. Submission of a report does not constitute an admission that medical personnel or the product caused or contributed to the event.

Please limit your submissions to those events that are serious. An event is classified as serious when the patient outcome is:

- Death
- Life-threatening
- Hospitalization (initial or prolonged)
- Disability or permanent damage
- Congenital anomaly/Birth defect
- Required medical or surgical intervention to prevent permanent impairment or damage (Devices)
- Other serious (Important medical events)

Please see instruction for block B2 for further information on each of these criteria.

Product problem (e.g. defects/malfunctions): Any report regarding the quality, performance, or safety of any medication, medical device or special nutritional product. In addition, please select this category when reporting device malfunctions that would lead to a death or serious injury if the malfunction were to recur. Product problem include, but are not limited to, such concerns as:

- Suspected counterfeit product
- Suspected contamination
- Questionable stability
- Defective components
- Therapeutic failures (product did not work)
- Product confusion (caused by name, labeling, design or packaging)
- Suspected superpotent or subpotent medication
- Labeling problems caused by printing errors/omissions.

Product use error:

Medication use error: Any report of a medication error regardless of patient involvement of outcome. Also report cirumstances or events that have the capacity to cause error (e.g. similar product appearance, similar packaging and labeling, sound-aloke/look-alike names, etc.).

Medication errors can and do originate in all stages of the medication use system, which includes selecting and procuring drugs, prescribing, preparing and dispensing, administering and monitoring. A medication error is defined as "any preventable event that may cause or lead to inappropriate medication use or patient harm while the medication is in the control of the health care professional, patient, or consumer. Such events may be related to professional practice, health care products, procedures, and systems, including prescribing, order communication, product labeling packaging, nomenclature, compounding, dispensing, distribution, administration, education, monitoring and use."

Medical device use error: Health care professionals, patients, and consumers can unintentionally cause harm to patients or to themselves when using medical devices. These problems can often arise due to problems with the design of the medical device or the manner in which the device is used. Often use-errors are caught and prevented before they can do harm (close call). Report use errors regardless of patient involvement or outcome. Also report circumstances or events that could cause use errors. Medical device use errors usually occur for one or more of the following reasons:

- Users expect devices to operate differently than they do.
- Product use is inconsistent with use's expectations or intuition
- Product use requires physical, perceptual, or cognitive abilities that exceed those of the user
- Devices are used in ways not anticipated by the manufacturer
- Product labeling or packaging is confusing or inadequate
- The environment adversely effects or influences device use.

Problem with different manufacturer of same medicine: Any incident, to include, but not limited to, differences in noted therapeutic response, suspected to have resulted from a switch, or change, from one manufacturer to another manufacturer of the **same** medicine or drug product. This could be changes from a brand name drug product to a generic manufacturer's same product, or from a genetic manufacturer's product to the same product as supplied by a different generic

Annexure 3C: Form FDA- 3500B

SECTION B: ADVERSE EVENT, PRODUCT PROBLEM, PRODUCT USE ERROR

manufacturer, or from a generic manufacturer's product to the same product as supplied by a different generic manufacturer, or from a generic manufacturer's product to a brand name manufacturer of the same product. In order to fully evaluate the incident, please include in **Section B5**. If available, specific information relative to the switch between different manufacturers of the same medicine, to include, but not limited to, the names of the manufacturers, length of treatment on each manufacture's product, product strength, and any relevant clinical data.

B2: Outcomes attributed to adverse event: Indicate all that apply to the reported event:

Death: Check only if you suspect that the death was an outcome of the adverse event, and include the date if known.

Do not check if:
- The patient died while using a medical product, but there was no suspected association between the death and the use of the product
- A fetus is aborted because of a congenital anomaly (birth defect), or is miscarried.

Life-threatening: Check if suspected that:
- The patient was at substantial risk of dying at the time of the adverse event, or
- Use or continued use of the device or other medical product might have resulted in the death of the patient.

Hospitalization (Initial or prolonged): Check if admission to the hospital or prolongation of hospitalization was a result of the adverse event.

Do not check if:
- A patient in the hospital received a medical product and subsequently developed an otherwise nonserious adverse event, unless the adverse event prolonged the hospital stay.

Do check if:
- A patient is admitted to the hospital for one or more days, even if released on the same day
- An emergency room visit results in admission to the hospital emergency room visits that do not result in admission to the hospital should be evaluated for one of the other serious outcomes (e.g. life-threatening; required intervention to prevent permanent impairment or damage; other serious (medically important event).

Disabiity or permanent damage: Check if the adverse event resulted in a substantial disruption of a person's ability to conduct normal life functions. Such would be the case if the adverse event resulted in a significant, persistent or permanent change, impairment, damage or disruption in the patient's body function/structure, physical activities and/or quality of life.

Congenital anomaly/birth defect: Check if you suspect that exposure to a medical product prior to conception or during pregnancy may have resulted in an adverse outcome in the child.

Required intervention to prevent permanent impairment or damage (Devices): Check if you believe that medical or surgical intervention was necessary to preclude permanent impairment of a body function, or prevent permanent damage to a body structure, either situation suspected to be due to the use of a medical product.

Other serious (important medical events): Check when the event does not fit the other outcomes, but the event may jeopardize the patient and may require medical or surgical intervention (treatment) to prevent one of the other outcomes. Examples include allergic brochospasm (a serious problem with breathing) requiring treatment in an emergency room, serious blood dyscrasias (blood disorders) or seizures/convulsions that do not result in hospitalization. The development of drug dependence of drug abuse would also be examples of important medical events.

B3: Date of Event
Provide the actual or best estimate of the date of first onset of the adverse event. If day is unknown, month and year are acceptable. If day and month are unknown, year is acceptable.
- When a newborn baby is found to have a congenital anomaly, the event onset date is the date of birth of the child.
- When a fetus is aborted because of a congenital anomaly, or is miscarried, the event onset date is the date pregnancy is terminated
- If information is available as to time during pregnancy when exposure occurred, indicate that information is narrative block **B5**.

B4: Date of this Report
The date the report is filled out.

B5: Describe event, problem or product user error
For an **adverse event:**

Describe the event in detail, including a description of what happened and a summary of all relevant clinical information (medical status prior to the event; signs and/or symptoms; differentials diagnosis for the event in question; clinical course; treatment; outcome, etc.). If available and if relevant, include synopses of any office visit notes or the

SECTION B: ADVERSE EVENT, PRODUCT PROBLEM, PRODUCT USE ERROR

hospital discharge summary. To save time and space (and if permitted by your institution), please attach copies of these records with any confidential information deleted. **Do not identify any patient, physician, or institution by name. The reporter's identity should be provided in full in Section G.**
Information as to any environmental conditions that may have influenced the event should be included, particularly when (but not exclusive to) reporting about a device.
- Results of relevant tests and laboratory data should be entered in block **B6**. (See instructions for **B6**)
- Pre-existing medical conditions and other relevant history belong in block **B7**. Be as complete as possible, including time courses for pre-existing diagnosis (see instruction for **B7**)

If it is determined that reuse of a medical device lebeled for single use may have caused or contributed to an adverse patient outcome, please report in block B5 the facts of the incident and the perceived contribution of reuse to the occurrence.

For a product problem: Describe the problem (quality, performance, or safety concern) in sufficient detail so that the circumstances surrounding the defect or malfunction of the medical product can be understood.
- If available, the results of any evaluation of a malfunctioning device and, if known, any relevant maintenance/service information should be included in this section
- For a medication or special nutritional product problem, please indicate if you have retained a sample that would be available to FDA.

For a product use error: Describe the sequence of events leading up to the error in sufficient detail so that the circumstances surrounding the error can be understood.
- **For medication use errors:** Include a description of the error, type of staff involved, work environment in which the error occurred, indicate causes or contributing factors to the error, location of the error, names of the products involved (including) the trade proprietary) and established (proper) name, manufacturer, dosage form, strength, concentration, and type and size of container.
- **For medical device use errors:** Report circumstances or events that could cause use errors. Medical device use errors usually occur for one or more of the following reasons:
  - Users expect devices to operate differently than they do
  - Product use is inconsistent with user's expectations or intuition
  - Product use requires physical, perceptual, or cognitive abilities that exceed those of the user
  - Devices are used in ways not anticipated by the manufacturer

- Product labeling or packaging is confusing or inadequate
- The environment adversely effects or influences device use.

For a problem with a different manufacturer of the same medicine:
Please include specific information relative to the switch between different manufacturers of the same medicine, to include, but not limited to, the names of the manufacturers, length of treatment on each manufacturer's product, product strength, and any relevant clinical data.

B6: Relevant tests/laboratory data, including dates
Please provide all appropriate information, including relevant negative tests and laboratory findings, in order to most completely convey how the medical work-up/assessment led to strong consideration of medical product-induced disease as etiology for clinical status, as other differential diagnostic considerations were being eliminated.

Please include:
- Any relevant baseline laboratory data prior to the administration or use of the medical product
- All laboratory data used in diagnosing the event
- Any available laboratory data/engineering analyses (for devices) that provide further information on the course of the event.

If available, please include:
- Any pre- and post-event medication levels and dates (if applicable)
- Synopses of any relevant autopsy, pathology, engineering, or laboratory reports.

If preferred, copies of any reports may be submitted as attachments, with all confidential information deleted.
Do not identify any patient, physician or institution by name. The initial's reporter's identity should be provided in full in **Section G**.

B7: Other relevant history, including pre-existing medical conditions
Knowledge of other risk factors can help in the evaluation of a reported adverse event. If available, provide information on:
- **Other known conditions in the patient, e.g.**
  - Hypertension (high blood pressure)
  - Diabetes mellitus
  - Liver or kidney problems
- **Significant history**
  - Race
  - Allergies
  - Pregnancy history
  - Smoking and alcohol use, drug abuse
  - Setting

Annexure 3C: Form FDA- 3500B

SECTION C: PRODUCT AVAILABILITY
Product available for evaluation: (Do not send the product to FDA)

To evaluate a reported problem with a medical product, it is often critical to be able to examine the product. Please indicate whether the product is available for evaluation. Also indicate if the product was returned to the manufacturer and, if so, the date of the return.

SECTION D: PRODUCT AVAILABILITY

For adverse event reporting:
A suspect product is one that your suspect is associated with the adverse event. In **Section F** enter other concomitant medical products (drug, biologics including human cells, tissues, and cellular and tissue-based products (HCT/Ps) medical devices, etc.) that the patient was using at the time of the event but which you do not think were involved in the event.

Up to two (2) suspect products may be reported on one form (#1 = first suspect product, #2 = second suspect product). Attach an additional form if there were more than two suspect products associated with the reported adverse event.

For product quality problem reporting:
A suspect product is the product that is the subject to the report. A separate form should be submitted for each individual product problem report.

Identification of the labeler/distributor and pharmaceutical manufacturer and labeled strength of the product is important for prescription or non-prescription products.

This section may also be used to report on special nutritional products (e.g. dietary supplements, infant formula or medical foods), cosmetics, human cells, tissues, or cellular and tissue-based products (HCT/Ps) or other products regulated by FDA.

If reporting on a special nutritional or a drug product quality problem, please attach labeling/packaging if available.

If reporting on a special nutritional only, please provide directions for use as listed on the product labeling.

D1: Name, strength, manufacturer

Use the trade/brand name. If the trade/brand name is not known or if there is no trade/brand name, use the generic product name and the name of the manufacturer or labeler. These names are usually found on the product packaging or labeling. Strength is the amount in each tablet or capsule, the concentration of an injectable, etc. (such as "10 mg", "100 units/cc", etc.).

For human cells, tissues, and cellular and tissue-based products (HCT/Ps), please provide the common name of the HCT/P. You can also indicate if the HCT/P has a proprietary or trade name. Examples, Achilles tendon, liac crest bone and Islet cells.

D2: Dose or Amount, Frequency, Route

Describe how the product was used by the patient (e.g. 500 mg QID orally or 10 mg every other day IV). For reports involving overdoses, the amount of product used in the overdose should be listed, not the prescribed amount (See **APPENDIX** for list of **Routes of Administration** on the next page).

D3: Dates of use

Provide the date administration was started (or best estimate) and the date stopped (or best estimate). If no dates are known, an estimated duration is acceptable (e.g. 2 years) or if therapy was less than one day, then duration is appropriate (e.g. 1 dose or 1 hour for an IV).

For human cells, tissues, and cellular and tissue-based products, provide the date of transplant and if applicable, the date of explanation.

D4: Diagnosis or reason for use (Indication)

Provide the reason or indication for which the product was prescribed or used in this particular patient.

D5: Event abated after use stopped or dose reduced

If available, this information is particularly useful in the evaluation of a suspected adverse event. In addition to checking the appropriate box, please provide supporting laboratory tests and dates, if available, in block B6.

D6: Lot #

If known, include the lot number(s) with all product quality problem reports, or any adverse event report with a biologic, or medication.

D7: Expiration date

Please include if available.

SECTION D: PRODUCT AVAILABILITY

D8: Event reappeared after reintroduction

This information is particularly useful in the evaluation of a suspected adverse event. In addition to checking the appropriate box, please provide a description of what happened when the drug was stopped and then restarted in block **B5**, and any supporting laboratory tests and dates in block **B6**.

D9: NDC # or unique identification

The National Drug Code (NDC #) is requested only when reporting a drug product problem. Zeros and dashes should be included as they appear on the label. NDC # can be found on the original product label and/or packaging, but is usually not found on dispensed pharmacy prescriptions.

If the product has a unique or distinct identification code, please provide this here. This is applicable to human cells, tissues, and cellular and tissue-based product (HCT/Ps).

APPENDIX: ROUTES OF ADMINISTRATION

Auricular (otic) 001	Intracerebral 018	Intrasynovial 035	Perineural 052
Buccal 002	Intracervical 019	Intratumor 036	Rectal 053
Cutaneous 003	Intracisternal 020	Intrathecal 037	Respiratory (Inhalation) 054
Dental 004	Intracorneal 021	Intrathoracic 038	Retrobulbar 055
Endocervical 005	Intracoronary 022	Intratracheal 039	Subconjunctival 056
Endosinusial 006	Intradermal 023	Intravenous bolus 040	Subcutaneous 057
Endotracheal 007	Intradiscal (intraspinal) 024	Intravenous drip 041	Subdermal 058
Epidural 008	Intrahepatic 025	Intravenous (not otherwise specified) 042	Sublingual 059
Extra-amniotic 009	Intralesional 026	Intravesical 043	Topical 060
Hemodialysis 010	Intralymphatic 027	Iontophoresis 044	Transdermal 061
Intracorpus cavernosum 011	Intramedullar (bone marrow) 028	Occlusive dressing technique 045	Transmammary 062
Intra-amniotic 012	Intrameningeal 029	Ophthalmic 046	Transplacental 063
Intra-arterial 013	Intramuscular 030	Oral 047	Unknown 064
Intra-articular 014	Intraocular 031	Oropharyngeal 048	Urethral 065
Intrauterine 015	Intrapericardial 032	Other 049	Vaginal 066
Intracardiac 016	Intraperitoneal 033	Parenteral 050	
Intracavernous 017	Intrapleural 034	Periarticular 051	

Annexure 3C: Form FDA- 3500B

SECTION E: SUSPECT MEDICAL DEVICE

The suspect medical device is (1) the device that may have caused or contributed to the adverse event or (2) the device that malfunctioned.

In **Section F**, report other concomitant medical products (drug, biologics including HCT/Ps, medical devices, etc.) that the patient was using at the time of the event but which you do not think were involved in the event.

If more than one suspect medical device was involved in the event, complete all of **Section E** for the first device and attach a separate completed **Section E** for each additional device.

If the suspect medical device is a single use device that has been reprocessed, then the reprocessor is now the device manufacturer.

E1: Brand Name

The trade or proprietary name of the suspect medical device as used in product labeling or in the catalog (e.g. Flo-easy Catheter, Reliable Heart Pacemaker, etc.). This information may (1) be on a label attached to a durable device, (2) be on a package of a disposable device, or (3) appear in labeling materials of an implantable device. Reprocessed single use devices may bear the original Equipment manufacturer (OEM) brand name. If the suspect device is a reprocessed single use device enter "NA".

E2: Common Device Name

The generic or common name of the suspect medical device or a generally descriptive name (e.g. urological catheter, heart pacemaker, patient restraint, etc.). Please do not use broad generic terms such as "catheter", "valve", "screw", etc.

E3: Manufacturer Name, City and State

If available, list the full name, city and state of the manufacturer of the suspected medical device. If the answer is Block E8 is "yes", then enter the name, city and state of the reprocessor.

E4: Model #, Catalog #, Serial #, Lot #, Expiration date, Other

If available, provide any or all identification numbers associated with the suspect medical device exactly as they appear on the device or device labeling. This includes spaces, hyphens, etc.

Model #
The exact model number found on the device label or accompanying packaging.

Catalog #
The exact number as it appears in the manufacturer's catalog, device labeling, or accompanying packaging.

Serial #
This number can be found on the device label or accompanying packaging; it is assigned by the manufacturer, and should be specific to each device.

Lot#:
This number can be found on the label or packaging material.

Expiration date (mm/dd/yyyy):
If available, this date can often be found on the device itself or printed on the accompanying packaging.

Other #:
Any other applicable identification number (e.g. component number, product number, part bar-coded product ID, etc.).

E5: Operator of Device

Indicate the type (not the name) of person operating or using the suspect medical device on the patient at the time of the event as follows:
- Health professional = physician, nurse, respiratory therapist, etc.
- Lay user/patient = person being treated, parent/spouse/friend of the patient
- Other = nurses aide, orderly, etc.

E6: If implanted, give date (mm/dd/yyyy)

For medical devices that are implanted in the patient, provide the implant date or your best estimate. If day is unknown, month and year are acceptable. If month and day are unknown, year is acceptable.

E7: If explanted, give date (mm/dd/yyyy)

If an implanted device was removed from the patient, provide the explantation date or your best estimate. If day is unknown, month and year are acceptable. If month and day are unknown, year is acceptable.

E8: Is this a single-use device that was return before reprocessed and reused on a patient?

Indicate "Yes" or "No"

E9: If yes to item no. 8, enter name and address of reprocessor:

Enter the name and address of the reprocessor of the single-use device. Anyone who reprocesses single-use devices for reuse in humans is the manufacturer of the reprocessed device.

SECTION F: OTHER (CONCOMITANT) MEDICAL PRODUCTS

Prorduct names and therapy dates (exclude treatment of event)

Information on the use of concomitant medical products can frequently provide insight into previously unknown interactions between products, or provide an alternative explanation for the observed adverse event. Please list and provide product names and therapy dates for any other medical products (drugs, biologics including HCT/Ps, medical devices, etc.) that the patient was using at the time of the event. Do not include products used to treat the event.

SECTION G: REPORTER

FDA recognize that confidentiality is an important concern in the context to adverse event reporting. The patient's identity is held in strict confidence by FDA and protected to the fullest extent of the law. However, to allow for timely follow-up in serious cases, the reporter's identity may be shared with the manufacturer unless specifically requested otherwise in block G5. The FDA will not disclose the reporter's identity in response to a request from the public, pursuant to the Freedom of Information Act.

G1: Name, address, phone #, e-mail
Please provide the name, mailing address, phone number and e-mail address of the person who can be contacted to provide information on the event if follow-up is necessary. While optional, providing the fax number would be most helpful, if available. This person will also receive an acknowledgment letter from FDA on receipt of the report.

G2: Health professional?
Please indicate whether you are a health professional (e.g. physician, pharmacist, nurse, etc.) or not.

G3: Occupation
Please indicate your occupation (particularly type of health professional), and include specialty, if appropriate.

G4: Also reported to
Please indicate whether you have also notified or submitted a copy of this report to the manufacturer and/or distributor of the product, or in the case of medical device reports only, to the user facility (institution) in which the event occurred. This information helps to track duplicate reports in the FDA database.

G5: Release of reporter's identify to the manufacturer
In the case of a serious adverse event, FDA may provide name, address and phone number of the reporter denoted in block **G1** to the manufacturer of the suspect product. If you do not want your identity released to the manufacturer, please put an X in this box.

ANNEXURE 4

First Information Report (FIR)

Section A — **FIRST INFORMATION REPORT (FIR)**
(To be completed by the person reporting the AEFI and sent to MO - Immediately)
(Only for Serious Adverse Events Following Immunization)

Serious AEFI category (Encircle): **Death / Hospitalized / Cluster* / Disability**

State	District
Block/ Ward	Village/ Urban Area

Address of the site:

Patient Name	
Age (in months) / Date of Birth	
Date of Vaccination	Time of Vaccination
Name of recent Vaccine(s) given:	
Date of first symptom	Time of first symptom
Current status (encircle)	**Death / Still Hospitalized / Recovered & Discharged / Left Against Medical Advice (LAMA)**
Date of Death	Time of Death
Additional Information:	

First Investigation Report (FIR)

Section B: **FIRST INVESTIGATION REPORT (FIR)**
(To be reported by MO to District HQ within 24 hours of AEFI case notification)
(Only for Serious Adverse Events Following Immunization)

AEFI Case ID (To be assigned by DIO):   IND (AEFI) /   State Code   /   District Code   /   Year   /   Serial No.

Reporting Medical Officer (Dr.) Name :   Date of filling FIR by MO :

Posted at: Designation: Mobile No.   Fax No.:

Land Line (with STD Code) :   Case Informed By :

If MO disagrees with information in Section A, please record details (with justification) here	
Patient Name	
Date of Birth	Age (in months) Sex Male Female
Date of Notification	Date of Investigation
Date of Vaccination	Time of Vaccination
Date of Onset	Time of Onset
Hospitalization No/ Yes Date	Time of Hospitalization
Name and Address of hospital:	
Outcome (encircle)	Death / Still Hospitalized / Recovered & Discharged / Left Against Medical Advice (LAMA)
If died, Date of Death	Time of Death
Post mortem done? (encircle)	Yes**/ No / Planned on (date) _____ If Yes, Date_____ Time_____

** Attach report (if available) with FIR

Details of vaccine, diluents & Vitamin-A given to the patient
(*In the doses administered column write the dose received by beneficiary like 1st, 2nd, 3rd, booster and any other)

Vaccine/Vit-A/ Diluent	*Dose Administered	Name of Manufacturer (in BLOCK Letters)	Batch No.	Manufacturing Date	Expiry Date
BCG					
BCG Diluent					
DPT					
OPV					
Measles					
Measles Diluent					
Hep-B					
DT					
TT					
Vit-A					
Others					

Annexure 4: First Investigation Report (FIR)

Place of vaccination   Govt. Health Facility /Outreach / Private Health Facility/ Other____   **Session**: SIA / Routine/ Other ___
Total number of beneficiaries immunized at session site: Pregnant women _____ Children _____
Number of other beneficiaries who received vaccine from the SAME VIAL:

Signature of Reporting Medical officer   Email id

Section C: The following information is to be completed by DIO &
                    forwarded to GoI and State within 24 hours of receiving the above information.

Proposed Date of District AEFI Review Committee Meeting for this Case.	D	D	M	M	Y	Y
Proposed date of preliminary investigation						

DIO/ District Nodal Person *(Officer forwarding this report)*

....Signature/ Seal

To be sent to : State Immunization Officer & Assistant commissioner
Immunization division of Govt. of India, MOHFW,
Nirman Bhawan, New Delhi – 110108. (Fax No. – 011 23062728   /   e mail: aefiindia@gmail.com**)**

ANNEXURE 5

Preliminary Investigation Report (PIR)

Section A

PRELIMINARY INVESTIGATION REPORT (PIR)
(To be reported to State & GoI within 7 days of submitting FIR)
(Only for Serious Adverse Events Following Immunization - Death / Hospitalized / Cluster / Disability)
DIO/RCHO/District Nodal Officer to complete all details in BLOCK letters only

State	District		Case ID	IND (AEFI) /	State Code /	District Code /	Year /	Serial No.

Block/ Ward		Village/ Urban Area	

Place of Vaccination *(encircle)* : Govt. Health Facility/ Private Health Facility/ Other Specify _____
Vaccination in *(encircle)* : SIA / Routine
Type of site *(encircle)* Outreach/ SC/ PHC/ CHC/ BPHC/ Dist Hospital State Hospital/ Medical College/ Other specify _____
Site Address:

Name of Reporting Officer :   Date of filling PIR :
Designation: Posted at:
Land Line (with STD Code) :   Mobile No.   Fax No.:

Patient Name*

* use separate form for each case in a cluster

Date of Birth	D	D	M	M	Y	Y	Y	Y	Age (in months)			Sex	Male	Female

Father's Name	
Mother's Name	

Complete Residential Address of the Case with landmarks *(Street name, house number, village, block, Tehsil, PIN No. etc.)*

P	I	N	-				P	H	O	N	E	-						

Details of vaccine, diluents & Vitamin-A given to the patient at this session site on the day of the event

Vaccine/Vit-A/ Diluent	*Dose Administered	Name of Manufacturer (in BLOCK Letters)	Batch No.	Manufacturing Date	Expiry Date
BCG	■				
BCG Diluent					
DPT					
OPV					
Measles					
Measles Diluent					
Hep-B					
DT	■				
TT					
Vit-A					
Others					

(*In the doses administered column write the dose received by beneficiary like 1st, 2nd, 3rd, booster and any other)

Date of First Information	D	D	M	M	Y	Y	Y	Y	Date of Preliminary Investigation	D	D	M	M	Y	Y	Y	Y
Date of Vaccination	D	D	M	M	Y	Y	Y	Y	Time of Vaccination	H	H	M	M	(	AM	PM	)
Date of first symptom	D	D	M	M	Y	Y	Y	Y	Time of first symptom	H	H	M	M	(	AM	PM	)
Date of Hospitalization	D	D	M	M	Y	Y	Y	Y	Time of Hospitalization	H	H	M	M	(	AM	PM	)

Outcome *(encircle)*	Death /Still Hospitalized /Discharged /Left Against Medical Advice (LAMA)/Not Hospitalized																
Date of Death	D	D	M	M	Y	Y	Y	Y	Time of Death	H	H	M	M	(	AM	PM	)

Post mortem done? *(encircle)*	Yes/ No / Planned on (date) _____	If Yes**, Date _____ Time _____ ** Attach report (if available) with FIR

Annexure 5: Preliminary Investigation Report (PIR)

Name _____ Case Id Number IND (AEFI) /State Code / District Code / Year / Serial No. PIR : Page 2/7

Section B	Relevant information of the patient prior to immunization:		
			If 'Yes', specify
Past H/o similar event		Yes / No	
Reaction after previous vaccination		Yes / No	
H/o allergy		Yes / No	
Pre-existing illness / disorder		Yes / No	
H/o hospitalization in last 30 days with cause		Yes / No	
Recent H/o trauma with date, time, site and mode		Yes / No	
For adult women			
	Currently pregnant?	Yes / No	
	Currently Breastfeeding	Yes / No	
Family History of any disease or allergy		Yes / No	
	Natal history	Full term / pre mature / post dated	
	Delivery	Normal / Caesarian / Assisted birth / any complication (specify)	
Was the patient on any concurrent medication for any illness (if Yes : name the drug, indication & Doses)		Yes / No /Unknown	

Section C	Details of first examination* of serious AEFI case

*Instructions – Attach copies of ALL available documents and then complete additional information NOT AVAILABLE in existing documents (case sheet, discharge summary, case notes, post mortem reports etc.) i.e.
 If Patient has taken medical care - <u>Attach copies of all available documents</u> (including case sheet, discharge summary, laboratory reports and post mortem reports - if available) <u>and complete only additional unavailable</u> information below
 If patient has not taken medical care – Complete this form fully

 If the investigator has disagreement with the findings in any of the document(s) mentioned above, the same may be expressed here with justification

Source of information (*encircle all that apply*): **Examination by the investigator/ Documents/ Verbal autopsy/ Other** _____

If from verbal autopsy, please mention the source (*encircle*)	Name of the person who first examined the child:_____
	Other sources (specify)

Signs and Symptoms in Chronological order:

The clinical details below are filled up by_____	Designation:
Date and time of onset of 1ˢᵗ symptoms:	Date and time of examination:

Findings on initial examination that are NOT documented in the available documents or if the investigator disagrees **with the information documented please record details (with justification) here**

Consciousness	Alert / drowsy / Unconscious other (specify)_____ Describe:
Vitals	Pulse Temperature Respiratory rate BP
Skin	Rash / cyanosis / petechiae / pallor / jaundice / others (specify)_____ Describe:
Eyes	Vision: Normal / Impaired Pupil : Normal / Constricted / Dilated / Reacting to light
Hearing Speech	Normal / Impaired (Describe) Normal / Abnormal (Describe)

Name   Case Id Number IND (AEFI) /State Code   / District Code   / Year   / Serial No.   PIR : Page 3/7

Neck	Neck Stiffness: Present / Absent
Chest	Auscultation Normal / Crepts / Rhonchi Heart sounds Normal / Murmur (Describe)
Respiratory	Normal / Cough / Shortness of breath / others (specify)_____ Describe:
GI	Pain abdomen / Vomiting / diarrhea / dysentery / others (specify)_____ Describe:
Abdomen	Normal / Distended / Tender Liver : Not palpable / Palpable (If palpable specify size) Spleen : Not palpable / Palpable (If palpable specify size) (Describe)

Limbs	Tone
	      Upper Limbs Normal / Increased / Decreased
	      Lower Limbs Normal / Increased / Decreased
	 Reflexes
	      Biceps Normal / Increased / Decreased / Absent
	      Triceps Normal / Increased / Decreased / Absent
	      Supinator Normal / Increased / Decreased / Absent
	 Plantar Extensor / Flexor

Any other abnormal signs.

Treatment provided:

Provisional diagnosis:

Add additional pages if needed

Annexure 5: Preliminary Investigation Report (PIR)

Name _____ Case Id Number IND (AEFI) /State Code / District Code / Year / Serial No.   PIR : Page 4/7

Section D — Details of immunization provided at the site on the day AEFI reported

Number of beneficiaries immunized for each antigen at session site. Attach record if available.	BCG	Hep-B1	OPV Birth	Hep B Birth	DPT-1	DPT-2	DPT-3	DPT-B1	DPT-B2	OPV-1	OPV-2
	OPV-3	OPV-B	Hep-B2	Hep-B3	Measles	DT	TT-1	TT-2	TT-B	Vit-A	Others

a) Number of beneficiaries immunized from the implicated vaccine vial/ampoule	
b) When was the patient immunized? *(encircle below)*	
Within the first vaccinations of the RI session / Within the last vaccinations of the RI session / Unknown	
Within the first few doses of the vial administered/ Within the last doses of the vial administered/ Unknown	
c) Number of OTHER beneficiaries immunized with the implicated vaccine vial in the same session	
d) Number of OTHER beneficiaries immunized with the implicated vaccine having the same batch number in the PHC/ CHC / district hospital/ other location specify _____	
c) Is this case a part of a cluster?	Yes / No
a. If yes, How many other cases have been detected in the cluster?	
b. Did all the cases receive vaccine from the same vial?	Yes / No
c. If No, Number of vials implicated	

Section E — Immunization practices at the location(s) where implicated vaccine was used
(fill up this section by asking & or observing practice)

Last vaccine storage point:

Temp of ILR (°C)		
Temp of deep freezer (°C)		
Correct procedure of storing vaccines, diluents and syringes followed?	Yes	No
Any other item (other than RI vaccines and diluents) in the ILR or freezer?	Yes	No
Partially used reconstituted vaccines in the ILR?	Yes	No
Unusable vaccines (expired, no label, VVM stage 3 & 4, frozen) in the ILR?	Yes	No
Unusable diluents (expired, manufacturer not matched, cracked, dirty ampoule) in the store?	Yes	No

Specific key findings/additional observations and comments:

Vaccine Transportation:

Type of vaccine carrier used		
Vaccine carrier sent to the RI site on the same day of vaccination?	Yes	No
Vaccination carrier returned from the RI site on the same day of vaccination?	Yes	No
Conditioned ice-pack used?	Yes	No

Specific key findings/additional observations and comments:

Syringes and Needles Used:

Are AD syringes used fro immunization?	Yes	No
If No, specify the type of syringes used: Glass/ Disposable/ Recycled disposable/ other specify _____		

Specific key findings/additional observations and comments:

Name _____ Case Id Number IND (AEFI) /State Code ___ / District Code ___ / Year ___ / Serial No. ___   PIR : Page 5/7

Reconstitution: (complete only if applicable, write NA if not applicable)

Reconstitution procedure (encircle)			
Same reconstitution syringe used for multiple vials of same vaccine?	Yes	No	NA
Same reconstitution syringe used for reconstituting different vaccines?	Yes	No	NA
Separate reconstitution syringe for each vaccine vial?	Yes	No	NA
Separate reconstitution syringe for each vaccination?	Yes	No	NA
Are the vaccines and diluents from the same manufacturer?	Yes	No	NA

Specific key findings/additional observations and comments:

Injection technique: (Observe another session in the same locality – same or different place)

Correct dose and route?	Yes	No
Time of reconstitution mentioned on vial (in case of BCG, Measles, JE)?	Yes	No
Non-touch technique followed?	Yes	No
Contraindication screened prior to vaccination?	Yes	No
How may AEFI reported from the centre that distributed the vaccine in last 30 days?		
Training on RI received by the vaccinator : (If Yes specify date of last training _____)	Yes	No

Specific key findings/additional observations and comments:

Private practitioner: (complete only if applicable, write NA for not applicable)

Source of vaccine (encircle)	Government Supply	Procured from manufacturer	Pharmacy (Chemist)	Others
Address of source from where vaccine was obtained for this patient				
Status of cold chain at private clinic (encircle)	Satisfactory***/ Unsatisfactory/ Not observed (specify why_____)			
Status of cold chain at procurement site (encircle)	Satisfactory***/ Unsatisfactory/ Not observed (specify why_____)			

***If it complies with ALL criteria in section E "Last vaccine storage point"

Additional observations and comments:

Section F   Community Investigation (Please visit locality and interview parents/ others)

Any similar events reported recently in the locality?   Yes / No
If Yes, Describe:

If Yes, How many events / Episodes?

Of those effected, How many are
 Vaccinated:_____
 Not Vaccinated:_____
 Unknown:_____

Annexure 5: Preliminary Investigation Report (PIR)

Name   Case Id Number IND (AEFI) /State Code   / District Code   / Year   / Serial No.   PIR : Page 6/7

Section G — District AEFI Committee Review & Investigation Report

a) District AEFI committee review held?				Yes	No
	If Yes, then date of review by district AEFI committee			D D M M Y Y	
b) Any implicated samples sent for testing following District AEFI committee review?				Yes	No

Details of Vaccine/ Diluent samples sent to CDL Kasauli

Vaccine/Diluent Name	Used Vial/Amp. Quantity	Batch no, Lot no, date of expiry	Date Sent	Unused Vial/Amp. Quantity	Batch no, Lot no, date of expiry	Date Sent

Details of Syringe/ Needle samples sent to CDL Kolkata

Type of Syringes	Quantity	Batch no, Lot no, date of expiry	Date Sent	Type of Needles	Quantity	Batch no, Lot no, date of expiry	Date Sent

c) Any **biological product** (CSF, Blood, Urine, etc) sent for testing?
If yes , specify details of the lab; attach copy of report if available   Yes   No

Note: for AEFI resulting within 28 days following JE vaccine , send sample of CSF, Serum to nearest NIV lab in Pune or Gorakhpur.

d) Was local drug inspector involved in collecting additional samples?   Yes   No

e) Other investigation, specify the findings and attach report.

Section H — Preliminary Assessment (working hypothesis of AEFI committee):

Probable underlying cause of the adverse event:

Type of Adverse Event suspected based on preliminary findings (encircle)	Programme Error	Vaccine Reaction*	Coincidental	Injection Reaction	Unknown

Specific reasons for suspecting the above:

Corrective actions/recommendations:

*If an event is suspected to be related to vaccine(s)/ diluent(s), immediate efforts should be initiated by DIO/ District Cold chain Officer to collate the information related to - Number of blocks supplied with the suspected batch and Number of beneficiaries vaccinated with the suspected batch.

| Name | Case Id Number IND (AEFI) /State Code | / District Code | / Year | / Serial No. | PIR : Page 7/7 |

Attached copies of reports / documents etc with this PIR:

1.
2.
3.
4.
5.
6.

District AEFI Committee that conducted the preliminary investigation

	Name	Designation	Phone #	Signature
1.				
2.				
3.				
4.				
5.				
6.				
7.				

Section I **DIO/ District Nodal Person** *(Officer forwarding this report)*

Name .... Designation................................Date of submission to state/ national level.....................

Mobile No.......................................Landline (with STD code).............................. Fax No. ....

Email id...................................... Complete Office address (with Pin code)...

....Signature/ seal............................Date

Please ensure that this PIR form (ALL 7 pages) reach:
State Immunization Officer & Assistant commissioner, Immunization division of Govt. of India, MOHFW, Nirman Bhawan, New Delhi – 110108.
(Fax No. – 011 23062728 / Email: aefiindia@gmail.com)

Important Laboratory Addresses:

Send Vaccines and Diluents to	Send syringes and needles to	Send Biological specimens to	
CDL Kasauli	**CDL Kolkata**	**NIV Gorakhpur**	**NIV Pune**
Director. Central Drugs Laboratory Central Research Institute Kasauli – 173204. Himachal Pradesh.	Director Central Drugs Laboratory Ministry of Health & Family Welfare Govt. of India 3, KYD Street Kolkata-700016	Director Officer In-Charge National Institute of Virology Gorakhpur Unit. BRD Medical College Campus Gorakhpur – 273013.	Director National Institute of Virology 20/ A, Dr. Ambedkar Road. Post Box No. 11, Pune - 411001 Maharashtra
Email : nclkasauli@bsnl.in	Email: cdlkol@gmail.com	Email: cdlkol@gmail.com	E-mail : nivicl@pn3.vsnl.net.in
Phone: 0179-2272046 0179-2272060	Phone: 033-22299021 033-22870513	Phone : 0551-2506698	Phone : 020-26127301 020-26006290
Fax: 0179-2272049 0179-2272016	Fax : 033-222 99380 033-222 99541	Fax : 0551-2506698	Fax: 020-26122669 020-26126399

For State level use only

Note: *If an event is suspected to be related to vaccine(s)/ diluent(s), then immediate efforts should be initiated by State Immunization Officer and State Cold chain Officer to collate the information related to the districts supplied with the suspected batch and number of beneficiaries vaccinated with the suspected batch. The consolidated data needs to be sent to the govt of India as early as possible*

ANNEXURE 6

Detailed Investigation Report (DIR)

Annex 3   DIR : Page 1/5

Section A

DETAILED INVESTIGATION REPORT (DIR)
(To be reported by district AEFI committee to State & GoI within 90 days of filling FIR)
(Only for Serious Adverse Events Following Immunization - Death / Hospitalized / Cluster / Disability)
DIO to fill page 1 to 4 and SEPIO to fill page 4 & 5 to complete all details in BLOCK letters only

State	District		Case ID	IND (AEFI) /	State Code	/	District Code	/	Year	/	Serial No.

Block/ Ward **Village/ Urban Area**

Place of Vaccination *(encircle)* : Govt. Health Facility/ Private Health Facility/ Other Specify _____
Vaccination in *(encircle)* : SIA / Routine
Type of site *(encircle)* Outreach/ SC/ PHC/ CHC/ BPHC/ Dist Hospital State Hospital/ Medical College/ Other specify _____
Site Address:

Name of Reporting Officer :   **Date of filling this DIR :**
Designation: **Posted at:**
Land Line (with STD Code) :   **Mobile No.**   **Fax No.:**

Patient Name*
* use separate form for each case in a cluster

Date of Birth	D	D	M	M	Y	Y	Y	Y	Age (in months)			Sex	Male	Female

Father's Name
Mother's Name
Complete Residential Address of the Case with landmarks *(Street name, house number, village, block, Tehsil, PIN No. etc.)*

P I N -   P H O N E -

Date of Vaccination	D	D	M	M	Y	Y	Y	Y	Time of Vaccination	H	H	M	M	(AM PM)
Date of Onset	D	D	M	M	Y	Y	Y	Y	Time of Onset	H	H	M	M	(AM PM)
Date of Hospitalization	D	D	M	M	Y	Y	Y	Y	Time of Hospitalization	H	H	M	M	(AM PM)

Outcome *(encircle)* Death/Still Hospitalized / Discharged / Left Against Medical Advice (LAMA)/ Not Hospitalized

| Date of Death | D | D | M | M | Y | Y | Y | Y | Time of Death | H | H | M | M | (AM PM) |
| Date of Post Mortem | D | D | M | M | Y | Y | Y | Y | Time of Post Mortem | H | H | M | M | (AM PM) |

Documents attached with this DIR: (Please retain the original and enclose ONLY COPIES)

Sl. No.	Documents	Date of submission/ completion	Attached with this document? *(encircle)*	Remarks (if any) and in case response is "No" then give reason
1.	First Information Report (FIR)		Yes / No	
2.	Preliminary Investigation Report (PIR)		Yes / No	
3.	Post Mortem Report done? *(in case of death)*		Yes / No	
4.	Result of any Pathology/Microbiology (Blood, CSF and Urine) Test done?		Yes / No	
5.	Doctor's prescription/treatment record for this AEFI		Yes / No	
6	Doctor's prescription/treatment record for other illness		Yes / No	
7.	Report of Laboratory test of vaccine/ diluent (if sent for testing)		Yes / No	

Patient Name	Case Id Number IND (AEFI) /State Code	/ District Code	/ Year	/ Serial No.	DIR : Page 2/5

8.	Report of Laboratory result of syringes/other drugs (if sent for testing)		Yes / No	
9.	Any other document relevant to case		Yes / No	If Yes, specify & attach report

Refer to FIR & PIR for writing the following case summary. Remember to include the following points, add additional sheet as necessary:

1. Detailed history of signs and symptoms and signs in chronological order
2. Additional relevant information prior to immunization:
3. Status of immunization on the day of AEFI reported (Completed doses before the event):
4. Vaccines administered on the day of the event:
5. Examination findings on first examination of serious AEFI case:
6. Any other abnormal signs (if any observed during initial examination). Add additional pages if needed:
7. Progress of the patient's condition, treatment provided and diagnosis:
8. Details of Community investigation if conducted:

CASE SUMMARY
Please add additional sheets to complete…

Please add additional sheets to complete…

Annexure 6: Detailed Investigation Report (DIR)

Patient Name .... Case Id Number IND (AEFI) /State Code / District Code / Year / Serial No. DIR : Page 3/5

DIO's report on District Assessment (working hypothesis of AEFI committee)

Probable underlying cause of the adverse event:

Type of Adverse Event suspected based on preliminary findings (encircle)	Programme Error	Vaccine Reaction*	Coincidental	Injection Reaction	Unknown

Specific reasons for suspecting the above:

Corrective actions/recommendations:

Details of District AEFI Committee members who conducted the preliminary investigation

	Name	Designation	Phone #
1.			
2.			
3.			
4.			
5.			
6.			
7.			

*If an event is suspected to be related to vaccine(s)/ diluent(s), then immediate efforts should be initiated by DIO/ District Cold chain Officer to collate the information related to - Number of blocks supplied with the suspected batch and Number of beneficiaries vaccinated with the suspected batch and the consolidated data needs to be reported in the following table:

Name of Vaccine/Diluent	Batch of suspected vaccine/diluent	Total number of blocks supplied with suspected vaccine/diluent in the district	Total number of beneficiaries vaccinated with suspected batch in the district	
			Children	Adults/ Preg women

DIO/ District Nodal Person (Officer forwarding this report)

Name .... Designation .... Date of submission to state/ national level.....................

Mobile No.................................... Landline (with STD code)........................... Fax No. ....

Email id................................... Complete Office address (with Pin code)...

....

....Signature/ seal.......................Date

Patient Name   **Case Id Number IND (AEFI)** /State Code   / District Code   / Year   / Serial No.   DIR : Page 4/5

Section B — To be completed at State Level
(Office of State Immunization Officer)

Date of receipt of this DIR at State	D	D	M	M	Y	Y	Y	Y

State/UT Causality Assessment Report

Note: State vaccine safety (AEFI) committee to complete causality assessment exercise and forward the report to GoI within 90 days of filling FIR.

Preparation for causality assessment check list for state EPI officer:

Sl. No.	List of document copies sent to the Govt of India	Availability (encircle)	Remarks (if any) / (if no why)
1.	First Information Report (FIR)	Yes / No	
2.	Preliminary Investigation Report (PIR)	Yes / No	
3.	Is the case summary completed in this DIR?	Yes / No	
4.	Report of Post Mortem Report done? (in case of death)	Yes / No	
5.	Report of any Pathology/Microbiology (Blood, CSF, Urine) Test done?	Yes / No	
6.	Doctor's prescription/treatment record for AEFI	Yes / No	
7.	Doctor's prescription/treatment record for other illness	Yes / No	
8.	Laboratory result of vaccine (if sent for testing)	Yes / No	
9.	Laboratory result of syringes/other drugs (if sent for testing)	Yes / No	
10.	Any other document relevant to case	Yes / No	If Yes, specify & attach report

Conclusion of State AEFI committee on causality

Probable underlying cause of the adverse event:

Type of Adverse Event suspected based on findings *** (encircle)	Programme Error	Vaccine Reaction	Coincidental	Injection Reaction	Unknown

***Causality: Very likely/Certain/ Probable/Possible/ Unlikely/Unrelated/Unclassifiable

(*** Refer to the relevant section on the Operational Guidelines on AEFI Surveillance – 2010 MoHFW – Government of India)

Specific reasons for suspecting the above:

Corrective actions/recommendations:

Annexure 6: Detailed Investigation Report (DIR)

Patient Name .... Case Id Number IND (AEFI) /State Code / District Code / Year / Serial No.   DIR : Page 5/5

Details of State AEFI Committee members who conducted the causality assessment			
Name	Designation	Phone #	Signature
1.			
2.			
3.			
4.			
5.			
6.			
7.			

Date of review of this case	D	D	M	M	Y	Y	Y	Y	Date of submission of report to GoI						

*If an event is suspected to be related to vaccine(s)/ diluent(s), then immediate efforts should be initiated by DIO/ District Cold chain Officer to collate the information related to - Number of blocks supplied with the suspected batch and Number of beneficiaries vaccinated with the suspected batch and the consolidated data needs to be reported in the following table:

Name of Vaccine/Diluent	Batch of suspected vaccine/diluent	Total number of blocks supplied with suspected vaccine/diluent in the district	Total number of beneficiaries vaccinated with suspected batch in the district	
			Children	Adults/ Preg women

State Nodal Person (Officer forwarding this report)

Name .... Designation............................Date of submission to national level.....................

Mobile No.................................... Landline (with STD code)........................... Fax No. ....

Email id....................... Complete Office address (with Pin code)...

....Signature/ seal...........................Date

Please ensure that this DIR form reaches:

Assistant Commissioner,
Immunization division of Govt. of India, MOHFW, Nirman Bhawan,
New Delhi – 110108.
(Fax No. – 011 23062728. or Email : aefiindia@gmail.com)

Section C	For use at National Level (Office of Assistant Commissioner- UIP)							
Date of receipt of DIR from District	D	D	M	M	Y	Y	Y	Y
Date of receipt of DIR from State (with Causality assessment report)	D	D	M	M	Y	Y	Y	Y

ANNEXURE 7

AEFI–Laboratory Requisition Form (LRF)

AEFI – LABORATORY REQUESITION FORM (LRF)
(To be completed by Drug Inspector/DIO. LRF should be accompanied with specimens)
(For Serious Adverse Events Following Immunization)

AEFI category (Encircle): **Death / Hospitalized / Cluster / Disability**

State		Case ID	IND (AEFI) / State Code / District Code / Year / Serial No.
District			
Block			

Name of Drug Inspector/DIO: Date of filling LRF :

Designation: Mobile No.:

Land Line (with STD Code) :   Fax No.:

Case Name	
Date of Birth	D D M M Y Y Y Y Age (in months) Sex Male / Female

Complete Address of the Case with landmarks *(Street name, house number, village, block, Tehsil, PIN No., Telephone No. etc.)*

P I N -   P H O N E -

Date of vaccination	D D M M Y Y Y Y	Date of Onset	D D M M Y Y Y Y
Date of collection of specimen	D D M M Y Y Y Y	Time of collection of specimen	H H M M (AM / PM)

1. Precise description of samples:

a) For vaccine/diluents specimens: (to be transported in reverse cold chain)

Mention vaccine/diluent	Quantity Sent	Name of Manufacturer (in BLOCK Letters)	Batch No.	Manufacturing Date	Expiry Date

b) For logistics specimens: (AD, Reconstitution, Disposable syringes)

Mention Logistics	Quantity Sent	Name of Manufacturer (in BLOCK Letters)	Batch No.	Manufacturing Date	Expiry Date

c) For Biological product specimen: (CSF, Blood, Urine, etc)

2. Test requested:

Annexure 7: AEFI–Laboratory Requisition Form (LRF) **315**

Name of AEFI Case:	Case ID IND (AEFI) /	State Code	/	District Code	/ Year	/ Serial No.

3. Preliminary clinical diagnosis (working hypotheses) of district AEFI committee:

4. Name & complete address of officials to whom laboratory results should be sent:

Send to	Complete address	Phone/Fax	Mobile	Email-ID
State Drug Controller				
State Cold Chain Officer				
State EPI Officer				
District Immunization Officer (DIO)				
Others (specify)				

To be completed by lab officials after receiving the specimen

Date of receipt of specimen at laboratory		D	D	M	M	Y	Y	Y	Y
Name of person receiving specimen(s) at laboratory								
Condition of specimen upon receipt at lab (*encircle*)		Good*			Poor			Unknown
Comments by pathologist, virologist or bacteriologist:								
Date specimen results sent from this lab		D	D	M	M	Y	Y	Y	Y
Name of laboratory professional								
Signature								
Landline No. :	Fax No.:				Email Id:			

* Criteria for "good" condition: Samples sent as per AEFI guidelines.

ANNEXURE 8

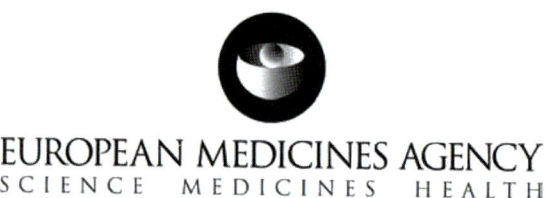

EUROPEAN MEDICINES AGENCY
SCIENCE MEDICINES HEALTH

30 March 2017
EMA/213497/2017

Guidelines on Good Pharmacovigilance Practices (GVP)

Introductory cover note, last updated with revision 2 of module V on risk management systems finalised post-public consultation, related revision 2 of module XVI and revision 2 of module II on pharmacovigilance system master file (PSMF)

- Background to GVP — 322
- History of the GVP development process and latest updates — 322
- Objectives of pharmacovigilance — 323
- Pharmacovigilance in the EU: roles of different actors — 323
- Legal basis, scope and process for GVP — 324
- Maintenance and Further Development of Gvp — 324
- Structure of GVP — 325
- Referencing of legal requirements in GVP — 325
- Practical advice for the public consultation — 326

BACKGROUND TO GVP

New legislation for pharmacovigilance applies in the European Union (EU) since July 2012, and to support its implementation, a set of guidelines for the conduct of pharmacovigilance in the EU has been developed which, as they have been adopted, replaced the previous set in Volume 9A of the Rules Governing Medicinal Products in the EU.

This new guidance on good pharmacovigilance practices (GVP) is organised into two types of chapters, namely Modules on pharmacovigilance processes and Product- or Population-Specific Considerations.

HISTORY OF THE GVP DEVELOPMENT PROCESS AND LATEST UPDATES

The first seven Modules on prioritised processes were consulted between 21 February and 18 April 2012 and revised, taking into account the comments received from stakeholders. They are available in their final versions which came into force on 2 July 2012.

Module III on pharmacovigilance inspections and Module X on processes for additional monitoring of medicinal products were released on 27 June 2012 for public consultation until 24 August 2012, and Module IV on pharmacovigilance audits and Module XV on safety communication were released on 26 July 2012 for public consultation until 21 September 2012. Modules III and IV were published in their final versions, together with the updated GVP Annexure I on definitions, on 13 December 2012. The final Module XV was published on 24 January 2013, together with a template for Direct Healthcare Professional Letters in the GVP Annexure II. On 25 April 2013, the final Module X on additional monitoring was published as final, taking into account latest additional legislation.

Since their first release as final, some Modules have been revised as final: Module II was published in its first revision, mainly to provide clarifications for herbal medicinal products, on 12 April 2013.

Module VIII Revision 1 and its Addendum Revision 1 as well as in Annexure II – Template for the PSUR Cover Page Revision 1 were published on 25 April 2013.

On 7 June 2013, the draft revision 1 of Module VI on the management and reporting of adverse reactions was released for public consultation, in order to provide more guidance on the clock state for reporting of valid case reports, reporting from post-authorisation safety studies as well as the handling of languages. Also on 7 June 2013, draft Module XVI on risk minimisation measures was released for public consultation. Both consultations closed on 5 August 2013. Module XVI was published in its final version on 28 February 2014; and revision 1 of Module VI was published as final on 15 September 2014.

On 12 December 2013, the first chapter with Product- or Population-Specific Considerations was provided in its final version, i.e. the chapter P.I on vaccines, following its public consultation launched on 12 April 2013. Also, revision 1 of Module VII on periodic safety update reports was provided in its final version following public consultation launched on 25 April 2013. This revision included updates for consistency with the recently finalised ICH-E2C (R2) guideline and on the operations in the EU.

On 8 January 2014, the definitions relating to vaccine pharmacovigilance, launched for public consultation on 12 April 2013, were published without any change post-consultation, together with other amendments to definitions and explanatory notes as detailed on page 2 of the GVP Annexure I on definitions in its revision 2.

On 25 April 2014, revision 1 of Module V on risk management system was published, mainly to amend the requirements of part VI of the RMP as published already in the updated RMP templates, to introduce amendments in line with the new requirements for variation applications and to align the definitions of Missing information and Safety concern and their explanatory notes with legal requirements, as well as to amend the definition for Risk minimisation activity. Annexure I on definitions was updated accordingly and published as revision 3, and likewise Module XVI on risk minimisation measures was published as revision 1.

On 15 September 2014, revision 1 of Module III was published with a reference to the new Union procedures for pharmacovigilance inspections.

On 27 April 2015, Addendum I to Module XVI on educational materials was published as a draft for public consultation, and published as final on 15 December 2015.

On 11 August 2015, revision 1 of the Module IV is published with a clarifying note what does not constitute an audit, and a public consultation was launched for revision 2 of Module VIII and its Addendum, in particular to clarify the link between the legislation on non-interventional post-authorisation safety studies (PASS) and categories 1-4 of non-interventional PASS for risk management planning and to update procedural and transmission requirements. These documents, having been amended in the light of their public consultations, were published as final on 8 August 2016.

On 15 December 2015, revision 1 of Module XV on safety communication, with revision 1 of the template for Direct Healthcare Professional Letters (DHPCs) and a new template for DHPC-Communication Plans in GVP Annexure II, and the second Product- or Population-Specific Considerations, namely on biological medicinal products, were released for public consultation until 29 February 2016. The Considerations P.II on biologicals were published as final, having been amended in the light of the public consultation, on 15 August 2016.

On 29 February 2016, revision 2 of Module V on risk management system was released for public consultation until 31 May 2016.

On 8 August 2016, draft revision 2 of Module VI on management and reporting of adverse reactions and draft revision 1 of Module IX on signal management with its Addendum were released for public consultation until 14 October 2016.

For timelines when the remaining new Considerations will be published for public consultation, please see the GVP webpage of the Agency's website: http://www.ema.europa.eu/ema/index.jsp?curl=pages/regulation/document_listing/document_listing_000345.jsp&mid=WC0b01ac058058f32c.

OBJECTIVES OF PHARMACOVIGILANCE

Pharmacovigilance has been defined by the World Health Organization (WHO) as the science and activities relating to the detection, assessment, understanding and prevention of adverse effects or any other medicine-related problem.

In line with this general definition, underlying objectives of the applicable EU legislation for pharmacovigilance are:
- Preventing harm from adverse reactions in humans arising from the use of authorised medicinal products within or outside the terms of marketing authorisation or from occupational exposure; and
- Promoting the safe and effective use of medicinal products, in particular through providing timely information about the safety of medicinal products to patients, healthcare professionals and the public.

Pharmacovigilance is therefore an activity contributing to the protection of patients' and public health.

PHARMACOVIGILANCE IN THE EU: ROLES OF DIFFERENT ACTORS

In the EU, a regulatory network, consisting of the competent authorities in Member States, the European Commission and the European Medicines Agency (in GVP referred to as "the Agency") is responsible for granting marketing authorisations and supervising medicinal products, including the conduct of pharmacovigilance. The Agency has a core role in coordinating these activities for the network.

In addition to the network's responsibilities, EU legislation imposes responsibility for pharmacovigilance, together with specific obligations (i.e. in terms of tasks and responsibilities), on marketing authorisation holders.

In the past, the role of healthcare professionals was mainly seen as contributing to pharmacovigilance through spontaneous reporting of suspected adverse reaction cases and as receiving, together with the patients, advice on minimising risks through updated product information or other information materials. However over time, participation of patients and healthcare professionals in EU regulatory processes, including those for pharmacovigilance, has steadily increased. A large number of Member States have established, over the last years, schemes for reporting of suspected adverse reactions by patients themselves. An EU legal framework for patient reporting in all Member States has now been introduced through the new pharmacovigilance legislation. The new legislation further increases public participation by including patient and healthcare professional representatives in the new Pharmacovigilance and Risk Assessment Committee (PRAC) and through public hearings on pharmacovigilance and benefit-risk matters at the Agency, involving all stakeholders.

LEGAL BASIS, SCOPE AND PROCESS FOR GVP

The legal framework for pharmacovigilance of medicinal products for human use in the EU is given in Regulation (EC) No 726/2004 and Directive 2001/83/EC on the Community code relating to medicinal products for human use, as amended in 2010 by Regulation (EU) No 1235/2010 and Directives 2010/84/EU and 2012/26/EU respectively, as well as by the Commission Implementing Regulation (EU) No 520/2012 on the Performance of Pharmacovigilance Activities Provided for in Regulation (EC) No 726/2004 and Directive 2001/83/EC. It should be noted that Chapter 3 of the Regulation (EC) No 726/2004 as amended, Title IX of the Directive 2001/83/EC as amended and the Implementing Regulation contain the majority of pharmacovigilance provisions in the legislation, however, other measures directly relevant to the conduct of pharmacovigilance are found in other Chapters and Titles of this Regulation and Directive.

The aforementioned amending legislation of 2010/12, together with the related Implementing Regulation, is commonly referred to as the new pharmacovigilance legislation in the EU. It was the outcome of a major review of the current pharmacovigilance system in the EU conducted by the European Commission, followed by a formal law-making process in the Council and European Parliament. The legislation has the primary aim to strengthen and rationalise pharmacovigilance and increase patient safety.

The pharmacovigilance legal requirements and GVP apply to all medicinal products authorised in the EU, whether centrally or nationally authorised. While risk proportionality underpins the new legislation, the requirements are generally the same for different types of product unless specific provision or exemptions apply as indicated in the GVP chapters.

GVP is drawn up to facilitate the performance of pharmacovigilance activities within the EU and applies to marketing authorisation holders in the EU, the Agency and competent authorities in Member States. Where in GVP reference is made to Member States of the EU, this should be read to include Iceland, Liechtenstein and Norway. These countries have, through the Agreement of the European Economic Area (EEA), adopted the complete Union acquis (i.e. the legislation at EU level, guidelines and judgements) on medicinal products, and are consequently parties to the EU procedures. The new pharmacovigilance Regulation (EU) No 1235/2010 and Directive 2010/84/EU have likewise been implemented in these countries.[1]

GVP is drawn up based on Article 108a(a) of Directive 2001/83/EC as amended, by the Agency in cooperation with competent authorities in Member States and interested parties.

GVP is being developed within a governance structure set up by the Agency and national competent authorities specifically for the implementation of the new pharmacovigilance legislation. This structure allows for the close collaboration of Member States, the Agency and the European Commission services, with regular stakeholder meetings an integral part of the implementation process.

Each draft chapter of GVP is prepared by a project team (Modules) or author team (Considerations) consisting of experts from Member States and the Agency, taking into account comments collected during the stakeholder meetings. The draft chapters are agreed by the Heads of Medicines Agencies' EU Network Pharmacovigilance Oversight Group (EU-POG) (until 2016 by the European Risk Management Strategy Facilitation Group (ERMS FG)) and are released for public consultation on behalf of the EU regulatory network. After public consultation, the chapters are finalised within the governance structure, addressing the comments from stakeholders, and then published by the Agency.

MAINTENANCE AND FURTHER DEVELOPMENT OF GVP

Proposals for corrections, revision/addition of guidance or new GVP chapters can be made by any member of the EU regulatory network as well as any other stakeholder. Members of the public and non-regulatory stakeholder organisations

---

1. The only exemption from this is that legally binding acts from the EU (e.g. Commission Decisions) do not directly confer rights and obligations but have first to be transposed into legally binding acts in Iceland, Liechtenstein and Norway.

can send proposals via http://www.ema.europa.eu/ema/index.jsp?curl=pages/about_us/landing/ask_ema_landing_page.jsp&mid.

There might not be an immediate, individual response, but all proposals will be reviewed regularly and prioritised within the governance structure set up by the Agency and national competent authorities for the implementation of the new pharmacovigilance legislation.

STRUCTURE OF GVP

Pharmacovigilance activities are organised by distinct but connected processes, and each GVP Module presents one major pharmacovigilance process. In addition, GVP provides guidance on the conduct of pharmacovigilance for specific product types or specific populations in which medicines are used. These GVP considerations apply in conjunction with the process-related guidance in the Modules.

While the development of GVP is ongoing, some guidelines developed under the previous legislation remain valid in principle (unless any aspect is not compatible with the new legislation) until they are revised at a later point in time for inclusion in GVP. They are published on the Agency's GVP webpage under GVP Annexure III.

Within each chapters, Section A provides the legal, technical and scientific context of the respective process. Section B gives guidance which, while based on EU legislation, reflects scientific and regulatory approaches, formats and standards agreed internationally in various for a; or, where such formal agreements or expert consensus do not exist, Section B describes approaches which are considered in line with general current thinking in the field. Section C focusses on the specifics of applying the approaches, formats and standards in the EU and other aspects of operating the respective process in the EU.

In particular in Sections B, the term "competent authority" is to be understood in its generic meaning of an authority regulating medicinal products and/or an authority appointed at national level for being in charge of all or individual pharmacovigilance processes. For the purpose of applying GVP in the EU, the term "competent authority" covers the competent authorities in Member States and the Agency.

A table of contents of GVP is kept up to date on the GVP webpage, accessible under: http://www.ema.europa.eu/ema/index.jsp?curl=pages/regulation/document_listing/document_listing_00034 5.jsp&mid=WC0b01ac058058f32c.

The overall structure of GVP was reviewed by the Implementation Group of above mentioned governance structure on 17 November 2015 and the following planned GVP Modules are not necessary anymore, given that other guidance has been made available since the initial planning of GVP: Module XI on public participation, Module XII on safety-related action, Module XIII on incident management and exchange of information exchange within the EU regulatory network and Module XIV on international collaboration. Where GVP chapters refer to Modules XI or XIV, one should now consult the Agency's webpage on Partners & Networks (http://www.ema.europa.eu/ema/index.jsp?curl=pages/partners_and_networks/general/general_content_00 0212.jsp&mid), and where GVP chapters refer to Module XII, one should now consult the post-authorisation section for human medicinal products of the Agency's website (http://www.ema.europa.eu/ema/index.jsp?curl=pages/regulation/document_listing/document_listing_0000 90.jsp&mid). Where GVP chapters refer to Module XIII, one should now consult the Agency's webpage on incident management (http://www.ema.europa.eu/ema/index.jsp?curl=pages/regulation/general/general_content_000544.jsp&mi d=WC0b01ac05805b713e).

REFERENCING OF LEGAL REQUIREMENTS IN GVP

In GVP, any reference to Regulation (EC) No 726/2004 and Directive 2001/83/EC refers to the Regulation and Directive respectively, always including their latest amendments. Where reference is made to specific Articles in square brackets "REG" means Regulation (EC) No 726/2004 as amended and "DIR" means Directive 2001/83/EC as amended. If reference is provided to any other Regulation or Directive, its full reference is provided.

Reference to specific Articles of the Commission Implementing Regulation (EU) No 520/2012 on the Performance of Pharmacovigilance Activities Provided for in Regulation (EC) No 726/2004 and Directive 2001/83/EC is provided in square brackets with the indication "IR".

Text in GVP describing legal requirements makes reference to the specific article in the legislation and uses the same modal verb as used in the article, which is usually "shall". Guidance for the implementation of legal requirements is presented with the modal verb "should".

PRACTICAL ADVICE FOR THE PUBLIC CONSULTATION

Those participating in the public consultation are asked to please submit comments by using the specific templates for each chapter (*see* page 1 of each draft chapter) and the Definition or Template Annexure, when these are under consultation too. Comments will only be processed if submitted as **completed templates in open word format**. Participants may additionally submit pdf-files of their comments, if they wish to do so, if they accompany them by a statement that the open and pdf-files are identical in content.

The public consultation relates to the guidance proposed for the practical implementation of the applicable legislation. Participants are therefore asked not to comment on the underlying legal requirements (identified in the draft chapters by reference to the respective Articles), as these cannot be altered through the GVP consultation process.

Participants should note that their comments will be published on the Agency's website, identifying the sender's organisation (but not the sender's name). Where a sender does not represent an organisation but submits comments as an individual, the sender's name will be published unless the sender objects against the publication. In the absence of a legitimate interest to oppose the publication of the name, the contribution will not be published nor will, in principle, its content be taken into account. Please consult the Agency's Privacy Policy (http://www.ema.europa.eu/ema/index.jsp?curl=pages/home/general/general_content_000516.jsp&mid) and the specific privacy statement for this consultation (http://www.ema.europa.eu/docs/en_GB/document_library/Other/2012/02/WC500123144.pdf).

The European Medicines Agency thanks all those participating in the public consultation for their contributions.

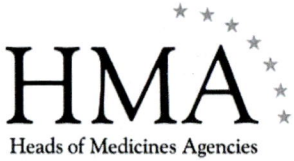
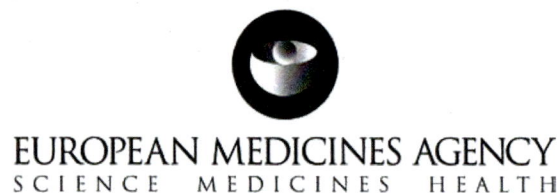

22 June 2012
EMA/541760/2011

GUIDELINE ON GOOD PHARMACOVIGILANCE PRACTICES (GVP)

Module I — Pharmacovigilance Systems and their Quality Systems

Draft finalised by the Agency in collaboration with Member States and submitted to ERMS FG	19 January 2012
Draft agreed by ERMS FG	24 January 2012
Draft adopted by Executive Director	20 February 2012
Released for consultation	21 February 2012
End of consultation (deadline for comments)	18 April 2012
Revised draft finalised by the Agency in collaboration with Member States	20 June 2012
Revised draft agreed by ERMS FG	21 June 2012
Revised draft adopted by Executive Director as final	22 June 2012
Date for coming into effect	2 July 2012

I.A. INTRODUCTION

This Module contains guidance for the establishment and maintenance of quality assured pharmacovigilance systems for marketing authorisation holders, competent authorities of Member States and the Agency. How the systems of these organisations interact while undertaking specific pharmacovigilance processes is described in each respective Module of GVP.

The definition of a pharmacovigilance system is provided in Article 1 of Directive 2001/83/EC as a system used by the marketing authorisation holder and by Member States to fulfil the tasks and responsibilities listed in Title IX and designed to monitor the safety of authorised medicinal products and detect any change to their risk-benefit balance. The Agency likewise maintains a pharmacovigilance system to fulfil its pharmacovigilance activities.

For performing their pharmacovigilance activities, marketing authorisation holders, competent authorities of Member States and the Agency shall establish and use quality systems that are adequate and effective for this performance. The legal requirement for quality systems was introduced by Directive 2010/84/EU amending Directive 2001/83/EC (the latter is referenced as DIR) and Regulation (EU) No 1235/2010 amending Regulation (EC) No 726/2004 (the latter is referenced as REG) to strengthen pharmacovigilance in the EU. The minimum requirements of these quality systems are set out in the Commission Implementing Regulation (EU) No 520/2012 on the Performance of Pharmacovigilance Activities Provided for in Regulation (EC) No 726/2004 and Directive 2001/83/EC (the Implementing Regulation is referenced as IR).

While there has to be compliance with these legal requirements, the implementation of a quality system should be adapted to the respective organisation.

By following the overall quality objectives in I.B.4. and the guiding principle in I.B.5. to meet the needs of patients, healthcare professionals and the public in relation to the safety of medicines, the application of the quality system should be adapted to how crucial each pharmacovigilance task is for fulfilling the quality objectives for each medicinal product covered by a quality system.

The guidance on quality systems in this Module is consistent with the general principles of the ISO 9000 Standards on good quality management practices, specifically the ISO 9001-2008 Standards on quality management systems, issued by the International Organization for Standardization (ISO). The general application of quality management to pharmacovigilance systems is described under I.B. and requirements specific to the operation of the EU network in I.C.

In this Module, all applicable legal requirements are referenced in the way explained in the GVP Introductory Cover Note and are usually identifiable by the modal verb "shall". Guidance for the implementation of legal requirements is provided using the modal verb "should".

I.B. STRUCTURES AND PROCESSES

I.B.1. Pharmacovigilance System

A pharmacovigilance system is defined as a system used by an organisation to fulfil its legal tasks and responsibilities in relation to pharmacovigilance and designed to monitor the safety of authorised medicinal products and detect any change to their risk-benefit balance [DIR Art 1(28d)].

A pharmacovigilance system, like any system, is characterised by its structures, processes and outcomes. For each specific pharmacovigilance process, including its necessary structures, a dedicated Module is included in GVP.

I.B.2. Quality, Quality Objectives, Quality Requirements and Quality System

For the purpose of GVP, which provides guidance on structures and processes of a pharmacovigilance system, the quality of a pharmacovigilance system can be defined as all the characteristics of the system which are considered to produce, according to estimated likelihoods, outcomes relevant to the objectives of pharmacovigilance.

In general terms, quality is a matter of degree and can be measured. Measuring if the required degree of quality has been achieved necessitates pre-defined quality requirements. Quality requirements are those characteristics of a system that are likely to produce the desired outcome, or quality objectives. The overall quality objectives for pharmacovigilance systems are provided under I.B.4.

Specific quality objectives and quality requirements for the specific structures and processes of the pharmacovigilance systems are provided in each Module of GVP as appropriate.

The quality system is part of the pharmacovigilance system and consists of its own structures and processes. It shall cover organisational structure, responsibilities, procedures, processes and resources of the pharmacovigilance system as well as appropriate resource management, compliance management and record management [IR Art 8(2)].

I.B.3. Quality Cycle

The quality system shall be based on all of the following activities:
- Quality planning: establishing structures and planning integrated and consistent processes;
- Quality adherence: carrying out tasks and responsibilities in accordance with quality requirements;
- Quality control and assurance: monitoring and evaluating how effectively the structures and processes have been established and how effectively the processes are being carried out; and
- Quality improvements: correcting and improving the structures and processes where necessary [IR Art 8(3)].

I.B.4. Overall Quality Objectives for Pharmacovigilance

The overall quality objectives of a pharmacovigilance system are:
- Complying with the legal requirements for pharmacovigilance tasks and responsibilities;
- Preventing harm from adverse reactions in humans arising from the use of authorised medicinal products within or outside the terms of marketing authorisation or from occupational exposure;
- Promoting the safe and effective use of medicinal products, in particular through providing timely information about the safety of medicinal products to patients, healthcare professionals and the public; and
- Contributing to the protection of patients' and public health.

I.B.5. Principles for Good Pharmacovigilance Practices

With the aim of fulfilling the overall quality objectives in I.B.4., the following principles should guide the design of all structures and processes as well as the conduct of all tasks and responsibilities:
- The needs of patients, healthcare professionals and the public in relation to the safety of medicines should be met.
- Upper management should provide leadership in the implementation of the quality system and motivation for all staff members in relation to the quality objectives.
- All persons within the organisation should be involved in and support the pharmacovigilance system on the basis of task ownership and responsibility in a degree according to their tasks and assigned responsibilities.
- All persons involved with the entire organisation should engage in continuous quality improvement following the quality cycle in I.B.3.
- Resources and tasks should be organised as structures and processes in a manner that will support the proactive, risk-proportionate, continuous and integrated conduct of pharmacovigilance.
- All available evidence on the risk-benefit balance of medicinal products should be sought and all relevant aspects, which could impact on the risk-benefit balance and the use of a product, should be considered for decision-making.
- Good cooperation should be fostered between marketing authorisation holders, competent authorities, public health organisations, patients, healthcare professionals, learned societies and other relevant bodies in accordance with the applicable legal provisions.

I.B.6. Responsibilities for the Quality System within an Organisation

A sufficient number of competent and appropriately qualified and trained personnel shall be available for the performance of pharmacovigilance activities [IR Art 10(1), Art 14(1)]. Their responsibility should include adherence to the principles defined in I.B.5.

For the purpose of a systematic approach towards quality in accordance with the quality cycle (*see* I.B.3.), managerial staff (i.e. staff with management responsibilities) in any organisation should be responsible for:
- Ensuring that the organisation documents the quality system as described in I.B.11.;
- Ensuring that the documents describing the quality system are subject to document control in relation to their creation, revision, approval and implementation;
- Ensuring that adequate resources are available and that training is provided (*see* I.B.7.);
- Ensuring that suitable and sufficient premises, facilities and equipment are available (*see* I.B.8.);
- Ensuring adequate compliance management (*see* I.B.9.);
- Ensuring adequate record management (*see* I.B.10.);
- Reviewing the pharmacovigilance system including its quality system at regular intervals in risk-based manner to verify its effectiveness (*see* I.B.12.) and introducing corrective and preventive measures where necessary;
- Ensuring that mechanisms exist for timely and effective communication, including escalation processes of safety concerns relating to medicinal products within an organisation;
- Identifying and investigating concerns arising within an organisation regarding suspected non-adherence to the requirements of the quality and pharmacovigilance systems and taking corrective, preventive and escalation action as necessary;
- Ensuring that audits are performed (*see* I.B.12.).

In relation to the management responsibilities described above, upper management within an organisation should provide leadership through:
- Motivating all staff members, based on shared values, trust and freedom to speak and act with responsibility and through recognition of staff members' contributions within the organisation; and
- Assigning roles, responsibilities and authorities to staff members according to their competencies and communicating and implementing these throughout the organisation.

For competent authorities, all persons involved in the procedures and processes of the quality system established for the performance of pharmacovigilance activities shall be responsible for the good functioning of that quality system and shall ensure a systematic approach towards quality and towards the implementation and maintenance of the quality system [IR Art 8(5)].

I.B.7. Training of Personnel for Pharmacovigilance

Achieving the required quality for the conduct of pharmacovigilance processes and their outcomes by an organisation is intrinsically linked with the availability of a sufficient number of competent and appropriately qualified and trained personnel (*see* I.B.6.).

All personnel involved in the performance of pharmacovigilance activities shall receive initial and continued training [IR Art 10(3), Art 14(2)]. For marketing authorisation holders, this training shall relate to the roles and responsibilities of the personnel [IR Art 10(3)].

The organisation shall keep training plans and records for documenting, maintaining and developing the competences of personnel [IR Art 10(3), Art 14(2)]. Training plans should be based on training needs assessment and should be subject to monitoring.

The training should support continuous improvement of relevant skills, the application of scientific progress and professional development and ensure that staff members have the appropriate qualifications, understanding of relevant pharmacovigilance requirements as well as experience for the assigned tasks and responsibilities. All staff members of the organisation should receive and be able to seek information about what to do if they become aware of a safety concern.

There should be a process in place within the organisation to check that training results in the appropriate levels of understanding and conduct of pharmacovigilance activities for the assigned tasks and responsibilities, or to identify unmet training needs, in line with professional development plans agreed for the organisations as well as the individual staff members.

Adequate training should also be considered by the organisation for those staff members to whom no specific pharmacovigilance tasks and responsibilities have been assigned but whose activities may have an impact on the pharmacovigilance system or the conduct of pharmacovigilance. Such activities include but are not limited to those related to clinical trials, technical product complaints, medical information, terminologies, sales and marketing, regulatory affairs, legal affairs and audits.

Appropriate instructions on the processes to be used in case of urgency, including business continuity (see I.B.11.3.), shall be provided by the organisation to their personnel [IR Art 10(4), Art 14(3)].

I.B.8. Facilities and Equipment for Pharmacovigilance

Achieving the required quality for the conduct of pharmacovigilance processes and their outcomes is also intrinsically linked with appropriate facilities and equipment used to support the processes. Facilities and equipment should include office space, information technology (IT) systems and (electronic) storage space. They should be located, designed, constructed, adapted and maintained to suit their intended purpose in line with the quality objectives for pharmacovigilance (see I.B.4.) and also be available for business continuity (see I.B.11.3.). Facilities and equipment which are critical for the conduct of pharmacovigilance (see I.B.11.3.) should be subject to appropriate checks, qualification and/or validation activities to prove their suitability for the intended purpose. There should be processes in place to keep awareness of the valid terminologies (see Module VI) in their valid versions and to keep the IT systems up-to-date accordingly.

I.B.9. Specific Quality System Procedures and Processes

I.B.9.1. Compliance Management by Marketing Authorisation Holders

For the purpose of compliance management, marketing authorisation holders shall have specific quality system procedures and processes in place in order to ensure the following:
- The continuous monitoring of pharmacovigilance data, the examination of options for risk minimisation and prevention and that appropriate measures are taken by the marketing authorisation holder [IR Art 11(1)(a)] (see Modules IX and XII);
- The scientific evaluation of all information on the risks of medicinal products as regards patients' or public health, in particular as regards adverse reactions in human beings arising from use of the product within or outside the terms of its marketing authorisation or associated with occupational exposure [IR Art 11(1)(b)] (see Modules VI, VII, VIII, IX);
- The submission of accurate and verifiable data on serious and non-serious adverse reactions to the competent authorities within the legally required time-limits [IR Art 11(1)(c)] (see Modules VI and IX);
- The quality, integrity and completeness of the information submitted on the risks of medicinal products, including processes to avoid duplicate submissions and to validate signals [IR Art 11(1)(d)] (see Modules V, VI, VII, VIII and IX);
- Effective communication by the marketing authorisation holder with competent authorities, including communication on new or changed risks (see Module XII and XV), the pharmacovigilance system master file (see Module II), risk management systems (see Module V), risk minimisations measures (see Modules V and XVI), periodic safety update reports (see Module VII), corrective and preventive actions (see Modules II, III and IV) and post-authorisation safety studies (see Module VIII) [IR Art 11(1)(e];
- The update of product information by the marketing authorisation holder in the light of scientific knowledge [IR Art 11(1)(f)] (see Module XII);
- Appropriate communication of relevant safety information to healthcare professionals and patients (see Module XII and XV) [IR Art 11(1)(g)].

I.B.9.2. Compliance Management by Competent Authorities

For the purpose of compliance management, competent authorities shall establish specific quality system procedures and processes in order to achieve all of the following objectives:

- Ensuring the evaluation of the quality, including completeness, of pharmacovigilance data submitted [IR Art 15(1)(a)];
- Ensuring the assessment of pharmacovigilance data and its processing in accordance with the legal timelines [IR Art 15(1)(b)];
- Ensuring independence in the performance of pharmacovigilance activities [IR Art 15(1)(c)];
- Ensuring effective communication with patients, healthcare professionals, marketing authorisation holders and the general public [IR Art 15(1)(d)];
- Conducting inspections, including pre-authorisation inspections [IR Art 15(1)(f)].

Independence in the performance of pharmacovigilance activities is interpreted in the sense that all regulatory decisions on medicinal products should be taken in the sole interest of patients' and public health.

I.B.10. Record Management

The organisation shall record all pharmacovigilance information and ensure that it is handled and stored so as to allow accurate reporting, interpretation and verification of that information [IR Art 12(1), Art 16(1)].

A record management system shall be put in place for all documents used for pharmacovigilance activities, ensuring their retrievability as well as traceability of the measures taken to investigate safety concerns, of the timelines for those investigations and of decisions on safety concerns, including their date and the decision-making process [IR Art 12(1), Art 16(1)].

The record management system should support:
- The management of the quality of pharmacovigilance data, including their completeness, accuracy and integrity;
- Timely access to all records;
- Effective internal and external communication; and
- The retention of documents relating to the pharmacovigilance systems and the conduct of pharmacovigilance for individual medicinal products, in accordance with the applicable retention periods.

In addition, marketing authorisation holders shall establish mechanisms enabling the traceability and follow-up of adverse reaction reports [IR Art 12(1)].

In this context, it should be ensured that the fundamental right to personal data protection is fully and effectively guaranteed in all pharmacovigilance activities in conformity with legal provisions. The purpose of safeguarding public health constitutes a substantial public interest and consequently the processing of personal data should be justified if identifiable personal data are processed only where necessary and only where the parties involved assess this necessity at every stage of the pharmacovigilance process (IR Recital 17). As part of a record management system, specific measures should therefore be taken at each stage in the storage and processing of pharmacovigilance data to ensure data security and confidentiality. This should involve strict limitation of access to documents and to databases to authorised personnel respecting the medical and administrative confidentiality of the data.

There should be appropriate structures and processes in place to ensure that pharmacovigilance data and records are protected from destruction during the applicable record retention period.

The record management system should be described in a record management policy.

I.B.11. Documentation of the Quality System

All elements, requirements and provisions adopted for the quality system shall be documented in a systematic and orderly manner in the form of written policies and procedures, such as quality plans, quality manuals and quality records [IR Art 8(4)].

A quality plan documents the setting of quality objectives and sets out the processes to be implemented to achieve them. A procedure is a specified way to carry out a process and may take the format of a standard operating procedure and other work instruction or quality manual. A quality manual documents the scope of the quality system, the processes of the quality system and the interaction between the two. A quality record is a document stating results achieved or providing evidence of activities performed.

In order to have a systematic approach, the organisation should define in advance:
- Quality objectives specific to their organisations in accordance with the overall quality objectives provided under I.B.4. and the structure- and process-specific quality objectives in accordance with each Module of GVP; and
- Methods for monitoring the effectiveness of the pharmacovigilance system (*see* I.B.12.).

The quality system shall be documented by:
- Documents on organisational structures and assignments of tasks to personnel (*see* I.B.11.1. and I.B.11.2.);
- Training plans and records (*see* I.B.7.) [IR Art 10(3), Art 14(2)];
- Instructions for the compliance management processes (*see* I.B.9.) [IR Art 11(1), Art 15(1)];
- Appropriate instructions on the processes to be used in case of urgency, including business continuity (*see* I.B.11.3.) [IR Art 10(4), Art 14(3)];
- Performance indicators where they are used to continuously monitor the good performance of pharmacovigilance activities [IR Art 9(1)];
- Reports of quality audits and follow-up audits, including their dates and results [IR Art 13(2), Art 17(2)].

Training plans and records shall be kept and made available for audit and inspection [IR Art 10(3), Art 14(2)].

It is recommended that the documentation of the quality system also includes:
- The methods of monitoring the efficient operation of the quality system and, in particular, its ability to fulfil the quality objectives;
- A record management policy;
- Records created as a result of pharmacovigilance processes which demonstrate that key steps for the defined procedures have been taken;
- Records and reports relating to the facilities and equipment including functionality checks, qualification and validation activities which demonstrate that all steps required by the applicable requirements, protocols and procedures have been taken;
- Records to demonstrate that deficiencies and deviations from the established quality system are monitored, that corrective and preventive actions have been taken, that solutions have been applied to deviations or deficiencies and that the effectiveness of the actions taken has been verified.

I.B.11.1. Additional Quality System Documentation by Marketing Authorisation Holders

In addition to the quality system documentation in accordance with I.B.11., marketing authorisation holders shall document:
- Their human resource management in the pharmacovigilance system master file (PSMF) (*see* Module II) [IR Art 2(5)(b)];
- Job descriptions defining the duties of the managerial and supervisory staff [IR Art 10(2)];
- An organisational chart defining the hierarchical relationships of managerial and supervisory staff [IR Art 10(2)];
- Instructions on critical processes (*see* I.B.11.3.) in the pharmacovigilance system master file (PSMF) (*see* Module II); and
- Their record management system in the pharmacovigilance system master file (PSMF) (*see* Module II) [IR Art 2(5)(c)].

It is recommended that the documentation of the quality system additionally includes the organisational structures and assignments of tasks, responsibilities and authorities to all personnel directly involved in pharmacovigilance tasks.

For the requirements of documenting the quality system in the pharmacovigilance system master file (PSMF) or its annexes, *see* Module II.

I.B.11.2. Additional Quality System Documentation by Competent Authorities

In addition to the quality system documentation in accordance with I.B.11., the organisational structures and the distribution of tasks and responsibilities shall be clear and, to the extent necessary, accessible [IR Art 14(1)].

It is recommended that the documentation of the quality system additionally includes the organisational structures and assignments of tasks, responsibilities and authorities to all personnel directly involved in pharmacovigilance tasks.

Contact points shall be established [IR Art 14(1)], in particular to facilitate interaction between competent authorities, marketing authorisation holders and persons reporting information on the risks of medicinal products as regards patients' or public health.

I.B.11.3. Critical Pharmacovigilance Processes and Business Continuity

The following pharmacovigilance processes should be considered as critical include:
- Continuous safety profile monitoring and benefit-risk evaluation of authorised medicinal products;
- Establishing, assessing and implementing risk management systems and evaluating the effectiveness of risk minimisation;
- Collection, processing, management, quality control, follow-up for missing information, coding, classification, duplicate detection, evaluation and timely electronic transmission of individual case safety reports (ICSRs) from any source;
- Signal management;
- Scheduling, preparation (including data evaluation and quality control), submission and assessment of periodic safety update reports;
- Meeting commitments and responding to requests from competent authorities, including provision of correct and complete information;
- Interaction between the pharmacovigilance and product quality defect systems;
- Communication about safety concerns between marketing authorisation holders and competent authorities, in particular notifying changes to the risk-benefit balance of medicinal products;
- Communicating information to patients and healthcare professionals about changes to the risk-benefit balance of products for the aim of safe and effective use of medicinal products;
- Keeping product information up-to-date with the current scientific knowledge, including the conclusions of the assessment and recommendations from the applicable competent authority;
- Implementation of variations to marketing authorisations for safety reasons according to the urgency required.

Business continuity plans should be established in a risk-based manner and should include:
- Provisions for events that could severely impact on the organisation's staff and infrastructure in general or on the structures and processes for pharmacovigilance in particular; and
- Back-up systems for urgent exchange of information within an organisation, amongst organisations sharing pharmacovigilance tasks as well as between marketing authorisation holders and competent authorities.

I.B.12. Monitoring of the Performance and Effectiveness of the Pharmacovigilance System and its Quality System

Processes to monitor the performance and effectiveness of a pharmacovigilance system and its quality system should include:
- Reviews of the systems by those responsible for management;
- Audits;
- Compliance monitoring;
- Inspections;
- Evaluating the effectiveness of actions taken with medicinal products for the purpose of minimising risks and supporting their safe and effective use in patients.

The organisation may use performance indicators to continuously monitor the good performance of pharmacovigilance activities [IR Art 9(1)] in relation to the quality requirements. The quality requirements for each pharmacovigilance process are provided in each Module of GVP as appropriate.

The requirements for the quality system itself are laid out in this Module and its effectiveness should be monitored by managerial staff, who should review the documentation of the quality system (see I.B.11.) at regular intervals, with the frequency and the extent of the reviews to be determined in a risk-based manner. Pre-defined programmes for the review of the system should therefore be in place. Reviews of the quality system should include the review of standard operating procedures and work instructions, deviations from the established quality system, audit and inspections reports as well as the use of the indicators referred to above.

Risk-based audits of the quality system shall be performed at regular intervals to ensure that it complies with the requirements for the quality system, the human resource management, the compliance management, the record management and the data retention and to ensure its effectiveness [IR Art 13(1), Art 17(1)]. Audits of the quality system should include audit of the pharmacovigilance system which is the subject of the quality system. The methods and processes for the audits are described in Module IV. In relation to the pharmacovigilance system of a marketing authorisation holder, a report shall be drawn up on the results for each quality audit and any follow-up audits be sent to the management responsible for the matters audited [IR Art 13(2)]. The report should include the results of audits of organisations or persons the marketing authorisation holder has delegated tasks to, as these are part of the marketing authorisation holder's pharmacovigilance system. For competent authorities, the audit report shall be sent to the management responsible for the matters audited [IR Art 17(2)].

As a consequence of the monitoring of the performance and effectiveness of a pharmacovigilance system and its quality system (including the use of audits), corrective and preventive measures should be implemented when deemed necessary. In particular as a consequence of audits, corrective action(s), including a follow-up audit of deficiencies, shall be taken where necessary [IR Art 13(2), Art 17(2)]. Additionally, the competent authorities should have in place arrangements for monitoring the compliance of marketing authorisations holders with legally required pharmacovigilance tasks and responsibilities. They shall further ensure compliance with the legal requirements by means of conducting inspections of marketing authorisation holders [DIR Art 111(1)] (*see* Module III). Guidance on compliance monitoring for each pharmacovigilance process is provided in each Module of GVP as appropriate.

Requirements and methods for evaluating the effectiveness of actions taken upon medicinal products for the purpose of minimising risks and supporting the safe and effective use of medicines in patients are described in Module XVI.

I.B.13. Preparedness Planning for Pharmacovigilance in Public Health Emergencies

Any pharmacovigilance system should be adaptable to public health emergencies and preparedness plans should be developed as appropriate.

For preparedness planning in the EU, *see* I.C.4..

I.C. OPERATION OF THE EU NETWORK

I.C.1. Overall Pharmacovigilance Responsibilities of the Applicant and Marketing Authorisation Holder in the EU

The marketing authorisation holder in the EU is responsible for the respective pharmacovigilance tasks and responsibilities laid down in Directive 2001/83/EC, Regulation (EC) No 726/2004 and the Commission Implementing Regulation (EU) No 520/2012 on the Performance of Pharmacovigilance Activities Provided for in Regulation (EC) No 726/2004 and Directive 2001/83/EC in order to assure responsibility and liability for its authorised medicinal products and to ensure that appropriate action can be taken, when necessary.

For this purpose, the marketing authorisation holder shall operate a pharmacovigilance system [DIR 104(1)] and shall establish and use a quality system that is adequate and effective for performing its pharmacovigilance activities [IR Art 8(1)].

There may be circumstances where a marketing authorisation holder may establish more than one pharmacovigilance system, e.g. specific systems for particular types of products (e.g. vaccines, products available without medical prescription).

A description of the pharmacovigilance system shall be developed by the applicant for a marketing authorisation in the format of a pharmacovigilance system master file (PSMF) and be maintained by the marketing authorisation holder for all authorised medicinal products (*see* Module II). The applicant or the marketing authorisation holder is also responsible for developing and maintaining product-specific risk management systems (*see* Module V).

Guidance on the structures and processes on how the marketing authorisation holder should conduct the pharmacovigilance tasks and responsibilities is provided in the respective GVP Modules.

I.C.1.1. Responsibilities of the Marketing Authorisation Holder in Relation to the Qualified Person Responsible for Pharmacovigilance in the EU

As part of the pharmacovigilance system, the marketing authorisation holder shall have permanently and continuously at its disposal an appropriately qualified person responsible for pharmacovigilance in the EU (QPPV) [DIR Art 104(3)(a)].

The marketing authorisation holder shall submit the name and contact details of the QPPV to the competent authorities in Member States and the Agency [DIR Art 104(3) last paragraph]. Changes to this information should be submitted in accordance with Regulation (EC) No 1234/2008 on variations to the terms of marketing authorisation and the Communication from the Commission - Guideline on the Details of the Various Categories of Variations to the Terms of Marketing Authorisations for Medicinal Products for Human Use and Veterinary Medicinal Products.[1]

The duties of the QPPV shall be defined in a job description [IR Art 10(2)]. The hierarchical relationship of the QPPV shall be defined in an organisational chart together with those of other managerial and supervisory staff [IR Art 10(2)].

Information relating to the QPPV shall be included in the pharmacovigilance systems master file (PSMF) [IR Art 2(1)] (*see* Module II).

Each pharmacovigilance system can have only one QPPV. A QPPV may be employed by more than one marketing authorisation holder, for a shared or for separate pharmacovigilance systems or may fulfil the role of QPPV for more than one pharmacovigilance system of the same marketing authorisation holder, provided that the QPPV is able to fulfil all obligations.

In addition to the QPPV, competent authorities in Member States are legally provided with the option to request the nomination of a pharmacovigilance contact person at national level reporting to the QPPV. Reporting in this context relates to pharmacovigilance tasks and responsibilities and not necessarily to line management. A contact person at national level may also be nominated as the QPPV.

The marketing authorisation holder shall ensure that the QPPV has sufficient authority to influence the performance of the quality system and the pharmacovigilance activities of the marketing authorisation holder [IR Art 10(2)]. The marketing authorisation holder should therefore ensure that the QPPV has access to the pharmacovigilance system master file (PSMF) as well as authority over it and is notified of any changes to it in accordance with Module II (*see* I.C.1.3). The authority over the pharmacovigilance system and the PSMF should allow the QPPV to implement changes to the system and to provide input into risk management plans (*see* Module V) as well as into the preparation of regulatory action in response to emerging safety concerns (*see* Module XII).

Overall, the marketing authorisation holder should ensure that structures and processes are in place, so that the QPPV can fulfil the responsibilities listed in I.C.1.3. In order to do this, the marketing authorisation holder should ensure that mechanisms are in place so that the QPPV receives all relevant information and that the QPPV can access all information the QPPV considers relevant, in particular on:

- Emerging safety concerns and any other information relating to the benefit-risk evaluation of the medicinal products covered by the pharmacovigilance system;
- Ongoing or completed clinical trials and other studies the marketing authorisation holder is aware of and which may be relevant to the safety of the medicinal products;
- Information from sources other than from the specific marketing authorisation holder, e.g. from those with whom the marketing authorisation holder has contractual arrangements; and
- The procedures relevant to pharmacovigilance which the marketing authorisation holder has in place at every level in order to ensure consistency and compliance across the organisation.

The outcome of the regular reviews of the quality system referred to in I.B.6. and I.B.12. and the measures introduced should be communicated by the managerial staff to the QPPV.

Compliance information should be provided to the QPPV on a periodic basis. Such information may also be used to provide assurance to the QPPV that commitments in the framework of risk management plans and post-authorisation safety systems are being adhered to.

---

1. See Volume 2C of the Rules Governing Medicinal Products in the EU; http://ec.europa.eu/health/documents/eudralex/vol-2/index_en.htm

The managerial staff should also inform the QPPV of scheduled pharmacovigilance audits. The QPPV should be able to trigger an audit where appropriate. The managerial staff should provide the QPPV with a copy of the corrective and preventive action plan following each audit relevant to the pharmacovigilance system the QPPV is responsible for, so that the QPPV can assure that appropriate corrective actions are implemented.

In particular with regard to its adverse reaction database (or other systems to collate adverse reaction reports), the marketing authorisation holder should implement a procedure to ensure that the QPPV is able to obtain information from the database, for example, to respond to urgent requests for information from the competent authorities or the Agency, at any time. If this procedure requires the involvement of other personnel, for example database specialists, then this should be taken into account in the arrangements made by the marketing authorisation holder for supporting the QPPV outside of normal working hours.

When a marketing authorisation holder intends to expand its product portfolio, for example, by acquisition of another company or by purchasing individual products from another marketing authorisation holder, the QPPV should be notified as early as possible in the due diligence process in order that the potential impact on the pharmacovigilance system can be assessed and the system be adapted accordingly. The QPPV may also have a role in determining what pharmacovigilance data should be requested from the other company, either pre- or post-acquisition. In this situation, the QPPV should be made aware of the sections of the contractual arrangements that relate to responsibilities for pharmacovigilance activities and safety data exchange and have the authority to request amendments.

When a marketing authorisation holder intends to establish a partnership with another marketing authorisation holder, organisation or person that has a direct or indirect impact on the pharmacovigilance system, the QPPV should be informed early enough and be involved in the preparation of the corresponding contractual arrangements (*see* I.C.1.5.) so that all necessary provisions relevant to the pharmacovigilance system are included.

I.C.1.2. Qualifications of the Qualified Person Responsible for Pharmacovigilance in the EU

The marketing authorisation holder shall ensure that the QPPV has acquired adequate theoretical and practical knowledge for the performance of pharmacovigilance activities [IR Art 10(1)]. The QPPV should have skills for the management of pharmacovigilance systems as well as expertise or access to expertise in relevant areas such as medicine, pharmaceutical sciences as well as epidemiology and biostatistics. Where the QPPV has not completed basic medical training in accordance with Article 24 of Directive 2005/36/EC, the marketing authorisation holder shall ensure that the QPPV is assisted by a medically trained person (i.e. in accordance with Article 24 of Directive 2005/36/EC) and this assistance shall be duly documented [IR Art 10(1)].

The expectation is that the applicant or marketing authorisation holder will assess the qualification of the QPPV prior to appointment by, for example, reviewing university qualifications, knowledge of EU pharmacovigilance requirements and experience in pharmacovigilance.

The applicant or marketing authorisation holder should provide the QPPV with training in relation to its pharmacovigilance system, which is appropriate for the role prior to the QPPV taking up the position and which is appropriately documented. Consideration should be given to additional training, as needed, of the QPPV in the medicinal products covered by the pharmacovigilance system.

I.C.1.3. Role of the Qualified Person Responsible for Pharmacovigilance in the EU

The qualified person responsible for pharmacovigilance in the EU (QPPV) is a natural[2] person.

The QPPV appointed by the marketing authorisation holder shall be appropriately

---

2. A natural person is a real human being, as distinguished from a corporation which is often treated at law as a fictitious person.

qualified (*see* I.C.1.2.) and shall be at the marketing authorisation holder's disposal permanently and continuously (*see* I.C.1.1.) [DIR Art 104 (3)(a)]. The QPPV shall reside and operate in the EU [DIR Art 104 (3) last paragraph]. Following European Economic Area (EEA) agreements, the QPPV may also reside and operate in Norway, Iceland or Liechtenstein. Back-up procedures in the case of absence of the QPPV shall be in place [IR Art 2(1)(d)] and should be accessible through the QPPV's contact details. The QPPV should ensure that the back-up person has all necessary information to fulfil the role.

The QPPV shall be responsible for the establishment and maintenance of the marketing authorisation holder's pharmacovigilance system [DIR Art 104 (3) last paragraph] and therefore shall have sufficient authority to influence the performance of the quality system and the pharmacovigilance activities [IR Art 10(2)] and to promote, maintain and improve compliance with the legal requirements [IR Art 2(1)(a)]. Hence, the QPPV should have access to the pharmacovigilance system master file (PSMF) (*see* Module II) and be in a position of authority to ensure and to verify that the information contained in the PSMF is an accurate and up-to-date reflection of the pharmacovigilance system under the QPPV's responsibility.

In relation to the medicinal products covered by the pharmacovigilance system, specific additional responsibilities of the QPPV should include:

- Having an overview of medicinal product safety profiles and any emerging safety concerns;
- Having awareness of any conditions or obligations adopted as part of the marketing authorisations and other commitments relating to safety or the safe use of the products;
- Having awareness of risk minimisation measures;
- Being aware of and having sufficient authority over the content of risk management plans;
- Being involved in the review and sign-off of protocols of post-authorisation safety studies conducted in the EU or pursuant to a risk management plan agreed in the EU;
- Having awareness of post-authorisation safety studies requested by a competent authority including the results of such studies;
- Ensuring conduct of pharmacovigilance and submission of all pharmacovigilance-related documents in accordance with the legal requirements and GVP;
- Ensuring the necessary quality, including the correctness and completeness, of pharmacovigilance data submitted to the competent authorities in Members States and the Agency;
- Ensuring a full and prompt response to any request from the competent authorities in Members States and from the Agency for the provision of additional information necessary for the benefit-risk evaluation of a medicinal product;
- Providing any other information relevant to the benefit-risk evaluation to the competent authorities in Members States and the Agency;
- Providing input into the preparation of regulatory action in response to emerging safety concerns (e.g. variations, urgent safety restrictions, and communication to patients and healthcare professionals);
- Acting as a single pharmacovigilance contact point for the competent authorities in Member States and the Agency on a 24-hour basis and also as a contact point for pharmacovigilance inspections.

This responsibility for the pharmacovigilance system means that the QPPV has oversight over the functioning of the system in all relevant aspects, including its quality system (e.g. standard operating procedures, contractual arrangements, database operations, compliance data regarding quality, completeness and timeliness of expedited reporting and submission of periodic update reports, audit reports and training of personnel in relation to pharmacovigilance). Specifically for the adverse reaction database, if applicable, the QPPV should be aware of the validation status of the database, including any failures that occurred during validation and the corrective actions that have been taken to address the failures. The QPPV should also be informed of significant changes that are made to the database (e.g. changes that could have an impact on pharmacovigilance activities).

The QPPV may delegate specific tasks, under supervision, to appropriately qualified and trained individuals, for example, acting as safety experts for certain products, provided that the QPPV maintains system oversight and overview of the safety profiles of all products. Such delegation should be documented.

I.C.1.4. Specific Quality System Processes of the Marketing Authorisation Holder in the EU

In applying the requirements set out in I.B.9.1. in the EU, the marketing authorisation holder shall put in place the following additional specific quality system processes for ensuring:
- The submission of adverse reaction data to EudraVigilance within the legal timelines [IR Art 11(c)];
- The monitoring of the use of terminology referred to in IR Art 25(1) either systematically or by regular random evaluation [IR Art 25(3)];
- The retention of minimum elements of the pharmacovigilance system master file (PSMF) (*see* IR Art 2 and Module II) as long as the system described in the PSMF exists and for at least further 5 years after it has been formally terminated by the marketing authorisation holder [IR Art 12(2)];
- The retention of pharmacovigilance data and documents relating to individual authorised medicinal products as long as the marketing authorisation exists and for at least further 10 years after the marketing authorisation has ceased to exist [IR Art 12(2)];
- That the product information is kept up-to-date by the marketing authorisation holder in the light of scientific knowledge, including the assessments and recommendations made public via the European medicines web-portal an on the basis of a continuous monitoring by the marketing authorisation holder of information published on the European medicines web-portal [IR Art 11(1)(g)].

The retention periods above apply unless the documents shall be retained for a longer period where EU or national law so requires [IR Art 12(2)].

During the retention period, retrievability of the documents should be ensured. Documents can be retained in electronic format, provided that the electronic system has been appropriately validated and appropriate arrangements exist for system security, access and back-up of data. If documents in paper format are transferred into an electronic format, the transfer process should ensure that all of the information present in the original format is retained in a legible manner and that the media used for storage will remain readable over time.

Documents transferred in situations where the business of the marketing authorisation holder is taken over by another organisation should be complete.

I.C.1.5. Quality System Requirements for Pharmacovigilance Tasks Subcontracted by the Marketing Authorisation Holder

The marketing authorisation holder may subcontract certain activities of the pharmacovigilance system to third parties [IR Art 6(1)], i.e. to another organisation or person (where the same requirements apply to a person as for an organisation). This may include the role of the QPPV. The marketing authorisation holder shall nevertheless retain full responsibility for the completeness and accuracy of the pharmacovigilance system master file (PSMF) (*see* Module II) [IR Art 6(1)]. The ultimate responsibility for the fulfilment of all pharmacovigilance tasks and responsibilities and the quality and integrity of the pharmacovigilance system always remains with the marketing authorisation holder.

Where a marketing authorisation holder has subcontracted some tasks of its pharmacovigilance tasks, it shall retain responsibility for ensuring that an effective quality system is applied in relation to those tasks [IR Art 11(2)]. All guidance provided in GVP is also applicable to the other organisation to which the tasks have been subcontracted.

When subcontracting tasks to another organisation, the marketing authorisation holder shall draw up subcontracts [IR Art 6(2)] and these should be detailed, up-to-date and clearly document the contractual arrangements between the marketing authorisation holder and the other organisation, describing arrangements for delegation and the responsibilities of each party. A description of the subcontracted activities and/or services shall be included in the pharmacovigilance system master file (PSMF) [IR Art 2(6)] and a list of the subcontracts shall be included in an annex to the PSMF, specifying the product(s) and territory(ies) concerned [IR Art 6(2)] (*see* Module II). The other organisation may be subject to inspection at the discretion of the competent or supervisory authority in the relevant Member State.

Contractual arrangements should be prepared with the aim of enabling compliance with the legal requirements by each party involved.

When preparing contractual arrangements, the marketing authorisation holder should include sufficiently detailed descriptions of the delegated tasks, the related interactions and data exchange, together with, for example, agreed definitions, tools, assignments and timelines. The contractual arrangements should also contain clear information on the practical management of pharmacovigilance as well as related processes, including those for the maintenance of pharmacovigilance databases. Further, they should indicate which processes are in place for checking whether the agreed arrangements are being adhered to on an ongoing basis. In this respect, regular risk-based audits of the other organisation by the marketing authorisation holder or introduction of other methods of control and assessment are recommended.

With respect to centrally authorised products, contractual arrangements between different marketing authorisation holders should also be in place in relation to separately authorised medicinal products with the application of Article 82(1) of Regulation (EC) No 726/2004 in order to ensure conduct of pharmacovigilance on the basis of complete worldwide data sets.

For responsibilities of the marketing authorisation holder towards the QPPV in this context, *see* I.C.1.1.

I.C.2. Overall Pharmacovigilance Responsibilities within the EU Regulatory Network

The competent authorities in Member States and the Agency are responsible for the respective pharmacovigilance tasks and responsibilities imposed on them by Directive 2001/83/EC, Regulation (EC) No 726/2004 and the Commission Implementing Regulation (EU) No 520/2012 on the Performance of Pharmacovigilance Activities Provided for in Regulation (EC) No 726/2004 and Directive 2001/83/EC in order to ensure that appropriate action can be taken, when necessary.

For this purpose each competent authority in a Member State as well as the Agency shall operate a pharmacovigilance system [DIR 101(1)] and shall establish and use an adequate and effective quality system for performing their pharmacovigilance activities [IR Art 8(1)].

The Agency and the Member States shall cooperate to continuously develop pharmacovigilance systems capable of achieving high standards of public health protection for all medicinal products, regardless of the routes of marketing authorisation, including the use of collaborative approaches, to maximise use of resources available within the EU [REG Art 28e].

The requirement in I.B.11.2. according to which competent authorities shall keep accessible clear descriptions of the organisational structures, assignment of tasks and responsibilities as well as contact points [IR Art 14(1)], should relate to the interaction between competent authorities in Member States, the Agency, the European Commission, marketing authorisation holders and persons reporting information on the risks of medicinal products.

Guidance on the structures and processes to enable the competent authorities in Member States and the Agency to conduct the pharmacovigilance tasks and responsibilities is provided in the respective Modules of GVP.

I.C.2.1. Role of the Competent Authorities in Member States

Each Member State shall designate a competent authority for the performance of pharmacovigilance [DIR Art 101(3)]. This authority is usually the same as the competent authority responsible for granting national marketing authorisations.

Each competent authority in a Member State must operate a pharmacovigilance system for the fulfilment of their pharmacovigilance tasks and their participation in EU pharmacovigilance activities [DIR Art 101(1)]. In this context, the competent authority in a Member State is responsible for the safety monitoring of each medicinal product, independent of its route of authorisation, in the territory of that Member State. In particular, the competent authority in each Member State shall be responsible for monitoring data originating in their territory [IR Art 18(4)].

For nationally authorised products, including those authorised through the mutual recognition or the decentralised procedure, the competent authority in a Member State is responsible for granting, varying, suspending and revoking a marketing authorisation. The pharmacovigilance tasks and responsibilities of competent authorities in Member States for each process in relation to such products, are detailed in the respective Modules of GVP.

For products authorised through the mutual recognition or the decentralised procedure, one Member State acts as the Reference Member State. For practical reasons, the competent authority of the Reference Member State should coordinate communication with the marketing authorisation holder on pharmacovigilance matters and monitor the compliance of the marketing authorisation holder with legal pharmacovigilance requirements. These arrangements do not replace the legal responsibilities of the marketing authorisation holder with respect to individual competent authorities and the Agency.

Nationally authorised products, including those authorised through the mutual recognition or the decentralised procedure, may become subject to regulatory procedures at EU level on pharmacovigilance grounds. If a Commission Decision for a nationally authorised product exists as an outcome of such a procedure, the competent authorities in Member States are responsible for the implementation of the Commission Decision and also for its follow-up, unless exceptionally further action by the Agency and the European Commission has been foreseen in the Commission Decision reflecting the outcome of the regulatory procedure (*see* Chapter 3 of the Notice to Applicants and the Agency's and HMA Procedural Advice on Referral Procedures for Safety Reasons).

The pharmacovigilance tasks and responsibilities of competent authorities in Member States in relation to centrally authorised products are also detailed in the respective Modules of GVP. They include the collaboration in signal detection (*see* Module IX) and implementation of Commission Decisions regarding risk management of centrally authorised products addressed to Member States (*see* Module V). Where urgent action is essential to protect human health or the environment, the competent authority in a Member State, on its own initiative or at the European Commission's request, may suspend the use of a centrally authorised product in its territory (*see* Modules XII).

Competent authorities in Member States are responsible for pharmacovigilance inspections of organisations in their territory in relation to medicinal products. This is independent of the route of marketing authorisation as well as which competent authority granted the marketing authorisation for the respective medicinal product (*see* Module III).

In relation to the various aspects of the role described above, each Member State's competent authority should ensure that all pharmacovigilance data are shared between competent authorities in other Member States, the European Commission and the Agency for each process in accordance with the legislation and the guidance in the respective GVP Modules.

I.C.2.2. Role of the European Commission

The European Commission is the competent authority for medicinal products authorised through the centralised procedure and is responsible for granting, varying, suspending and revoking their marketing authorisations by adoption of Commission Decisions on the basis of Opinions adopted by the Committee for Medicinal Products for Human Use (CHMP) (*see* I.C.2.3.3.).

Further, the European Commission adopts Commission Decisions in relation to nationally authorised medicinal products subject to regulatory procedures at EU level, including on pharmacovigilance grounds. The European Commission may also initiate such procedures (*see* Chapter 3 of the Notice to Applicants and the Agency's and HMA Procedural Advice on Referral Procedures for Safety Reasons).

I.C.2.3. Role of the European Medicines Agency

I.C.2.3.1. General role of the Agency and the role of the Agency's secretariat

The role of the Agency is to coordinate the monitoring of medicinal products for human use authorised in the EU and to provide advice on the measures necessary to ensure their safe and effective use, in particular, by coordinating the evaluation and implementation of legal pharmacovigilance requirements and the monitoring of such implementation. The tools established and maintained by the Agency for the coordination are presented in the GVP Modules for each process.

The Agency provides coordination and technical, scientific and administrative support to the Pharmacovigilance Risk Assessment Committee (PRAC) (*see* I.C.2.3.2.) and the Committee for Medicinal Products for Human Use (CHMP) (*see* I.C.2.3.3.) and coordination and technical and administrative support to the Coordination Group for Mutual Recognition and Decentralised Procedures - Human (CMDh) (*see* I.C.2.3.4.), as well as coordination between the committees and the CMDh.

Pharmacovigilance for centrally authorised products is conducted by the Agency with the involvement of the Rapporteurs, the PRAC and the CHMP. The Agency should take the lead for communicating with the marketing authorisation holders of centrally authorised products. The respective responsibilities for each pharmacovigilance process are detailed in the GVP Modules.

For nationally authorised products, the Agency coordinates regulatory procedures at EU level on pharmacovigilance grounds through providing support to the CMDh and CHMP (*see* Chapter 3 of the Notice to Applicants and the Agency's and HMA Procedural Advice on Referral Procedures for Safety Reasons).

The Agency also cooperates with other EU bodies as necessary.

Specific pharmacovigilance tasks of the Agency include:

- Running the EudraVigilance database [REG Art 57(d)];
- Monitoring selected medical literature for reports of suspected adverse reactions to medicinal products containing certain active substances [REG Art 27] (*see* Module VI);
- Running processes for the EU coordination of the assessment of periodic safety update reports (*see* Module VII) and oversight of post-authorisation safety studies (*see* Module VIII);
- Tasks relating to signal detection [REG Art 28a(1)(c), IR Art 18-24] (*see* Module IX);
- Tracking of follow-up of safety concerns and other pharmacovigilance matters at EU level (*see* Module XII);
- Assisting Member States with the rapid communication of information on safety concerns to healthcare professionals and coordinating the safety announcements of the national competent authorities [REG Art 57(e)] (*see* Module XV);
- Distributing appropriate information on safety concerns to the general public, in particular by setting up and maintaining the European medicines web-portal [REG Art 57(f)] (*see* Module XV);
- Coordination of safety announcements between national competent authorities for active substances contained in medicinal products authorised in more than one Member State, including providing timetables for the publication of information [DIR 106a(3)] (*see* Module XV); and specifically in relation to centrally authorised products;
- Assessing updates to risk management systems [REG Art 28a(1)(b)] (*see* Module V);
- Monitoring the outcome of risk minimisation measures [REG Art 28a(1)(a)] (*see* Module XVI).

I.C.2.3.2. Role of the Pharmacovigilance Risk Assessment Committee (PRAC)

The Pharmacovigilance Risk Assessment Committee (PRAC) is responsible for providing recommendations to the Committee for Medicinal Products for Human Use (CHMP) and the Coordination Group for Mutual Recognition and Decentralised Procedures - Human (CMDh) on any question relating to pharmacovigilance activities in respect of medicinal products for human use and on risk management systems, including the monitoring of the effectiveness of those risk management systems [REG Art 56(1)(aa)]. The Details on the responsibilities for each process are presented in the respective GVP Modules. The Mandate and Rules of Procedure of the PRAC are published on the Agency's website.[3]

I.C.2.3.3. Role of the Committee for Medicinal Products for Human Use (CHMP)

The Committee for Medicinal Products for Human Use (CHMP) is responsible for evaluating applications and formulating Opinions serving as a basis for granting, varying, suspending or withdrawing marketing authorisations for centrally authorised products. The CHMP also prepares Opinions on safety concerns emerging

---
3. http://www.ema.europa.eu

after a marketing authorisation has been granted for centrally authorised products or, for nationally authorised products, including those through the mutual recognition or the decentralised procedure, in the framework of regulatory procedures at EU level in which at least one centrally authorised product is involved (*see* Chapter 3 of the Notice to Applicants and the Agency's and HMA Procedural Advice on Referral Procedures for Safety Reasons), procedures for the assessment of periodic safety update reports (PSURs) (*see* Module VII) and procedures for post-authorisation safety studies (*see* Module VIII). For questions related to pharmacovigilance activities and risk management systems, the CHMP relies on the recommendations from the Pharmacovigilance Risk Assessment Committee (PRAC). The specific responsibilities of each party for each pharmacovigilance process are described in the GVP Modules. The Rules of Procedure of the CHMP are published on the Agency's website.[4]

I.C.2.3.4. Role of the Coordination Group for Mutual Recognition and Decentralised Procedures - Human (CMDh)

The Coordination Group for Mutual Recognition and Decentralised Procedures - Human (CMDh) is responsible for examining any question relating to marketing authorisations for medicinal products authorised through the mutual recognition or the decentralised procedure and questions on the variation of marketing authorisations granted by the Member States as well as questions arising for nationally authorised products from assessments of periodic safety update reports (*see* Module VII), post-authorisation safety studies (*see* Module VIII) and during regulatory procedures at EU level. The CMDh shall reach a position, based on a PRAC recommendation, on regulatory procedures at EU level when only nationally authorised products, including those authorised through the mutual recognition or the decentralised procedure, are involved [DIR Art 107k](*see* Chapter 3 of the Notice to Applicants and the Agency's and HMA Procedural Advice on Referral Procedures for Safety Reasons). The responsibilities of the CMDh for each pharmacovigilance process are described in the respective GVP Modules. The Rules of Procedure of the CMDh and the Functions and Tasks for CMDh are published on the HMA website.[5]

I.C.2.4. Specific Quality System Processes of the Quality Systems of Competent Authorities in Member States and the Agency

In applying the requirements set out in I.B.9.2. in the EU, the competent authorities in Member States and the Agency shall put in place the following additional specific quality system processes for:

- Monitoring and validating the use of terminology referred to in IR Art 25(1), either systematically or by regular random evaluation [IR Art 25(3)];
- Assessing and processing pharmacovigilance data in accordance with the timelines provided by legislation [IR Art 15(1)(b)];
- Ensuring effective communication within the EU regulatory network in accordance with the provisions on safety announcements in Article 106a of Directive 2001/83/EC [IR Art 15(1)(d)] (*see* Module XV);
- Guaranteeing that competent authorities in Member States and the Agency inform each other and the European Commission of their intention to make announcements relating to the safety of a medicinal product or an active substance contained in a medicinal product authorised in several Member State (*see* Modules XII and XV) [IR Art 15(1)(e)];
- Arranging for the essential documents describing their pharmacovigilance systems to be kept as long as the system exists and for at least further 5 years after they have been formally terminated [IR Art 16(2)];
- Ensuring that pharmacovigilance data and documents relating to individual authorised medicinal products are retained as long as the marketing authorisation exists or for at least further 10 years after the marketing authorisation has expired [IR Art 16(2)].

---

4. http://www.ema.europa.eu/ema/index.jsp?curl=pages/about_us/general/general_content_000095.jsp&murl=menus/about_us/about_us.jsp&mid=WC0b01ac0580028c7a
5. http://www.hma.eu/205.html

In this context, documents relating to a medicinal product include documents of a reference medicinal product where this is applicable.

The retention periods above apply unless the documents shall be retained for a longer period where EU or national law so requires [IR Art 16(2)].

During the retention periods referred to above, retrievability of the documents should be ensured.

Documents can be retained in electronic format, provided that the electronic system has been appropriately validated and appropriate arrangements exist for system security, access and back-up of data. If pharmacovigilance documents in paper format are transferred into an electronic format, the transfer process should ensure that all of the information present in the original format is retained in a legible manner and that the media used for storage will remain readable over time.

The legal requirements for record management (*see* I.B.10.) imply accessibility to the records from within the EU, preferably at a single point.

In addition to the above, competent authorities in Member States shall establish procedures for collecting and recording all suspected adverse reactions that occur in their territory (*see* Module VI) [IR Art 15(2)].

In addition to the above, the Agency shall establish procedures for literature monitoring in accordance with Article 27 of Regulation (EC) No 726/2004 (*see* Module VI) [IR Art 15(3)].

In addition to the quality system documentation in accordance with I.B.11. and I.B.11.2., competent authorities in Member States and the Agency shall clearly determine, and to the extent necessary, keep accessible the organisational structures and the distribution of tasks and responsibilities [IR Art 14(1)] as well as establish contact points [IR Art 14(1)], in particular to facilitate interaction between competent authorities in Member States, the Agency, marketing authorisation holders and persons reporting information on the risks of medicinal products as regards patients' or public health.

Quality audits of the Member States' and Agency's pharmacovigilance systems (*see* I.B.12.) shall be performed according to a common methodology [IR Art 17(1)]. The results of audits shall be reported by competent authorities in Member States in accordance with Article 101(2) of Directive 2001/83/EC and by the Agency in accordance with Article 28f of Regulation (EC) No 726/2004 (*see* Module IV).

I.C.2.5. Quality System Requirements for Pharmacovigilance Tasks Delegated or Transferred by Competent Authorities in Member States

A competent authority in a Member State may delegate any pharmacovigilance task to another Member State subject to a written agreement of the latter Member State [DIR Art 103]. The written agreement should be reflected by exchange of letters, defining the scope of the delegation.

A competent authority in a Member State may transfer any or all of the pharmacovigilance tasks to another organisation, but the ultimate responsibility for the fulfilment of all pharmacovigilance tasks and responsibilities and the quality and integrity of the pharmacovigilance system always remains with the competent authority in a Member State.

Where tasks are transferred to another organisation, the competent authority in a Member State should ensure that the tasks are subject to a quality system compliant with the legal requirements applicable to their own organisation.

I.C.2.6. Transparency of the Quality System of the EU Regulatory Network

The European Commission (EC) shall publish every three years a report on the performance of pharmacovigilance based on the reports submitted by the competent authorities in Member States (first EC report due on 21 July 2015) and by the Agency (first EC report due on 2 January 2014) on the results of their regular pharmacovigilance system audits (*see* Module IV) [DIR Art 101(2), Art 108b, REG Art 28f, Art 29].

I.C.3. Data Protection in the EU

All legal requirements of the IR, including those relating to the record management described in I.B.10., shall apply without prejudice to the obligations of national competent authorities and marketing authorisation holders relating to their processing of personal data under Directive 95/46/EC or the obligations of the Agency relating to its processing of personal data under Regulation (EC) No 45/2001 [IR Art 39].

I.C.4. Preparedness Planning in the EU for Pharmacovigilance in Public Health Emergencies

The pharmacovigilance systems of marketing authorisation holders, competent authorities in Member States and the Agency should be adaptable to public health emergencies. Preparedness plans should be developed as appropriate (*see* I.B.13.).

A public health emergency is a public health threat duly recognised either by the World Health Organization (WHO) or the Community in the framework of Decision No. 2119/98/EC of the European Parliament and of the Council.

Pharmacovigilance requirements for public health emergencies should be considered by the competent authorities in Member States, the European Commission and the Agency on a case-by-case basis and appropriately notified to marketing authorisation holders and the public. The Agency publishes its notifications on the Agency's website.

Annexure 8: Guidelines on Good Pharmacovigilance Practices (GVP) 341

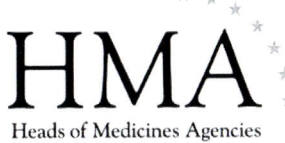
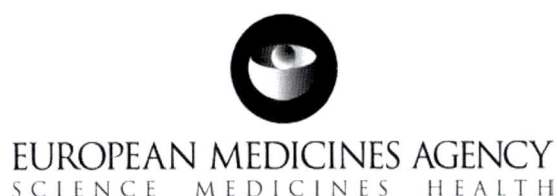

28 March 2017
EMA/816573/2011 Rev 2*

GUIDELINE ON GOOD PHARMACOVIGILANCE PRACTICES (GVP)

Module II Pharmacovigilance System Master File (Rev 2)

Date for coming into effect of first version	2 July 2012
Date for coming into effect of Revision 1	12 April 2013
Draft Revision 2* finalised by the Agency in collaboration with Member States	9 March 2017
Draft Revision 2 agreed by the EU Network Pharmacovigilance Oversight Group (EU-POG)	23 March 2017
Draft Revision 2 adopted by Executive Director as final	28 March 2017
Date for coming into effect of Revision 2	31 March 2017

*__Note:__ Revision 2 contains the following:
- Deletion of text in II.A. referring to transition period as this is not applicable anymore;
- Clarification in II.B. that the content of the PSMF should reflect global availability of safety information for medicinal products authorised in the EU, presenting information on the pharmacovigilance system applied at global, regional and local levels;
- Deletion of text in II.A. not applicable anymore and rearrangement of sections in II.B.2.1., II.B.2.2., II.B.2.3. and II.C.1.1. to put emphasis on requirements for the submission of the summary of the applicant's pharmacovigilance system at the moment of the initial marketing authorisation application, the requirement for the initial electronic submission of QPPV/contact details and PSMF location information via the Article 57 database (PSMF location registration) and updates to the Article 57 database only, without the need to submit a type IAIN variation (QPPV and PSMF location information maintenance);
- Clarification in II.B.4.7. on the inclusion of corrective and preventative action plan(s) that have not yet been agreed for a particular audit or finding in the note required in the PSMF, in order to address queries received from the public;
- Addition in II.B.4.8. of the legal reference on the information to be included in the product list regarding the marketing status of the medicinal product.

This revision of the Module was not subject to public consultation because it concerns only updates and clarifications without changes to the content.

II.A. INTRODUCTION

The legal requirement for marketing authorisation holders to maintain and make available upon request a pharmacovigilance system master file (PSMF) was introduced by Directive 2010/84/EU amending, as regards pharmacovigilance, Directive 2001/83/EC (see Recitals (7) and (35), Article 23(4), Article 104(3)(b) of Directive 2010/84/EU) and Regulation (EU) No 1235/2010 amending, as regards pharmacovigilance of medicinal products for human use, Regulation (EC) No 726/2004 (see Recitals (22) and (25), Article 16(3a) of Regulation (EU) No 1235/2010), to harmonise and strengthen the conduct of pharmacovigilance activities in the EU.

The PSMF definition is provided in Article 1(28e) of Directive 2001/83/EC and the minimum requirements for its content and maintenance are set out in the Commission Implementing Regulation (EU) No 520/2012 on the performance of pharmacovigilance activities provided for in Regulation (EC) No 726/2004 and Directive 2001/83/EC. The detailed requirements provided by the Commission Implementing Regulation are further supported by the guidance in this GVP Module.

Regulation (EC) No 726/2004, Directive 2001/83/EC and Commission Implementing Regulation (EU) No 520/2012 are hereinafter referred to as REG, DIR and IR, respectively.

The PSMF shall be located either at the site in the EU where the main pharmacovigilance activities of the marketing authorisation holder are performed or at the site in the EU where the qualified person responsible for pharmacovigilance operates [IR Art 7(1)].

It is a requirement of the marketing authorisation application that summary information about the pharmacovigilance system is submitted to the competent authorities [DIR Art 8(3)(ia)]. This summary includes information on the location of the PSMF (see II.B.2.1.).

This Module provides detailed guidance regarding the requirements for the PSMF, including its maintenance, content and associated submissions to competent authorities.

In this Module, all applicable legal requirements are referenced in the way explained in the GVP Introductory Cover Note and are usually identifiable by the modal verb "shall". Guidance for the implementation of legal requirements is provided using the modal verb "should".

II.B. STRUCTURES AND PROCESSES

The PSMF is a legal requirement in the EU. This guidance concerns the requirements for the PSMF and is applicable for any medicinal product authorised in the EU, irrespective of the marketing authorisation procedure. The required content and management of the PSMF applies irrespective of the organisational structure of a marketing authorisation holder, including any subcontracting or delegation of activities, or their location. Irrespective of the location of other activities, the qualified person for pharmacovigilance (QPPV's) residence, the location at which he/she carries out his/her tasks and the PSMF location must be within the EU. Following European Economic Area (EEA) agreements, the QPPV may also reside and operate in Norway, Iceland or Liechtenstein.

The content of the PSMF should reflect global availability of safety information for medicinal products authorised in the EU, presenting information on the pharmacovigilance system applied at global, regional and local levels.

II.B.1. Objectives

The PSMF shall describe the pharmacovigilance system and support/document its compliance with the requirements. As well as fulfilling the requirements for a PSMF laid down in the legislation and guidance, it shall also contribute to the appropriate planning and conduct of audits by the applicant or marketing authorisations holder(s), the fulfilment of supervisory responsibilities of the QPPV, and of inspections or other verification of compliance by national competent authorities. The PSMF provides an overview of the pharmacovigilance system, which may be requested and assessed by national competent authorities during marketing authorisation application(s) or post-authorisation.

Through the production and maintenance of the PSMF, the marketing authorisation holder and the QPPV should be able to:
- Gain assurance that a pharmacovigilance system has been implemented in accordance with the requirements;

- Confirm aspects of compliance in relation to the system;
- Obtain information about deficiencies in the system, or non-compliance with the requirements;
- Obtain information about risks or actual failure in the conduct of specific aspects of pharmacovigilance.

The use of this information should contribute to the appropriate management of and improvement(s) to the pharmacovigilance system.

The requirements for submission of a summary of the marketing authorisation holder's pharmacovigilance system, provision of the content of PSMF and the history of changes to the relevant authority(ies) should enable the appropriate coordination of inspections by the Agency, and the planning and effective conduct of inspections by national competent authorities, based on a risk assessment approach.

Responsibilities, in terms of the PSMF, for marketing authorisation holders and applicants, national competent authorities and the Agency are described in detail in Section C (see II.C.1.).

II.B.2. Registration and Maintenance

II.B.2.1. Summary of the Applicant's Pharmacovigilance System

Article 8(3)(ia) of Directive 2001/83/EC requires a summary of the applicant's pharmacovigilance system to be included in the marketing authorisation application, which shall include the following elements in module 1.8.1 of the dossier:
- Proof that the applicant has at his disposal a qualified person responsible for pharmacovigilance;
- The Member States in which the qualified person resides and carries out his/her tasks;
- The contact details of the qualified person;
- A statement signed by the applicant to the effect that the applicant has the necessary means to fulfil the tasks and responsibilities listed in Title IX;
- A reference to the location where the PSMF for the medicinal product is kept.

Applicants for, and holders of simplified registrations of traditional herbal medicinal products are not required to submit a pharmacovigilance system summary, however, they are required to operate a pharmacovigilance system and prepare, maintain and make available on request a PSMF [based on DIR Art 16g(1)].

For other herbal medicinal products, not falling within the scope of the traditional-use registration, the requirements to operate a pharmacovigilance system, to prepare, maintain and make available on request a PSMF and to submit a summary of the pharmacovigilance system apply.

For homeopathic medicinal products registered via the simplified registration procedure the requirements to operate a pharmacovigilance system, to maintain and make available on request a PSMF and to submit a summary of the pharmacovigilance system do not apply [DIR Art 16(3)].

For other homeopathic medicinal products, not falling within the scope of the simplified registration, the requirements to operate a pharmacovigilance system, to prepare, maintain and make available on request a PSMF and to submit a summary of the pharmacovigilance system apply [DIR Art 16(3)].

II.B.2.2. Location, Registration and Maintenance

The PSMF shall be located within the EU, either at the site where the main pharmacovigilance activities are performed or at the site where the qualified person responsible for pharmacovigilance operates [IR Art 7(1)], irrespective of the format (paper-based or electronic format file). Following European Economic Area (EEA) agreements, the PSMF may also be located in Norway, Iceland or Liechtenstein.

At the time of marketing authorisation application, the applicant should submit electronically the PSMF location information using the agreed format [IR Art26 1(a)], and subsequently include in the application, the PSMF reference number, which is the unique code assigned by the EudraVigilance (EV) system to the master file when the EudraVigilance Medicinal Product Report Message (XEVPRM) is processed (see[1]). Further to the granting of a marketing authorisation, the PSMF will be linked by the marketing authorisation holder to the EVMPD product code(s). All PSMFs must be registered in the Article 57 database.

---
1. ema.europa.eu, Data submission on medicines (Article 57) webpage

Marketing authorisation holders shall continue to ensure that their entries in the Article 57 database for medicinal products for human use are up-to-date, including the information about the qualified person responsible for pharmacovigilance (QPPV), name and contact details (telephone and fax numbers, postal address and email addresses) and PSMF location information [based on IR Art 4(4)]. Upon a change in the QPPV or location of the PMSF information, the Article 57 database shall be updated by the marketing authorisation holder immediately and no later than 30 calendar days, in order to have the information in the Article 57 database and on the European medicines web-portal referred to in Article 26(1) of Regulation (EC) No 726/2004 updated and to allow continuous supervision by the competent authorities [based on IR Art 4(4), REG Art 57(2)(c)] (see[2]).

The required location information for the PSMF is a physical office address of the marketing authorisation holder or a contracted third party. Where the PSMF is held in electronic form, the location stated must be a site where the data stored can be directly accessed, and this is sufficient in terms of a practical electronic location [IR Art 7(3)].

When determining the main site of pharmacovigilance activity, the marketing authorisation holder should consider the most relevant EU site for the pharmacovigilance system as a whole, since the relative importance of particular activities may vary according to products and fluctuate in the short term. The marketing authorisation holder should have an appropriate rationale for the location decision. In the situation where the main activities take place outside the EU, or where a main site cannot be determined, the location should default to the site where the QPPV operates.

II.B.2.3. Transfers of Responsibilities for the Pharmacovigilance System Master File

The pharmacovigilance system may change with time. Transfer or delegation of responsibilities and activities concerning the master file should be documented (see II.B.4.2. and II.B.4.8.) and managed to ensure that the marketing authorisation holder fulfils their responsibilities. Since a specific QPPV has responsibility for the pharmacovigilance system, changes to the PSMF should also be notified to the QPPV in order to support their authority to make improvements to the system. The types of changes that should be routinely and promptly notified to the QPPV are:

- Updates to the PSMF or its location that are notified to the competent authorities;
- The addition of corrective and/or preventative actions to the PSMF (e.g. following audits and inspections). The QPPV should also be able to access information about deviations from the processes defined in the quality management system for pharmacovigilance;
- Changes to content that fulfil the criteria for appropriate oversight of the pharmacovigilance system (in terms of capacity, functioning and compliance);
- Changes in arrangements for the provision of the PSMF to competent authorities;
- Transfer of significant services for pharmacovigilance to a third party (e.g. outsourcing of PSUR production);
- Inclusion of products into the pharmacovigilance system for which the QPPV is responsible;
- Changes for existing products which may require a change or increased workload in relation to pharmacovigilance activity, e.g. new indications, studies or the addition of territories.

Any recipient QPPV should explicitly accept the following changes in writing:

- Transfer of responsibility for a pharmacovigilance system to a QPPV.

The QPPV should be in a position to ensure and to verify that the information contained in the PSMF is an accurate and up to date reflection of the pharmacovigilance system under his/her responsibility (see GVP Module I).

II.B.3. The Representation of Pharmacovigilance Systems

The PSMF, as per definition in Article 1(28e) of Directive 2001/83/EC, shall describe the pharmacovigilance system for one or more medicinal products of the marketing authorisation holder. For different categories of medicinal products the marketing authorisation holder may,

---

2. ema.europa.eu, EudraVigilance webpage

if appropriate, apply separate pharmacovigilance systems. Each such system shall be described in a separate PSMF. Those files shall cumulatively cover all medicinal products of the marketing authorisation holder for which a marketing authorisation has been issued in accordance with Directive 2001/83/EC or an authorisation has been granted in accordance with Regulation (EC) No 726/2004.

- It is anticipated that there will be circumstances where a single marketing authorisation holder may establish more than one pharmacovigilance system, e.g. specific systems for particular types of products (vaccines, consumer health, etc.), or that the pharmacovigilance system may include products from more than one marketing authorisation holder. In either case, a single and specific PSMF shall be in place to describe each system.
- In accordance with Articles 8 and 104 of Directive 2001/83/EC, a single QPPV shall be appointed to be responsible for the establishment and maintenance of the pharmacovigilance system described in the PSMF.
- Where a pharmacovigilance system is shared by several marketing authorisation holders each marketing authorisation holder is responsible ensuring that a PSMF exists to describe the pharmacovigilance system applicable for his products. For a particular product(s) the marketing authorisation holder may delegate through written agreement (e.g. to a licensing partner or contractor) part or all of the pharmacovigilance activity for which the marketing authorisation holder is responsible. In this case the PSMF of the marketing authorisation holder may cross refer to all or part of the PSMF managed by the system of the party to whom the activity has been delegated subject to agreement on access to that system's information for the marketing authorisation holder and the authorities. The marketing authorisation holder should be able to assure the content of the referenced file(s) in relation to the pharmacovigilance system applicable to their product(s). Activities for maintaining the PSMF in a current and accessible state can be delegated.
- Where applicable, a list of all PSMFs held by the same marketing authorisation holder shall be provided in the annex (see II.B.4.8.) [IR Art 3(7)]; this includes their location(s), details of the responsible QPPV(s) and the relevant product(s).
- Submission of summary information to competent authorities cannot contain multiple locations for a single PSMF. The address of the location of the PSMF provided to fulfil the requirement of Article 8(3) of Directive 2001/83/EC (and within the Article 57 database) should be an office address which reflects either the site in the EU where the main pharmacovigilance activities of the marketing authorisation holder are performed or the site where the qualified person responsible for pharmacovigilance operates. This address may be different to that of the applicant/marketing authorisation holder, for example, a different office of the marketing authorisation holder or when a third party undertakes the main activities.
- Similarly, the QPPV details aligned to a product in the Article 57 database may be those of a contract QPPV responsible for the pharmacovigilance system for a particular medicinal product, and not necessarily a QPPV directly employed by the marketing authorisation holder.
- When delegating any activities concerning the pharmacovigilance system and its master file, the marketing authorisation holder retains ultimate responsibility for the pharmacovigilance system, submission of information about the PSMF location, maintenance of the PSMF and its provision to competent authorities upon request [IR Art 6]. Detailed written agreements describing the roles and responsibilities for PSMF content, submissions and management, as well as to govern the conduct of pharmacovigilance in accordance with the legal requirements, should be in place [based on IR Art 6].
- When a pharmacovigilance system is shared, it is advised that the partners agree on how to mutually maintain the relevant sections within their own PSMFs. Accessibility of the PSMF to all the applicable marketing authorisation holder(s), and its provision to competent authorities should be defined in written agreements. It is vital that marketing

authorisation holder(s) can gain assurance that the pharmacovigilance system used for its products is appropriate and compliant.

II.B.4. Information to be Contained in the Pharmacovigilance System Master File

The PSMF shall contain at least all of the documents listed in Article 2 of Commission Implementing Regulation (EU) No 520/2012.

The PSMF shall include documents to describe the pharmacovigilance system. The content of the PSMF should reflect the global availability of safety information for medicinal products authorised in the EU. The content shall be indexed to allow for efficient navigation around the document and follow the modular system described in the following sections and the annex headings described in II.B.6.1. The main principle for the structure of the content of the PSMF is that the primary topic sections contain information that is fundamental to the description of pharmacovigilance system. Detailed information is required to fully describe the system, and, since this may change frequently, it should be referred to and contained in the Annexes. The control associated with change of content is described in section II.B.5.

It is accepted that, where no marketing authorisation (and master file) previously existed in the EU, there may be information that cannot be initially provided, for example, compliance information, however, descriptions of what will be implemented should be provided instead.

II.B.4.1. PSMF Section on Qualified Person Responsible for Pharmacovigilance (QPPV)

For the QPPV, contact details shall be provided in the marketing authorisation application [DIR Art 8(3)(ia)] and/or via the Article 57 database.

The information relating to the QPPV provided in the PSMF [IR Art 2(1)] shall include:

- A description of the responsibilities guaranteeing that the qualified person has sufficient authority over the pharmacovigilance system in order to promote, maintain and improve compliance;
- A summary curriculum vitae with the key information on the role of the qualified person responsible for pharmacovigilance, including proof of registration with the EudraVigilance database;
- Contact details;
- Details of back-up arrangements to apply in the absence of the qualified person responsible for pharmacovigilance; and
- Responsibilities of the contact person for pharmacovigilance issues where such a person has been nominated at national level in accordance with Article 104(4) of Directive 2001/83/EC, including contact details.

A list of tasks that have been delegated by the qualified person for pharmacovigilance shall also be included in the Annexes (see II.B.4.8.). This should outline the activities that are delegated and to whom, and include the access to a medically qualified person if applicable (GVP Module I and [IR Art 10(1)]). This list may be supplied as a copy of a written procedural document provided the required content is covered.

The details provided in relation to the QPPV should also include the description of the QPPV qualifications, experience and registrations relevant to pharmacovigilance (including registration with EudraVigilance). The contact details supplied should include name, postal address, telephone, fax and e-mail and represent the usual working address of the QPPV, which may therefore be different to a marketing authorisation holder address. If the QPPV is employed by a third party, even if the usual working address is an office of the marketing authorisation holder, this should be indicated and the name of the company the QPPV works for provided.

II.B.4.2. PSMF Section on the Organisational Structure of the Marketing Authorisation Holder

A description of the organisational structure of the marketing authorisation holder relevant to the pharmacovigilance system must be provided. The description should provide a clear overview of the company(ies) involved, the main pharmacovigilance departments and the relationship(s) between organisations and operational units relevant to the fulfilment of pharmacovigilance obligations. This

should include third parties. Specifically, the PSMF shall describe:
- The organisational structure of the marketing authorisation holder(s), showing the position of the QPPV in the organisation.
- The site(s) where the pharmacovigilance functions are undertaken covering individual case safety report collection, evaluation, safety database case entry, periodic safety update report production, signal detection and analysis, risk management plan management, pre- and post-authorisation study management, and management of safety variations to product particulars [IR Art 2(2)].

Diagrams may be particularly useful; the name of the department or third party should be indicated.

Delegated activities: The PSMF, where applicable, shall contain a description of the activities and/or services subcontracted by the marketing authorisation holder [IR Art 2 (6)] relating to the fulfillment of pharmacovigilance obligations. This includes arrangements with other parties in any country, Worldwide and if applicable, to the pharmacovigilance system applied to products authorised in the EU.

Links with other organisations, such as co-marketing agreements and contracting of pharmacovigilance activities should be outlined. A description of the location and nature of contracts and agreements relating to the fulfilment of pharmacovigilance obligations should be provided. This may be in the form of a list/table to show the parties involved, the roles undertaken and the concerned product(s) and territories. The list should be organised according to: service providers (e.g. medical information, auditors, patient support programme providers, study data management, etc.), commercial arrangements (distributors, licensing partners, co-marketing etc.) and other technical providers (hosting of computer systems, etc.). Individual contractual agreements shall be made available at the request of national competent authorities and the Agency or during inspection and audit and the list provided in the Annexes (*see* II.B.4.8.).

II.B.4.3. PSMF Section on the Sources of Safety Data

The description of the main units for safety data collection should include all parties responsible, on a global basis, for solicited and spontaneous case collection for products authorised in the EU. This should include medical information sites as well as affiliate offices and may take the form of a list describing the country, nature of the activity and the product(s) (if the activity is product specific) and providing a contact point (address, telephone and e-mail) for the site. The list may be located in the Annexes of the PSMF. Information about third parties (licence partners or local distribution/marketing arrangements) should also be included in the section describing contracts and agreements (*see* II.B.4.2. and II.B.4.8.).

Flow diagrams indicating the main stages, timeframes and parties involved may be used. However represented, the description of the process for ICSRs from collection to reporting to competent authorities should indicate the departments and/or third parties involved.

For the purposes of inspection and audit of the pharmacovigilance system, sources include data arising from study sources, including any studies, registries, surveillance or support programmes sponsored by the marketing authorisation holder through which ICSRs could be reported. MAHs should be able to produce and make available a list of such sources to support inspection, audit and QPPV oversight. In the interests of harmonisation, it is recommended that the list should be comprehensive for products authorised in the EU, irrespective of indication, product presentation or route of administration. The list should describe, on a worldwide basis, the status of each study/programme, the applicable country(ies), the product(s) and the main objective. It should distinguish between interventional and non-interventional studies and should be organised per active substance. The list should be comprehensive for all studies/programmes and should include ongoing studies/programmes as well as studies/programmes completed in the last two years and may be located in an Annex or provided separately.

II.B.4.4. PSMF Section on Computerised Systems and Databases

The location, functionality and operational responsibility for computerised systems and databases used to receive, collate, record and report safety information and an assessment of their fitness for purpose shall be described in the PSMF [IR Art 2(3)].

Where multiple computerised systems/databases are used, the applicability of these to pharmacovigilance activities should be described in such a way that a clear overview of the extent of computerisation within the pharmacovigilance system can be understood. The validation status of key aspects of computer system functionality should also be described; the change control, nature of testing, back-up procedures and electronic data repositories vital to pharmacovigilance compliance should be included in summary, and the nature of the documentation available described. For paper-based systems (where an electronic system may only be used for expedited submission of ICSRs), the management of the data, and mechanisms used to assure the integrity and accessibility of the safety data, and in particular the collation of information about adverse drug reactions, should be described.

II.B.4.5. PSMF Section on Pharmacovigilance Processes

An essential element of any pharmacovigilance system is that there are clear written procedures in place. GVP Module I describes the required minimum set of written procedures for pharmacovigilance. A description of the procedural documentation available (standard operating procedures, manuals, at a global and/or National level, etc.), the nature of the data held (e.g. the type of case data retained for ICSRs) and an indication of how records are held (e.g. safety database, paper file at site of receipt) should be provided in the PSMF.

A description of the process, data handling and records for the performance of pharmacovigilance, covering the following aspects shall be included in the PSMF:

- Continuous monitoring of product risk-benefit profile(s) applied and the result of evaluation and the decision making process for taking appropriate measures; this should include signal generation, detection and evaluation. This may also include several written procedures and instructions concerning safety database outputs, interactions with clinical departments, etc.
- Risk management system(s) and monitoring of the outcome of risk minimisation measures; several departments may be involved in this area and interactions should be defined in written procedures or agreements;
- ICSR collection, collation, follow-up, assessment and reporting; the procedures applied to this area should clarify what are local and what are global activities;
- PSUR scheduling, production and submission, if applicable (see GVP Module VII);
- Communication of safety concerns to consumers, healthcare professionals and the competent authorities;
- Implementation of safety variations to the summary of product characteristics (SmPC) and patient information leaflets; procedures should cover both internal and external communications [based on IR Art 2(4)].

In each area, the marketing authorisation holder should be able to provide evidence of a system that supports appropriate and timely decision making and action.

The description must be accompanied by the list of processes referred to in Article 11(1) of Commission Implementing Regulation (EU) No 520/2012 under the topic compliance management, as well as interfaces with other functions. Interfaces with other functions include, but are not limited to, the roles and responsibilities of the QPPV, responding to competent authority requests for information, literature searching, safety database change control, safety data exchange agreements, safety data archiving, pharmacovigilance auditing, quality control and training. The list, which may be located in the Annexes, should comprise the procedural document reference number, title, effective date and document type (for all standard operating procedures, work instructions, manuals, etc.). Procedures belonging to service providers and other third parties should be clearly identified. Documents relating to specific local/country procedures need not be listed, but a list may be requested on a per country basis. If no or only some countries use specific local procedures, this should be indicated (and the names of the applicable countries provided).

II.B.4.6. PSMF Section on Pharmacovigilance System Performance

The PSMF should contain evidence of the ongoing monitoring of performance of the pharmacovigilance system including compliance of the main outputs of pharmacovigilance. The PSMF should include a description of the monitoring methods applied and contain as a minimum:
- An explanation of how the correct reporting of ICSRs is assessed. In the annex, figures/graphs should be provided to show the timeliness of 15-day and 90-day reporting over the past year;
- A description of any metrics used to monitor the quality of submissions and performance of pharmacovigilance. This should include information provided by competent authorities regarding the quality of ICSR reporting, PSURs or other submissions;
- An overview of the timeliness of PSUR reporting to competent authorities in the EU (the annex should reflect the latest figures used by the marketing authorisation holder to assess compliance);
- An overview of the methods used to ensure timeliness of safety variation submissions compared to internal and competent authority deadlines, including the tracking of required safety variations that have been identified but not yet been submitted;
- Where applicable, an overview of adherence to risk management plan commitments, or other obligations or conditions of marketing authorisation(s) relevant to pharmacovigilance.

Targets for the performance of the pharmacovigilance system shall be described and explained. A list of performance indicators must be provided in the Annex to the PSMF [IR Art 3(6) and Art 9], alongside the results of (actual) performance measurements.

II.B.4.7. PSMF Section on Quality System

A description of the quality management system should be provided, in terms of the structure of the organisation and the application of the quality to pharmacovigilance. This shall include:

Document and record control: A description of the archiving arrangements for electronic and/or hardcopy versions of the PSMF should be provided, as well as an overview of the procedures applied to other quality system and pharmacovigilance records and documents (*see* also GVP Module I).

Procedural documents:
- A general description of the types of documents used in pharmacovigilance (standards, operating procedures, work instructions, etc.), the applicability of the various documents at global, regional or local level within the organisation, and the controls that are applied to their accessibility, implementation and maintenance.
- Information about the documentation systems applied to relevant procedural documents under the control of third parties.

A list of specific procedures and processes related to the pharmacovigilance activities and interfaces with other functions, with details of how the procedures can be accessed must be provided [IR Art 2(5)(a)] and the detailed guidance for the inclusion of these is in section II.B.4.5.

Training:
- A description of the resource management for the performance of pharmacovigilance activities:
  – The organisational chart giving the number of people (full time equivalents) involved in pharmacovigilance activities, which may be provided in the section describing the organisational structure (*see* II.B.4.3.)
- Information about sites where the personnel are located (this is described under sections II.B.4.2. and II.B.4.3.);
- Whereby the sites are provided in the PSMF in relation to the organisation of specific pharmacovigilance activities and in the Annexes which provide the list of site contacts for sources of safety data. However, a description should be provided in order to explain the training organisation in relation to the personnel and site information;
- A summary description of the training concept, including a reference to the location training files.

Staff should be appropriately trained for performing pharmacovigilance related activities and this includes not only staff within pharmacovigilance departments but also any individual that may receive safety reports.

Auditing: Information about quality assurance auditing of the pharmacovigilance system should be included in the PSMF. A description of the approach used to plan audits of the pharmacovigilance system and the reporting mechanism and timelines should be provided, with a current list of the scheduled and completed audits concerning the pharmacovigilance system maintained in the annex referred to II.B.4.8. [IR Art 3(5)]. This list should describe the date(s) (of conduct and of report), scope and completion status of audits of service providers, specific pharmacovigilance activities or sites undertaking pharmacovigilance and their operational interfaces relevant to the fulfilment of the obligations in the Directive 2001/83/EC, and cover a rolling 5 year period.

The PSMF shall also contain a note associated with any audit where significant findings are raised. This means that the presence of findings that fulfil the EU criteria for major or critical findings must be indicated (*see* GVP Module IV). The audit report must be documented within the quality system; in the PSMF it is sufficient to provide a brief description of the corrective and/or preventative action(s) associated with the significant finding, the date it was identified and the anticipated resolution date(s), with cross reference to the audit report and the documented corrective and preventative action plan(s). In case corrective and preventative action plan(s) have not yet been agreed for a particular audit or finding, the PSMF should include the note required and stating that "corrective and preventative action plan(s) are to be agreed". In the annex, in the list of audits conducted, those associated with unresolved notes in the PSMF, should be identified. The note and associated corrective and preventative action(s), shall be documented in the PSMF until the corrective and/or preventative action(s) have been fully implemented, that is, the note is only removed once corrective action and/or sufficient improvement can be demonstrated or has been independently verified [DIR Art 104(2)]. The addition, amendment or removal of the notes must therefore be recorded in the logbook.

As a means of managing the pharmacovigilance system, and providing a basis for audit or inspection, the PSMF should also describe the process for recording, managing and resolving deviations from the quality system. The master file shall also document deviations from pharmacovigilance procedures, their impact and management until resolved [IR Art 4(3)]. This may be documented in the form of a list referencing a deviation report, and its date and procedure concerned.

II.B.4.8. Annex to the PSMF

An annex to the PSMF shall contain the following documents:
- A list of medicinal products covered by the PSMF including the name of the medicinal product, the international non-proprietary name of the active substance(s), and te Member State(s) in which the authorisation is valid [IR Art 3];

The list of medicinal products authorised in the EU should also include the authorisation number(s) including, per authorisation:
- The type of procedure for authorisation and procedure number (e.g. centrally authorised, nationally authorised products, including those authorised through the mutual recognition or the decentralised procedure);
- The Rapporteur country or Reference Member State;
- The presence on the market in the EU [DIR Art 23(a), REG Art 13(4)];
- Other (non EU) territories where the product is authorised or on the market.

The list should be organised per active substance and, where applicable, should indicate what type of product specific safety monitoring requirements exist (for example, risk minimisation measures contained in the risk management plan or laid down as conditions of the marketing authorisation, non-standard PSUR periodicity, referral under Article 31 of Directive 2001/83/EC, or included in the list described in Article 23 of Regulation (EC) No 726/2004). The monitoring information may be provided as a secondary list.

For marketing authorisations that are included in a different pharmacovigilance system, for example, because the MAH has more than one pharmacovigilance system or

Annexure 8: Guidelines on Good Pharmacovigilance Practices (GVP)

third party agreements exist to delegate the system, reference to the additional PSMF(s) should also be provided as a separate list in the Annexes, such that, for a MAH, the entire product portfolio can be related to the set of PSMFs.

Where pharmacovigilance systems are shared, all products that utilise the pharmacovigilance system should be included, so that the entire list of products covered by the file is available. The products lists may be presented separately, organised per MAH. Alternatively, a single list may be used, which is supplemented with the name of the MAH(s) for each product, or a separate note can be included to describe the product(s) and the MAH(s) covered;

- A list of written policies and procedures for the purpose of complying with Article 11(1) of Commission Implementing Regulation (EU) 520/2012 [IR Art 3(2)];
- A list of contractual agreements covering delegated activities including the medicinal products and territory(ies) concerned in accordance with Article 6(2) of Commission Implementing Regulation (EU) No 520/2012 (see II.B.4.3.) [IR Art 3(3)];
- A list of tasks that have been delegated by the qualified person for pharmacovigilance [IR Art 3(4)];
- A list of all completed audits, for a period of five years, and a list of audit schedules [IR Art 3(5)];
- Where applicable, a list of performance indicators in accordance with Article 9 of Commission Implementing Regulation (EU) No 520/2012 [IR Art 3(6)];
- Where applicable, a list of other PSMFs held by the same marketing authorisation holder [IR Art 3(7)];

This list should include the PSMF number(s), and the name of MAH of the QPPV responsible for the pharmacovigilance system used. If the pharmacovigilance system is managed by another party that is not a marketing authorisation holder, the name of the service provider should also be included.

- A logbook in accordance with Article 5(4) of Commission Implementing Regulation (EU) No 520/2012 [IR Art 3(8)]. Other change control documentation should be included as appropriate. Documented changes shall include at least the date, person responsible for the change and the nature of the change [IR Art 5(4)].

II.B.5 Change Control, Logbook, Versions and Archiving

It is necessary for marketing authorisation holders to implement change control systems and to have robust processes in place to continuously be informed of relevant changes in order to maintain the PSMF accordingly. The competent authorities may solicit information about important changes to the pharmacovigilance system, such as, but not limited to:

- Changes to the pharmacovigilance safety database(s), which could include a change in the database itself or associated databases, the validation status of the database as well as information about transferred or migrated data;
- Changes in the provision of significant services for pharmacovigilance, especially major contractual arrangements concerning the reporting of safety data;
- Organisational changes, such as takeovers, mergers, the sites at which pharmacovigilance is conducted or the delegation/transfer of PSMF management.

In addition to these changes being documented in the PSMF for the purpose of change control (in the logbook), the QPPV should always been kept informed of these changes.

Changes to the PSMF should be recorded, such that a history of changes is available (specifying the date and the nature of the change), changes to the PSMF must be recorded in the logbook described in Article 5(4) of Commission Implementing Regulation No 520/2012. Descriptive changes to the content of the master file must be recorded in the logbook.

Change history for the information contained in the Annexes may be 'on demand', in which case the logbook would indicate the date of the revision of PSMF content and/or Annex update(s), the history of changes for Annex content would also be updated. Information that is being regularly updated and is contained in the Annexes, such as product and standard operating procedure lists or compliance figures, may include outputs from controlled systems (such as electronic document management systems or regulatory databases). The superseded versions of such content may be managed outside of the PSMF content itself, provided that the history of changes is maintained and available to competent authorities and the agency on request. If the PSMF has not been requested, or has remained unchanged for a period of time (for example, if the changes in the content of Annexes are managed outside of the PSMF), it is recommended that a review is conducted periodically. Marketing authorisations holders need to ensure that the obligations concerning the timely provision of the PSMF can be met. It is also noted that the QPPV must be able to gain access to current and accurate information about the pharmacovigilance system, hence permanent access to the PSMF must be enabled, including the information contained in the Annexes (either via the pharmacovigilance master file itself or via access to the systems used to generate the Annex content).

Marketing authorisation holders should be able to justify their approach and have document control procedures in place to govern the maintenance of the PSMF. As a basis for audit and inspections, the PSMF provides a description of the pharmacovigilance system at the current time, but the functioning and scope of the pharmacovigilance system in the past may need to be understood.

Changes to the PSMF should also account for shared pharmacovigilance systems and delegated activities. A record of the date and nature of notifications of the changes made available to the competent authorities, the QPPV and relevant third parties should be kept in order to ensure that change control is fully implemented.

The PSMF should be retained in a manner that ensures its legibility and accessibility [IR Art 5 and Art 7].

II.B.6. Pharmacovigilance System Master File Presentation

The PSMF shall be continuously accessible to the QPPV [IR Art 7(2)] and to the competent authorities on request [REG Art 16(3a), DIR Art 23(4), IR Art 7]. The information shall be succinct, accurate and reflect the current system in place, which means that whatever format is used, it must be possible to keep the information up to date and, when necessary, to revise to take account of experience gained, technical and scientific progress and amendments to the legislative requirements [IR Art 4(1)]. Although provision of the document within 7 days of request by a competent authority is stated in Article 23(4) of Directive 2001/83/EC, marketing authorisation holders should be aware that immediate access to the PSMF may also be required by the competent authorities, at the stated PSMF location or QPPV site (if different).

II.B.6.1. Format and Layout

The PSMF may be in electronic form on condition that a clearly arranged printed copy can be made available to competent authorities if requested [IR Art 5(3)]. In any format, the PSMF should be legible, complete, provided in a manner that ensures all documentation is accessible and allow full traceability of changes. Therefore, it may be appropriate to restrict access to the PSMF in order to ensure appropriate control over the content and to assign specific responsibilities for the management of PSMF in terms of change control and archiving.

The PSMF should be written in English (unless the marketing authorisation holder only holds approvals in one Member State when it can be written in the EU official language for that territory), indexed in a manner consistent with the headings described in this Module [IR Art 5(2)], and allow easy navigation to the contents. In general, embedded documents are discouraged. The use of electronic book-marking and searchable text is recommended. Documents such as copies of signed statements or agreements should be included as appendices and described in the index.

The documents and particulars of the PSMF shall be presented with the following headings and, if hardcopy, in the order outlined:

Cover page to include:
- The unique number assigned by the EV System to the PSMF when the XEVPRM is processed in the XEVMPD (Article 57 database).
- The name of the MAH, the MAH of the QPPV responsible for the pharmacovigilance system described (if different), as well as the relevant QPPV third party company name (if applicable).
- The name of other concerned MAH(s) (sharing the pharmacovigilance system).

- The list of PSMFs for the MAH (concerning products with a different pharmacovigilance system).

The date of preparation/last update. The headings used in II.B.4. should be used for the main content of the PSMF. The minimum required content of the Annexes is outlined in II.B.4.8., and additional information may be included in the Annexes, provided that the requirements for the content of the main sections (II.B.1.-7.) are also met. The positioning of content in the Annexes is further outlined; the bulleted points are descriptions of possible content (and not required headings):

- The qualified person responsible for pharmacovigilance, Annex A
  - The list of tasks that have been delegated by the QPPV, or the applicable procedural document
  - The curriculum vitae of the QPPV and associated documents
  - Contact details supplementary to those contained in Article 57 database, if appropriate
- The Organisational Structure of the MAH, Annex B
  - The lists of contracts and agreements
- Sources of safety data, Annex C
  - Lists associated with the description of sources of safety data, e.g. affiliates and third party contacts
- Computerised systems and Databases, Annex D
- Pharmacovigilance Process, and written procedures, Annex E
  - Lists of procedural documents
- Pharmacovigilance System Performance, Annex F
  - Lists of performance indicators
  - Current results of performance assessment in relation to the indicators
- Quality System, Annex G
  - Audit schedules
  - List of audits conducted and completed
- Products, Annex H
  - List(s) of products covered by the pharmacovigilance system
  - Any notes concerning the MAH per product
- Document and Record Control, Annex I
  - Logbook
  - Documentation of history of changes for Annex contents, indexed according to the Annexes A-H and their content if not provided within the relevant annex itself.

Documentation to support notifications and signatures concerning the PSMF, as required. Where there is no content for an Annex, there is no need to provide blank content pages with headings, however, the Annexes that are provided should still be named according to the format described. For example, Annex E should not be renamed to Annex D in circumstances where no Annex concerning computerised systems and databases is used, Annex D should simply be described as 'unused' in the indexing, in order that recipients of the PSMF are assured that missing content is intended.

II.C. OPERATION OF THE EU NETWORK

II.C.1. Responsibilities

II.C.1.1. Marketing Authorisation Holders and Applicants

Marketing authorisation holders shall have a pharmacovigilance system in place to ensure the monitoring and supervision of one or more medicinal products. They are also responsible for introducing and maintaining a PSMF that records the pharmacovigilance system in place with regard to one or more authorised products [DIR Art 23(4), Art 104(3)(b), REG Art 16(3a)]. In accordance with Articles 8(3)(ia) and 104(3) of Directive 2001/83/EC a single QPPV shall be appointed to be responsible for the establishment and maintenance of the pharmacovigilance system described in the PSMF.

Applicants are required, at the time of initial marketing authorisation application, to have in place a summary of the pharmacovigilance system that records the system that will be in place and functioning at the time of granting of the marketing authorisation and placing of the product on the market. During the evaluation of a marketing authorisation application the applicant may be requested to provide a copy of the PSMF for review.

The applicant/marketing authorisation holder is responsible for establishing the PSMF in an EU country (at any marketing authorisation holder or contractual partner site including the site of a contractor or marketing partner) and for registering the master file location with the competent authorities in the marketing authorisation application (as applicable) and in the Article 57 database. The PSMF shall describe the pharmacovigilance system in place at the current time. Information about elements of the system to be implemented in future may be included, but these should be clearly described as planned rather than established or current.

The PSMF creation, maintenance in a current and accessible state (permanently available for audit and inspection purposes) and provision to competent authorities can be outsourced to a third party, but the marketing authorisation holder retains ultimate responsibility for compliance with the legal requirements.

Marketing authorisation holders are responsible for notifying the Agency immediately of any change in the QPPV details and the PSMF location details. The Agency shall update accordingly the EudraVigilance database referred to in Article 24(1) of Regulation (EC) No 726/2004 and, where necessary, the European medicines web-portal referred to in Article 26(1) of Regulation (EC) No 726/2004 [IR Art 4(4)].

II.C.1.2. National Competent Authorities

The national competent authorities are obliged to supervise the pharmacovigilance systems of marketing authorisation holders [Recital 7 of Directive 2010/84/EU]. As part of this requirement, they will review the summary information about the pharmacovigilance system included in the marketing authorisation application. The full PSMF may be requested at any time, for example, to review the summary of the pharmacovigilance system of an applicant that has not previously held a marketing authorisation in the EU or where specific concerns about the pharmacovigilance system and/or the product safety profile exist, and in preparation for an inspection (*see* GVP Module III). Information concerning changes to the summary information or content of the PSMF will also be used to inform inspection planning and conduct.

For centrally authorised products, the Member State where the master file is located will become the supervisory authority [Recital 22 of Regulation (EU) No 1235/2010, REG Art 18(3)]. For pharmacovigilance systems that include centrally authorised products, as well as nationally authorised products, including those authorised through the mutual recognition or the decentralised procedure, national competent authorities will supervise the pharmacovigilance system in co-operation with the supervisory authority and the Agency. For pharmacovigilance systems that do not include centrally authorised products, individual national competent authorities remain responsible for supervision of the pharmacovigilance system and will work together to minimise duplication of effort.

National competent authorities will share information about pharmacovigilance systems and use the information to inform national risk-based inspection programmes. Inspectors from national competent authorities will report non-compliance with the requirements of legislation and guidance, including both non-compliance with the requirements for the PSMF and the pharmacovigilance system (*see* GVP Module III).

II.C.1.3. The European Medicines Agency

For centrally authorised products, the Agency co-ordinates the inspections of marketing authorisation holders or their service providers. Supervision of the pharmacovigilance system is based on the location of the PSMF, with the Member State where the master file is held becoming the supervisory authority [REG Art 18(3)]. The Agency may request the PSMF in order to fulfil its co-ordination role.

The main responsibility of the Agency, in relation to PSMFs, is the maintenance of EU wide databases, dissemination of information and coordination of EU wide activities. To this effect, the Agency, in collaboration with the Member States and the European Commission, is responsible for the set up and maintenance of the European medicines web-portal for the dissemination of information on medicinal products authorised in the EU [REG Art 26]. The Agency will manage the product list described in Article 57 of Regulation (EC) No 726/2004 which provides a practical mechanism for maintaining up-to-date information about the location of the PSMF, the QPPV contact information and the products relevant to the pharmacovigilance system described in the PSMF. The list of the locations in the EU where PSMFs are kept will be made public via the web-portal [REG Art 26(1)(e)].

II.C.2. Accessibility of the Pharmacovigilance System Master File

The PSMF shall be kept up to date and be permanently available to the QPPV [IR Art 4(1) and Art 7(2)]. It shall also be permanently available for inspection, at the site where it is kept [IR Art 7(3)] (the stated location), irrespective of whether the inspection has been notified in advance or is unannounced.

According to Article 104(3)(b) of Directive 2001/83/EC the marketing authorisation holder shall maintain and make available on request a copy of the PSMF. The marketing authorisation holder must submit the copy 7 days at the latest after receipt of the request from a national competent authority or the Agency. The PSMF should be submitted in a readable electronic format or clearly arranged printed copy.

In the situation where the same PSMF is used by more than one marketing authorisation holder (where a common pharmacovigilance system is used) the concerned PSMF should be accessible to each, as any of the applicable marketing authorisation holders shall be able to provide the file to the competent authorities within 7 days, upon request [DIR Art 23(4), IR Art 7(4)].

The PSMF should not routinely be requested during the assessment of new marketing authorisation applications (i.e. pre-authorisation), but may be requested on an ad hoc basis, particularly if a new pharmacovigilance system is being implemented, or if product specific safety concerns or issues with compliance with pharmacovigilance requirements have been identified.

II.C.3. Transparency

Information on the PSMF location should be made available to the public via the European medicines web-portal [REG Art 26(1)(e)] for transparency and communication purposes.

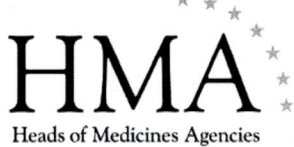
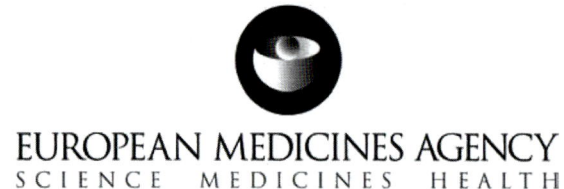

8 September 2014
EMA/119871/2012 Rev 1*

GUIDELINE ON GOOD PHARMACOVIGILANCE PRACTICES (GVP)

Module III Pharmacovigilance Inspections (Rev 1)

Draft finalised by the Agency in collaboration with Member States and submitted to ERMS FG	25 May 2012
Draft agreed by ERMS FG	30 May 2012
Draft adopted by Executive Director	22 June 2012
Start of public consultation	27 June 2012
End of consultation (deadline for comments)	24 August 2012
Revised draft in collaboration with Member States	23 November 2012
Revised draft agreed by ERMS FG	6 December 2012
Revised draft adopted by Executive Director as final	12 December 2012
Date for coming into effect	13 December 2012
Draft Revision 1* adopted by Executive Director as final	8 September 2014
Date for coming into effect of Revision 1	16 September 2014

***Note:** Revision 1 contains the following:
- Reference to the new Union procedures for pharmacovigilance inspections in III.B.5.

III.A. INTRODUCTION

This Module contains guidance on the planning, conduct, reporting and follow-up of pharmacovigilance inspections in the EU and outlines the role of the different parties involved. General guidance is provided under III.B., while III.C. covers the overall operation of pharmacovigilance inspections in the EU.

In order to determine that marketing authorisation holders comply with pharmacovigilance obligations established within the EU, and to facilitate compliance, competent authorities of the Member States concerned shall conduct, in cooperation with the Agency, pharmacovigilance inspections of marketing authorisation holders or any firms employed to fulfil marketing authorisation holder's pharmacovigilance obligations. Such inspections shall be carried out by inspectors appointed by the national competent authorities and empowered to inspect the premises, records, documents and pharmacovigilance system master file (PSMF) of the marketing authorisation holder or any firms employed by the marketing authorisation holder to perform the activities described in Title IX of Directive 2001/83/EC in accordance with Articles 111(1) and 111(1)(d) (Directive is referenced as DIR). In particular, marketing authorisation holders are required to provide, on request, the pharmacovigilance system master file, which will be used to inform inspection conduct [DIR Art 23(4) and Regulation (EC) No 726/2004 Article 16(4) (Regulation is referenced as REG) (*see* Module II).

The objectives of pharmacovigilance inspections are:
- To determine that the marketing authorisation holder has personnel, systems and facilities in place to meet their pharmacovigilance obligations;
- To identify, record and address non-compliance which may pose a risk to public health;
- To use the inspection results as a basis for enforcement action, where considered necessary.

For marketing authorisation holders of centrally authorised products, it is the responsibility of the supervisory authority for pharmacovigilance to verify, on behalf of the EU, that the marketing authorisation holder for the medicinal product satisfies the pharmacovigilance requirements laid down in Directive 2001/83/EC [REG Art 19]. The supervisory authority for pharmacovigilance shall be the competent authority of the Member State in which the pharmacovigilance system master file is located [REG Art 18(3)]. According to Article 7(1) of the Commission Implementation Regulation (EU) No 520/2012 (Implementing Regulation is referenced as IR) the pharmacovigilance system master file shall be located either at the site in the Union where the main pharmacovigilance activities of the marketing authorisation holder are performed or at the site in the Union where the qualified person responsible for pharmacovigilance operates. The supervisory authority may conduct pre-authorisation inspections to verify the accuracy and successful implementation of the existing or proposed pharmacovigilance system [REG Art 18(3)].

For marketing authorisation holders of non-centrally authorised products (i.e. nationally authorised products, including those authorised through the mutual recognition or the decentralised procedure), it is the responsibility of the competent authority of the Member State concerned, in cooperation with the Agency, to ensure by means of inspection that the legal requirements governing medicinal products are complied with. This cooperation shall consist of the sharing of information between national competent authorities and the Agency concerning inspections that are planned and those that have been conducted [DIR Art 111(1)].

Pharmacovigilance inspection programmes will be implemented, which will include routine inspections scheduled according to a risk-based approach and will also incorporate "for cause" inspections, which have been triggered to examine suspected non-compliance or potential risks, usually with impact on a specific product(s).

There shall be cooperation between national competent authorities and the Agency to minimise duplication and maximise the use of available resources. National competent authorities and the Agency will make use of the shared information on planned and conducted inspections to facilitate this and to adapt the scope and/or timing of their inspections.

The results of an inspection will be provided to the inspected entity [DIR Art 111(3) and 111(8)], who will be given the opportunity to comment on any non-compliance identified [DIR Art 111(8)]. Any non-compliance should also be rectified by the marketing authorisation holder in a timely manner through the implementation of a corrective and preventive action plan.

If the outcome of the inspection is that the marketing authorisation holder does not comply with the pharmacovigilance obligations, the Member State concerned shall inform the other Member States, the Agency and the Commission in accordance with section III.C.1 [DIR Art 111(8)].

Sharing of information and communication between inspectors and assessors from the Pharmacovigilance Risk Assessment Committee (PRAC) and from the Committee for Medicinal Products for Human Use (CHMP), is very important in relation to issues of Union interest and, where considered appropriate, for the proper follow-up of inspections and the provision of recommendations on actions to be taken.

Where appropriate, the Member State concerned shall take the necessary measures to ensure that a marketing authorisation holder is subject to effective, proportionate and dissuasive penalties [DIR Art 111(8)]. Regulation (EC) No 658/2007 also empowers the Commission to impose financial penalties on marketing authorisations holders to ensure the enforcement of certain obligations connected with marketing authorisations for medicinal products granted in accordance with Regulation (EC) No 726/2004.

Information on the conduct and outcome of pharmacovigilance inspections and the follow-up and evaluation of the consequences may be made publicly available as part of the overall transparency of pharmacovigilance activities.

III.B. STRUCTURES AND PROCESSES

III.B.1. Inspection Types

III.B.1.1. System and Product-related Inspections

Pharmacovigilance system inspections are designed to review the procedures, systems, personnel, and facilities in place and determine their compliance with regulatory pharmacovigilance obligations. As part of this review, product specific examples may be used to demonstrate the operation of the pharmacovigilance system.

Product-related pharmacovigilance inspections are primarily focused on product-related pharmacovigilance issues, including product-specific activities and documentation, rather than a general system review. Some aspects of the general system may still be examined as part of a product-related inspection (e.g. the system used for that product).

III.B.1.2. Routine and "for cause" Pharmacovigilance Inspections

Routine pharmacovigilance inspections are inspections scheduled in advance as part of inspection programmes. There is no specific trigger to initiate these inspections, although a risk-based approach to optimize supervisory activities should be implemented. These inspections are usually system inspections but one or more specific products may be selected as examples to verify the implementation of the system and to provide practical evidence of its functioning and compliance. Particular concerns, e.g. raised by assessors, may also be included in the scope of a routine inspection, in order to investigate the specific issues.

For cause pharmacovigilance inspections are undertaken when a trigger is recognised, and an inspection is considered an appropriate way to examine the issues. For cause inspections are more likely to focus on specific pharmacovigilance processes or to include an examination of identified compliance issues and their impact for a specific product. However, full system inspections may also be performed resulting from a trigger. For cause inspections may arise when, for example, one or more of the triggers listed below are identified:

- Risk-benefit balance of the product:
  - Change in the risk-benefit balance where further examination through an inspection is considered appropriate;
  - Delays or failure to identify or communicate a risk or a change in the risk-benefit balance;
  - Communication of information on pharmacovigilance concerns to the general public without giving prior or simultaneous notification to the national competent authorities or Agency, as applicable;
  - Non-compliance or product safety issues identified during the monitoring

of pharmacovigilance activities by the national competent authorities and/or the Agency;
- Suspension or product withdrawal with no advance notice to the competent authorities;
- Reporting obligations (expedited and periodic):
  - Delays or omissions in reporting;
  - Poor quality or incomplete reports;
  - Inconsistencies between reports and other information sources;
- Requests from competent authorities:
  - Failure to provide the requested information or data within the deadline specified by the competent authorities;
  - Poor quality or inadequate provision of data to fulfil requests for information from the competent authorities;
- Fulfilment of commitments:
  - Concerns about the status or fulfilment of risk management plan (RMP) commitments;
  - Delays or failure to carry out specific obligations relating to the monitoring of product safety, identified at the time of the marketing authorisation;
  - Poor quality of reports requested as specific obligations;
- Inspections:
  - Delays in the implementation or inappropriate implementation of corrective and preventive actions;
  - Information such as non-compliance or product safety issues from other types of inspections (GCP, GMP, GLP and GDP);
  - Inspection information received from other authorities (EU or non-EU), which may highlight issues of non-compliance;
- Others:
  - Concerns following review of the pharmacovigilance system master file;
  - Non-inspection related information received from other authorities, which may highlight issues of non-compliance;
  - Other sources of information or complaints.

III.B.1.3. Pre-authorisation Inspections

Pre-authorisation pharmacovigilance inspections are inspections performed before a marketing authorisation is granted. These inspections are conducted with the intent of examining the existing or proposed pharmacovigilance system as it has been described by the applicant in support of the marketing authorisation application [REG Art 19]. Pre-authorisation inspections are not mandatory, but may be requested in specific circumstances. Principles and procedures for requesting pre-authorisation inspections should be developed to avoid performing unnecessary inspections which may delay the granting of a marketing authorisation. The following aspects shall be considered during the validation phase and/or early during the assessment phase:
- The applicant has not previously operated a pharmacovigilance system within the EU or is in the process of establishing a new pharmacovigilance system;
- Previous information (e.g. inspection history and non-compliance notifications or information from other authorities) indicates that the applicant has a poor history or culture of compliance. If the marketing authorisation holder has a history of serious and/or persistent pharmacovigilance non-compliance, a pre-authorisation pharmacovigilance inspection may be one mechanism to confirm that improvements have been made to the system before a new authorisation is granted;
- Due to product-specific safety concerns, it may be considered appropriate to examine the applicant's ability:
  - To implement product specific risk-minimisation activities; or
  - To meet specific safety conditions which may be imposed; or
  - To manage routine pharmacovigilance for the product of concern (e.g. anticipated significant increase in adverse reaction reports when compared to previous products).

In most cases, a risk assessment based on a combination of product-specific and system-related issues should be performed before a pre-authorisation pharmacovigilance inspection is requested.

If the outcome of the pre-authorisation inspection raises concerns about the applicant's ability to comply with the requirements laid down in the Regulation and the Directive, the following recommendations may be considered:
- Non-approval of the marketing authorisation;

- A re-inspection prior to approval of the marketing authorisation to confirm that critical findings and recommendations have been addressed;
- Granting of the marketing authorisation with the recommendation to perform an early post-authorisation pharmacovigilance inspection. In this case, the findings would influence the timing of an inspection conducted as part of the EU routine programme of pharmacovigilance inspections (*see* III.B.2.);
- Imposition of safety conditions to the marketing authorisation based on DIR Art 21a and REG Art 14.8.

III.B.1.4. Post-authorisation Inspections

Post-authorisation pharmacovigilance inspections are inspections performed after a marketing authorisation is granted and are intended to examine whether the marketing authorisation holder complies with its pharmacovigilance obligations. They can be any of the types mentioned under III.B.1.1 and III.B.1.2.

III.B.1.5. Announced and Unannounced Inspections

It is anticipated that the majority of inspections will be announced i.e. notified in advance to the inspected party, to ensure the availability of relevant individuals for the inspection. However, on occasion, it may be appropriate to conduct unannounced inspections or to announce an inspection at short notice (e.g. when the announcement could compromise the objectives of the inspection or when the inspection is conducted in a short timeframe due to urgent safety reasons).

III.B.1.6. Re-inspections

A re-inspection may be conducted on a routine basis as part of a routine inspection programme. Risk factors will be assessed in order to prioritise re-inspections. Early re-inspection may take place where significant non-compliance has been identified and where it is necessary to verify actions taken to address findings and to evaluate ongoing compliance with the obligations, including evaluation of changes in the pharmacovigilance system. Early re-inspection may also be appropriate when it is known from a previous inspection that the inspected party had failed to implement appropriately corrective and preventive actions in response to an earlier inspection.

III.B.1.7. Remote Inspections

These are pharmacovigilance inspections performed by inspectors remote from the premises of the marketing authorisation holder or firms employed by the marketing authorisation holder. Communication mechanisms such as the internet or telephone may be used in the conduct of the inspection. For example, in cases where key sites for pharmacovigilance activities are located outside the EU or a third party service provider is not available at the actual inspection site, but it is feasible to arrange interviews of relevant staff and review of documentation, including the safety database, source documents and pharmacovigilance system master file, via remote access. This approach may also be taken where there are logistical challenges to an on-site inspection during exceptional circumstances (e.g. a pandemic outbreak or travel restrictions). Such approaches are taken at the discretion of the inspectors and in agreement with the body commissioning the inspection. The logistical aspects of the remote inspection should be considered following liaison with the marketing authorisation holder. Where feasible, a remote inspection may lead to a visit to the inspection site if it is considered that the remote inspection has revealed issues which require on-site inspection or if the objectives of the inspection could not be met by remote inspection.

III.B.2. Inspection Planning

Pharmacovigilance inspection planning should be based on a systematic and risk-based approach to make the best use of surveillance and enforcement resources whilst maintaining a high level of public health protection. A risk-based approach to inspection planning will enable the frequency, scope and breadth of inspections to be determined accordingly.

In order to ensure that inspection resources are used in an efficient way, the scheduling and conduct of inspections will be driven by the preparation of inspection programmes. Sharing of information and communication between inspectors and assessors is important to ensure successful prioritisation and targeting of these inspections.

Factors which may be taken into consideration, as appropriate, by the competent authorities when establishing pharmacovigilance inspection programmes include, but are not limited to:
- Inspection related:
  - Compliance history identified during previous pharmacovigilance inspections or other types of inspections (GCP, GMP, GLP and GDP);
  - Re-inspection date recommended by the inspectors or assessors as a result of a previous inspection;
- Product related:
  - Product with additional pharmacovigilance activities or risk-minimisation activities;
  - Authorisation with conditions associated with safety, e.g. requirement for post-authorisation safety studies (PASS) or designation for additional monitoring;
  - Product(s) with large sales volume, i.e. products associated with large patient exposure in the EU;
  - Product(s) with limited alternative in the market place;
- Marketing authorisation holder related:
  - Marketing authorisation holder that has never been subject to a pharmacovigilance inspection;
  - Marketing authorisation holder with many products on the market in the EU;
  - Resources available to the marketing authorisation holder for the pharmacovigilance activities they undertake;
  - Marketing authorisation holder with no previous marketing authorisations in the EU;
  - Negative information and/or safety concerns raised by competent authorities, other bodies outside the EU or other areas (i.e. GCP, GMP, GLP and GDP);
  - Changes in the marketing authorisation holder organisation, such as mergers and acquisitions;
- Pharmacovigilance system related:
  - Marketing authorisation holder with sub-contracted pharmacovigilance activities (function of the qualified person responsible for pharmacovigilance in the EU (QPPV), reporting of safety data, etc.) and/or multiple firms employed to perform pharmacovigilance activities;
  - Change of QPPV since the last inspection;
  - Changes to the pharmacovigilance safety database(s), which could include a change in the database itself or associated databases, the validation status of the database as well as information about transferred or migrated data;
  - Changes in contractual arrangements with pharmacovigilance service providers or the sites at which pharmacovigilance is conducted;
  - Delegation or transfer of pharmacovigilance system master file management.

National competent authorities and the Agency may solicit information from marketing authorisation holders for risk-based inspection planning purposes if it is not readily available elsewhere.

III.B.3. Sites to be Inspected

Any party carrying out pharmacovigilance activities in whole or in part, on behalf of, or in conjunction with the marketing authorisation holder may be inspected, in order to confirm their capability to support the marketing authorisation holder's compliance with pharmacovigilance obligations.

The sites to be inspected may be located in the EU (e.g. EU QPPV site) or outside the EU. Inspections of sites outside the EU might be appropriate where the main pharmacovigilance centre, databases and/or activities are located outside the EU and it would be otherwise inefficient or impossible to confirm compliance from a site within the EU. Member States and the Agency shall cooperate in the coordination of inspections in third countries [DIR Art 111(1)].

The type and number of sites to be inspected should be selected appropriately to ensure that the key objectives within the scope of the inspection are met.

III.B.4. Inspection Scope

The inspection scope will depend on the objectives of the inspection as well as the coverage of any previous inspections by competent authorities of Member States and whether it is a system or product-related inspection (a description of the types of inspection, inspection triggers and points to consider for the different types of inspection is provided in III.B.1.).

The following elements should be considered when preparing the scope of the inspection, as applicable:
- Information supplied in the pharmacovigilance system master file;
- Information concerning the functioning of the pharmacovigilance system, e.g. compliance data available from the Agency such as EudraVigilance reporting and data quality audits;
- Specific triggers (see III.B.1.2. for examples of triggers);

It may be appropriate for additional data to be requested in advance of an inspection in order to select appropriate sites or clarify aspects of the pharmacovigilance system.

III.B.4.1. Routine Pharmacovigilance Inspections

Routine pharmacovigilance inspections conducted on behalf of the EU should examine compliance with EU legislation and guidance, and the scope of such inspections should include the following elements, as appropriate:
- Individual case safety reports (ICSRs):
  - Collecting, receiving and exchanging reports - from all types of sources, sites and departments within the pharmacovigilance system, including from those firms employed to fulfil marketing authorisation holder's pharmacovigilance obligations and departments other than drug safety;
  - Assessment, including mechanisms for obtaining and recording reporter assessments, company application of event terms, seriousness, expectedness and causality. In addition to examples of ICSRs from within the EU, examples of ICSRs reported from outside the EU should be examined as part of this review (if applicable);
  - Follow-up and outcome recording, for example final outcome of cases of exposure in pregnancy and medical confirmation of consumer reported events;
  - Reporting according to the requirements for various types of reported ICSRs, including onward reporting to the relevant bodies and timeliness of such reporting;
  - Record keeping and archiving for ICSRs;
- Periodic safety update reports (PSURs), (as applicable):
  - Completeness and accuracy of the data included, appropriateness of decisions concerning data that are not included;
  - Addressing safety topics, providing relevant analyses and actions;
  - Formatting according to requirements;
  - Timeliness of submissions;
- Ongoing safety evaluation;
  - Use of all relevant sources of information for signal detection;
  - Appropriately applied methodology concerning analysis;
  - Appropriateness of investigations and follow-up actions, e.g. the implementation of recommendations following data review;
  - Implementation of the RMP, or other commitments, e.g. conditions of marketing authorisation;
  - Timely identification and provision of complete and accurate data to the competent authority(ies), in particular in response to specific requests for data;
  - Implementation of approved changes to safety communications and product information, including internal distribution and external publication;
- Interventional (where appropriate) and non-interventional clinical trials:
  - Reporting suspected unexpected serious adverse reactions (SUSARs) according to Directive 2001/20/EC and non-interventional study cases according to Directive 2001/83/EC;
  - Receiving, recording and assessing cases from interventional and non-interventional trials (see ICSRs);
  - Submission of study results and relevant safety information (e.g. development safety update reports (DSURs) and information included in PSURs), where applicable, PASS or post-authorisation efficacy studies (PAES) submissions, particularly when associated with specific obligations or RMP commitments;

- Appropriate selection of reference safety information, maintenance of investigator brochures and patient information with respect to safety;
- The inclusion of study data in ongoing safety evaluation;
• Pharmacovigilance system:
  - QPPV roles and responsibilities, e.g. access to the quality system, the pharmacovigilance system master file, performance metrics, audit and inspection reports, and their ability to take action to improve compliance;
  - The roles and responsibilities of the marketing authorisation holder in relation to the pharmacovigilance system;
  - Accuracy, completeness and maintenance of the pharmacovigilance system master file;
  - Quality and adequacy of training, qualifications and experience of staff;
  - Coverage and adherence to the quality system in relation to pharmacovigilance, including quality control and quality assurance processes;
  - Fitness for purpose of computerised systems;
  - Contracts and agreements with all relevant parties appropriately reflect responsibilities and activities in the fulfilment of pharmacovigilance, and are adhered to.

The inspection may include the system for the fulfilment of conditions of a marketing authorisation and the implementation of risk–minimisation activities, as they relate to any of the above safety topics.

III.B.4.2. For Cause Inspections

The scope of the inspection will depend on the specific trigger(s). Some, but not all of the elements listed in III.B.4.1 and below, may be relevant:
• QPPV involvement and awareness of product-specific issues;
• In-depth examination of processes, decision-making, communications and actions relating to a specific trigger and/or product.

III.B.4.3. Re-inspections

For the scope of a re-inspection, the following aspects should be considered:
• Review of the status of the system and/or corrective and preventive action plan(s) resulting from previous pharmacovigilance inspection(s);
• Review of significant changes that have been made to the pharmacovigilance system since the last pharmacovigilance inspection (e.g. change in the pharmacovigilance database, company mergers or acquisitions, significant changes in contracted activities, change in QPPV);
• Review of process and/or product-specific issues identified from the assessment of information provided by the marketing authorisation holder, or not covered in a prior inspection.

The scope of re-inspection will depend on inspection history. It may be appropriate to conduct a complete system review, for example if a long time has elapsed since the previous inspection, in which case the elements listed in III.B.4.1. may be considered for the inspection scope, as appropriate.

III.B.5. Inspection Process

Pharmacovigilance inspections should be planned, coordinated, conducted, reported on, followed-up and documented in accordance with inspection procedures consistent with agreed Union pharmacovigilance inspection procedures developed by the PhVIWG to support harmonisation for the mutual recognition of pharmacovigilance inspections within the EU. The Union procedures on pharmacovigilance inspections are published on the webpage "Pharmacovigilance inspection procedures: human" of the Agency's website[1]. Improvement and harmonisation of inspection conduct is promoted by agreed processes and procedures, joint inspection(s) and sharing of experience and training by national competent authority inspectorates.

The Union procedures on pharmacovigilance inspections cover, at least, the following processes:

---
1. See: http://www.ema.europa.eu/ema/index.jsp?curl=pages/regulation/document_listing/document_listing_000164.jsp&mid=WC0b01ac0580029754

- Sharing of information;
- Inspection planning;
- Pre-authorisation inspections;
- Coordination of pharmacovigilance inspections in the EU;
- Coordination of third country inspections (including inspections of contractors in third countries);
- Preparation of pharmacovigilance inspections;
- Conduct of pharmacovigilance inspections;
- Reporting of pharmacovigilance inspections and inspection follow-up;
- Communication and prioritisation of pharmacovigilance inspections and findings;
- Interaction with PRAC in relation to inspections and their follow-up;
- Record-keeping and archiving of documents obtained or resulting from pharmacovigilance inspections;
- Unannounced inspections;
- Sanctions and enforcement in case of serious non-compliance;
- Recommendations on the training and experience of inspectors performing pharmacovigilance inspections.

These procedures will be revised and updated as deemed necessary. New procedures may also be developed when the need is identified in relation to the inspection process.

III.B.6. Inspection Follow-up

When non-compliance with pharmacovigilance obligations is identified during an inspection, follow-up will be required until a corrective and preventive action plan is completed. The following follow-up actions should be considered, as appropriate:
- Review of the marketing authorisation holder's corrective and preventive action plan;
- Review of the periodic progress reports, when deemed necessary;
- Re-inspection to assess appropriate implementation of the corrective and preventive action plan;
- Requests for submission of previously unsubmitted data; submission of variations, e.g. to amend product information; submission of impact analyses, e.g. following review of data that were not previously considered during routine signal detection activities;
- Requests for issuing safety communications, including amendments of marketing and/or advertising information;
- Requests for a meeting with the marketing authorisation holder to discuss the deficiencies, the impact of the deficiencies and action plans;
- Communication of the inspection findings to other regulatory authorities (including outside the EU);
- Other product-related actions depending on the impact of the deficiencies and the outcome of follow-up actions (this may include recalls or actions relating to the marketing authorisations or clinical trial authorisations).

Sharing information and communication between inspectors and assessors is important for the proper follow-up of inspections. Details of the processes relating to interaction between inspectors and assessors and inspection follow-up will be elaborated further in the compilation of Union procedures on pharmacovigilance inspections mentioned in III.B.5.

III.B.7. Regulatory Actions and Sanctions

Under EU legislation, in order to protect public health, competent authorities are obliged to ensure compliance with pharmacovigilance obligations. When non-compliance with pharmacovigilance obligations is detected, the necessary action will be judged on a case-by-case basis. What action is taken will depend on the potential negative public health impact of the non-compliance(s), but any instance of non-compliance may be considered for enforcement action. Action may be taken by the Agency, the Commission or the competent authorities of the Member States as appropriate. As stated in Article 111(8) of Directive 2001/83/EC, where appropriate, the Member State concerned shall take the necessary measures to ensure that a marketing authorisation holder is subject to effective, proportionate and dissuasive penalties. Moreover Regulation (EC) No 658/2007 also empowers the Commission, to impose financial penalties on the holders of marketing authorisations to ensure the enforcement of certain obligations connected with marketing authorisations for medicinal products granted in accordance with Regulation (EC) No 726/2004.

In the event of non-compliance, possible regulatory options include the following, in accordance with guidance and, as applicable, rules set in legislation:
- Education and facilitation: national competent authorities may communicate with marketing authorisation holder representatives (e.g. in a meeting) to summarise the identified non-compliances, to clarify the legal requirements and the expectations of the regulator, and to review the marketing authorisation holder's proposals for corrective and preventive actions;
- Provision of information to other competent authorities, the Agency or third country regulators under the framework of confidentiality arrangements;
- Inspection: non-compliant marketing authorisation holders may be inspected to determine the extent of non-compliance and then re-inspected to ensure compliance is achieved;
- Warning letter, non-compliance statement or infringement notice: these are non-statutory or statutory instruments in accordance with national legislation which competent authorities may issue stating the legislation and guideline that has been breached, reminding marketing authorisation holders of their pharmacovigilance obligations or specifying the steps that the marketing authorisation holder must take and in what timeframe in order to rectify the non-compliance and in order to prevent a further case of non-compliance;
- Competent authorities may consider making public a list of marketing authorisation holders found to be seriously or persistently non-compliant;
- Actions against a marketing authorisation(s) or authorisation application(s), e.g.
  - Urgent Safety Restriction;
  - Variation of the marketing authorisation;
  - Suspension or revocation of the marketing authorisation;
  - Delays in approvals of new marketing authorisation applications until corrective and preventive actions have been implemented or the addition of safety conditions to new authorisations;
  - Requests for pre-authorisation inspections;
- Product recalls, e.g. where important safety warnings have been omitted from product information;
- Action relating to marketing or advertising information;
- Amendments or suspension of clinical trials due to product-specific safety issues;
- Administrative penalties, usually fixed fines or based on company profits or levied on a daily basis;
- Referral for criminal prosecution with the possibility of imprisonment (in accordance with national legislation).

III.B.8. Record Management and Archiving

The principles and requirements to be followed will be described in the Union procedure on Record Keeping and Archiving of Documents Obtained or Resulting from the Pharmacovigilance Inspections referred to in III.B.5.

III.B.9. Qualification and Training of Inspectors

Inspectors who are involved in the conduct of pharmacovigilance inspections requested by their Member States or by the CHMP should be officials of, or appointed by, the Member State in accordance with national regulation and follow the provisions of the national competent authority.

It is recommended that inspectors are appointed based upon their experience and the minimum requirements defined by the national competent authority. In addition, consideration should be given to the recommendations for training and experience described in the compilation of Union procedures on pharmacovigilance inspections mentioned in III.B.5.

The inspectors should undergo training to the extent necessary to ensure their competence in the skills required for preparing, conducting and reporting inspections. They should also be trained in pharmacovigilance processes and requirements in such way that they are able, if not acquired by their experience, to comprehend the different aspects of a pharmacovigilance system.

Documented processes should be in place in order to ensure that inspection competencies are maintained. In particular, inspectors should be kept updated with the current status of pharmacovigilance legislation and guidance.

Training and experience should be documented individually and evaluated according to the requirements of the applicable quality system of the concerned competent authority.

III.B.10. Quality Management of Pharmacovigilance Inspection Process

Quality of the pharmacovigilance inspection process is managed by the national competent authorities and covered by their pharmacovigilance systems and associated quality systems, meaning that the process is also subject to audit. Guidance on establishment and maintenance of a quality assured pharmacovigilance system is provided in Module I.

Quality and consistency of the inspections is facilitated by the Union procedures for pharmacovigilance inspections developed by the PhVIWG to support the mutual recognition of inspections within the EU mentioned in III.B.5.

III.C. OPERATION OF THE EU NETWORK

III.C.1. Sharing of Information

The Agency and the Member States shall cooperate to facilitate the exchange of information on inspections and in particular:
- Information on inspections planned and conducted in order to avoid unnecessary repetition and duplication of activities in the EU and optimise the inspection resources;
- Information on the scope of the inspection in order to focus future inspections;
- Information on the outcome of the inspection, in particular when the outcome is that the marketing authorisation holder does not comply with the requirements laid down in legislation and relevant guidance. A summary of the critical and/or major findings and a summary of the corresponding corrective and preventive actions with their follow-up(s) should be exchanged.

Tools and procedures will be developed at EU level to facilitate and optimise the exchange and sharing of information and the communication across the Union.

III.C.2. Role of the European Medicines Agency

III.C.2.1. General Role of the Agency

Regarding the monitoring of compliance with regulatory pharmacovigilance obligations and pharmacovigilance inspections, the roles of the Agency are set out in Article 57(1)(c) and Article 57(1)(i) of Regulation (EC) No 726/2004 and can be summarised as follows:
- Coordination of the monitoring of medicinal products for human use which have been authorised within the Union, in particular by coordinating the evaluation and implementation of pharmacovigilance obligations and systems and the monitoring of such implementation;
- Coordination of the verification of compliance with pharmacovigilance obligations.

Pharmacovigilance inspections coordinated by the Agency are performed by the supervisory authority concerned as outlined in III.C.3.2. The supervisory authority may be assisted by other national competent authorities, when required.

As part of this coordination role the Agency is responsible for:
- Establishing and maintaining processes through the PhVIWG to support the consistency and quality of pharmacovigilance inspections of marketing authorisation holders with centrally authorised products conducted by inspectorates of the national competent authorities;
- Coordinating and ensuring the implementation of a risk-based programme for routine pharmacovigilance inspections of marketing authorisation holders with centrally authorised products (*see* III.B.2.) enabling the timely sharing of information on planned and conducted pharmacovigilance inspections between Member States, with the aim of reducing duplication of inspection activity and facilitating mutual recognition of inspection findings;
- Coordinating "for cause" inspections, as requested by the CHMP. If a "for cause" inspection has been or will be conducted in a similar timeframe as a routine one, it may replace the need for the planned routine

inspection and the programme shall be revised to reflect this;
- Coordinating third country inspections: according to Article 111(1) of the Directive 2001/83/EC, the Agency shall cooperate in the coordination of inspections in third countries. Member States should liaise with the Agency when the need for an inspection of a third country site is identified in order to ensure productive use of pharmacovigilance inspection resource in the interests of the Union;
- Communication and follow-up of inspections of Union interest across the Agency, the PRAC, the CHMP, the CMD(h), the EU regulatory network and with third country regulators, whenever confidentiality arrangements are in place to facilitate this.

III.C.2.2. Role of the PRAC

The PRAC may make recommendations on the need and scope of "for cause" pharmacovigilance inspections related to medicinal products of Union interest.

The PRAC may, in relation to issues of Union interest and where considered appropriate, review the outcome of pharmacovigilance inspections and assess marketing authorisation holder-related corrective and preventive action plan submission(s) in order to make or endorse further recommendations on actions to be taken and their follow-up.

The PRAC is also responsible for providing input in the preparation of and agreeing on the risk-based programme for routine pharmacovigilance inspections of marketing authorisation holders with centrally authorised products outlined in III.B.2 and III.C.3.3.

III.C.2.3. Role of the CHMP

The CHMP is responsible for the request of pharmacovigilance inspections in the context of the centralised procedure and for the endorsement of the recommendations made by the PRAC in relation to the outcome of these inspections and their follow-up. The CHMP is also responsible for the adoption of the risk-based programme for routine pharmacovigilance inspections outlined in III.B.2. and III.C.4.3.

III.C.3. Role of the European Commission

For medicinal products authorised under Regulation (EC) No 726/2004, the European Commission may request at any point in time the Agency to coordinate the conduct of a pharmacovigilance inspection if public health information in the possession of the Commission so mandates.

III.C.4. Role of the Member States

III.C.4.1. General Considerations

Member States should establish the legal and administrative framework within which pharmacovigilance inspections operate, including the definition of the rights of inspectors for inspecting pharmacovigilance sites and access to pharmacovigilance data.

Member States should provide sufficient resources and appoint adequately qualified inspectors to ensure effective determination of compliance with good pharmacovigilance practice. The inspector(s) appointed may be accompanied, when needed, by expert(s) on relevant areas. A Member State may also request assistance from another Member State, in which case, access to the inspection sites and data by the Member State providing assistance is desirable.

Pharmacovigilance inspections should be planned, coordinated, conducted, reported on, followed-up and documented in accordance with inspection procedures consistent with agreed Union pharmacovigilance inspection procedures developed by the PhVIWG to support harmonisation for the mutual recognition of pharmacovigilance inspections within the EU as mentioned in section III.B.5.

The scheduling and conduct of these inspections will be driven by the preparation of inspection programmes based on a systematic and risk-based approach as outlined in III.B.2. and III.C.4.3.

The national competent authorities, when preparing inspection programmes, should verify the inspection status of the marketing authorisation holders they plan to inspect by considering the information shared on planned or conducted inspections under the programmes in other Member States in order to assure coordination of inspection activities, prevent unnecessary duplication and to make the most efficient use of inspection resources.

When the pharmacovigilance system a national competent authority plans to inspect is the same as that already inspected by another national competent authority, sharing of information on the scope and outcomes of previous inspections and consideration of the national supervisory requirements, can help to define the objective, scope and timing of that national inspection.

A common repository, accessible to all Member States, the Agency and the Commission, should be created to facilitate this information sharing on pharmacovigilance inspections.

III.C.4.2. Role of the Supervisory Authority

The concept of the supervisory authority applies only in relation to centrally authorised products. According to Article 18 of Regulation (EC) 726/2004, the supervisory authority for the conduct of pharmacovigilance inspections shall be the competent authority of the Member State in which the pharmacovigilance system master file is located.

The supervisory authorities for pharmacovigilance are responsible for verifying on behalf of the Union that the marketing authorisation holder for the medicinal product satisfies the pharmacovigilance requirements laid down in Directive 2001/83/EC and Regulation 726/2004/EC. They may, if this is considered necessary, conduct pre-authorisation inspections to verify the accuracy and successful implementation of the existing or proposed pharmacovigilance system [REG Art 19].

Where the sites selected to be inspected are located outside the EU, the same supervisory authority as above will be responsible for the inspection on behalf of the Union. Where relevant or on request, and in particular for product-specific issues, the inspection may be conducted or assisted by inspector(s) from the Rapporteur or Co-Rapporteur Member State and/or expert(s) from the Rapporteur or Co-Rapporteur Member State or from other Member States as appropriate.

III.C.4.3. Inspection Programmes

A programme for routine inspections for centrally authorised products will be determined by the Agency in conjunction with the supervisory authorities of the Member States, the PhVIWG, the PRAC and the CHMP. These inspections will be prioritised based on the potential risk to public health, considering the factors listed in III.B.5.. As a general approach, a marketing authorisation holder should be inspected on the basis of risk-based considerations, but at least once every 4 years.

If the same pharmacovigilance system is used for a variety of authorisation types (centralised and national, mutual recognition and decentralised), then the results of a supervisory authority inspection may be applicable for all products covered by that system.

This routine inspection programme will be separate from any "for cause" inspections, but if a "for cause" inspection takes place it may replace the need for one under this programme, dependent on its scope.

Member States are also responsible for the planning and coordination of pharmacovigilance inspections within their territory in relation to products authorised nationally or via the mutual recognition or decentralised procedures in order to ensure compliance with the legislation within their own Member States and to verify the effectiveness of the marketing authorisation holder's pharmacovigilance system at national level.

As indicated in III.C.4.1., based on the information from other inspections, the national competent authority will prioritise the inspections in its national programme and will use the information for the preparation of an appropriate scope for the national inspection. For example, national competent authorities may seek to verify the fulfilment of requirements concerning the national implementation of specific risk-minimisation measures, national communications concerning safety, locally conducted safety studies, or issues linked to national health care systems. A broader examination of pharmacovigilance applied to particular products of national interest may also be appropriate if this was not covered within the scope of a supervisory authority inspection.

III.C.5. Role of Marketing Authorisation Holders and Applicants

Marketing authorisation holders with authorised products and applicants who have submitted new applications under the centralised procedure are subject to pharmacovigilance inspections (*see* III.B.1.). Therefore both have responsibilities in relation to inspections, including but not limited to the following:

- Always to be inspection-ready as inspections may be unannounced;
- To maintain and make available to the inspectors on request, no later than 7 calendar days after the receipt of a request, the pharmacovigilance system master file as required by Article 23(4) of Directive 2001/83/EC and Article 16(4) of Regulation (EU) 726/2004;
- To ensure that the sites selected for inspection, which may include firms employed by the marketing authorisation holder to perform pharmacovigilance activities, agree to be inspected before the inspection is performed;
- To make available to the inspectors any information and/or documentation required for the preparation of the inspection within the deadline given or during the conduct of the inspection;
- To ensure that relevant staff involved in pharmacovigilance activities or related activities are present and available during the inspection for interviews or clarification of issues identified;
- To ensure that relevant pharmacovigilance data is accessible from at least one point in the Union [DIR Art 107(1)];
- To ensure that appropriate and timely corrective and preventive action plans are implemented to address findings observed during an inspection, with appropriate prioritisation of critical and/or major findings.

III.C.6. Inspection Fees

For inspections requested by the CHMP, an inspection fee(s) (and inspectors' expenses where applicable) will be charged in accordance with the Council Regulation (EC) No 297/95 on fees payable to the European Agency for the Evaluation of Medicinal Products as amended and implementing rules applicable at the time. For pharmacovigilance inspections performed in the context of national, mutual recognition and decentralised procedures similar fees may or may not apply depending on the legal requirements of the Member State carrying out the inspection.

III.C.7. Transparency

Information on the conduct and outcome of pharmacovigilance inspections and their follow-up may be made publicly available. This will then be elaborated further in the compilation of Union procedures on pharmacovigilance inspections mentioned in III.B.5.

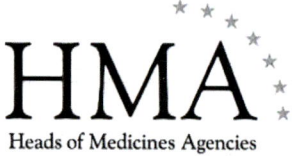
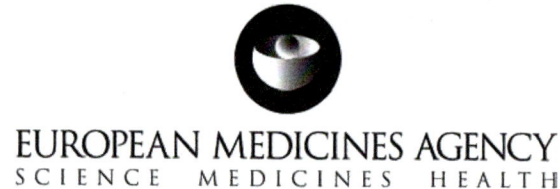

3 August 2015
EMA/228028/2012 Rev 1*

GUIDELINE ON GOOD PHARMACOVIGILANCE PRACTICES (GVP)

Module IV   Pharmacovigilance audits (Rev 1)

Draft finalised by the Agency in collaboration with Member States and submitted to ERMS FG	12 July 2012
Draft agreed by ERMS FG	20 July 2012
Draft adopted by Executive Director	25 July 2012
Start of public consultation	26 July 2012
End of consultation (deadline for comments)	21 September 2012
Revised draft finalised by the Agency in collaboration with Member States	5 December 2012
Revised draft agreed by ERMS FG	6 December 2012
Revised draft adopted by Executive Director as final	12 December 2012
Date for coming into effect	13 December 2012
Draft Revision 1* finalised by the Agency in collaboration with Member States	2 July 2015
Draft Revision 1 agreed by the European Risk Management Facilitation Group (ERMS FG)	16 July 2015
Draft Revision 1 adopted by Executive Director as final	3 August 2015
Date for coming into effect of Revision 1	12 August 2015

*__Note:__ Revision 1 contains the following:
- Addition of an explanatory note for the definition of audit in footnote 3
- Editorial improvements in line with the overall GVP style.

IV.A. INTRODUCTION

The entry into force of the new legislation on pharmacovigilance in July 2012, established legal requirements for competent authorities in the Member States and the European Medicines Agency (the Agency) and marketing authorisation holders to perform audits of their pharmacovigilance systems [DIR Art 101(2), Art 104(2), REG Art 28f], including risk based audits of their quality systems [IR Art 13 (1), Art 17 (1)].

For the purposes of this Module reference to pharmacovigilance audit(s) and pharmacovigilance audit activity(ies) are deemed to include pharmacovigilance system audits and audit(s) of the quality system for pharmacovigilance activities.

The minimum requirements of the pharmacovigilance systems and the quality system are set out in the Commission Implementing Regulation (EU) No 520/2012 (IR) on the performance of pharmacovigilance activities provided for in Regulation (EC) No 726/2004 and Directive 2001/83/EC. Risk-based audits of the pharmacovigilance system should cover all areas listed in Directive 2001/83/EC (DIR) and Regulation (EC) 726/2004 (REG). The specificities of the risk-based audits of the quality system [for pharmacovigilance activities] are as described in the Implementing Measures [IR Art 8,10, 11,12,13(1) for marketing authorisation holders, and IR Art 8,14,15,16,17(1) for the competent authorities in Member States and the Agency].

The overall description and objectives of pharmacovigilance systems and quality systems for pharmacovigilance activities are referred to in GVP Module I, while the specific pharmacovigilance processes are described in each respective Module of GVP.

In this Module, all applicable legal requirements are referenced in the way explained in the GVP Introductory Cover Note and are usually identifiable by the modal verb "shall". Guidance for the implementation of legal requirements is provided using the modal verb "should".

This Module provides guidance on planning and conducting the legally required audits, and in respect of the operation of the EU regulatory network, the role, context and management of pharmacovigilance audit activity. This Module is intended to facilitate the performance of pharmacovigilance audits, especially to promote harmonisation, and encourage consistency and simplification of the audit process. The principles in this Module are aligned with internationally accepted auditing standards, issued by relevant international auditing standardisation organisations[1] and support a risk-based approach to pharmacovigilance audits.

Section IV.B. outlines the general structures and processes that should be followed to identify the most appropriate pharmacovigilance audit engagements and describes the steps which can be undertaken by marketing authorisation holders, competent authorities in Member States and the European Medicines Agency, to plan, conduct and report upon an individual pharmacovigilance audit engagements. This Section also provides an outline of the general quality system and record management practices for pharmacovigilance audit processes.

Section IV.C. provides an outline of the operation of the EU network in respect of pharmacovigilance audits.

IV.A.1. Terminology

Audit, Audit findings, Audit plan, Audit programme, Audit recommendations,

Upper management: see in GVP Annex I.

Auditee: [entity] being audited [ISO 19011 (3.7)[2]].

Compliance: Conformity and adherence to policies, plans, procedures, laws, regulations, contracts, or other requirements (IIA International Standards for the Professional Practice of Internal Auditing[2]).

Control(s): Any action taken by management and other parties to manage risk and increase the

---

1. For more details regarding The Institute of Internal Auditors (IIA) *see* www.theiia.org; the International Organisation for Standardisation (ISO) *see* www.iso.org; Information Systems Audit and Control Association (ISACA) *see* www.isaca.org; The International Auditing and Assurance Standards Board (IAASB) *see* www.ifac.org; The International Organisation of Supreme Audit Institutions (INTOSAI) *see* www.issai.org.
2. *See* The Institute of Internal Auditors (IIA), www.theiia.org.

likelihood that established objectives and goals will be achieved. Management plans, organises, and directs the performance of sufficient actions to provide reasonable assurance that objectives and goals will be achieved (IIA International Standards for the Professional Practice of Internal Auditing[2]).

Evaluation (of audit activities): Professional auditing bodies promote compliance with standards, including in quality assurance of their own activities, and codes of conduct, which can be used to address adequate fulfilment of the organisation's basic expectations of Internal Audit activity and its conformity to internationally accepted auditing standards.

Finding(s): see Audit findings

Head of the organisation: see Upper management

Auditors' independence: The freedom from conditions that threaten objectivity or the appearance of objectivity. Such threats to objectivity must be managed at the individual auditor, engagement, functional and organisational levels (IIA International Standards for the Professional Practice of Internal Auditing[2]).

Internal Control: Internal control is an integral process that is effected by an entity's management and personnel and is designed to address risk and provide reasonable assurance that in pursuit of the entity's mission, the following general objectives are being achieved: executing orderly, ethical, economical, efficient and effective operations, fulfilling accountability obligations, complying with applicable laws and regulations and safeguarding resources against loss, misuse and damage (for further information refer to COSO standards).

International Auditing Standards: issued by International Auditing Standardisation Organisations.

International Auditing Standardisation Organisations: More details can be found at: regarding The Institute of Internal Auditors (IIA) Standards at http://www.theiia.org/guidance/standards-and-guidance/ippf/standards/full-standards; the International Organisation for Standardisation (ISO) standard 19011 Guidelines for Quality and/or Environmental Management Systems Auditing at http://www.iso.org/iso/home.html; Information Systems Audit and Control Association (ISACA) Standards at http://www.isaca.org/Standards; The International Auditing and Assurance Standards Board (IAASB) Standards at http://www.ifac.org/auditing-assurance/clarity-center/clarified-standards; The International Organisation of Supreme Audit Institutions (INTOSAI) Standards at http://www.issai.org/composite-347.htm.

Auditors' objectivity: An unbiased mental attitude that allows internal auditors to perform engagements in such a manner that they have an honest belief in their work product and that no significant quality compromises are made. Objectivity requires internal auditors not to subordinate their judgment on audit matters to that of others (IIA International Standards for the Professional Practice of Internal Auditing[2]).

IV.B. STRUCTURES AND PROCESSES

IV.B.1. Pharmacovigilance Audit and its Objective

Pharmacovigilance audit activities should verify, by examination and evaluation of objective evidence, the appropriateness and effectiveness of the implementation and operation of a pharmacovigilance system, including its quality system for pharmacovigilance activities.

In general, an audit is a systematic, disciplined, independent and documented process for obtaining evidence and evaluating the evidence objectively to determine the extent to which the audit criteria are fulfilled, contributing to the improvement of risk management, control and governance processes.[3]

Audit evidence consists of records, statements or other information, which are relevant to the audit criteria and verifiable. Audit criteria are, for each audit objective, the standards of performance and control against which the auditee and its activities will be assessed. In the context of pharmacovigilance, audit criteria should reflect the requirements for the pharmacovigilance system, including its quality system for pharmacovigilance activities, as found in the legislation and guidance.

---

3. Benchmarking, reviews of qualifications, risk assessment questionnaires, surveys or other activities in which evidence of fulfilment of pharmacovigilance requirements is not independently obtained and evaluated, would not be regarded as an audit.

IV.B.2. The Risk-based Approach to Pharmacovigilance Audits

A risk-based approach is one that uses techniques to determine the areas of risk, where risk is defined as the probability of an event occurring that will have an impact on the achievement of objectives, taking account of the severity of its outcome and/or likelihood of non-detection by other methods. The risk-based approach to audits focuses on the areas of highest risk to the organisation's pharmacovigilance system, including its quality system for pharmacovigilance activities. In the context of pharmacovigilance, the risk to public health is of prime importance. Risk can be assessed at the following stages:

- Strategic level audit planning resulting in an audit strategy (long term approach), which should be endorsed by upper management;
- Tactical level audit planning resulting in an audit programme, setting audit objectives, and the extent and boundaries, often termed as scope, of the audits in that programme; and
- Operational level audit planning resulting in an audit plan for individual audit engagements, prioritising audit tasks based on risk and utilising risk-based sampling and testing approaches, and reporting of audit findings in line with their relative risk level and audit recommendations in line with the suggested grading system (see IV.B.2.3.1.).

Risk assessment should be documented appropriately for the strategic, tactical and operational planning of pharmacovigilance audit activity in the organisation (see IV.B.2.1., IV.B.2.2. and IV.B.2.3. respectively).

IV.B.2.1. Strategic Level Audit Planning

The audit strategy is a high level statement of how the audit activities will be delivered over a period of time, longer than the annual programme, usually for a period of 2-5 years. The audit strategy includes a list of audits that could reasonably be performed. The audit strategy is used to outline the areas highlighted for audit, the audit topics as well as the methods and assumptions (including e.g. risk assessment) on which the audit programme is based.

The audit strategy should cover the governance, risk management and internal controls of all parts of the pharmacovigilance system including:

- All pharmacovigilance processes and tasks;
- The quality system for pharmacovigilance activities;
- Interactions and interfaces with other departments, as appropriate;
- Pharmacovigilance activities conducted by affiliated organisations or activities delegated to another organisation (e.g. regional reporting centres, MAH affiliates or third parties, such as contract organisations and other vendors).

This is a non-prioritised, non-exhaustive list of examples of risk factors that could be considered for the purposes of a risk assessment:

- Changes to legislation and guidance;
- Major re-organisation or other re-structuring of the pharmacovigilance system, mergers, acquisitions (specifically for marketing authorisation holders, this may lead to a significant increase in the number of products for which the system is used);
- Change in key managerial function(s);
- Risk to availability of adequately trained and experienced pharmacovigilance staff, e.g. due to significant turn-over of staff, deficiencies in training processes, re-organisation, increase in volumes of work;
- Significant changes to the system since the time of a previous audit, e.g. introduction of a new database(s) for pharmacovigilance activities or of a significant upgrade to the existing database(s), changes to processes and activities in order to address new or amended regulatory requirements;
- First medicinal product on the market (for a marketing authorisation holder);
- Medicinal product(s) on the market with specific risk minimisation measures or other specific safety conditions such as requirements for additional monitoring;
- Criticality of the process, e.g.:
  - For competent authorities: how critical is the area/process to proper functioning of the pharmacovigilance system and the overall objective of safeguarding public health;
  - For marketing authorisation holders: how critical is the area/process to proper functioning of the pharmacovigilance system. When deciding when to audit an affiliate or third party, the marketing authorisation holder should consider

the nature and criticality of the pharmacovigilance activities that are being performed by an affiliate or third party on behalf of the marketing authorisation holder, in addition to considering the other factors included in this list;
- Outcome of previous audits, e.g. has the area/process ever been audited (if not, then this may need to be prioritised depending on criticality); if the area/process has previously been audited, the audit findings are a factor to consider when deciding when to re-audit the area/process, including the implementation of agreed actions;
- Identified procedural gaps relating to specific areas/processes;
- Other information relating to compliance with legislation and guidance, for example:
  - For competent authorities: information from compliance metrics (as described in the Commission Implementing Regulation on the Performance of Pharmacovigilance Activities Provided for in Regulation (EC) No 726/2004 and Directive 2001/83/EC), from complaints, from external sources, e.g. audits/assessments of the competent authority conducted by external bodies;
  - For marketing authorisation holders: information from compliance metrics (as described in the Commission Implementing Regulation on the Performance of Pharmacovigilance Activities Provided for in Regulation (EC) No 726/2004 and Directive 2001/83/EC), from inspections (see GVP Module III), from complaints, from other external sources, e.g. audits;
- Other organisational changes that could negatively impact on the area/process, e.g. if a change occurs to a support function (such as information technology support) this could negatively impact upon pharmacovigilance activities.

IV.B.2.2. Tactical Level Audit Planning

An audit programme is a set of one or more audits planned for a specific timeframe, normally for a year. It should be prepared in line with the long term audit strategy. The audit programme should be approved by upper management with overall responsibility for operational and governance structure.

The risk-based audit programme should be based on an appropriate risk assessment and should focus on:
- The quality system for pharmacovigilance activities;
- Critical pharmacovigilance processes (see e.g. GVP Module I and IR Art 11, 15);
- Key control systems relied on for pharmacovigilance activities;
- Areas identified as high risk, after controls have been put in place or mitigating action taken.

The risk-based audit programme should also take into account historical areas with insufficient past audit coverage, and high risk areas identified by and/or specific requests from management and/or persons responsible for pharmacovigilance activities.

The audit programme documentation should include a brief description of the plan for each audit to be delivered, including an outline of scope and objectives.

The rationale for the timing, periodicity and scope of the individual audits which form part of the audit programme should be based on the documented risk assessment. However, risk-based pharmacovigilance audit(s) should be performed at regular intervals, which are in line with legislative requirements.

Changes to the audit programme may happen and will require proper documentation.

IV.B.2.3. Operational Level Audit Planning and Reporting

IV.B.2.3.1. Planning and Fieldwork

The organisation should ensure that written procedures are in place regarding the planning and conduct of individual audits that will be delivered. Timeframes for all the steps required for the performance of an individual audit should be settled in the relevant audit related procedures, and the organisation should ensure that audits are conducted in accordance with the written procedures, in line with this GVP Module.

Individual pharmacovigilance audits should be undertaken in line with the approved risk-based audit programme (see IV.B.2.2.). When planning individual audits, the auditor identifies and assesses the risks relevant to the area under review and employs the most appropriate risk-based sampling and testing methods, documenting the audit approach in an audit plan.

IV.B.2.3.2. Reporting

The findings of the auditors should be documented in an audit report and should be communicated to management in a timely manner. The audit process should include mechanisms for communicating the audit findings to the auditee and receiving feedback, and reporting the audit findings to management and relevant parties, including those responsible for pharmacovigilance systems, in accordance with legal requirements and guidance on pharmacovigilance audits. Audit findings should be reported in line with their relative risk level and should be graded in order to indicate their relative criticality to risks impacting the pharmacovigilance system, processes and parts of processes. The grading system should be defined in the description of the quality system for pharmacovigilance, and should take into consideration the thresholds noted below which would be used in further reporting under the legislation as set out in IV.C.2.:

- **Critical** is a fundamental weakness in one or more pharmacovigilance processes or practices that adversely affects the whole pharmacovigilance system and/or the rights, safety or well-being of patients, or that poses a potential risk to public health and/or represents a serious violation of applicable regulatory requirements.
- **Major** is a significant weakness in one or more pharmacovigilance processes or practices, or a fundamental weakness in part of one or more pharmacovigilance processes or practices that is detrimental to the whole process and/or could potentially adversely affect the rights, safety or well-being of patients and/or could potentially pose a risk to public health and/or represents a violation of applicable regulatory requirements which is however not considered serious.
- **Minor** is a weakness in the part of one or more pharmacovigilance processes or practices that is not expected to adversely affect the whole pharmacovigilance system or process and/or the rights, safety or well-being of patients.

Issues that need to be urgently addressed should be communicated in an expedited manner to the auditee's management and the upper management.

IV.B.2.4. Actions Based on Audit Outcomes and Follow-up of Audits

Actions referenced in this section of the guideline, i.e., immediate action, prompt action, action within a reasonable timeframe, issues that need to be urgently addressed, or communicated in an expedited manner, are intended to convey timelines that are appropriate, relevant, and in line with the relative risk to the pharmacovigilance system. Corrective and preventive actions to address critical and major issues should be prioritised. The precise timeframe for action(s) related to a given critical finding, for example, may differ depending on nature of findings and the planned action(s).

The management of the organisation is responsible for ensuring that the organisation has a mechanism in place to adequately address the issues arising from pharmacovigilance audits. Actions should include root cause analysis and impact analysis of identified audit findings and preparation of a corrective and preventive action plan, where appropriate.

Upper management and those charged with governance, should ensure that effective action is implemented to address the audit findings. The implementation of agreed actions should be monitored in a systematic way, and the progress of implementation should be communicated on a periodic basis proportionate to the planned actions to upper management.

Evidence of completion of actions should be recorded in order to document that issues raised during the audit have been addressed.

Capacity for follow-up audits should be foreseen in the audit programme. They should be carried out as deemed necessary, in order to verify the completion of agreed actions. [IR Art 13(2), Art 17(2)]

IV.B.3. Quality System and Record Management Practices

IV.B.3.1. Competence of Auditors and Quality Management of Audit Activities

IV.B.3.1.1. Independence and Objectivity of Audit Work and Auditors

The organisation should assign the specific responsibilities for the pharmacovigilance audit activities. Pharmacovigilance audit activities should be independent. The organisation's management should ensure this independence and objectivity in a structured manner and document this.

Auditors should be free from interference in determining the scope of auditing, performing pharmacovigilance audits and communicating audit results. The main reporting line should be to the upper management with overall responsibility for operational and governance structure that allows the auditor(s) to fulfil their responsibilities and to provide independent, objective audit opinion. Auditors can consult with technical experts, personnel involved in pharmacovigilance processes, and with the person responsible for pharmacovigilance; however auditors should maintain an unbiased attitude that allows them to perform audit work in such a manner that they have an honest belief in their work product and that no significant quality compromises are made. Objectivity requires auditors not to subordinate their judgement on audit matters to that of others.

IV.B.3.1.2. Qualifications, Skills and Experience of Auditors and Continuing Professional Development

Auditors should demonstrate and maintain proficiency in terms of the knowledge, skills and abilities required to effectively conduct and/or participate in pharmacovigilance audit activities. The proficiency of audit team members will have been gained through a combination of education, work experience and training and, as a team, should cover knowledge, skills and abilities in:
- Audit principles, procedures and techniques;
- Applicable laws, regulations and other requirements relevant to pharmacovigilance;
- Pharmacovigilance activities, processes and system(s);
- Management system(s);
- Organisational system(s).

IV.B.3.1.3. Evaluation of the Quality of Audit Activities

Evaluation of audit work can be undertaken by means of ongoing and periodic assessment of all audit activities, auditee feedback and self-assessment of audit activities (e.g. quality assurance of audit activities, compliance to code of conduct, audit programme, and audit procedures).

IV.B.3.2. Audits Undertaken by Outsourced Audit Service Providers

Ultimate responsibility for the operation and effectiveness of the pharmacovigilance system resides within the organisation (i.e. within the Agency, competent authority or marketing authorisation holder). Where the organisation decides to use an outsourced audit service provider to implement the pharmacovigilance audit requirements on the basis of this GVP Module and perform pharmacovigilance audits:
- The requirements and preparation of the audit risk assessment, the audit strategy and audit programme and individual engagements should be specified to the outsourced service providers, by the organisation, in writing;
- The scope, objectives and procedural requirements for the audit should be specified to the outsourced service provider, by the organisation, in writing;
- The organisation should obtain and document assurance of the independence and objectivity of outsourced service providers;
- The outsourced audit service provider should also follow the relevant parts of this GVP Module.

IV.B.3.3. Retention of Audit Reports

Retention of the audit report and evidence of completion of action needs to be in line with the requirements stipulated in GVP Module I.

IV.C. PHARMACOVIGILANCE AUDIT POLICY FRAMEWORK AND ORGANISATIONAL STRUCTURE

IV.C.1. Marketing Authorisation Holders in the EU

IV.C.1.1. Requirement to Perform an Audit

The marketing authorisation holder in the EU is required to perform regular risk-based audit(s) of their pharmacovigilance system [DIR Art 104(2)], including audit(s) of its quality system to ensure that the quality system complies with the quality system requirements [IR Art 8,10,11,12,13(1)]. The dates and results of audits and follow-up audits shall be documented [IR Art 13(2)]

See IV.C.2. for further details of the requirements for audit reporting by the marketing authorisation holder.

IV.C.1.1.1. The Qualified Person Responsible for Pharmacovigilance in the EU (QPPV)

The responsibilities of the QPPV in respect of audit are provided in GVP Module I. Furthermore, the QPPV should receive pharmacovigilance audit reports, and provide information to the auditors relevant to the risk assessment, including knowledge of status of corrective and preventive actions.

The QPPV should be notified of any audit findings relevant to the pharmacovigilance system in the EU, irrespective of where the audit was conducted.

IV.C.1.2. Competent Authorities in Member States and the European Medicines Agency

IV.C.1.2.1. Requirement to Perform an Audit

The Agency shall perform regular independent audits of its pharmacovigilance tasks [REG Art 28f] and competent authorities in Member States shall perform a regular audit of their pharmacovigilance system [DIR Art 101(2)]. Included in their obligation to perform audits of their pharmacovigilance system/tasks, competent authorities in the Member States and the Agency shall perform risk-based audits of the quality system as well, at regular intervals according to a common methodology to ensure that the quality system complies with the requirements [IR Art 8,14,15,16,17(1)]. The dates and results of audits and follow-up audits shall be documented [IR Art 17(2)].

IV.C.1.2.2. Common Methodology

In order to have a useful audit system, all audits at the competent authorities in the Member States and the European Medicines Agency should have a common ground in terms of methodology. This should ensure harmonised planning, implementation and reporting by every competent authority in Member States and at the Agency.

IV.C.1.2.3. The Pharmacovigilance Risk Assessment Committee (PRAC)

The mandate of the Pharmacovigilance Risk Assessment Committee (PRAC) shall cover all aspects of the risk management of the use of medicinal products for human use, having due regard to the design and evaluation of pharmacovigilance audits [REG Art 61a(6)].

IV.C.2. Requirements for Audit Reporting in the EU

IV.C.2.1. Reporting by the Marketing Authorisation Holder

The marketing authorisation holder shall place a note concerning critical and major audit findings of any audit relating to the pharmacovigilance system in the pharmacovigilance system master file (PSMF) (*see* GVP Module II). Based on the audit findings, the marketing authorisation holder shall ensure that an appropriate plan detailing corrective and preventative action is prepared and implemented. Once the corrective and preventive actions have been fully implemented, the note may be removed [DIR Art 104(2), IR Art 13(2)]. Objective evidence is required in order that any note of audit findings can be removed from the pharmacovigilance system master file (*see* GVP Module II).

The marketing authorisation holders should ensure that a list of all scheduled and completed audits is kept in the annex to the pharmacovigilance system master file [IR Art 3(5)] and that they comply with reporting commitments in line with the legislation, GVP guidance and their internal reporting policies. The dates and results of audits and follow-up audits shall be documented [IR Art 13(2)].

IV.C.2.2. Reporting by Competent Authorities in Member States and the Agency

Competent authorities in Member States, and the Agency should ensure that they comply with reporting commitments in line with the legislation, GVP guidance and their internal reporting policies.

Competent authorities in Member States shall report the results [of their pharmacovigilance system audits] to the Commission on 21 September 2013 at the latest and then every 2 years thereafter [DIR Art 101(2)].

The Agency shall report the results [of its pharmacovigilance system audits] to its

Management Board on a 2-yearly basis [REG Art 28f].

The reports to the European Commission will follow an agreed format.

IV.C.3. Confidentiality

Documents and information collected by the internal auditor should be treated with appropriate confidentiality and discretion, and also respect Directive 95/46/EC [Regulation (EC) No. 45/2001 for Community institutions and bodies] and national legislation on the protection of individuals with regard to the processing of personal data and on the free movement of such data.

IV.C.4. Transparency

The European Commission shall make public a report on the performance of pharmacovigilance tasks by the Agency on 2 January 2014 at the latest and subsequently every 3 years thereafter [REG Art 29] and on the performance of pharmacovigilance tasks by the competent authorities in Member States on 21 July 2015 at the latest and then every 3 years thereafter [DIR Art 108(b)].

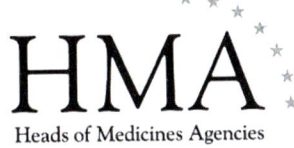
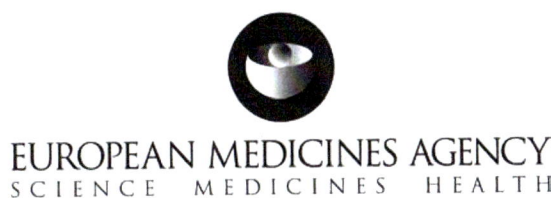

3 August 2015
EMA/228028/2012 Rev 1*

GUIDELINE ON GOOD PHARMACOVIGILANCE PRACTICES (GVP)

Module V Risk Management Systems (Rev 2)

Date for coming into effect of first version	2 July 2012
Date for coming into effect of Revision 1	28 April 2014
Draft Revision 2* finalised by the Agency in collaboration with Member States	16 February 2016
Draft Revision 2 agreed by the European Risk Management Facilitation Group (ERMS FG)	23 February 2016
Draft Revision 2 adopted by Executive Director	24 February 2016
Release for public consultation	29 February 2016
End of consultation (deadline for comments)	31 May 2016
Revised draft Revision 2 finalised by the Agency in collaboration with Member States	9 March 2017
Revised draft Revision 2 agreed by the EU Network Pharmacovigilance Oversight Group (EU-POG)	23 March 2017
Revised draft Revision 2 adopted by Executive Director as final	28 March 2017
Date for coming into effect of Revision 2*	31 March 2017

Note: RMPs submitted for initial marketing authorisation applications and D121 responses applying GVP Module V Rev 1 will be accepted for a further 6 months, and all other RMP submissions (including D91 responses for an initial application under accelerated assessment) will be accepted for one further year until 31 March 2018.

* **Note:** Revision 2 is a major revision with modifications throughout and contains the following:
- Further clarification of what RMPs should focus on in relation to an important identified or important potential risk and missing information;
- Removal of duplication within GVP Module V;
- Removal of duplication of information in other guidance documents;
- Further guidance on the expected changes in the RMP during the life cycle of the product;
- Updated requirements for different types of initial marketing authorisation applications, with the aim to create risk-proportionate RMPs.

The guidance is updated in parallel to an amended RMP template for initial marketing authorisation application.

V.A. INTRODUCTION

A medicinal product is authorised on the basis that in the specified indication(s), at the time of authorisation, the risk-benefit balance is judged to be positive for the target population. Generally, a medicinal product will be associated with adverse reactions and these will vary in terms of severity, likelihood of occurrence, effect on individual patients and public health impact. However, not all adverse reactions and risks will have been identified at the time when an initial marketing authorisation is granted and some will only be discovered and characterised in the post-authorisation phase. The aim of a risk management plan (RMP) is to document the risk management system considered necessary to identify, characterise and minimise a medicinal product's important risks. To this end, the RMP contains:

1. the identification or characterisation of the safety profile of the medicinal product, with emphasis on important identified and important potential risks and missing information, and also on which safety concerns need to be managed proactively or further studied (the 'safety specification');
2. the planning of pharmacovigilance activities to characterise and quantify clinically relevant risks, and to identify new adverse reactions (the 'pharmacovigilance plan');
3. the planning and implementation of risk minimisation measures, including the evaluation of the effectiveness of these activities (the 'risk minimisation plan').

As knowledge regarding a medicinal product's safety profile increases over time, so will the risk management plan change.

Regulation (EC) No 726/2004, Directive 2001/83/EC and Commission Implementing Regulation (EU) No 520/2012 (hereinafter referred to as REG, DIR and IR) include provisions for post-authorisation safety studies and post-authorisation efficacy studies to be a condition of the marketing authorisation in certain circumstances [REG Art 9(4)(cb) and (cc), REG Art 10a(1)(a) and (b), DIR Art 21a(b) and (f), DIR Art 22a(1)(a) and (b)] and for these studies to be included in the risk management system [REG 14a, DIR Art 22c(1), IR Art 30(1)(d)]. The legislation also includes provisions for additional risk minimisation activities to be included in the risk management system as a condition to the marketing authorisation [REG Art 9(4)(ca), DIR Art 21a(a)]. Marketing authorisation applicants are encouraged to plan from very early on in a product's life cycle how they will further characterise and minimise the risks associated with the product in the post-authorisation phase. Guidance on templates and submission of RMPs is kept up-to-date on the Agency's website[1]. This Module includes the principles of risk minimisation and should be read in conjunction with GVP Module XVI and GVP Module XVI Addendum I on educational materials.

In this Module, all applicable legal requirements are referenced in the way explained in the GVP Introductory Cover Note and are usually identifiable by the modal verb "shall". Guidance for the implementation of legal requirements is provided using the modal verb "should".

The following articles provide the main references in relation to the legal basis for risk management but additional articles may also be relevant:

- DIR: Article 8(3)(ia) and (iaa), Article 21a, Article 22a(1), Article 22c(1), Article 104(3), Article 106(c), Article 127a;
- REG: Article 6(1), Article 9(4)(c), (ca), (cb), (cc), Article 10a(1), Article 14a, Article 26(1)(c);
- IR: Article 30, Article 31, Article 32, Article 33, Annex I;
- Regulation (EC) No 1901/2006 Article 34(2);
- Regulation (EC) No 1394/2007 Article 14(2).

V.A.1. Terminology

The definitions from GVP Annex I apply also for the purpose of this GVP Module. However, the RMP should focus on those risks that are relevant for the risk management activities for the authorised medicinal product.

From the **identified risks** of the medicinal product, the RMP should address only the risks that are undesirable clinical outcomes and for which there is sufficient scientific evidence that they are caused by the medicinal product. Reports of adverse reactions may be derived from multiple sources such as non-clinical findings confirmed by clinical data, clinical trials, epidemiological studies, and spontaneous data sources, including published

---
1. See www.ema.europa.eu

literature. They may be linked to situations such as off label use, medication errors or drug interactions. Not all reported adverse reactions are necessarily considered a relevant risk of the product in a given therapeutic context.

From the **potential risks** of the medicinal product, the RMP should address only the risks that are undesirable clinical outcomes and for which there is scientific evidence to suspect the possibility of a causal relationship with the medicinal product, but where there is currently insufficient evidence to conclude that this association is causal.

The RMP should focus on the **important identified risks** that are likely to have an impact on the risk-benefit balance of the product. An important identified risk to be included in the RMP would usually warrant:

- Further evaluation as part of the pharmacovigilance plan (e.g. to investigate frequency, severity, seriousness and outcome of this risk under normal conditions of use, which populations are particularly at risk);
- Risk minimisation activities: product information advising on specific clinical actions to be taken to minimise the risk (*see* V.B.8.), or additional risk minimisation activities.

The **important potential risks** to be included in the RMP are those important potential risks that, when further characterised and if confirmed, would have an impact on the risk-benefit balance of the medicinal product. Where there is a scientific rationale that an adverse clinical outcome might be associated with off-label use, use in populations not studied, or resulting from the long-term use of the product, the adverse reaction should be considered a potential risk, and if deemed important, should be included in the list of safety concerns as an important potential risk. Important potential risks included in the RMP would usually require further evaluation as part of the pharmacovigilance plan.

Missing information relevant to the risk management planning refers to gaps in knowledge about the safety of a medicinal product for certain anticipated utilisation (e.g. long-term use) or for use in particular patient populations, for which there is insufficient knowledge to determine whether the safety profile differs from that characterised so far. The absence of data itself (e.g. exclusion of a population from clinical studies) does not automatically constitute a safety concern. Instead, the risk management planning should focus on situations that might differ from the known safety profile. A scientific rationale is needed for the inclusion of that population as missing information in the RMP.

V.B. STRUCTURES AND PROCESSES

V.B.1. Principles of Risk Management

The overall aim of risk management is to ensure that the benefits of a particular medicinal product exceed the risks by the greatest achievable margin. The primary aim and focus of the RMP remains that of appropriate risk management planning throughout a medicinal product's life cycle. The risk management system shall be proportionate to the identified risks and the potential risks of the medicinal product, and the need for post-authorisation safety data [DIR Art 8(3)].

The RMP is a dynamic document that should be updated throughout the life cycle of the product(s). This includes the addition of safety concerns where required, but also, as the safety profile is further characterised, the removal or reclassification of safety concerns.

The guidance on risk classification in this document may facilitate that during the life cycle of the products the list of safety concerns in the RMP will be reduced (*see* also V.A.1. and V.B.5.8.):

- It may be that important potential risks can be removed from the safety specification in the RMP (e.g. when accumulating scientific and clinical data do not support the initial supposition, the impact to the individual has been shown to be less than anticipated resulting in the potential risk not being considered important, or when there is no reasonable expectation that any pharmacovigilance activity can further characterise the risk), or they need to be reclassified to 'important identified risks' (e.g. if scientific and clinical data strengthen the association between the risk and the product).
- In certain circumstances, where the risk is fully characterised and appropriately managed, important identified risks may be removed from the safety specification (e.g. for products marketed for a long time for which there are no outstanding additional pharmacovigilance activities and/or the risk minimisation activities recommending specific clinical measures to address the risk have become fully integrated

into standard clinical practice, such as inclusion into treatment protocols or clinical guidelines).
- Given the overall aim of obtaining more information regarding the risk-benefit balance in certain populations excluded in the pre-authorisation phase, it is expected that as the product matures, the classification as missing information might not be appropriate anymore once new data become available, or when there is no reasonable expectation that the existing or future feasible pharmacovigilance activities could further characterise the safety profile of the product with respect to the areas of missing information.

With the exception of some patient registries, it is expected that over time the additional pharmacovigilance activities in the RMP will be completed and thus removed from the RMP.

The need to continue additional risk minimisation activities may change, as the recommendations for specific clinical measures to address the risk become part of the routine practice such as inclusion into standard treatment protocols in the EU, or in response to the findings of effectiveness of risk minimisation evaluations (i.e. they may need to be replaced with more effective activities). Some risk minimisation activities might be needed to be retained for the lifetime of the medicinal product (e.g. pregnancy prevention programmes).

V.B.2. Responsibilities for Risk Management

The principal organisations directly involved in medicinal products' risk management planning are applicants/marketing authorisation holders and the competent authorities who regulate the medicinal products.

An applicant/marketing authorisation holder is responsible for:
- Having an appropriate risk management system in place [DIR 8(3)(iaa); DIR Art 104(3)(c)];
- Ensuring that the knowledge and understanding on the product's safety profile, following its use in clinical practice, are critically reviewed. The marketing authorisation holder should monitor pharmacovigilance data to determine whether there are new risks or whether risks have changed or whether there are changes to the risk-benefit balance of medicinal products [Dir Art 104(3)(e)], and update the risk management system and the RMP accordingly, as described below. The critical review of the safety profile of the product is a continuous activity and is reflected in data submitted with periodic safety update reports (PSUR) (see GVP Module VII), where an RMP submission may or may not be warranted. In addition, there are two specific milestones when the marketing authorisation holders of products approved following full initial marketing authorisation applications are advised to reflect on the need to review the list of safety concerns and the planned and ongoing pharmacovigilance and risk minimisation activities:
- With the (first) 5-year renewal;
- In the time period when the first PSUR following the first 5 year renewal is due for submission. It is anticipated that this PSUR submission would occur approximately 8-9 years following the granting of the marketing authorisation, at the time when the assessment of the initial marketing authorisation applications for generic products for the active substance commences. As such, the safety profile of the medicinal product is likely to be sufficiently well characterised to allow for a critical review and update of the list of safety concerns.

V.B.3. Overview of the Format and Content of the Risk Management Plan (RMP)

The RMP consists of seven parts. The submitted RMP shall follow the RMP template [IR Annex I]. Part II of the RMP - Safety specification is subdivided into modules [IR Annex I], so the content can be tailored to the specifics of the medicinal product. RMP part II modules generally follow the section titles in the safety specification of ICH-E2E (see GVP Annex IV). The modular structure aims to facilitate the update of the RMP; in addition, in specific circumstances certain RMP modules may have reduced content requirements (see V.C.1.1.). However, the RMP document is expected to be submitted as one single document including all modules and annexes, as relevant.

Table V.1: Overview of the RMP parts and modules

Part I	Product(s) overview
Part II	Safety specification
Module SI	Epidemiology of the indication(s) and target population(s)
Module SII	Non-clinical part of the safety specification
Module SIII	Clinical trial exposure
Module SIV	Populations not studied in clinical trials
Module SV	Post-authorisation experience
Module SVI	Additional EU requirements for the safety specification
Module SVII	Identified and potential risks
Module SVIII	Summary of the safety concerns
Part III	Pharmacovigilance plan (including post-authorisation safety studies)
Part IV	Plans for post-authorisation efficacy studies
Part V	Risk minimisation measures (including evaluation of the effectiveness of risk minimisation activities)
Part VI	Summary of the risk management plan
Part VII	Annexes

An overview of the parts and modules of the RMP is provided in Table V.1. [IR Annex I]:

The amount of information, particularly in RMP part II, should be proportionate to the identified risk and the potential risk, and will depend on the type of medicinal product, its risks, and where it is situated in its life cycle [by reference to DIR Art 8(3)].

Article 14(2) of Regulation (EC) No 1394/2007 provides for a specific framework for RMP for advanced therapy medicinal products (ATMP). The marketing authorisation applicants/holders should adapt the risk management plans of ATMP, considering and discussing the anticipated post-authorisation follow-up needs, focusing on particularities of these medicinal products. The specific RMP content requirements for ATMP should be discussed with the competent authority before the submission. Further guidance on the safety and efficacy follow-up and risk management requirements for ATMP is provided on the Agency's website[2].

It is recommended, where appropriate, that the RMP document includes all relevant medicinal products from the same applicant/marketing authorisation holder containing the same active substance(s) (i.e. the RMP is an active substance-based document) [IR Art 30(2)].

Information in the RMP should be provided in enough detail whilst avoiding unnecessary text that distracts from the key issues to be considered for risk management of the product. However, the safety specifications in the RMP should not be a duplication of data submitted elsewhere in the dossier, unless the sections are intended to be common modules with other documents such as the PSUR. Where applicable, the information in the RMP should provide an integrated overview/discussion focusing on the most important risks that have been identified or are anticipated based on pre-clinical, clinical and post-marketing data presented in other modules of the eCTD. Any data included in the RMP should be consistent with other sections of the dossier. Links or references to relevant sections of the non-clinical and clinical overviews and summaries should be included in the RMP.

For new RMP submissions for nationally authorised products with limited safety data in the dossier, the RMP may contain the relevant safety data and discussion, to support the risk identification discussion.

To aid consistency between the information provided in the dossier and the RMP, Table V.2. indicates where information from the eCTD is likely to be discussed in the RMP. The eCTD data refers to the submission containing the RMP (e.g. initial marketing authorisation applications and major variations) or to historical data already included in the dossier with previous submissions.

In the context of a centralised procedure, the RMP should be submitted as part of an eCTD submission; however, for non-centralised procedures the RMP submission might still be part of a CTD submission. eCTD data/submissions in this Module should be read as eCTD or CTD

---

2. *See* www.ema.europa.eu; further ATMP-specific guidance is being developed

Table V.2: Mapping between RMP modules and information in eCTD

RMP Module	eCTD
Part I Product(s) overview	Module 2.3 Quality overall summary Module 3 Quality
Module SI Epidemiology of the indication(s) and target population(s)	Module 2.5 Clinical overview
Module SII Non-clinical part of the safety specification	Module 2.4 Non-clinical overview Module 2.6 Non-clinical written and tabulated summaries Module 4 Non-clinical study reports
Module SIII Clinical trial exposure	Module 2.7 Clinical summary Module 5 Clinical Study reports
Module SIV Populations not studied in clinical trials	Module 2.5 Clinical overview
Module SV Post-authorisation experience	Module 2.5 Clinical overview
Module SVI "Additional EU requirements for the safety specification"	Data not presented elsewhere in eCTD
Module SVII Identified and potential risks	Module 2.5 Clinical overview (including benefit-risk conclusion) Module 2.7 Clinical summary (SPC)
Module SVIII Summary of the safety concerns	Module 2.5 Clinical overview Module 2.7 Clinical summary
Part III Pharmacovigilance plan (including post-authorisation safety studies)	Module 2.5 Clinical overview Module 2.7 Clinical summary
Part IV Plans for post-authorisation efficacy studies	Module 2.5 Clinical overview Module 2.7 Clinical summary
Part V Risk minimisation measures (including evaluation of the effectiveness of risk minimisation activities)	Module 2.5 Clinical overview Module 2.7 Clinical summary

data/submission, corresponding to the type of submission to the competent authority.

Only key literature referenced in the RMP should be included in RMP annex 7. This should be in the format of electronic links or references if already included elsewhere in eCTD (*see* V.B.10.).

The description of the parts and modules of an RMP in V.B.4. provides guidance on the main topics to be addressed within each specific area. However, some sections may not be relevant to all medicinal products and there may be additional topics that need to be included but are not mentioned in this guidance. The RMP is part of the scientific dossier of a product and as such should be scientifically based and should not include any element of a promotional nature.

The preliminary section of the RMP should include the following administrative information about the RMP document:
- Data lock point of the current RMP;
- Sign off date and the version number of the RMP;
- List of all parts and modules. For RMP updates, modules version number and date of approval (opinion date) should be tabulated in this section. High level comment on the rationale for creating the update should be included for significant changes to each module;
- The evidence of oversight from the qualified person for pharmacovigilance (QPPV) is not needed for versions submitted for assessment. The QPPV's actual signature or the evidence that the RMP was reviewed and approved by the QPPV should be included in the finalised approved version of the document; for eCTD submissions this would be the RMP with the last eCTD sequence of the procedure (e.g. closing sequence). The evidence of QPPV oversight can take the form of a statement that the RMP has been reviewed and approved by the marketing

authorisation holder/applicant's QPPV and that the electronic signature is on file.

V.B.4. RMP Part I "Product(s) Overview"

This should provide the administrative information on the RMP and an overview of the product(s). The information presented should be current and accurate in relation to the ongoing application as it is anticipated to appear in the marketing authorisation. The information should include:

Active substance information:
- Active substance(s);
- Pharmacotherapeutic group(s) (ATC code);
- Name of the:
  - Marketing authorisation applicant- for initial marketing authorisation applications; or
  - Marketing authorisation holder - for RMPs submitted with post-authorisation procedures;
- For mutual recognition/decentralised procedures applications: the name(s) of the expected future marketing authorisation holder(s) in the reference Member State, if known at the time of the application;
- Medicinal product(s) to which this RMP refers.
- Authorisation procedure(s) (centralised, mutual recognition, decentralised, national);
- Invented name(s) in the European Economic Area (EEA);
- Brief description of the product including:
  - Chemical class;
  - Summary of mode of action;
  - Important information about its composition (e.g. origin of active substance of biologicals, relevant adjuvants or residues for vaccines);
- eCTD link to the proposed product information, as appropriate;
- Indications: approved and proposed (if RMP submitted with an extension/restriction of indication);
- Dosage (summary information – only related to main population; not a duplication of SmPC section 4.2);
- Pharmaceutical forms and strengths;
- Whether the product is subject to additional monitoring in the EU (at initial marketing authorisation application conclusion or with RMP updates).

V.B.5. RMP Part II "Safety Specification"

The purpose of the safety specification is to provide an adequate discussion on the safety profile of the medicinal product(s), with focus on those aspects that need further risk management activities. It should include a summary of the important identified risks of a medicinal product, important potential risks, and missing information. It should also address the populations potentially at risk (where the product is likely to be used, i.e. both as authorised and off-label use), and any outstanding safety questions that warrant further investigation to refine the understanding of the risk-benefit balance during the post-authorisation period. The safety specification forms the basis of the pharmacovigilance plan and the risk minimisation plan.

The safety specification consists of eight RMP modules, of which RMP modules SI-SV, SVII and SVIII correspond to safety specification headings in ICH-E2E. RMP module SVI includes additional elements required to be submitted in the EU.

Although the elements outlined in V.B.5.2. to V.B.5.9. serve as a guide only, it is recommended that applicants/ marketing authorisation holders follow the structure provided when compiling the safety specification.

Details of specific requirements for initial marketing authorisation applications are included in V.C.1.1..

V.B.5.1. General Considerations for Generic Products and Advanced Therapy Medicinal Products

V.B.5.1.1. Generics
For generic medicinal products the expectation is that the safety specification is the same as that of the reference product or of other generic products for which an RMP is in place. If discrepancies exist between approved RMPs for such products, then the applicant is expected to propose and justify the most appropriate safety specification for their product. Exceptionally, the applicant for a new generic medicinal product may add or remove

safety concerns compared with the safety profile of the reference product if this is appropriately justified (for example, when there is a more up to date understanding of the current safety profile or when there are differences in product characteristics compared with the reference product, e.g. there is a risk associated with an excipient present only in some of the products containing the same active substance).

V.B.5.1.2. Advanced Therapy Medicinal Products
Under Regulation (EC) No 1394/2007, certain products for human medicinal use are categorised within the EU as advanced therapy medicinal products. These products are fully defined in the above Regulation but broadly comprise:
- Gene therapy medicinal products;
- Somatic cell therapy medicinal products;
- Tissue engineered products.

Because of the nature of these products, risks may occur that are not normally a concern with other medicinal products including risks to living donors, risks of germ line transformation and transmission of vectors. These risks need to be taken into consideration when developing the safety specification for ATMPs (see V.B.5.8.).

V.B.5.2. RMP Part II, Module SI "Epidemiology of the Indication(s) and Target Population(s)"

This RMP module should include incidence, prevalence, outcome of the (untreated) target disease (i.e. indications) and relevant co-morbidity, and should when relevant for assessment of safety and risk management be stratified by age, gender, and ethnic origin. Risk factors for the disease and the main existing treatment options should also be described. The emphasis should be on the epidemiology of the proposed indication in the EU. Differences in the epidemiology in different regions should be discussed (where epidemiology varies across regions).

This section should also describe the relevant adverse events to be anticipated in the (untreated) target population in EU, their frequency and characteristics. The text should help anticipate and interpret any potential signals and help identify opportunities for risk minimisation. The text should be kept concise and should not include any element of a promotional nature.

V.B.5.3. RMP Part II, Module SII "Non-clinical Part of the Safety Specification"

This RMP module should present a high-level summary of the significant non-clinical safety findings, for example:
- Toxicity (key issues identified from acute or repeat-dose toxicity, reproductive/developmental toxicity, genotoxicity, carcinogenicity);
- Safety pharmacology (e.g. cardiovascular system, including QT interval prolongation, nervous system);
- Other toxicity-related information or data.

What constitutes an important non-clinical safety finding will depend upon the medicinal product, the target population and experience with other similar compounds or therapies in the same class. Normally, significant areas of toxicity (by target organ system) and the relevance of the findings to the use in humans should be discussed. Also, quality aspects if relevant to safety (e.g. genotoxic impurities) should be discussed. If a product is intended for use in women of childbearing age, data on the reproductive/developmental toxicity should be explicitly mentioned and the implications for use in this population discussed. Where the non-clinical safety finding could constitute an important potential risk to the target population, it should be included as a safety concern in RMP module SVIII. Where the non-clinical safety finding is not considered relevant for human beings, provision of a brief explanation is required, but the safety finding is not expected to be carried forward to SVII and SVIII as a safety concern.

If, based on the assessment of the non-clinical or clinical data, additional non-clinical studies are considered warranted and proposed to be part of the pharmacovigilance plan, this should be briefly discussed here.

Final conclusions on this section should be aligned with content of module SVII and any safety concerns should be carried forward to module SVIII.

The content of this section should be assessed for relevance over time. Post-authorisation, this section would only be expected to be updated when new non-clinical data impact the list of safety concerns. Safety concerns identified on the basis of non-clinical data which are no longer relevant and/or have not been confirmed when sufficient relevant post-marketing experience and evidence are gathered, can be removed from the list of safety concerns.

V.B.5.4. RMP Part II, Module SIII "Clinical Trial Exposure"

In this RMP module, in order to assess the limitations of the human safety database, summary information on the patients studied in clinical trials should be provided in an appropriate format (e.g. tables/graphs) at time of submission of the initial RMP or when there is a major update due to new exposure data from clinical studies (e.g. in a new indication). The content of this section should be assessed for relevance over time and, in the absence of new significant clinical trial exposure data, this section does not need to be updated.

The size of the study population should be detailed using both numbers of patients and, where appropriate, patient time exposed to the medicinal product. This should be stratified for relevant categories; stratifications would normally include:
- Age and gender;
- Indication;
- Dose;
- Other stratifications should be provided where this adds meaningful information for risk management planning purposes (e.g. ethnic origin).
- Paediatric data should be divided by age categories (e.g. ICH-E11[3]); similarly the data on older people should be stratified into age categories reflecting the target population (e.g. 65-74, 75-84 and 85 years and above).

Unless clearly relevant and duly justified, data should not be presented by individual trial, but pooled. Totals should be provided for each table/graph as appropriate. Where patients have been enrolled in more than one trial (e.g. open label extension study following a trial) they should only be included once in the age/gender/ethnic origin tables. Reasons for differences in the total numbers of patients between tables should be explained.

When the RMP is being submitted with an application for a new indication, a new pharmaceutical form or route of administration, the clinical trial data specific to the application should be presented separately at the start of the module as well as being pooled across all indications.

V.B.5.5. RMP Part II, Module SIV "Populations Not Studied in Clinical Trials"

Populations that are considered under missing information should be described in this RMP module.

Information on the low exposure of special populations or the lack thereof (e.g. pregnant women, breast-feeding women, patients with renal impairment, hepatic impairment or cardiac impairment, populations with relevant genetic polymorphisms, immuno-compromised patients and populations of different ethnic origins) should be provided where available and as appropriate. The degree of renal, hepatic or cardiac impairment should be specified as well as the type of genetic polymorphism, as available.

If the product is expected to be used in populations not studied and if there is a scientific rationale to suspect a different safety profile, but the available information is insufficient to determine whether or not the use in these circumstances could constitute a safety concern, then this should be included as missing information in the RMP. Excluded populations from the clinical trial development programme should be included as missing information only when they are relevant for the approved and proposed indications, i.e. "on-label", and if the use in such populations might be associated with risks of clinical significance. In discussing differences between target populations and those exposed in clinical trials it should be noted that some differences may arise through trial setting (e.g. hospital or general practice) rather than through explicit inclusion/exclusion criteria. When such populations are proposed as missing information, then RMP module SIV should also include a discussion on the relevant subpopulations.

If there is evidence that use in excluded populations is associated with an undesirable clinical outcome, then the outcome should be included as an important (potential) risk.

---

3. See http://www.ema.europa.eu/ema/index.jsp?curl=pages/regulation/general/general_content_000429.jsp&mid=WC0b01ac0580029590

V.B.5.6. RMP Part II, Module SV "Post-authorisation Experience"

If post-marketing data are available from post-authorisation experience in other regions outside EU, where the product is already authorised or from other authorised products containing the same active substance, from the same marketing authorisation holder, the data should be discussed in this RMP module.

It should only provide an overview of experience in the post-authorisation phase that is helpful for risk management planning purposes. It is not the intention to duplicate information from the PSUR.

Additionally, a discussion on how the medicinal product is being used in practice and on-label and off-label use, including use in the special populations mentioned in RMP module SIV, can also be included when relevant for the risk identification discussion in module SVII.

Where appropriate and relevant for the discussion in SVII, data on use in markets outside the EU from indications not authorised in EU should also be summarised, and the implications for the authorisation in the EU should be discussed.

V.B.5.7. RMP Part II, Module SVI "Additional EU Requirements for the Safety Specification"

In addition to safety topics required by ICH-E2E (see GVP Annex IV), the following should be addressed in the EU-RMP: the potential for misuse for illegal purposes, and, where appropriate, the proposed risk minimisation measures, e.g. limited pack size, controlled access programme, special medical prescription [DIR Art 71(2)] (see also V.B.8.).

V.B.5.8. RMP Part II, Module SVII "Identified and Potential Risks"

This RMP module should provide a focussed discussion on the identification of important identified and important potential risks, and missing information (i.e. safety concerns).

The following safety topics derived from specific situations/data sources are thought to be of particular interest for the risk identification discussion in module SVII, and should be discussed when they lead to risks of the product:

- *Potential harm from overdose*, whether intentional or accidental, for example in cases where there is a narrow therapeutic margin or potential for major dose-related toxicity, and/or where there is a high risk of intentional overdose in the treated population (e.g. in depression). Where harm from overdose has occurred during clinical trials this should be explicitly mentioned and, where relevant, the important risks following overdose should be included as safety concerns in RMP module SVIII and appropriate risk minimisation proposed in RMP part V;

- *Potential for risks resulting from medication errors*, defined as an unintended failure in the drug treatment process that leads to, or has the potential to lead to, harm to the patient. Medication errors leading to important risks, identified during product development including clinical trials, should be discussed and information on the errors, their potential cause(s) and possible remedies given. Where applicable an indication should be given of how these have been taken into account in the final product design. Further guidance on medication errors is provided in Good Practice Guide on Risk Minimisation and Prevention of Medication Errors, Annex 2 - Design features which should be considered to reduce the risk of medication error[4] which includes an extensive list of potential medication errors and the consequence to the patients. Important risks related to medication errors in the post marketing period should be discussed in the updated RMP and ways of limiting the errors proposed;

- *Potential for transmission of infectious agents* due to the nature of the manufacturing process or the materials involved. For live attenuated vaccines any potential for transmission of mutated live vaccine virus, and the potential of causing the disease in immunocompromised contacts of the vaccine should be discussed with the view of considering them as important potential risks;

- *Potential for off-label use*, when differences in safety concerns between the target and the off-

---

4. *See* www.ema.europa.eu, EMA/606103/2014

label population are anticipated, the potential risks arising from the off-label use of the product should be considered for inclusion in the safety specifications;
- If an important identified or potential risk common to other members of the pharmacological class is not thought to be an important identified or important potential risk with the concerned medicinal product, the evidence to support this should be provided and discussed;
- *Important risks* related to identified and potential pharmacokinetic and pharmacodynamic interactions should be discussed in relation to the treatments for the condition, but also in relation to commonly used medications in the target population. The evidence supporting the interaction and possible mechanism should be summarised, the potential health risks discussed for different indications and populations, and plans to further characterise and minimise the risks described. Important risks derived from interactions should be included as a safety concern;
- *Risks in pregnant and lactating women*, e.g. teratogenic risk - direct or through exposure to semen: contraception recommendations can be considered as risk minimisation measures. Further guidance on risk management in case of exposure of the embryo / foetus to teratogenic agents can be found in the GVP P.III. and GVP Module XVI;
- *Effect on fertility* - appropriate risk minimisation measures should be considered, e.g. routine risk communication and/or additional activities recommending fertility preservation: sperm cryopreservation in men and embryo and oocyte cryopreservation in women;
- Risks associated with the disposal of the used product (e.g. transdermal patches with remaining active substance or remains of radioactive diagnostics);
- Risks related to the administration procedure (e.g. risks related to the use of a medical device (malfunction which impacts on the dose administered, risk of variability in complex administrations);
- Paediatric safety issues that are particular causes of concern in paediatric population,

as described in section 5 of annex I of the PIP opinion (Potential long-term safety/efficacy issues in relation to paediatric use for consideration in the RMP/Pharmacovigilance activities).

For RMPs of ATMPs, the applicants should also consider the possible specific risks in drafting the safety specifications (*see* Guideline on Safety and Efficacy Follow-up – Risk Management of Advanced Therapy Medicinal Products[5]).

V.B.5.8.1. RMP Part II, Module SVII Section "Identification of Safety Concerns in the Initial Rmp Submission"

This RMP section should contain the initial identification of safety concerns and is expected to be populated with the initial submission of an RMP, either at the time of the initial marketing authorisation (MA) application or post-authorisation (i.e. for approved products that previously did not have an RMP).

This section is expected to be "locked" and not change after the approval of the initial RMP.

V.B.5.8.1.a. RMP Part II, Module SVII Sections "Risk Considered Important for Inclusion in the List of Safety Concerns" and "Risk not Considered Important for Inclusion in the List of Safety Concerns"

In this RMP section the following information should be summarised and discussed:
- Risk seriousness;
- Risk frequency;
- The risk-benefit impact of the risks.

For risks not taken forward as safety concerns, the information can be grouped by reasons for not including them as safety concerns.

V.B.5.8.2. RMP Part II, Module SVII Section "New Safety Concerns and Reclassification with a Submission of an Updated RMP"

In the post-authorisation phase, it is expected that new identified and potential risks of the product are presented in the safety section of the dossier (with e.g. signal evaluation, periodic benefit-risk evaluation, or safety variations procedures) together with an evaluation on whether the risks should be considered important and added in the safety specification in the RMP. This discussion should not be duplicated in the RMP, but the details

---
5. *See* www.ema.europa.eu

of any new important identified or potential risk should be included in the RMP section described in V.B.5.8.3..

When an important identified or potential risk or missing information is re-classified or removed, a justification should be provided in this RMP section, with appropriate reference to the safety data. The information included in this section may take the form of a statement describing a previous regulatory request, with a reference to the procedure where such request was formulated.

V.B.5.8.3. RMP Part II, Module SVII Section "Details of Important Identified Risks, Important Potential Risks, and Missing Information"

For RMPs containing multiple products, if there are significant differences between products (e.g. fixed dose combination products) it is appropriate to make it clear which safety concerns relate to which product.

This RMP section applies to all stages of the product's life cycle.

Presentation of important identified risks and important potential risks data:
- Name of the risk (using MedDRA terms when appropriate);
- Potential mechanism;
- Evidence source(s) and strength of the evidence (i.e. the scientific basis for suspecting the association);
- Characterisation of the risk: e.g. frequency, absolute risk, relative risk, severity, reversibility, long-term outcomes, impact on quality of life;
- Risk factors and risk groups (including patient factors, dose, at risk period, additive or synergistic factors);
- Preventability (i.e. predictability of a risk; whether risk factors have been identified that can be minimised by routine or additional risk minimisation activities other than general awareness using the PI; possibility of detection at an early stage which could mitigate seriousness);
- Impact on the risk-benefit balance of the product;
- Public health impact (e.g. absolute risk in relation to the size of the target population and consequently actual number of individuals affected, or overall outcome at population level).

Presentation of missing information data:
- Name of the missing information (using MedDRA terms when appropriate);
- Evidence that the safety profile is expected to be different than in the general target population;
- Description of a population in need of further characterisation, or description of the risk anticipated in the population not studied, as appropriate.

V.B.5.9. RMP Part II, Module SVIII "Summary of the Safety Concerns"

In this RMP module, a list of safety concerns should be provided with the following categories:
- Important identified risks;
- Important potential risks;
- Missing information.

V.B.6. RMP Part III "Pharmacovigilance Plan (Including Post-authorisation Safety Studies)"

The purpose of the pharmacovigilance plan in part III of the RMP is to present an overview and discuss how the applicant/marketing authorisation holder plans to further characterise the safety concerns in the safety specification. It provides a structured plan for:
- The investigation of whether a potential risk is confirmed as an identified risk or refuted;
- Further characterisation of safety concerns including severity, frequency, and risk factors;
- How missing information will be sought;
- Measuring the effectiveness of risk minimisation measures.

It does not include actions intended to reduce, prevent or mitigate risks; these are discussed in RMP part V.

The pharmacovigilance plan should focus on the safety concerns summarised in RMP module SVIII of the safety specifications and should be proportionate to the benefits and risks of the product. Early discussions between competent authorities and the applicant/marketing authorisation holder are recommended to identify whether, and which, additional pharmacovigilance activities are needed and consequently milestones should be agreed.

Pharmacovigilance activities can be divided into routine and additional pharmacovigilance activities.

V.B.6.1. RMP Part III Section "Routine Pharmacovigilance Activities"

Routine pharmacovigilance is the primary/minimum set of activities required for all medicinal products as per the obligations set out in DIR and REG. Signal detection, which is part of routine pharmacovigilance, is an important element in identifying new risks for all products. The descriptions of these activities in the pharmacovigilance system master file (*see* GVP Module II) are not required to be repeated in the RMP.

The Pharmacovigilance Risk Assessment Committee (PRAC), the Committee for Medicinal Products for Human Use (CHMP), the Coordination Group for Mutual recognition and Decentralised Procedures – Human (CMDh), or national competent authorities may make recommendations for specific activities related to the collection, collation, assessment and reporting of spontaneous reports of adverse reactions which differ from the normal requirements for routine pharmacovigilance (*see* GVP Module I). If these recommendations include recording of tests (including in a structured format) that would form part of standard clinical practice for a patient experiencing the adverse reaction, then this requirement would still be considered routine. The routine pharmacovigilance section of the pharmacovigilance plan should be used in these circumstances to explain how the applicant will modify its routine pharmacovigilance activities to fulfil any special PRAC, CHMP, CMDh, and national competent authority recommendations on routine pharmacovigilance.

However, if the recommendation includes the submission of tissue or blood samples to a specific laboratory (e.g. for antibody testing) that is outside standard clinical practice, then this would constitute an additional pharmacovigilance activity.

This RMP section should describe only the routine pharmacovigilance activities beyond adverse reaction reporting and signal detection.

V.B.6.1.1. Specific Adverse Reaction Follow-Up Questionnaires

Where an applicant/marketing authorisation holder is requested, or plans, to use specific questionnaires to obtain structured information on reported suspected adverse reactions of special interest, the use of these materials should be described in the routine pharmacovigilance activities section and copies of these forms should be provided in RMP annex 4.

Without prejudice to the originality of the format of the questionnaire(s), it is in the interest of public health that questionnaire(s) used by different applicants/marketing authorisation holders for the same adverse event should be kept as similar as possible, in order to deliver a consistent message and to provide useful data for the analysis of the reports, which are relevant for regulatory decisions, while decreasing the burden on healthcare professionals. Therefore, marketing authorisation holders are strongly encouraged to share the content of their questionnaire(s) upon request from other marketing authorisation holders.

V.B.6.1.2. Other Forms of Routine Pharmacovigilance Activities

The description of the planned other forms of routine pharmacovigilance activities should be described in this section, e.g. the high level description of the enhanced passive surveillance system, observed versus expected analyses, cumulative reviews of adverse events of interest.

V.B.6.2. RMP Part III Section "Additional pharmacovigilance Activities"

The applicant/marketing authorisation holder should list in this RMP section their planned additional pharmacovigilance activities, detailing what information is expected to be collected that can lead to a more informed consideration of the risk-benefit balance.

Additional pharmacovigilance activities are pharmacovigilance activities that are not considered routine. They may be non-clinical studies, clinical trials or non-interventional studies. Examples include long-term follow-up of patients from the clinical trial population or a cohort study to provide additional characterisation of the long-term safety of the medicinal product. When any doubt exists about the need for additional pharmacovigilance activities, consultation with a competent authority should be considered.

Studies in the pharmacovigilance plan aim to identify and characterise risks, to collect further data where there are areas of missing information or to evaluate the effectiveness of additional risk minimisation activities. They should relate to the safety concerns identified in the safety specification, be feasible and should not include any element of a promotional nature.

Studies in the pharmacovigilance plan should be designed and conducted according to the respective legislation in place, and recommendations in the GVP Module VIII.

Study protocols may be included for evaluation in an RMP update only when the studies are included in the pharmacovigilance plan and the protocols submission has been requested by the competent authority. Reviewed and approved protocols for studies in the pharmacovigilance plan should be provided in RMP annex 3 – part C (or electronic links or references to the protocol included in other section of the eCTD dossier). Other category 3 studies protocols, submitted for information only, may also be included in RMP annex 3 – part C. Protocols of completed studies should be removed from RMP annex 3 once the final study reports are submitted to the competent authority for assessment and the study is removed from the parmacovigilance plan (see V.B.10.3.).

The milestones for the final study report submission to the competent authority should be included for all studies in the pharmacovigilance plan.

Marketing authorisation holders may also submit to EMA or national competent authorities protocols of post-authorisation safety studies (PASS) for scientific advice.

V.B.6.3. RMP Part III Section "Summary Table of Additional Pharmacovigilance Activities"

This RMP section outlines the pharmacovigilance activities designed to identify and characterise risks associated with the use of a medicinal product. Some may be imposed as conditions to the marketing authorisation, either because they are key to the risk-benefit profile of the product (category 1 studies in the pharmacovigilance plan), or because they are specific obligations in the context of a conditional marketing authorisation or a marketing authorisation under exceptional circumstances (category 2 studies in the pharmacovigilance plan). If the condition or the specific obligation is a non-interventional PASS, it will be subject to the supervision set out in DIR Art 107m-q and the format and content of such non-interventional PASS should be as described in IR Annex III (see GVP Module VIII).

Other studies might be required in the RMP to investigate a safety concern or to evaluate the effectiveness of risk minimisation activities. Such studies included in the pharmacovigilance plan are also legally enforceable (category 3 studies in the pharmacovigilance plan). The summary table of the pharmacovigilance plan should provide clarity to all stakeholders as to which category an activity in the pharmacovigilance plan falls under (see Table V.3.).

Studies required in jurisdictions outside the EU should not be included in the RMP unless they are also imposed as a condition to the marketing authorisation or as a specific obligation, or required by the Agency or a national competent authority. Studies not required by the EMA or a national competent authority should not be included in the pharmacovigilance plan in the RMP. This is without prejudice to safety concerns arising from any such studies, which should be reported as per the applicable legislation.

For generic products, the pharmacovigilance plan will reflect the outstanding needs for pharmacovigilance investigations at the time of their approval. In some cases, ongoing or planned PASS for the originator product would also be required to be conducted for the generic products (e.g. registries may need to be in place to include most/all patients treated with the medicine, be it generic or originator products). Where applicable, the marketing authorisation holders are encouraged to set up joint PASS, for instance in the case of registries or when a referral has resulted in an imposed PASS for all authorised medicinal products containing a named substance in a specified indication.

V.B.7. RMP Part IV "Plans for Post-Authorisation Efficacy Studies"

This RMP part should include a list of post-authorisation efficacy studies (PAES) imposed as conditions to the marketing authorisation or when included as specific obligations in the context of a conditional marketing authorisation or a marketing authorisation under exceptional circumstances. If no such studies are required, RMP Part IV may be left empty.

Table V.3: Attributes of additional pharmacovigilance activities

	Type of activity	In annex II of MA (CAPs only)	Study category (PhV plan)	Status	Supervised under Article 107m	Supervised under Article 107 n-q
Imposed PASS	"Interventional"*	Yes, in annex IID	1	Mandatory and subject to penalties	No	No
	Non-interventional	Yes, in annex IID			Yes	Yes
Specific obligation	"Interventional"*	Yes, in annex IIE	2	Mandatory and subject to penalties	No	No
	Non-interventional	Yes, in annex IIE			Yes	Yes
Required	"Interventional"*	No	3	Legally enforceable	No	No
	Non-interventional	No			Yes	No

*Clinical interventional studies are subject to the requirements of Directive 2001/20/EC. Non-clinical interventional studies are subject to the legal and ethical requirements related to the protection of laboratory animals, and Good Laboratory Practice as appropriate.

V.B.8. RMP Part V "Risk Minimisation Measures (Including Evaluation of the Effectiveness of Risk Minimisation Activities)"

Part V of the RMP should provide details of the risk minimisation measures which will be taken to reduce the risks associated with respective safety concerns.

For active substances where there are individual products with substantially different indications or target populations, it may be appropriate to have a risk minimisation plan specific to each product. i.e. products where the indications lie in different medical specialities and have different safety concerns associated; products where risks differ according to the target population; products with different legal status for the supply of medicinal products to patients.

The need for continuing risk minimisation measures should be reviewed at regular intervals and the effectiveness of risk minimisation activities assessed (*see* V.B.8.). Guidance on additional risk minimisation measures and the assessment of the effectiveness of risk minimisation measures is provided in GVP Module XVI and GVP Module XVI Addendum I – Educational materials.

Routine risk minimisation activities
Routine risk minimisation activities are those which apply to every medicinal product. These relate to:

- The summary of product characteristics;
- The labelling (e.g. on inner and outer carton);
- The package leaflet;
- The pack size(s);
- The legal status of the product.

Even the formulation itself may play an important role in minimising the risk of the product.

Summary of product characteristics (SmPC) and package leaflet (PL)

The summary of product characteristics and the package leaflet are important tools for risk minimisation as they constitute a controlled and standardised format for informing healthcare professionals and patients about the medicinal product. The Guideline on Summary of Product Characteristics provides guidance on how information should be presented.

Both materials provide routine risk minimisation recommendations; however, there are two types of messages the SmPC and PL can provide:

- **Routine risk communication messages:** usually found in section 4.8 of the SmPC or section 4 of the PL; these messages communicate to healthcare professionals and patients the undesirable effects of the medicinal product, so that an informed decision on the treatment can be made;
- **Routine risk minimisation activities recommending specific clinical measures to address the risk:** usually found in sections

4.2 and 4.4 of the SmPC but can also be found in sections 4.1, 4.3, 4.5, 4.6, 4.7 and 4.9, and sections 2 and 3 of the PL; warning and precaution messages and recommendations in the SmPC will include information on addressing the risk of the product by e.g.:
- Performing a test before the start of treatment;
- Monitoring of laboratory parameters during treatment;
- Monitoring for specific signs and symptoms;
- Adjusting the dose or stopping the treatment when adverse events are observed or laboratory parameters change;
- Performing a wash-out procedure after treatment interruption;
- Providing contraception recommendations;
- Prohibiting the use of other medicines while taking the product;
- Treating or preventing the risk factors that may lead to an adverse event of the product;
- Recommending long-term clinical follow-up to identify in early stages delayed adverse events.

Pack size

Since every pack size is specifically authorised for a medicinal product, planning the number of "dosage units" within each pack and the range of pack sizes available can be considered a form of routine risk management activity. In theory, controlling the number of "dosage units" should mean that patients will need to *see* a healthcare professional at defined intervals, thus increasing the opportunity for testing and reducing the length of time a patient is without review. In extreme cases, making units available in only one pack size to try to link prescribing to the need for review may be considered.

A small pack size can also be useful, especially if overdose or diversion are thought to be major risks.

Legal status

Controlling the conditions under which a medicinal product may be made available can reduce the risks associated with its use or misuse.

The marketing authorisation must include details of any conditions or restrictions imposed on the supply or the use of the medicinal product, including the conditions under which a medicinal product may be made available to patients. This is commonly referred to as the "legal status" of a medicinal product. Typically it includes information on whether or not the medicinal product is subject to medical prescription [DIR Art 71(1)]. It may also restrict where the medicinal product can be administered (e.g. in a hospital) or by whom it may be prescribed (e.g. specialist).

For medicinal products only available on prescription, additional conditions may be imposed by classifying them into those available only upon either a restricted medical prescription, or upon a special medical prescription.

Restricted medical prescription

This may be used to control who may initiate treatment, prescribe the medicinal product and the setting in which the medicinal product can be given or used. According to EU legislation, when considering classification of a medicinal product as subject to restricted medical prescription, the following factors shall be taken into account [DIR Art 71(3)]:
- The medicinal product, because of its pharmaceutical characteristics or novelty or in the interests of public health, is reserved for treatments which can only be followed in a hospital environment.
- The medicinal product is used in the treatment of conditions which must be diagnosed in a hospital environment or in institutions with adequate diagnostic facilities, although administration and follow-up may be carried out elsewhere.
- The medicinal product is intended for outpatients but its use may produce very serious adverse reactions requiring a prescription drawn up as required by a specialist and special supervision throughout the treatment.

Special medical prescription

For classification as 'subject to special medical prescription', the following factors shall be taken into account [DIR Art 71(2)]:
- The medicinal product contains, in a non-exempt quantity, a substance classified as a narcotic or a psychotropic substance within the meaning of the international conventions in force, such as the United Nations Conventions of 1961 and 1971;
- The medicinal product is likely, if incorrectly used, to present a substantial risk of medicinal abuse, to lead to addiction or be misused for illegal purposes, or

- The medicinal product contains a substance which, by reason of its novelty or properties, could be considered as belonging to the group envisaged in the second indent as a precautionary measure.

Categorisation at Member State level
There is the possibility of implementing sub-categories at Member State level, which permits the Member States to tailor the above-mentioned classifications to their national situation. The definitions and therefore also the implementation vary in those Member States where the sub-categories exist.

Additional risk minimisation activities
Additional risk minimisation activities should only be suggested when essential for the safe and effective use of the medicinal product. If additional risk minimisation activities are proposed, these should be detailed and a justification of why they are needed provided. The need for continuing with such measures should be periodically reviewed.

Where relevant, key messages of additional risk minimisation activities should be provided in RMP annex 6 – Details of proposed additional risk minimisation activities.

For medicinal products approved non-centrally, in situations where the need for additional risk minimisation may vary across Member States, the RMP can reflect that the need for (and content of) additional risk minimisation can be agreed at a national level.

Further guidance on additional risk minimisation measures is provided in GVP Module XVI.

Evaluation of the effectiveness of risk minimisation activities
When the RMP is updated, the risk minimisation plan should include a discussion of the impact of additional risk minimisation activities. Where relevant, such information may be presented by EU region.

A discussion on the results of any formal assessment(s) of risk minimisation activities should be included when available. If a particular risk minimisation strategy proves ineffective, or to be causing an excessive or undue burden on patients or the healthcare system then consideration should be given to alternative activities. The marketing authorisation holder should comment in the RMP on whether additional or different risk minimisation activities are needed for each safety concern or whether in their view the (additional) risk minimisation measures may be removed (e.g. when risk minimisation measures have become part of standard clinical practice).

If a study to evaluate the effectiveness of risk minimisation activities is required or imposed by the competent authority, the study should be included in the pharmacovigilance plan, part III of the RMP.

Guidance on monitoring the effectiveness of risk minimisation activities is included in the GVP Module XVI.

V.B.8.1. RMP Part V Section "Risk Minimisation Plan"

In the RMP section on the risk minimisation plan, for each safety concern in the safety specification, the following information should be provided:
- Routine risk minimisation activities, including details of whether only inclusion in the SmPC and PL is foreseen or any other routine risk minimisation activities are proposed;
- Additional risk minimisation activities (if any), including individual objectives and justification of why needed, and how their effectiveness will be measured.

V.B.8.2. RMP Part V Section "Summary of Risk Minimisation Measures"

A table listing the routine and additional risk minimisation activities by safety concern should be provided in this RMP section (e.g. the SmPC section number where the risk appears in the SmPC, the list of educational materials). A further summary of pharmacovigilance activities should be included, as described in the EMA Guidance on Format of the Risk Management Plan in the EU[6].

V.B.9. RMP Part VI "Summary of the Risk Management Plan"

A summary of the RMP for each authorised medicinal product shall be made publicly available

---
6. *See* www.ema.europa.eu

and shall include the key elements of the risk management plan [REG Art 26(1)(c), DIR Art 106(c), IR Art 31(1)].

Part VI of the RMP shall be provided by the marketing authorisation applicant/holder for medicinal products which have an RMP, regardless of whether they are centrally or nationally authorised in the EU. Based on the information contained in part VI of the RMP, for centrally authorised medicinal products, the Agency should publish the RMP summary on the EMA website at the time of the European Commission decision together with the other documents of the European public assessment report (EPAR) of that medicinal product. For nationally authorised medicinal products, a summary of the RMP should be published on the national competent authorities' websites.

The RMP summary should be updated when important changes are introduced into the full RMP. Changes should be considered important if they relate to the following:
- New important identified or potential risks or important changes to or removal of a safety concern;
- Inclusion or removal of additional risk minimisation measures or routine risk minimisation activities recommending specific clinical measures to address the risk;
- Major changes to the pharmacovigilance plan (e.g. addition of new studies or completion of ongoing studies).

The audience of RMP summaries is very broad. To ensure that the summary can satisfy the different needs, it should be written and presented clearly, using a plain-language approach[7]. However, this does not mean that technical terms should be avoided. The document should clearly explain its purpose and how it relates to other information, in particular the product information (i.e. the SmPC, the PL and the labelling).

The summary of the RMP part VI should be consistent with the information presented in RMP part II modules SVII, SVIII and RMP parts III, IV and V. It should contain the following information:
- The medicinal product and what it is authorised for;
- Summary of safety concerns and missing information;
- Routine and additional risk minimisation measures;
- Additional pharmacovigilance activities.

V.B.10. RMP Part VII "Annexes to the Risk Management Plan"

The RMP should contain the annexes listed below (if applicable). If the RMP applies to more than one medicinal product, usually it would be expected that the annexes will be relevant for all products. Particular aspects not applicable to all medicinal products in the RMP should be highlighted (e.g. a follow-up form in annex 4 might only be applicable to the products containing the active substance that is causally linked to the event).

V.B.10.1. RMP Annex 1

Annex 1 of the RMP is the structured electronic representation of the EU risk management plan. It is not required to be submitted in eCTD, the electronic file should be submitted in accordance to V.C.2. and the applicable guidance[8]. This annex can be left empty in the RMP document.

V.B.10.2. RMP Annex 2: Tabulated Summary of Planned, on-Going, and Completed Pharmacovigilance Study Programme

This annex should include a tabulation of studies included in the pharmacovigilance plan (current

---

7. Plain-language approach includes organising information logically (and giving priority to action points), breaking information into digestible chunks, and using layout that improves readability of a document. *See* http://www.plainenglish.co.uk/campaigning/past-campaigns/legal/drafting-in-plain-english.html and Office of Disease Prevention and Health Promotion. Plain language: a promising strategy for clearly communicating health information and improving health literacy. US Department of Health and Human Services, Rockville. Accessible at: http://health.gov/communication/literacy/plainlanguage/IssueBrief.pdf (accessed 1 Sep 2015).

8. *See* http://www.ema.europa.eu/ema/index.jsp?curl=pages/regulation/general/general_content_000683.jsp&mid=WC0b01ac058067a113

or in previous RMP versions; category 1, 2 and 3 studies), as follows:
- Planned and ongoing studies, including objectives, safety concern addressed, and the planned dates of submission of intermediate and final results.
- Completed studies, including objectives, safety concern addressed, and the date of submission of results to the competent authorities (effective, planned, or state the reason for not submitting the results).

V.B.10.3. RMP Annex 3: Protocols for Proposed, on-Going, and Completed Studies in the Pharmacovigilance Plan

Annex 3 should not include protocols of studies not imposed nor requested by the competent authority (i.e. not in the pharmacovigilance plan). This annex may include the electronic links or references to other modules of the eCTD dossier where the protocols are included, instead of the full protocol documents.

V.B.10.3.1. RMP Annex 3 – part A: Requested protocols of studies in the pharmacovigilance plan, submitted for regulatory review with this updated version of the RMP

If protocols have been requested to be submitted for review by the competent authority, and the marketing authorisation holder choses to submit for assessment a study protocol within the same procedure as the RMP submission, part A should include this protocol; alternatively the protocol might be reviewed in a stand-alone procedure, and once agreed, included in the RMP annex 3 – part C. The regulatory pathway for the protocol submission should be agreed with the competent authority.

V.B.10.3.2. RMP Annex 3 – Part B: Requested Amendments of Previously Approved Protocols of Studies in the Pharmacovigilance Plan, Submitted for Regulatory Review with this Updated Version of the RMP

If protocols amendments have been requested to be submitted for review by the competent authority, and the marketing authorisation holder choses to submit for assessment the study protocol amendment within the same procedure as the RMP submission, part B should include the updated protocol; alternatively the protocol amendment might be reviewed in a stand-alone procedure, and once agreed, included in the RMP annex 3 – part C. The regulatory pathway for the protocol submission should be agreed with the competent authority.

Once approved, protocols from parts A or B should be moved to part C, with the next warranted RMP update.

V.B.10.3.3. RMP Annex 3 – Part C: Previously Agreed Protocols for on-Going Studies and Final Protocols not Reviewed by the Competent Authority

Previously agreed protocols for on-going studies and final protocols not reviewed by the competent authority should be included in this part C of RMP annex 3, as follows:
- The full protocols that have been previously assessed by the competent authority and agreed (i.e. no protocol resubmission was requested). The protocols should be accompanied by the name of the procedure when the protocol was approved and date of the outcome. This may include the electronic link or reference to other modules of the eCTD dossier where the protocols have been previously submitted, instead of the full protocol documents.
- The final protocols of other category 3 studies: protocols that were not requested to be reviewed by the competent authorities and are submitted by the marketing authorisation holder for information only.

Protocols of completed studies should be removed from this annex once the final study reports are submitted to the competent authority for assessment.

V.B.10.4. RMP Annex 4: Specific Adverse Event Follow-up forms

This annex should include all follow-up forms used by the marketing authorisation holder to collect additional data on specific safety concerns. The usage of follow-up forms included in this annex should be detailed in the pharmacovigilance plan in the RMP, as routine pharmacovigilance activities.

The forms that should be included in this annex are sometimes known as "event follow-up questionnaire", "adverse event data capture/collection aid" or "adverse reaction follow-up form".

V.B.10.5. RMP Annex 5: Protocols for Proposed and on-going Studies in RMP Part IV

This annex should include links or reference to other parts of the eCTD dossier, where the protocols for an imposed efficacy study are already included, for studies included in RMP part IV.

V.B.10.6. RMP Annex 6: Details of Proposed Additional Risk Minimisation Activities

If applicable, this annex should include the proposed draft (and approved, if applicable) key messages of the additional risk minimisation activities.

V.B.10.7. RMP Annex 7: Other Supporting Data (Including Referenced Material)

When applicable, to avoid duplication of the materials presented as references, this annex should include eCTD links or reference to other documents included in other modules of the dossier.

V.B.10.8. RMP Annex 8: "Summary of Changes to the Risk Management Plan Over Time"

A list of all significant changes to the RMP in chronological order should be provided in this annex. This should include a brief description of the changes and the date and version number of the RMPs when:

- Safety concerns were added, removed or reclassified;
- Studies were added or removed from the pharmacovigilance plan;
- Risk minimisation activities recommending specific clinical measures to address the risks or additional risk minimisation activities were modified in the risk minimisation plan.

V.B.11. The Relationship Between the Risk Management Plan and the Periodic Safety Update Report

The primary post-authorisation pharmacovigilance documents for safety surveillance are the RMP and the PSUR. Although there is some overlap between the documents, the main objectives of the two are different and the situations when they are required are not always the same. Regarding objectives, the main purpose of the PSUR is retrospective, integrated, post-authorisation risk-benefit assessment whilst that of the RMP is prospective pre- and post-authorisation risk-benefit management and planning. As such, the two documents are complementary.

When a PSUR and an RMP are submitted together, the RMP should reflect the conclusions of the accompanying PSUR. For example, if a new signal is discussed in the PSUR and the PSUR concludes that this is an important identified or important potential risk to be added in the RMP, the important risk can be added in the updated RMP submitted with the PSUR. The pharmacovigilance plan and the risk minimisation plan should be updated to reflect the marketing authorisation holder's proposals to further investigate the safety concern and minimise the risk.

Table V.4: Periodic safety update report and risk management plan modules containing similar information (however, may not be in identical format and may not be interchangeable)

RMP section	PSUR section
Part II, module SIII – "Clinical trial exposure"	Sub-section 5.1 "Cumulative subject exposure in clinical trials"
Part II, module SV – "Post-authorisation experience"	Sub-section 5.2 "Cumulative and interval patient exposure from marketing experience"
Part II, module SVII – "Identified and potential risks" and part II, module SVIII – "Summary of the safety concerns"	Sub-sections 16.1 "Summaries of safety concerns" and 16.4 "Characterisation of risks"
Part V – "Risk minimisation measures", section "Evaluation of the effectiveness of risk minimisation activities"	Sub-section 16.5 "Effectiveness of risk minimisation (if applicable)"

V.B.12. Quality Systems and Record Management

Although many experts may be involved in writing the RMP, the final responsibility for its quality, accuracy and scientific integrity lies with the marketing authorisation applicant/holder. As such the QPPV should be aware of, and have sufficient authority over the content. The marketing authorisation holder is responsible for updating the RMP when new information becomes available and should apply the quality principles detailed in GVP Module I. The marketing authorisation holder should maintain records of when RMPs were submitted to competent authorities and the significant changes between RMP versions. These records, the RMPs and any documents relating to information within the RMP may be subject to audit and inspection by pharmacovigilance inspectors.

V.C. OPERATION OF THE EU NETWORK

V.C.1. Requirements for the Applicant/Marketing Authorisation Holder in the EU

For all new marketing applications, the applicant shall submit the risk management plan describing the risk management system, together with a summary thereof [DIR Art 8(3)(iaa)].

In the post-authorisation phase, an RMP update or a new RMP may need to be submitted at any time:
- At the request of the Agency or a competent authority in a Member State when there is a concern about a risk affecting the risk-benefit balance.
- With an application involving a change to an existing marketing authorisation when the data included leads to a change in the list of the safety concerns, or when a new additional pharmacovigilance activity or a new risk minimisation activity is needed or is proposed to be removed. The RMP update may be warranted as a result of data submitted with applications such as new or significant change to the indication, a new dosage form, a new route of administration, a new manufacturing process of a biotechnologically-derived product.

The need for an RMP or an update to the RMP should be discussed with the Agency or a competent authority in a Member State, as appropriate, well in advance of the submission of an application involving a significant change to an existing marketing authorisation.

V.C.1.1. Risk Management Plans with Initial Marketing Authorisation Applications

For full initial marketing authorisation applications, all parts of an RMP should be submitted (see V.B.4.). For other types of initial marketing authorisation applications, the requirements for the RMP content follow the concept of proportionality to the identified risks and potential risks of the medicinal product, and the need for post-authorisation safety data [DIR Art 8(3)]; therefore certain parts or modules may have reduced content requirements or may be left empty, where not applicable.

V.C.1.1.1. New Applications Under Article 10(1), i.e. "Generic"

The elements for new applications under DIR Art 10(1) are as follows:
- RMP part I: The elements are the same as for initial marketing authorisation application for a full application;
- RMP part II: there are 3 situations possible:
1. The originator product has an RMP: RMP modules SI-SVII may not be applicable. Module SVIII should include the summary of the safety concerns, in line with the originator product. If the applicant considers that the available evidence justifies the removal or the change of a safety concern, then data in module SVII should also be included to address the safety concern and detailing the applicant's arguments. Similarly, if the applicant has identified a new safety concern specific to the generic product (e.g. risks associated with a new excipient or a new safety concern raised from any clinical data generated), this should be discussed and the new safety concern detailed in module SVII.

Table V.5: Summary of minimum RMP requirements for initial marketing authorisation applications (for full description see text below)

Product	Part I	Part II								Part III	Part IV	Part V	Part VI
		SI	SII	SIII	SIV	SV	SVI	SVII	SVIII				
0. Full MA application	√	√	√	√	√	√	√	√	√	√	√	√	√
1. Generic product	√							‡	√	√	*	∫	√
2. Informed consent product	√	√	√	√	√	√	√	√	√	√	√	√	√
3. Hybrid product	√	†		†				†	√	√	√	∫	√
4.a. Fixed combination product – new active substance	√	T	T	T	T	T	T	√	√	√	√	√	√
4.b. ixed combination product – no new active substance	√		†	†				‡	√	√	*	∫	√
5. Well established medicinal use product	√							√	√	√	√	√	√
6. Biosimilar product	√		√	√	√	√	√	√	√	√	√	√	√

√ = applicable/relevant
‡ = relevant only if "originator" product does not have an RMP and its safety profile is not published on CMDh website
* = relevant only when a PAES was imposed for the "originator" product
∫ = statement of alignment of safety information in PI is sufficient
† = requirements based on risk proportionality principle, addressing new data generated or differences with the "originator" product
T = focus on the new active substance

2. The originator product does not have an RMP but the safety concerns of the substance are published on the CMDh website[9]. The elements under point 1 above should be followed. If more than one list of safety concerns published on CMDh website apply for the same active substance, the applicant should justify the choice of proposed safety concerns in module SVIII.
3. The originator product does not have an RMP and the safety concerns of the substance are not published on the CMDh website: Full modules SVII and SVIII should be included in the RMP. Module SVII should critically analyse available relevant information (e.g. own pre-clinical and clinical data, scientific literature, originator product's product information) and propose a list of important identified and potential risks as well as missing information.

- RMP part III: This should include a description of the routine pharmacovigilance activities, as detailed in V.B.6.1.

The applicant is strongly encouraged to contribute to and participate in the planned or ongoing studies performed by the marketing authorisation holder of the originator product, when it is important that all available (prospective) data are collected in one study. This may be the case for instance when data from patients using the new product are important to further characterise the safety profile of the substance and enrolling patients in separate studies with the same or similar objectives creates an unnecessary burden on patients, clinicians or investigators (e.g. pregnancy registries, disease registries, any PASS evaluating long-term use).

The competent authority may also consider imposing studies to be conducted for generic

---

9. See www.hma.eu/464.html

products as applicable (e.g. within the context of referrals when generic products are involved or as consequence of the outcome of a referral imposing a study to the originator product).
- RMP part IV: This part of the RMP may be left empty unless a PAES has been imposed to be conducted for the generic product (e.g. following a referral).
- RMP part V: When the originator product does not have additional risk minimisation activities, a statement that the safety information in the product information of the generic product is aligned with the originator product is sufficient for RMP part V. Where new risks have been identified for the generic product, the risk minimisation activities for such safety concerns should be presented in part V, following the same elements as for a full marketing authorisation application.

If the originator product does have additional risk minimisation activities, a full part V is required for the generic product.
- RMP part VI: The elements are the same as for a full initial marketing authorisation application, to the extent of data requested and provided in other parts of the RMP, as per above.
- RMP part VII: The elements are the same for a full initial marketing authorisation application. For RMP annexes 4 and 5, the applicant is strongly encouraged to use materials as similar, in content, as possible to the originator product.

V.C.1.1.2. New Applications Under Article 10c, i.e. "Informed Consent"

For new applications under DIR Art 10c, the RMP should be the same as the RMP of the cross-referred medicinal product. An RMP will still be required even if the cross-referred product does not have an RMP. If the marketing authorisation holder is the same as for the authorised product, the marketing authorisation holder is encouraged to put in place only one RMP document for their products with the same active substance.

V.C.1.1.3. New Applications Under Article 10(3), i.e. "Hybrid"

For new applications under DIR Art 10(3), the RMP elements are the same as for a generic product. However, for changes in the active substance(s), therapeutic indications, strength, pharmaceutical form or route of administration, the applicant should discuss in RMP module SVII whether this results in the addition or deletion of a safety concern. Clinical trial data generated to support the application should be discussed in the RMP, as appropriate (e.g. RMP part II, modules SI, SIII). Other parts of the RMP should also be aligned (e.g. parts V and VI).

V.C.1.1.4. New Applications Under Article 10B, i.e. Involving "Fixed Combination" Medicinal Products

For new applications for fixed dose combinations, there are two situations:
1. The combination contains a new active substance: A full RMP, following the elements as for full initial marketing authorisation application, should be submitted. RMP modules SI-SVI should focus on the new active substance.
2. The combination does not contain a new active substance: The RMP should follow the elements for a generic product. For the purpose of establishing the elements of RMP part II, "the originator product" should be read as "any/all authorised products containing the same active substances included in the new product".

In addition, new data generated with the fixed combination should be provided in modules SII and SIII.

V.C.1.1.5. New Applications Under Article 10A, i.e. "Well Established Medicinal Use"

For new applications under DIR Art 10a, RMP elements are as follows:
- RMP part I: The elements are the same as for a full initial marketing authorisation application.
- RMP part II: Only RMP modules SVII and SVIII might be applicable. The applicant is required to justify the proposed safety concerns, or the lack of any thereof, using available evidence from published scientific literature (information available in the public domain).
- RMP parts III-VII: The elements are the same as for a full initial marketing authorisation application.

V.C.1.1.6. New Applications Under Article 10(4), i.e. "Biosimilar Products"

For new applications for biosimilar products, the RMP elements are described in GVP P.II.

V.C.1.1.7. New Applications for Homeopathic and Herbal Products not Falling Within the Scope of the Simplified Registration

New applications for homeopathic and herbal medicinal products not falling within the scope of the simplified registration are subject to standard marketing authorisation; therefore the RMP elements are the same as defined by the type of the marketing authorisation application (i.e. legal basis).

V.C.1.2. Risk Management Plans First Submitted Post-authorisation

V.C.1.2.1. New Risk Management Plans at the Request of a Competent Authority to Address One or More Safety Concerns

The elements are the same as those applicable to a generic product where the originator product does not have an RMP (see V.C.1.1.1.).
Two possible scenarios are envisaged:
1. Marketing authorisation holders may be requested to submit an RMP with a RMP module SVII focused on the safety concern(s) evaluated in the procedure. Other safety concerns should be included as needed.
2. Marketing authorisation holders may be requested to submit an RMP based on a comprehensive identification of safety concerns.

It is left to the discretion of the competent authority, which is the most appropriate in given circumstances.

V.C.1.2.2. Unsolicited Risk Management Plan Submission in Post-Authorisation Phase

This RMP follows the elements of the type of marketing authorisation under which this medicinal product was initially submitted (i.e. full marketing authorisation application, generic medicinal products, "informed consent" applications, etc., see V.C.1.1.).

V.C.2. Submission of a Risk Management Plan to Competent Authorities In the EU

For centrally authorised medicinal products, the RMP should be submitted as PDF files within the eCTD submission. Following a Commission decision where the procedure has involved the submission of an RMP, marketing authorisation holders should submit the RMP annex 1 in XML format within a specified timescale. RMP annex 1 provides the key information regarding the RMP in a structured electronic format which, following validation at the Agency, is uploaded into an Agency database that is accessible and searchable by the Agency and the competent authorities in the Member States. The system for nationally authorised medicinal products varies across Member States and the national requirements should be followed.

Details of new submission requirements and the electronic format will be provided on the Agency and Member State's websites, as appropriate, and may in future replace the requirements in the paragraph above.

The initial RMP should be submitted as part of the initial marketing authorisation, or if required, for those products that do not have an RMP, through the appropriate post-authorisation procedure.

V.C.2.1. Risk Management Plans Updates

An RMP update is expected to be submitted at any time when there is a change in the list of the safety concerns, or when there is a new or a significant change in the existing additional pharmacovigilance or additional risk minimisation activities. The significant changes of the existing additional pharmacovigilance and risk minimisation activities may include removing such activities from the RMP. For example, a change in study objectives, population or due date of final results, or addition of a new safety concern in the key messages of the educational materials would be expected to be reflected in an updated RMP with the procedure triggering those changes.

An update of the RMP might be considered when data submitted in the procedure results or is expected to result in changes of routine pharmacovigilance activities beyond adverse reaction reporting and signal detection activities, or of routine risk minimisation activities recommending specific clinical measures to address the risk. For example, an RMP update might also be warranted with a significant change of the plans for annual enhanced safety surveillance (routine pharmacovigilance activity), or when monitoring of renal function is added as a recommendation in the Special warnings and precautions for use section 4.4 of the SmPC (routine risk minimisation activity). The need to update the plans to evaluate the effectiveness of risk minimisation activities should also be considered with such updates. When an emerging safety issue is still under assessment (as defined in GVP Module VI), in particular in the context of a signal or potential risk that could be an important identified risk, an RMP update may be required if the emerging safety issue is confirmed and the important identified or potential risk requires to be added to the list of safety concerns in the RMP.

Unless requested otherwise, a track-changes RMP document should be included with every RMP update, showing changes introduced in the latest update (as applicable), as well as compared with the "current" approved version of the RMP.

A medicinal product can only have one "current" approved version of an RMP. If several updates to the RMP are submitted during the course of a procedure, the version considered as the "current" approved RMP for future updates and track-changes purposes shall be the one submitted with the closing sequence of the procedure.

When an RMP update is submitted with a procedure, the RMP is considered approved at the end of the procedure, when all changes are considered acceptable.

In the post-authorisation phase, submission of a new or updated RMP outside of another regulatory procedure constitutes a variation in accordance with the Guidelines on Variations[10]. For detailed guidance on relevant variation categories and their classification, please also refer to the EMA Practical Questions and Answers to Support the Implementation of the Variations Guidelines in the Centralised Procedure[11].

RMP management with parallel procedures
If a medicinal product has more than one concurrently on-going procedure which requires submission of an RMP, ideally a combined RMP should be submitted with appropriate separation of data in RMP module SIII. The best regulatory path for the RMP update in case of multiple procedures potentially impacting on the RMP content should be discussed with the competent authority before submission.

RMP updates with the PSUR
If, when preparing a PSUR, there is a need for changes to the RMP as a result of new safety concerns, or other data presented in the PSUR, then an updated RMP should be submitted at the same time. In this case no stand-alone RMP variation is necessary. Should only the timing for submission of both documents coincide, but the changes are not related to each other, then the RMP submission should be handled as a stand-alone variation.

However, in the context of a PSUR EU single assessment (PSUSA), submission of RMP updates cannot be accepted together with the PSURs of medicinal products (centrally and/or nationally authorised). Marketing authorisation holders should take the opportunity of another upcoming procedure to update their RMP. Alternatively, marketing authorisation holders should submit a separate variation to update their RMP.

For nationally authorised medicinal products, RMP updates should be submitted to the competent authorities in the Member States for assessment.

V.C.3. Assessment of the Risk Management Plan within the EU Regulatory Network

Within the EU, the regulatory oversight of RMPs for medicinal products authorised centrally lies with the Pharmacovigilance Risk Assessment Committee (PRAC). For the RMP assessment, the PRAC appoints a PRAC rapporteur who works closely with the (Co-)Rapporteur(s) appointed by the CHMP and Committee for Advanced Therapies (CAT) (for ATMPs) or with the Reference Member State, as appropriate. The EMA may, on a case-by-case basis, consult healthcare professionals and patients

---

10. Guidelines on the details of the various categories of variations, on the operation of the procedures laid down in Chapters II, IIa, III and IV of Commission Regulation (EC) No 1234/2008 of 24 November 2008 concerning the examination of variations to the terms of marketing authorisations for medicinal products for human use and veterinary medicinal products and on the documentation to be submitted pursuant to those procedures.
11. *See* http://www.ema.europa.eu/ema/index.jsp?curl=pages/regulation/document_listing/document_listing_000104.jsp&mid=WC0b01ac0580025b88

during the assessment of RMPs to gather their input on proposed risk minimisation measures.

For medicinal products authorised nationally, the national competent authorities are responsible of the assessment of the RMP. The national competent authority may impose an obligation on a marketing authorisation holder to operate a risk management system for each medicinal product, as referred to in DIR Art 104(3)(c), if there are concerns about the risks affecting the risk-benefit balance of an authorised medicinal product. In that context, the national competent authority shall also oblige the marketing authorisation holder to submit a detailed description of the risk-management system which he intends to introduce for the medicinal product concerned [DIR Art 104a(2)].

For centrally authorised medicinal products, only risk minimisation measures recommended by the PRAC and subsequently agreed by the CHMP should be included in the risk minimisation plan as additional risk minimisation activities. Additional risk minimisation measures are conditions to the marketing authorisation; key elements are detailed in annex II to the Commission decision. In addition, exceptionally, certain conditions or restrictions with regard to the safe and effective use of the medicinal product may be imposed to the Member States through a Commission decision in accordance with DIR Art 127a for their implementation at national level.

When necessary, the competent authorities should ensure that all marketing authorisation holders of medicinal products containing the same active substance make similar changes to their risk minimisation measures when changes are made to those of the reference medicinal product.

V.C.4. Transparency

The Agency and Member States shall make publically available, by means of the European medicines web-portal and the national medicines web-portals, public assessment reports and summaries of risk management plans [REG Art 26(1)(c), DIR Art 106(c)].

For centrally authorised medicinal products the Agency:
- Makes public a summary of the RMP;
- Includes tables relating to the RMP in the EPAR including the product information and any conditions to the marketing authorisation.

The national competent authorities will provide details of how they intend to implement the transparency measures at national level [by reference to DIR Art 106].

Annexure 8: Guideline on Good Pharmacovigilance Practices (GVP)

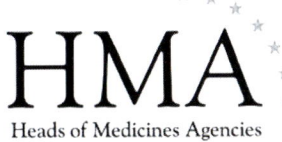

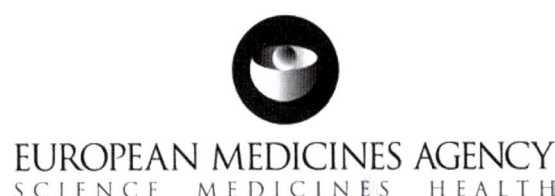

8 september 2014
EMA/873138/2011 Rev 1*

GUIDELINE ON GOOD PHARMACOVIGILANCE PRACTICES (GVP)

Module VI Management and Reporting of Adverse Reactions to Medicinal Products (Rev 1)

Date for coming into effect of first version	2 July 2012
Draft Revision 1* finalised by the Agency in collaboration with Member States	28 May 2013
Draft Revision 1 agreed by ERMS FG	29 May 2013
Draft Revision 1 adopted by Executive Director	6 June 2013
Released for public consultation	7 June 2013
End of consultation (deadline for comments)	5 August 2013
Revised draft Revision 1 finalised by the Agency in collaboration with Member States	16 July 2014
Revised draft Revision 1 agreed by ERMS FG	31 August 2014
Revised draft Revision 1 adopted by Executive Director as final	8 September 2014
Date for coming into effect of Revision 1	16 September 2014

Note: New requirements for non-interventional post-authorisation studies will become mandatory for any new study started after 1 January 2015. Implementation for new or ongoing studies started before that date is optional.

Note: Revision 1 contains the following:
- Revisions in VI.A.2.1.1. (Causality), VI.A.2.4. (Seriousness), VI.B.1.2. (Solicited reports), VI.B.3. (Follow-up of reports), VI.B.6.3. (Reports of overdose, abuse, off-label use, misuse, medication error or occupational exposure), VI.C.1. (Reporting rules for clinical trials and post-authorisation studies in the EU), VI.C.2.2.2. (Solicited reports), VI.C.6.2.3.7. (Reports of suspected adverse reactions originating from organised data collection systems and other systems);
- Clarifications on the clock start for the reporting of valid ICSRs in VI.B.7.;
- Clarifications on the handling of ICSRs when reported in an official language in VI.C.6.2.2.9.;
- Replacements of tables highlighting interim arrangements applicable to marketing authorisation holders in VI. App.3.1.1.;
- Correction in VI.C.2.2.9. (Period during a public health emergency).

VI.A. INTRODUCTION

VI.A.1. Scope

This Module of GVP addresses the legal requirements detailed in Title IX of Directive 2001/83/EC [DIR] and chapter 3 of Regulation (EC) No 726/2004 [REG], which are applicable to competent authorities in Member States, marketing authorisation holders and the Agency as regards the collection, data management and reporting of suspected adverse reactions (serious and non-serious) associated with medicinal products for human use authorised in the European Union (EU). Recommendations regarding the reporting of emerging safety issues or of suspected adverse reactions occurring in special situations are also presented in this Module. The requirements provided in chapters IV, V and IX of the Commission Implementing Regulation (EU) No 520/2012 [IR] shall be applied in this Module.

The guidance provided in this Module does not address the collection, management and reporting of events or patterns of use, which do not result in suspected adverse reactions (e.g. asymptomatic overdose, abuse, off-label use, misuse or medication error) or which do not require to be reported as individual case safety report or as emerging safety issues. This information may however need to be collected and presented in periodic safety update reports for the interpretation of safety data or for the benefit risk evaluation of medicinal products. In this aspect, guidance provided in Module VII applies.

All applicable legal requirements detailed in this Module are referenced in the way explained in the GVP Introductory Cover Note and are usually identifiable by the modal verb "shall". Guidance for the implementation of legal requirements is provided using the modal verb "should".

VI.A.2. Terminology

The definitions provided in Article 1 of Directive 2001/83/EC shall be applied for the purpose of this Module; of particular relevance are those provided in this Section. Some general principles presented in the ICH-E2A and ICH-E2D guidelines (*see* GVP Annex IV) should also be adhered to; they are included as well in this Section (*see* GVP Annex I for all definitions applicable to GVP).

VI.A.2.1. Adverse Reaction

An adverse reaction is a response to a medicinal product which is noxious and unintended [DIR Art 1]. This includes adverse reactions which arise from:
- The use of a medicinal product within the terms of the marketing authorisation;
- The use outside the terms of the marketing authorisation, including overdose, off-label use, misuse, abuse and medication errors;
- Occupational exposure.

VI.A.2.1.1. Causality

In accordance with ICH-E2A (*see* GVP Annex IV), the definition of an adverse reaction implies at least a reasonable possibility of a causal relationship between a suspected medicinal product and an adverse event. An adverse reaction, in contrast to an adverse event, is characterised by the fact that a causal relationship between a medicinal product and an occurrence is suspected. For regulatory reporting purposes, as detailed in ICH-E2D (*see* GVP Annex IV), if an event is spontaneously reported, even if the relationship is unknown or unstated, it meets the definition of an adverse reaction. Therefore, all spontaneous reports notified by healthcare professionals[1] or consumers[2] are considered suspected adverse reactions, since they convey the suspicions of the primary sources, unless the reporters specifically state that they believe the events to be unrelated or that a causal relationship can be excluded.

VI.A.2.1.2. Overdose, Off-Label Use, Misuse, Abuse, Occupational exposure

a. Overdose

This refers to the administration of a quantity of a medicinal product given per administration or cumulatively, which is above the maximum recommended dose according to the authorised product information. Clinical judgement should always be applied.

b. Off-label use

This relates to situations where the medicinal product is intentionally used for a medical purpose not in accordance with the authorised product information.

c. Misuse

This refers to situations where the medicinal product is intentionally and inappropriately used

---

1. *See* VI.A.2.3.for definition of primary source

not in accordance with the authorised product information.

d. Abuse

This corresponds to the persistent or sporadic, intentional excessive use of a medicinal product, which is accompanied by harmful physical or psychological effects [DIR Art 1].

e. Occupational exposure

This refers to the exposure to a medicinal product (as defined in [DIR Art 1]), as a result of one's professional or non-professional occupation.

VI.A.2.2. Medicinal Product

A medicinal product is characterised by any substance or combination of substances:
- Presented as having properties for treating or preventing disease in human beings;or
- Which may be used in or administered to human beings either with a view to restoring, correcting or modifying physiological functions by exerting a pharmacological, immunological or metabolic action, or to making a medical diagnosis [DIR Art1].

In accordance with Article 107 of Directive 2001/83/EC, the scope of this module is not only applicable to medicinal products authorised in the EU but also to any such medicinal products commercialised outside the EU by the same marketing authorisation holder (see VI.C.2.2.). Given that a medicinal product is authorised with a defined composition, all the adverse reactions suspected to be related to any of the active substances being part of a medicinal product authorised in the EU should be managed in accordance with the requirements presented in this module. This is valid independently of the strengths, pharmaceutical forms, routes of administration, presentations, authorised indications, or trade names of the medicinal product.

The guidance provided in this Module also applies, subject to amendments where appropriate, to medicinal products supplied in the context of compassionate use (see VI.C.1.2.2.) as defined in Article 83(2) of Regulation (EC) No 726/2004. As the case may be, this guidance may also apply to named patient use as defined under Article 5(1) of Directive 2001/83/EC.

VI.A.2.3. Primary Source

The primary source of the information on a suspected adverse reaction(s) is the person who reports the facts. Several primary sources, such as healthcare professionals and/or a consumer, may provide information on the same case. In this situation, all the primary sources' details, including the qualifications, should be provided in the case report, with the "Primary source(s)" section repeated as necessary in line with ICH-E2B(R2) (see GVP Annex IV)[2].

In accordance with the ICH-E2D (see GVP Annex IV),
- A healthcare professional is defined as a medically-qualified person such as a physician, dentist, pharmacist, nurse, coroner or as otherwise specified by local regulations;
- A consumer is defined as a person who is not a healthcare professional such as a patient, lawyer, friend, relative of a patient or carer.

Medical documentations (e.g. laboratory or other test data) provided by a consumer that support the occurrence of the suspected adverse reaction, or which indicate that an identifiable healthcare professional suspects a reasonable possibility of causal relationship between a medicinal product and the reported adverse event, are sufficient to consider the spontaneous report as confirmed by a healthcare professional.

If a consumer initially reports more than one reaction and at least one receives medical confirmation, the whole report should be documented as a spontaneous report confirmed by a healthcare professional and be reported accordingly. Similarly, if a report is submitted by a medically qualified patient, friend, relative of the patient or carer, the case should also be considered as a spontaneous report confirmed by a healthcare professional.

VI.A.2.4. Seriousness

As described in ICH-E2A (see GVP Annex IV), a serious adverse reaction corresponds to any untoward medical occurrence that at any dose results in death, is life-threatening, requires inpatient hospitalisation or prolongation of existing hospitalisation, results in persistent or significant disability or incapacity, or is a congenital anomaly/birth defect.

The characteristics/consequences should be considered at the time of the reaction to determine the seriousness of a case. For example, life-threatening refers to a reaction in which the patient was at risk of death at the time of the reaction; it does not refer to a reaction that hypothetically might have caused death if more severe.

Medical judgement should be exercised in deciding whether other situations should be considered as serious reactions. Some medical events may jeopardise the patient or may require an intervention to prevent one of the above characteristics/consequences. Such important medical events should be considered as serious.[3] The EudraVigilance Expert Working Group has co-ordinated the development of an important medical event (IME) terms list based on the Medical Dictionary for Regulatory Activities (MedDRA) (*see* GVP Annex IV). This IME list aims to facilitate the classification of suspected adverse reactions, the analysis of aggregated data and the assessment of the individual case safety reports (ICSRs) in the framework of the day-to-day pharmacovigilance activities. The IME list is intended for guidance purposes only and is available on the EudraVigilance web site[4] to stakeholders who wish to use it for their pharmacovigilance activities. It is regularly updated in line with the latest version of MedDRA.

VI.A.2.5. Individual Case Safety Report (ICSR)

This refers to the format and content for the reporting of one or several suspected adverse reactions in relation to a medicinal product that occur in a single patient at a specific point of time. A valid ICSR should include at least one identifiable reporter, one single identifiable patient, at least one suspect adverse reaction and at least one suspect medicinal product.

VI.B. STRUCTURES AND PROCESSES

Section B of this Module highlights the general principles in relation to the collection, recording and reporting of reports of suspected adverse reactions associated with medicinal products for human use, which are applicable to competent authorities and marketing authorisation holders. The definitions and recommendations provided in VI.A. should be followed. EU requirements are presented in VI.C.

VI.B.1. Collection of Reports

Competent authorities and marketing authorisation holders should take appropriate measures in order to collect and collate all reports of suspected adverse reactions associated with medicinal products for human use originating from unsolicited or solicited sources.

For this purpose, a pharmacovigilance system should be developed to allow the acquisition of sufficient information for the scientific evaluation of those reports.

The system should be designed so that it helps to ensure that the collected reports are authentic, legible, accurate, consistent, verifiable and as complete as possible for their clinical assessment.

All notifications that contain pharmacovigilance data should be recorded and archived in compliance with the applicable data protection requirements (*see* VI.C.6.2.2.8. for EU requirements).

The system should also be structured in a way that allows for reports of suspected adverse reactions to be validated (*see* VI.B.2.) in a timely manner and exchanged between competent authorities and marketing authorisation holders within the legal reporting time frame (*see* VI.B.7.1.).

In accordance with the ICH-E2D (*see* GVP Annex IV), two types of safety reports are distinguished in the post-authorisation phase; reports originating from unsolicited sources and those reported as solicited.

VI.B.1.1. Unsolicited Reports

VI.B.1.1.1. Spontaneous Reports

A spontaneous report is an unsolicited communication by a healthcare professional, or consumer to a competent authority, marketing authorisation holder or other organisation (e.g.

---

2. *See* VI.C.6 as regards the electronic reporting of ICSRs in the EU.
3. Examples are provided in section II.B of ICH-E2A (*see* GVP Annex IV).
4. http://eudravigilance.ema.europa.eu/human/textforIME.asp.

Regional Pharmacovigilance Centre, Poison Control Centre) that describes one or more suspected adverse reactions in a patient who was given one or more medicinal products and that does not derive from a study or any organised data collection systems where adverse events reporting is actively sought, as defined in VI.B.1.2.

Stimulated reporting that occurs consequent to a direct healthcare professional communication (*see* Module XV), publication in the press, questioning of healthcare professionals by company representatives, communication from patients' organisations to their members, or class action lawsuits should be considered spontaneous reports.

Unsolicited consumer adverse reactions reports should be handled as spontaneous reports irrespective of any subsequent "medical confirmation".

The reporting modalities and applicable time frames for spontaneous reports are described in VI.B.7.and VI.B.8.

VI.B.1.1.2. Literature Reports

The scientific and medical literature is a significant source of information for the monitoring of the safety profile and of the risk-benefit balance of medicinal products, particularly in relation to the detection of new safety signals or emerging safety issues. Marketing authorisation holders are therefore expected to maintain awareness of possible publications through a systematic literature review of widely used reference databases (e.g. Medline, Excerpta Medica or Embase) no less frequently than once a week. The marketing authorisation holder should ensure that the literature review includes the use of reference databases that contain the largest reference of articles in relation to the medicinal product properties.[5] In addition, marketing authorisation holders should have procedures in place to monitor scientific and medical publications in local journals in countries where medicinal products have a marketing authorisation, and to bring them to the attention of the company safety department as appropriate.

Reports of suspected adverse reactions from the scientific and medical literature, including relevant published abstracts from meetings and draft manuscripts, should be reviewed and assessed by marketing authorisation holders to identify and record ICSRs originating from spontaneous reports or non-interventional post-authorisation studies.

If multiple medicinal products are mentioned in the publication, only those which are identified by the publication's author(s) as having at least a possible causal relationship with the suspected adverse reaction should be considered by the concerned marketing authorisation holder(s).

Valid ICSRs should be reported according to the modalities detailed in VI.B.7.and VI.B.8.

One case should be created for each single patient identifiable based on characteristics provided in VI.B.2. Relevant medical information should be provided and the publication author(s) should be considered as the primary source(s).

EU specific requirements, as regards medicinal products and scientific and medical publications, which are not monitored by the Agency and for which valid ICSRs shall be reported by marketing authorisation holders, are provided in VI.C.2.2.3.

VI.B.1.1.3. Reports from Other Sources

If a marketing authorisation holder becomes aware of a report of suspected adverse reactions originating from a non-medical source, for example, the lay press or other media, it should be handled as a spontaneous report. Every attempt should be made to follow-up the case to obtain the minimum information that constitutes a valid ICSR. The same reporting time frames should be applied as for other spontaneous reports.

VI.B.1.1.4. Information on Suspected Adverse Reactions from the Internet or Digital media

Marketing authorisation holders should regularly screen internet or digital media[6] under their management or responsibility, for potential reports of suspected adverse reactions. In this aspect, digital media is considered to be company sponsored if it is owned, paid for and/or controlled by the marketing authorisation holder.[7] The frequency of the screening should allow for potential valid ICSRs to be reported to the competent authorities within the appropriate reporting time frame based on the

---

5. *See* VI. Appendix 2.for the detailed guidance on the monitoring of medical and scientific literature.
6. Although not exhaustive, the following list should be considered as digital media: web site, web page, blog, vlog, social network, internet forum, chat room, health portal.
7. A donation (financial or otherwise) to an organisation/site by a marketing authorisation holder does not constitute ownership, provided that the marketing authorisation holder does not control the final content of the site.

date the information was posted on the internet site/digital medium. Marketing authorisation holders may also consider utilising their websites to facilitate the collection of reports of suspected adverse reactions (see VI.C.2.2.1.).

If a marketing authorisation holder becomes aware of a report of suspected adverse reaction described in any non-company sponsored digital medium, the report should be assessed to determine whether it qualifies for reporting.

Unsolicited cases of suspected adverse reactions from the internet or digital media should be handled as spontaneous reports. The same reporting time frames as for spontaneous reports should be applied (see VI.B.7.).

In relation to cases from the internet or digital media, the identifiability of the reporter refers to the existence of a real person, that is, it is possible to verify the contact details of the reporter (e.g. an email address under a valid format has been provided). If the country of the primary source is missing, the country where the information was received, or where the review took place, should be used as the primary source country.

VI.B.1.2. Solicited reports

As defined in ICH-E2D (see GVP Annex IV), solicited reports of suspected adverse reactions are those derived from organised data collection systems, which include clinical trials, non-interventional studies, registries, post-approval named patient use programmes, other patient support and disease management programmes, surveys of patients or healthcare providers, compassionate use or name patient use, or information gathering on efficacy or patient compliance. Reports of suspected adverse reactions obtained from any of these data collection systems should not be considered spontaneous. This is with the exception of:
- Suspected adverse reactions in relation to those adverse events for which the protocol of non- interventional post-authorisation studies provides differently and does not require their systematic collection (see VI.C.1.2.1.),
- Suspected adverse reactions originating from compassionate use or named patient use conducted in Member States where the active collection of adverse events occurring in these programmes is not required (see VI.C.1.2.2.).

For the purpose of safety reporting, solicited reports should be classified as study reports, and should have an appropriate causality assessment, to consider whether they refer to suspected adverse reactions and therefore meet the criteria for reporting. General reporting rules for suspected adverse reactions occurring in organised data collection systems conducted in the EU under the scope of Directive 2001/83/EC, Regulation (EC) No 726/2004 or Directive 2001/20/EC, are presented in VI.C.1.

VI.B.2. Validation of Reports

Only valid ICSRs qualify for reporting. All reports of suspected adverse reactions should therefore be validated before reporting them to the competent authorities to make sure that the minimum criteria for reporting are included in the reports [see ICH-E2D (see GVP Annex IV)]. These are:
- One or more identifiable reporter (primary source), characterised by qualification (e.g. physician, pharmacist, other healthcare professional, lawyer, consumer or other non-healthcare professional) name, initials or address.[8] Whenever possible, contact details for the reporter should be recorded so that follow-up activities can be performed. However, if the reporter does not wish to provide contact details, the ICSR should still be considered as valid providing the organisation who was informed of the case was able to confirm it directly with the reporter. All parties providing case information or approached for case information should be identifiable, not only the initial reporter.
- One single identifiable patient characterised by initials, patient identification number, date of birth, age, age group or gender. The information should be as complete as possible[9].
- One or more suspected substance/medicinal product (see VI.A.2.2.).
- One or more suspected adverse reaction (see VI.A.2.1.). If the primary source has made an explicit statement that a causal relationship between the medicinal product and the

---
8. Local data privacy laws regarding patient's and reporter's identifiability might apply.
9. See Footnote 9.

adverse event has been excluded and the receiver (competent authority or marketing authorisation holder) agrees with this, the report does not qualify as a valid ICSR since the minimum information is incomplete.[10] The report does not also qualify as a valid ICSR if it is reported that the patient experienced an unspecified adverse reaction and there is no information provided on the type of adverse reaction experienced. Similarly, the report is not valid if only an outcome (or consequence) is notified and (i) no further information about the clinical circumstances is provided to consider it as a suspected adverse reaction, or (ii) the primary source has not indicated a possible causal relationship with the suspected medicinal product. For instance a marketing authorisation holder is made aware that a patient was hospitalised or died, without any further information. In this particular situation, medical judgement should always be applied in deciding whether the notified information is an adverse reaction or an event. For example, a report of sudden death would usually need to be considered as a case of suspected adverse reaction and reported.

The lack of any of these four elements means that the case is considered incomplete and does not qualify for reporting. Competent authorities and marketing authorisation holders are expected to exercise due diligence in following up the case to collect the missing data elements. Reports, for which the minimum information is incomplete, should nevertheless be recorded within the pharmacovigilance system for use in on-going safety evaluation activities. Recommendations on the electronic reporting of valid ICSRs, when missing information has been obtained, are provided in VI.C.6.2.3.8.

When collecting reports of suspected adverse reactions via the internet or digital media, the term "identifiable" refers to the possibility of verification of the existence of a reporter and a patient (*see* VI.B.1.1.4.).

When one party (competent authority or a marketing authorisation holder) is made aware that the primary source may also have reported the suspected adverse reaction to another concerned party, the report should still be considered as a valid ICSR. All the relevant information necessary for the detection of the duplicate case should be included in the ICSR.[11]

A valid case of suspected adverse reaction initially submitted by a consumer cannot be downgraded to a report of non-related adverse event if the contacted healthcare professional (nominated by the consumer for follow-up information) disagrees with the consumer's suspicion (*see* VI.A.2.1.1.). In this situation, the opinions of both the consumer and the healthcare professional should be included in the ICSR. Guidance on the reporting of the medical confirmation of a case, provided in ICH-E2B(R2) Section A.1.14 ("Was the case medically confirmed, if not initially from a healthcare professional?") (*see* GVP Annex IV), should be followed.

For solicited reports of suspected adverse reactions (*see* VI.B.1.2.), where the receiver disagrees with the reasonable possibility of causal relationship between the suspected medicinal product and the adverse reaction expressed by the primary source, the case should not be downgraded to a report of non-related adverse event. The opinions of both, the primary source and the receiver, should be recorded in the ICSR.

The same principle applies to the ICSR seriousness criterion, which should not be downgraded from serious to non-serious if the receiver disagrees with the seriousness reported by the primary source.

VI.B.3. Follow-up of Reports

When first received, the information in suspected adverse reactions reports may be incomplete. These reports should be followed-up as necessary to obtain supplementary detailed information significant for the scientific evaluation of the cases. This is particularly relevant for monitored events of special interest, prospective reports of pregnancy, cases notifying the death of a patient, cases reporting new risks or changes in the known risks. This is in addition to any effort to collect missing minimum information (*see* VI.B.2.). Any attempt

---

10. There is no suspected adverse reaction.
11. For further guidance on reporting of other duplicate ICSRs, refer to section A.1.11 "Other case identifiers in previous transmission" of ICH-E2B(R2) (*see* GVP Annex IV).

to obtain follow-up information should be documented.

Follow-up methods should be tailored towards optimising the collection of missing information. This should be done in ways that encourage the primary source to submit new information relevant for the scientific evaluation of a particular safety concern. The use of targeted specific forms in the local language should avoid requesting the primary source to repeat information already provided in the initial report and/or to complete extensive questionnaires, which could discourage future spontaneous reporting. Therefore, consideration should be given to pre-populating some data fields in those follow-up report forms to make their completion by the primary source easy.

When information is received directly from a consumer suggesting that an adverse reaction may have occurred, if the information is incomplete, attempts should be made to obtain consent to contact a nominated healthcare professional to obtain further follow-up information. When such a case, initially reported by a consumer, has been confirmed (totally or partially) by a healthcare professional, this information should be clearly highlighted in the ICSR.[12]

For suspected adverse reactions relating to biological medicinal products, the definite identification of the concerned product with regard to its manufacturing is of particular importance. Therefore, all appropriate measures should be taken to clearly identify the name of the product and the batch number. A business process map in relation to the mandatory follow-up of information for the identification of suspected biological medicinal products is presented in VI. Appendix 1.

For cases related to vaccines, GVP P.I. should also be followed as appropriate.

VI.B.4. Data Management

Electronic data and paper reports of suspected adverse reactions should be stored and treated in the same way as other medical records with appropriate respect for confidentiality regarding patients' and reporters' identifiability and in accordance with local data privacy laws. Confidentiality of patients' records including personal identifiers, if provided, should always be maintained. Identifiable personal details of reporting healthcare professionals should be kept in confidence. With regards to patient's and reporter's identifiability, case report information should be transmitted between stakeholders (marketing authorisation holders or competent authorities) in accordance with local data privacy laws (see VI.C.6.2.2.8. for the processing of personal data in ICSRs in the EU).

In order to ensure pharmacovigilance data security and confidentiality, strict access controls should be applied to documents and to databases to authorised personnel only. This security extends to the complete data path. In this aspect, procedures should be implemented to ensure security and non-corruption of data during data transfer.

When transfer of pharmacovigilance data occurs within an organisation or between organisations having concluded contractual agreements, the mechanism should be such that there is confidence that all notifications are received; in that, a confirmation and/or reconciliation process should be undertaken.

Correct data entry, including the appropriate use of terminologies, should be verified by quality assurance auditing, either systematically or by regular random evaluation. Data entry staff should be instructed in the use of the terminologies, and their proficiency confirmed.

Data received from the primary source should be treated in an unbiased and unfiltered way and inferences as well as imputations should be avoided during data entry or electronic transmission. The reports should include the verbatim text as used by the primary source or an accurate translation of it. The original verbatim text should be coded using the appropriate terminology as described in VI.B.8. In order to ensure consistency in the coding practices, it is recommended to use, where applicable, the translation of the terminology in the local language to code the verbatim text.

Electronic data storage should allow traceability (audit trail) of all data entered or modified, including dates and sources of received data, as well as dates and destinations of transmitted data.

A procedure should be in place to account for identification and management of duplicate cases at data entry and during the generation of aggregated reports (see VI.C.6.2.4.).

---

12. For further guidance on reporting this information, refer to ICH-E2B(R2), section A.1.14 ("Was the case medically confirmed, if not initially from a healthcare professional?") (see GVP Annex IV).

VI.B.5. Quality Management

Competent authorities and marketing authorisation holders should have a quality management system in place to ensure compliance with the necessary quality standards at every stage of case documentation, such as data collection, data transfer, data management, data coding, case validation, case evaluation, case follow-up, ICSR reporting and case archiving (see VI.C.6.2.4.and Module I).

Conformity of stored data with initial and follow-up reports should be verified by quality control procedures, which permit for the validation against the original data or images thereof. In this aspect, the source data (e.g. letters, e-mails, records of telephone calls that include details of an event) or an image of the source data should be easily accessible.

Clear written standard operating procedures should guarantee that the roles and responsibilities and the required tasks are clear to all parties involved and that there is provision for proper control and, when needed, change of the system. This is equally applicable to activities that are contracted out to third parties, whose procedures should be reviewed to verify that they are adequate and compliant with applicable requirements.

Staff directly performing pharmacovigilance activities, should be appropriately trained in applicable pharmacovigilance legislation and guidelines in addition to specific training in report processing activities for which they are responsible and/or undertake. Other personnel who may receive or process safety reports (e.g. clinical development, sales, medical information, legal, quality control) should be trained in adverse event collection and reporting in accordance with internal policies and procedures.

VI.B.6. Special Situations

VI.B.6.1. Use of a Medicinal Product During Pregnancy or Breastfeeding

a. Pregnancy

Reports, where the embryo or foetus may have been exposed to medicinal products (either through maternal exposure or transmission of a medicinal product via semen following paternal exposure), should be followed-up in order to collect information on the outcome of the pregnancy and development of the child after birth. The recommendations provided in the Guideline on the Exposure to Medicinal Products during Pregnancy: Need for Post-Authorisation Data (see GVP Annex III) should be considered as regard the monitoring, collection and reporting of information in these specific situations in order to facilitate the scientific evaluation. When an active substance (or one of its metabolites) has a long half-life, this should be taken into account when assessing the possibility of exposure of the embryo, if the medicinal product was taken before conception.

Not infrequently, pregnant women or healthcare professionals will contact either competent authorities or marketing authorisation holders to request information on the teratogenicity of a medicinal product and/or experience of use during pregnancy. Reasonable attempts should be made to obtain information on any possible medicinal product exposure to an embryo or foetus and to follow-up on the outcome of the pregnancy.

Reports of exposure to medicinal products during pregnancy should contain as many detailed elements as possible in order to assess the causal relationships between any reported adverse events and the exposure to the suspected medicinal product. In this context the use of standard structured questionnaires is recommended.

Individual cases with an abnormal outcome associated with a medicinal product following exposure during pregnancy are classified as serious reports and should be reported, in accordance with the requirements outlined in VI.B.7.[13]

This especially refers to:
- Reports of congenital anomalies or developmental delay, in the foetus or the child;
- Reports of foetal death and spontaneous abortion; and
- Reports of suspected adverse reactions in the neonate that are classified as serious.

Other cases, such as reports of induced termination of pregnancy without information on congenital malformation, reports of pregnancy exposure without outcome data or reports which have a normal outcome, should not be reported since there is no suspected adverse reaction. These

---
13. See VI.C.6.2.3.1 for electronic reporting recommendations in the EU.

reports should however be collected and discussed in the periodic safety update reports (*see* Module VII).

However, in certain circumstances, reports of pregnancy exposure with no suspected reactions may necessitate to be reported. This may be a condition of the marketing authorisation or stipulated in the risk management plan; for example pregnancy exposure to medicinal products contraindicated in pregnancy or medicinal products with a special need for surveillance because of a high teratogenic potential (e.g. thalidomide, isotretinoin).

A signal of a possible teratogen effect (e.g. through a cluster of similar abnormal outcomes) should be notified immediately to the competent authorities in accordance with the recommendations presented in VI.C.2.2.6.

b. Breastfeeding
Suspected adverse reactions which occur in infants following exposure to a medicinal product from breast milk should be reported in accordance with the criteria outlined in VI.B.7.[14].

VI.B.6.2. Use of A Medicinal Product in A Paediatric or Elderly Population

The collection of safety information in the paediatric or elderly population is important. Reasonable attempts should therefore be made to obtain and submit the age or age group of the patient when a case is reported by a healthcare professional, or consumer in order to be able to identify potential safety signals specific to a particular population.

As regards the paediatric population, the guidance published by the Agency[15] on the conduct of pharmacovigilance in this population should be followed.

VI.B.6.3. Reports of Overdose, Abuse, Off-Label Use, Misuse, Medication Error or Occupational exposure

For the purpose of this Module, medication error refers to any unintentional error in the prescribing, dispensing, or administration of a medicinal product while in the control of the healthcare professional or consumer.

Reports of overdose, abuse, off-label use, misuse, medication error or occupational exposure with no associated adverse reaction should not be reported as ICSRs. They should be considered in periodic safety update reports as applicable. When those reports constitute safety issues impacting on the risk-benefit balance of the medicinal product, they should be notified to the competent authorities in accordance with the recommendations provided in VI.C.2.2.6.

Reports associated with suspected adverse reactions should be subject to reporting in accordance with the criteria outlined in VI.B.7. and with the electronic reporting requirements described in VI.C.6.2.3.3. They should be routinely followed-up to ensure that the information is as complete as possible with regards to the symptoms, treatments, outcomes, context of occurrence (e.g. error in prescription, administration, dispensing, dosage, unauthorised indication or population, etc.).

VI.B.6.4. Lack of Therapeutic Efficacy

Reports of lack of therapeutic efficacy should be recorded and followed-up if incomplete. They should not normally be reported, but should be discussed in periodic safety update reports as applicable.

However, in certain circumstances, reports of lack of therapeutic efficacy may require to be reported within a 15-day time frame (*see* VI.C.6.2.3.4. as regards electronic reporting in the EU). Medicinal products used in critical conditions or for the treatment of life-threatening diseases, vaccines, contraceptives are examples of such cases. This applies unless the reporter has specifically stated that the outcome was due to disease progression and was not related to the medicinal product.

Clinical judgement should be used when considering if other cases of lack of therapeutic efficacy qualify for reporting. For example, an antibiotic used in a life-threatening situation where the medicinal product was not in fact appropriate for the infective agent should not be reported. However, a life-threatening infection, where the lack of therapeutic efficacy appears to be due to the development of a newly resistant strain of a

---
14. *See* Footnote 16.
15. Guideline on conduct of pharmacovigilance for medicines used by the paediatric population.

bacterium previously regarded as susceptible, should be reported within 15 days.

For vaccines, cases of lack of therapeutic efficacy should be reported, in particular with the view to highlight potential signals of reduced immunogenicity in a sub-group of vaccinees, waning immunity, or strain replacement. With regard to the latter, it is considered that spontaneously reported cases of lack of therapeutic efficacy by a healthcare professional may constitute a signal of strain replacement. Such a signal may need prompt action and further investigation through post-authorisation safety studies as appropriate. General guidance regarding the monitoring of vaccines failure, provided in the Report of CIOMS/WHO Working Group on Vaccine Pharmacovigilance,[16] may be followed.

VI.B.7. Reporting of Individual Case Safety Reports (ICSRs)

Only valid ICSRs (see VI.B.2.) should be reported. The clock for the reporting of a valid ICSR starts as soon as the information containing the minimum reporting criteria has been brought to the attention of the national or regional pharmacovigilance centre of a competent authority or of any personnel of the marketing authorisation holder, including medical representatives and contractors. This date should be considered as day zero. It is the first day when a receiver gains knowledge of a valid ICSR, irrespective of whether the information is received during a weekend or public holiday. Reporting timelines are based on calendar days.

Where the marketing authorisation holder has set up contractual arrangements with a person or an organisation, explicit procedures and detailed agreements should exist between the marketing authorisation holder and the person/organisation to ensure that the marketing authorisation holder can comply with the reporting obligations. These procedures should in particular specify the processes for exchange of safety information, including timelines and regulatory reporting responsibilities and should avoid duplicate reporting to the competent authorities.

For ICSRs described in the scientific and medical literature (see VI.B.1.1.2.), the clock starts (day zero) with awareness of a publication containing the minimum information for reporting. Where contractual arrangements are made with a person/organisation to perform literature searches and/or report valid ICSRs, detailed agreements should exist to ensure that the marketing authorisation holder can comply with the reporting obligations.

When additional significant information is received for a previously reported case, the reporting time clock starts again for the submission of a follow-up report from the date of receipt of the relevant follow-up information. For the purpose of reporting, significant follow-up information corresponds to new medical or administrative information that could impact on the assessment or management of a case or could change its seriousness criteria; non-significant information includes updated comments on the case assessment or corrections of typographical errors in the previous case version. See also VI.C.6.2.2.7. as regards the distinction between significant and non-significant follow-up information.

VI.B.7.1. Reporting Time Frames

In general, the reporting of serious valid ICSRs is required as soon as possible, but in no case later than 15 calendar days after initial receipt of the information by the national or regional pharmacovigilance centre of a competent authority or by any personnel of the marketing authorisation holder, including medical representatives and contractors. This applies to initial and follow-up information. Where a case initially reported as serious becomes non-serious, based on new follow-up information, this information should still be reported within 15 days; the reporting time frame for non-serious reports should then be applied for the subsequent follow-up reports.

Information as regards the reporting time frame of non-serious valid ICSRs in the EU is provided in VI.C.3.

VI.B.8. Reporting Modalities

Taking into account the international dimension of adverse reactions reporting and the need to achieve harmonisation and high quality between

---

16. Council for International Organizations of Medical Sciences (CIOMS). Definition and application of terms of vaccine pharmacovigilance (report of CIOMS/WHO Working Group on Vaccine Pharmacovigilance). Genève: CIOMS; 2012. http://www.cioms.ch/

all involved parties, ICSRs should be submitted electronically as structured data with the use of controlled vocabularies for the relevant data elements where applicable. In this aspect, with regard to the content and format of electronic ICSRs, competent authorities and marketing authorisation holders should adhere to the following internationally agreed ICH[17] guidelines and standards:

- ICH M1 terminology: Medical Dictionary for Regulatory Activities (MedDRA) (*see* GVP Annex IV);
- MedDRA Term selection: Points to Consider Document: The latest version of the ICH-endorsed Guide for MedDRA Users (*see* GVP Annex IV);
- ICH M2 EWG: Electronic Transmission of Individual Case Safety Reports Message Specification (*see* GVP Annex IV);
- ICH E2B (R2): Maintenance of the ICH Guideline on Clinical Safety Data Management: Data Elements for Transmission of Individual Case Safety Reports (*see* GVP Annex IV);
- ICH E2B Implementation Working Group: Questions & Answers (R5) (March 3, 2005) (*see* GVP Annex IV).

As technical standards evolve over time, the above referred documents may require revision and maintenance. In this context, the latest version of these documents should always be taken into account.

Information regarding EU specific reporting modalities is provided in VI.C.4.

VI.C. OPERATION OF THE EU NETWORK

Section C of this Module highlights the EU specific requirements, as defined in Directive 2001/83/EC and Regulation (EC) No 726/2004, in relation to the collection, management and reporting of reports of suspected adverse reactions (serious and non-serious) associated with medicinal products for human use authorised in the EU, independently of their condition of use. They are applicable to competent authorities in Member States and/or to marketing authorisation holders. Section C should be read in conjunction with the definitions and general principles detailed in VI.A and VI.B of this Module and with the requirements provided in chapters IV, V and IX of the Commission Implementing Regulation (EU) No 520/2012 [IR].

VI.C.1. Reporting Rules for Clinical Trials and Post-Authorisation Studies in the EU

The pharmacovigilance rules laid down in Directive 2001/83/EC and Regulation (EC) No 726/2004 do not apply to investigational medicinal products and non-investigational medicinal products[18] used in clinical trials conducted in accordance with Directive 2001/20/EC.[19]

Post-authorisation safety or efficacy studies requested by competent authorities in Member States or the Agency in accordance with Directive 2001/83/EC or Regulation (EC) No 726/2004, or conducted voluntarily by marketing authorisation holders, can either be clinical trials or non-interventional post-authorisation studies as shown in Figure VI.1. The safety reporting falls therefore either under the scope of Directive 2001/20/EC for any clinical trials or under the provisions set out in Directive 2001/83/EC and Regulation (EC) No 726/2004 for any non-interventional post-authorisation studies. Suspected adverse reactions should not be reported under both regimes, that is Directive 2001/20/EC as well as Regulation (EC) No 726/2004 and Directive 2001/83/EC as this creates duplicate reports.

Further guidance on post-authorisation safety studies is provided in Module VIII.

The different types of studies and clinical trials which can be conducted in the EU are illustrated in Figure VI.1. The safety reporting for clinical trials corresponding to sections A, B, C and D of Figure VI.1. follows the requirements of Directive 2001/20/EC. The safety reporting for non-interventional post-authorisation studies corresponding to section E and F follows the requirements of Directive 2001/83/EC and Regulation (EC) No 726/2004. The reporting rules of reports of suspected adverse

---

17. http://www.ich.org/
18. For guidance on these terms, *see* The Rules Governing Medicinal Products in the European Union, Volume 10, Guidance Applying to Clinical Trials, Guidance on Investigational Medicinal Products and Non-Investigational Medicinal Products (NIMPs) (Ares(2011)300458 - 18/03/2011).
19. *See* DIR Art 3(3), Art 107(1) third subparagraph.

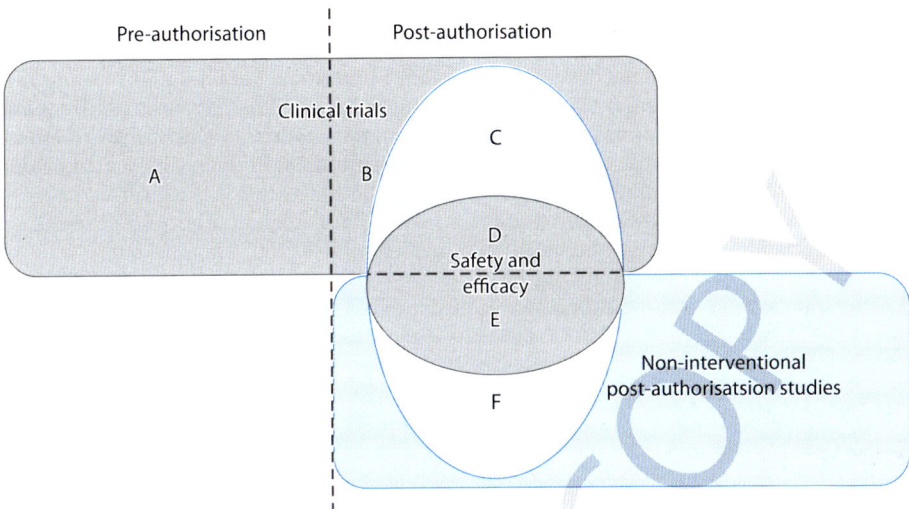

SECTION A: Clinical trials, which fall under the scope of Directive 2001/20/EC and which are conducted when no marketing authorisation exists in the EU.
SECTION B: Clinical trials, which fall under the scope of Directive 2001/20/EC and which are conducted in the post- authorisation period, e.g. for new indication.
SECTION C: Post-authorisation clinical trials conducted in accordance with the summary of product characteristics (SmPC) indication and condition of use, but which fall under the scope of Directive 2001/20/EC due to the nature of the intervention.
SECTION D: Post-authorisation safety or efficacy clinical trials requested in accordance with Directive 2001/83/EC or Regulation (EC) No 726/2004 or conducted voluntarily by marketing authorisation holders, but which fall under the scope of Directive 2001/20/EC due to the nature of the intervention.
SECTION E: Non-interventional post-authorisation safety or efficacy studies requested in accordance with Directive 2001/83/EC or Regulation (EC) No 726/2004 or conducted voluntarily by the marketing authorisation holders and which follow the same legal requirements.
SECTION F: Non-interventional post-authorisation studies conducted in accordance with SmPC indication and condition of use and which fall under the scope of Directive 2001/83/EC or Regulation (EC) No726/2004.

Fig. VI.1: Diagram illustrating different types of clinical trials and studies in the EU.

reactions to the EudraVigilance database modules are dependent on the types of organised collection systems where they occurred; recommendations provided in VI.C.6.2.1 Should be followed.

VI.C.1.1. Reporting Rules for Clinical Trials

A suspected adverse reaction to an investigational medicinal product occurring in a clinical trial which falls under the scope of Directive 2001/20/EC is only to be addressed by the sponsor based on the requirements detailed in that Directive. It is therefore excluded from the scope of this Module even if the clinical trial where the suspected adverse reaction occurred is a post-authorisation safety or efficacy study, requested in accordance with Directive 2001/83/EC or Regulation (EC) No 726/2004, or conducted voluntarily.

If a clinical trial, conducted under the scope of Directive 2001/20/EC, yields safety concerns which impact on the risk-benefit balance of an authorised medicinal product, the competent authorities in the Member States where the medicinal product is authorised and the Agency should be notified immediately in accordance with the modalities detailed in VI.C.2.2.6. This applies as well if a safety concern arises from a clinical trial conducted exclusively outside the EU.

The safety data from clinical trials to be presented in the relevant sections of the periodic safety update report of the authorised medicinal product are detailed in Module VII.

Where an untoward and unintended response originating from a clinical trial conducted in accordance with Directive 2001/20/EC, is suspected to be related only to a non-investigational medicinal product (or another medicinal product, which is not part of the clinical trial protocol) and does not result from a possible interaction with the investigational medicinal product, it does not follow the expedited reporting requirements of Directive

2001/20/EC, which apply only to the investigational medicinal product. The investigator or the sponsor is encouraged to report the case to the competent authority in the Member State where the reaction occurred or to the marketing authorisation holder of the suspected medicinal product, but not to both to avoid duplicate reporting.[20] Where made aware of such case, the competent authority or the marketing authorisation holder should apply the reporting requirements described in VI.C.3, VI.C.4, and VI.C.6. As regards electronic reporting, the recommendations detailed in VI.C.6.2.3.7 should be followed.

VI.C.1.2. Reporting Rules for Non-Interventional Post-Authorisation Studies, Compassionate Use and Named Patient use

This Section applies to non-interventional post-authorisation studies, compassionate use and named patient use. For these organised data collection schemes, a system should be put in place to record and document complete and comprehensive case information on solicited adverse events[21] which need to be collected as specified in VI.C.1.2.1. and in VI.C.1.2.2. These adverse events should be systematically assessed to determine whether they are possibly related to the studied (or supplied) medicinal products [see ICH-E2D (see GVP Annex IV)]. A method of causality assessment should be applied for assessing the causal role of the studied (or supplied) medicinal products in the solicited adverse events (for example, the WHO-UMC system for standardised case causality assessment). An adverse event should be classified as an adverse reaction, if there is at least a reasonable possibility of causal relationship. Only valid ICSRs (see VI.B.2.) of adverse reactions, which are suspected to be related to the studied (or supplied) medicinal product by the primary source or the receiver of the case, should be reported in accordance with the requirements provided in VI.C.3., VI.C.4. and VI.C.6.2.3.7. Other reports of adverse events should be summarised as part of any interim safety analysis and in the final study report, where applicable. In situations where adverse reactions are suspected to be related to medicinal products other than the studied (or supplied) medicine, these reports should be managed, classified and reported as spontaneous ICSRs. They should be notified by the primary source to the competent authority in the Member State where the reactions occurred or to the marketing authorisation holder of the suspected medicinal product, but not to both (to avoid duplicate reporting).

Where made aware, in the frame of these organised data collection schemes, of events which affect the known risk-benefit balance of the studied (or supplied) medicinal product and/or impact on public health, the marketing authorisation holder should notify the concerned competent authorities and the Agency in accordance with the modalities detailed in VI.C.2.2.6.

Further guidance on post-authorisation studies conducted by marketing authorisation holders is provided in VI.C.2.2.2.

The requirements provided in this Module do not apply to non-interventional post-authorisation studies conducted by organisations such as academia, medical research charities or research organisations in the public sector. These organisations should follow local requirements as regards the reporting of cases of suspected adverse reactions to the competent authority in the Member State where the reaction occurred. However, where a study conducted by one of these organisations is directly initiated, managed, financed, or where its design is controlled by a marketing authorisation holder (voluntarily or pursuant to obligations imposed in accordance with Articles 21a or 22a of Directive 2001/83/EC and Articles 10 or 10(a) of Regulation 726/2004), the requirements provided in this Module are applicable.[22] In this context, contractual agreements should be in place to clearly define the role and responsibilities for implementing these requirements (see Module I).

VI.C.1.2.1. Non-Interventional Post-Authorisation Studies

Non-interventional post-authorisation studies[23] should be distinguished between those with primary data collection directly from healthcare professionals or consumers and study designs which are based on the secondary

---

20. See The Rules Governing Medicinal Products in the European Union, Volume 10, Detailed guidance on the collection, verification and presentation of adverse event/reaction reports arising from clinical trials on medicinal products for human use ('CT-3'), (2011/C 172/01).
21. See GVP Annex I for definition of adverse event.

Annexure 8: Guideline on Good Pharmacovigilance Practices (GVP)

Table VI.1: Non-interventional post-authorisation studies with primary data collection: Requirements concerning adverse events collection and suspected adverse reactions reporting.

	Adverse events for which the protocol does not provide differently and those with fatal outcomes
Collection requirements	• Collect comprehensive and high quality information • Perform causality assessment
Reporting requirements for suspected adverse reactions	• Cases of adverse reactions, which are suspected to be related to the studied medicinal product by the primary source or the receiver of the case, should be reported in the form of valid ICSRs in line with the appropriate timeframes (See VI.C.3) • In certain circumstances, fatal outcome may not be subject to expedited reporting as ICSRs. A justification should always be provided in the protocol
Reporting requirements for adverse events	• Summarise all collected adverse events as part of any interim safety analysis and in the final study report

use of data. Depending on the study design, the requirements provided hereafter apply.[24] In case of doubt, the reporting requirements should be clarified with the concerned competent authorities in Member States. National legislation should be followed as applicable regarding the obligations towards local ethics committees.

a. Non-interventional post-authorisation studies with primary data collection

Information on all adverse events should be collected from healthcare professionals or consumers in the course of the study unless the protocol provides differently with a due justification for not collecting certain adverse events. For all collected adverse events, comprehensive and high quality information should be sought in a manner which allow for valid ICSRs to be reported within the appropriate timeframes (see VI.C.3.).

For all collected adverse events, cases of adverse reactions, which are suspected to be related to the studied medicinal product by the primary source or the receiver of the case, should be reported in accordance with the requirements provided in VI.C.3. and VI.C.4. Valid ICSRs should be classified as solicited reports (see VI.C.2.2.2. and VI.C.6.2.3.7.). See summary in Table VI.1.

All fatal outcomes should be considered as adverse events which should be collected. In certain circumstances, suspected adverse reactions with fatal outcome may not be subject to expedited reporting as ICSRs, for example, because they refer to study outcomes (efficacy end points), because the patients included in the study have a disease with high mortality, or because the fatal outcomes have no relation to the objective of the study. For these particular situations, the rational for not reporting certain adverse reactions with fatal outcomes should be clearly described in the protocol.

All collected adverse events should be summarised as part of any interim safety analysis and in the final study report.

For adverse events for which the protocol provides differently and does not require their systematic collection, healthcare professionals and consumers should be informed in the protocol (or other study documents) of the possibility to report adverse reactions (for which they suspect a causal role of a medicine) to the marketing authorisation holder of the suspected medicinal product (studied or not) or to the concerned competent authorities via the national spontaneous reporting system. Valid ICSRs should be managed, classified and reported as spontaneous by the receiver of the

---

22. This does not concern donation of a medicinal product for research purpose if the marketing authorisation holder has no control on the study.
23. See GVP Annex I for definition of non-interventional study.
24. For combined study designs with primary and secondary data collection, the same requirements as for studies with primary data collection should befollowed.

reports. When made aware of them, these reports should also be summarised in the relevant study reports.

b. Non-interventional post-authorisation studies based on secondary use of data

The design of such studies is characterised by the secondary use of data previously collected from consumers or healthcare professionals for other purposes. Examples include medical chart reviews (including following-up on data with healthcare professionals), analysis of electronic healthcare records, systematic reviews, meta-analyses.

For these studies, the reporting of suspected adverse reactions in the form of ICSRs is not required. Reports of adverse events/reactions should be summarised as part of any interim safety analysis and in the final study report unless the protocol provides for different reporting.

VI.C.1.2.2. Compassionate Use and Named Patient use

The guidance provided in this Module applies, subject to amendments where appropriate, to medicinal products supplied in the context of compassionate use as defined in Article 83(2) of Regulation (EC) No 726/2004. As the case may be, this guidance may also apply to named patient use as defined under Article 5(1) of Directive 2001/83/EC. Local requirements should be followed as applicable.

Where an organisation[25] or a healthcare professional, supplying a medicinal product under compassionate use or named patient use, is notified or becomes aware of an adverse event, it should be managed as follows depending on the requirements in the concerned Member State:

- For compassionate use and named patient use conducted in Member States where the active collection of adverse events occurring in these programmes is required, reports of adverse reactions, which are suspected to be related to the supplied medicinal product by the primary source or the receiver of the case, should be reported. They should be considered as solicited reports (see VI.C.2.2.2. and VI.C.6.2.3.7.).
- For compassionate use and named patient use conducted in Member States where the active collection of adverse events occurring in these programmes is not required, any notified noxious or unintended response to the supplied medicinal product should be reported. It should be considered as a spontaneous report of suspected adverse reaction.

VI.C.2. Collection of Reports

VI.C.2.1. Responsibilities of Member States

Each Member State shall have in place a system for the collection and recording of unsolicited and solicited reports of suspected adverse reactions that occur in its territory and which are brought to its attention by healthcare professionals, consumers, or marketing authorisation holders[26] [DIR Art 101(1) and 107a(1)]. In this context, competent authorities in Member States shall establish procedures for collecting and recording all reports of suspected adverse reactions that occur in their territory [IR Art 15 (2)]. The general principles detailed in VI.B, together with the reporting modalities presented in VI.C.3, VI.C.4 and VI.C.6 should be applied to those reports. Pharmacovigilance data and documents relating to individual authorised medicinal products shall be retained as long as the product is authorised and for at least 10 years after the marketing authorisation has expired. However, the documents shall be retained for a longer period where Union law or national law so requires [IR Art 16(2)].

Each Member State shall take all appropriate measures to encourage healthcare professionals and consumers in their territory to report suspected adverse reactions to their competent authority. In addition, the competent authority in a Member State may impose specific obligations on healthcare professionals. To this end, competent authorities in Member States shall facilitate in their territory the reporting of suspected adverse reactions by means of alternative straightforward reporting systems, accessible to healthcare professionals and consumers, in addition to web-based formats [DIR Art 102]. Information on the different ways of reporting suspected adverse reactions related to

---

25. E.g. sponsor, applicant, marketing authorisation holder, hospital or wholesaler.
26. Marketing authorisation holders shall report ICSRs to the competent authorities in Member States in accordance with the transitional provisions set out in Article 2(4) and Article 2(5) of Directive 2010/84/EU and further detailed in VI.C.4.1.

medicinal products, shall be made publicly available including by means of national medicines web-based portals [DIR 106(e)]. To increase awareness of the reporting systems, organisations representing consumers and healthcare professionals may be involved as appropriate [DIR Art 102].

Standard web-based structured forms for the reporting of suspected adverse reactions by healthcare professionals and consumers shall be developed by the Agency in collaboration with Member States in order to collect across the EU harmonised information relevant for the evaluation of suspected adverse reactions, including errors associated with the use of medicinal products [REG Art 25]. In this context, core data fields for reporting will be made available by the Agency to the competent authorities in Member States for use in their national reporting systems as applicable.

The reports of suspected adverse reactions received from healthcare professionals and consumers should be acknowledged where appropriate and further information should be provided to the reporters as requested and when available.

For reports submitted by a marketing authorisation holder, Member States on whose territory the suspected adverse reaction occurred may involve the marketing authorisation holder in the follow-up of the reports [DIR Art 107a(2)].

Each Member State shall ensure that the competent authority responsible for medicinal products within that Member State is informed of any suspected adverse reaction, brought to the attention of any other authority, body, institution or organisation responsible for patient safety within that Member State, and that valid ICSRs are made available to the EudraVigilance database. Therefore, where reports of suspected adverse reactions are sent directly to other authorities, bodies, organisations and/or institutions within a Member State, the competent authority in that Member State shall have data exchange agreements in place so that these reports are brought to its attention and are made available to EudraVigilance in a timely manner[DIR Art 107a(5)]. This applies as well to reports of suspected adverse reactions arising from an error associated with the use of a medicinal product.

Those error reports of suspected adverse reactions for which a competent authority in a Member State is made aware of, including those received from the EudraVigilance database in accordance with Article 24(4) of Regulation (EC) No 726/2004, shall also be brought to the attention of other authorities, bodies, organisations and/or institutions responsible for patient safety within that Member State [DIR Art107a(5)].

Unless there are justifiable grounds resulting from pharmacovigilance activities, individual Member States shall not impose any additional obligations on marketing authorisation holders for the reporting of suspected adverse reactions [DIR Art 107a(6)].

VI.C.2.2. Responsibilities of the Marketing Authorisation Holder in the EU

Each marketing authorisation holder shall have in place a system for the collection and recording of all reports of suspected adverse reactions which are brought to its attention, whether reported spontaneously by healthcare professionals or consumers or occurring in the context of a post-authorisation study [DIR Art 104(1), Art 107(1)]. Marketing authorisation holders shall not refuse to consider reports of suspected adverse reactions received electronically or by any other appropriate means from patients and healthcare professionals [Art 107(2)]. All those reports shall be accessible at a single point within the Union [Dir Art 107(1)].

Marketing authorisation holders shall establish mechanisms enabling the traceability and follow-up of adverse reaction reports while complying with the data protection legislation [IR Art 12 (1)]. Pharmacovigilance data and documents relating to individual authorised medicinal products shall be retained as long as the product is authorised and for at least 10 years after the marketing authorisation has ceased to exist. However, the documents shall be retained for a longer period where Union law or national law so requires [IR Art 12 (2)].

With regard to the collection and recording of reports of suspected adverse reactions, marketing authorisation holders responsibilities apply to reports related to medicinal products (*see* VI.A.2.2.) for which ownership cannot be excluded on the basis of one the following criteria: medicinal product name, active substance name, pharmaceutical form, batch number or route of administration.

Exclusion based on the primary source country or country of origin of the adverse reaction is possible if the marketing authorisation holder can demonstrate that the suspected medicinal product has never been supplied or placed on the market in that territory or that the product is not a travel medicine (e.g. anti-malarial medicinal product).

The marketing authorisation holder shall ensure that any information on adverse reactions, suspected to be related to at least one of the active substances of its medicinal products authorised in the EU, is brought to its attention by any company outside the EU belonging to the same mother company (or group of companies).[27] The same applies to the marketing authorisation holder when having concluded a commercial agreement with a company outside the EU for one of its medicinal product authorised in the EU. The clock for reporting (see VI.B.7.) starts when a valid ICSR is first received by one of these companies outside the EU.

In addition to the requirements presented in this Section, the general principles detailed in Section VI.B., together with the reporting modalities presented in VI.C.3., VI.C.4.and VI.C.6. should be applied by marketing authorisation holders to all reports of suspected adverse reactions.

VI.C.2.2.1. Spontaneous Reports

Marketing authorisation holders shall record all reports of suspected adverse reactions originating from within or outside the EU, which are brought to their attention spontaneously by healthcare professionals, or consumers. This includes reports of suspected adverse reactions received electronically or by any other appropriate means [DIR Art 107(1), Art 107(2)]. In this context, marketing authorisation holders may consider utilising their websites to facilitate the collection of reports of suspected adverse reactions by providing adverse reactions forms for reporting, or appropriate contact details for direct communication (see VI.B.1.1.4.).

VI.C.2.2.2. Solicited Reports

In accordance with Art 107(1) of Directive 2001/83/EC, marketing authorisation holders shall record all reports of suspected adverse reactions originating from within or outside the EU, which occur in post-authorisation studies, initiated, managed, or financed by them.[28] For non-interventional post-authorisation studies, this requirement applies to study designs based on primary data collection and the guidance provided in VI.C.1.2.1. should be followed. For all solicited reports (see VI.B.1.2.), marketing authorisation holders should have mechanisms in place to record and document complete and comprehensive case information and to evaluate that information, in order to allow meaningful assessment of individual cases and reporting of valid ICSRs (see VI.B.2.) related to the studied (or supplied) medicinal product. Marketing authorisation holders should therefore exercise due diligence in establishing such system, in following-up those reports (see VI.B.3.) and in seeking the view of the primary source as regard the causal role of the studied (or supplied) medicinal product on the notified adverse event. Where this opinion is missing, the marketing authorisation holder should exercise its own judgement based on the information available in order to decide whether the report is a valid ICSR, which should be reported to the competent authorities. This requirement does not apply to study designs based on secondary use of data since reporting of ICSRs is not required (see VI.C.1.2.1.). Safety data from solicited reports to be presented in the relevant sections of the periodic safety update report of the authorised medicinal product are detailed in Module VII.

VI.C.2.2.3. Case Reports Published in the Scientific Literature

General principles in relation to the monitoring for individual cases of suspected adverse reactions described in the scientific and medical literature are provided in VI.B.1.1.2. As regards the screening of the scientific and medical literature, the requirements provided in this Module are part of the wider literature searches which need to be conducted for periodic safety update reports (see Module VII).

In accordance with Article 107(3) of Directive 2001/83/EC, in order to avoid the reporting of duplicate ICSRs, marketing authorisation holders shall only report those ICSRs described in the scientific and medical literature which is

---

27. As outlined in the Commission Communication on the Community Marketing Authorization Procedures for Medicinal Products (98/C229/03).
28. This does not concern donation of a medicinal product for research purpose if the marketing authorisation holder has no control on the study.

not reviewed by the Agency, for all medicinal products containing active substances which are not included in the list monitored by the Agency pursuant to Article 27 of Regulation (EC) No 726/2004. Until such lists of scientific and medical literature and active substance names are published by the Agency, marketing authorisation holders should monitor all the active substances for which they hold a marketing authorisation in the EU by accessing a widely used systematic literature review and reference database, in line with the principles detailed in VI.B.1.1.2.and in VI. Appendix 2.

Articles can be excluded from the reporting of ICSRs by the marketing authorisation holder if another company's branded medicinal product is the suspected medicinal product. In the absence of a specified medicinal product source and/or invented name, ownership of the medicinal product should be assumed for articles about an active substance, unless alternative reasons for exclusion detailed hereafter apply:

- Where ownership of the medicinal product by the marketing authorisation holder can be excluded on the basis of the criteria detailed in VI.C.2.2.;
- For individual case safety reports identified in the scientific and medical literature that originate in a country where a company holds a marketing authorisation but has never commercialised the medicinal product;
- For literature ICSRs which are based on an analysis from a competent authority database within the EU. The reporting requirements remain for those ICSRs which are based on the analysis from a competent authority database outside the EU;
- For literature articles, which present data analyses from publicly available databases or, which summarise results from post-authorisation studies (see VI.C.1.2.). This type of literature article describes adverse reactions, which occur in a group of patients with a designated medicinal product with the aim of identifying or quantifying a safety hazard related to a medicinal product, and aggregated data on patients are often presented in tables or line listings. The main objective of those studies is to detect/evaluate specific risks that could affect the overall risk-benefit balance of a medicinal product.

New and significant safety findings presented in these articles, for which reporting is not required, should however be discussed in the relevant sections of the concerned periodic safety update report (see Module VII) and analysed as regards their overall impact on the medicinal product risk-benefit profile. In addition, any new safety information, which may impact on the risk-benefit profile of a medicinal product, should be notified immediately to the competent authorities in Member States where the medicinal product is authorised and to the Agency in accordance with the recommendations provided in VI.C.2.2.6.

A detailed guidance on the monitoring of the scientific and medical literature has been developed in accordance with Article 27(3) of Regulation (EC) No 726/2004; it is included in VI. Appendix 2.

The electronic reporting recommendations regarding suspected adverse reactions reports published in the scientific and medical literature are provided in VI.C.6.2.3.2.

VI.C.2.2.4. Suspected Adverse Reactions Related to Quality Defect or Falsified Medicinal Products

When a report of suspected adverse reactions is associated with a suspected or confirmed falsified medicinal product or quality defect of a medicinal product, a valid ICSR should be reported. The seriousness of the ICSR is linked to the seriousness of the reported suspected adverse reactions in accordance with the definitions provided in VI.A.2.4. Electronic reporting recommendations provided in VI.C.6.2.3.5. should be followed.

In addition in order to protect public health, it may become necessary to implement urgent measures such as the recall of one or more defective batch(es) of a medicinal product from the market. Therefore, marketing authorisation holders should have a system in place to ensure that reports of suspected adverse reactions related to falsified medicinal products or to quality defects of a medicinal products are investigated in a timely fashion and that confirmed quality defects are notified separately to the manufacturer and to competent authorities in accordance with the provisions described in Article 13 of Directive 2003/94/EC.

VI.C.2.2.5. Suspected Transmission via a Medicinal Product of an Infectious agent

For the purposes of reporting, any suspected transmission of an infectious agent via a medicinal product should be considered as a serious adverse reaction and such cases should be reported within 15 days in accordance with the requirements outlined in VI.C.4.[29] If no other criterion is applicable, the seriousness of this ICSR should be considered as important medical event (*see* VI.A.2.4.). This also applies to vaccines. Electronic reporting recommendations provided in VI.C.6.2.3.6. should be followed.

In the case of medicinal products derived from human blood or human plasma, haemovigilance procedures may also apply in accordance with Directive 2002/98/EC. Therefore the marketing authorisation holder should have a system in place to communicate suspected transmission via a medicinal product of an infectious agent to the manufacturer, the relevant blood establishment(s) and national competent authorities in Member States.

Any organism, virus or infectious particle (e.g. prion protein transmitting transmissible spongiform encephalopathy), pathogenic or non-pathogenic, is considered an infectious agent.

A transmission of an infectious agent may be suspected from clinical signs or symptoms, or laboratory findings indicating an infection in a patient exposed to a medicinal product.

Emphasis should be on the detection of infections/infectious agents known to be potentially transmitted via a medicinal product, but the occurrence of unknown agents should also always be considered.

In the context of evaluating a suspected transmission of an infectious agent via a medicinal product, care should be taken to discriminate, whenever possible, between the cause (e.g. injection/administration) and the source (e.g. contamination) of the infection and the clinical conditions of the patient at the time of the infection (immunosuppressed /vaccinee).

Confirmation of contamination (including inadequate inactivation/attenuation of infectious agents as active substances) of the concerned medicinal product increases the evidence for transmission of an infectious agent and may therefore be suggestive of a quality defect for which the procedures detailed in VI.C.2.2.4. should be applied.

Medicinal products should comply with the recommendations provided in the Note for Guidance on Minimising the Risk of Transmitting Animal Spongiform Encephalopathy Agents via Human and Veterinary Products.[30] For advanced therapy medicinal products, Article 14(5) of Regulation (EC) No 1394/2007 and the Guideline on Safety and Efficacy Follow-up—Risk Management of Advanced Therapy Medicinal Products,[31] should also be followed as appropriate.

VI.C.2.2.6. Emerging Safety Issues

Events may occur, which do not fall within the definition of reportable valid ICSRs, and thus are not subject to the reporting requirements, even though they may lead to changes in the known risk-benefit balance of a medicinal product and/or impact on public health. Examples include:

- Major safety findings from a newly completed non-clinical study;
- Major safety concerns identified in the course of a non-interventional post-authorisation study or of a clinical trial;
- Signal of a possible teratogen effect or of significant hazard to public health;
- Safety issues published in the scientific and medical literature;
- Safety issues arising from the signal detection activity (*see* Module IX) or emerging from a new ICSR and which impact on the risk-benefit balance of the medicinal product and/or have implications for public health;
- Safety issues related to the use outside the terms of the marketing authorisation;
- Safety issues due to misinformation in the product information;
- Marketing authorisation withdrawal, non-renewal, revocation or suspension outside the EU for safety-related reasons;
- Urgent safety restrictions outside the EU;

---

29. *See* VI.C.6.2.3.6. for electronic reporting recommendations.
30. Latest revision. (Ref.: EMA/410/01).
31. Ref.: EMEA/149995/2008

- Safety issues in relation to the supply of raw material;
- Lack of supply of medicines.

These events/observations, which may affect the risk-benefit balance of a medicinal product, are not to be submitted as ICSRs. They should be notified as emerging safety issues in writing to the competent authorities in Member States where the medicinal product is authorised and to the Agency via email (P-PV-emerging-safety-issue@ema.europa.eu); this should be done immediately when becoming aware of them. The document should indicate the points of concern and the actions proposed in relation to the marketing application/authorisation for the concerned medicinal product. Those safety issues should also be analysed in the relevant sections of the periodic safety update report of the authorised medicinal product.

VI.C.2.2.7. Period between the Submission of the Marketing Authorisation Application and the Granting of the Marketing authorisation

In the period between the submission of the marketing authorisation application and the granting of the marketing authorisation, information (quality, non-clinical, clinical) that could impact on the risk- benefit balance of the medicinal product under evaluation may become available to the applicant.[32] It is the responsibility of the applicant to ensure that this information is immediately submitted in accordance with the modalities described in VI.C.2.2.6. to the competent authorities in the Member States where the application is under assessment (including Reference Member State and all concerned Member States for products assessed under the mutual recognition or decentralised procedures) and to the Agency. For applications under the centralised procedure, the information should also be provided to the (Co-) Rapporteur.

In the situation where a medicinal product application is under evaluation in the EU while it has already been authorised in a third country, valid ICSRs from outside the EU, originating from unsolicited reports (*see* VI.B.1.1.) or solicited reports (*see* VI.B.1.2.), should be reported in accordance with the requirements provided in VI.C.3., and VI.C.6.

VI.C.2.2.8. Period after suspension, revocation or withdrawal of marketing authorisation

The marketing authorisation holder shall continue to collect any reports of suspected adverse reactions related to the concerned medicinal product following the suspension of a marketing authorisation. The reporting requirements outlined in VI.C.4. remain.

Where a marketing authorisation is withdrawn or revoked, the former marketing authorisation holder is encouraged to continue to collect spontaneous reports of suspected adverse reactions originating within the EU to for example facilitate the review of delayed onset adverse reactions or of retrospectively notified cases.

VI.C.2.2.9. Period during a public health emergency

A public health emergency is a public health threat duly recognised either by the World Health Organization (WHO) or the Community in the framework of Decision No. 2119/98/EC as amended of the European Parliament and of the Council. In the event of a public health emergency, regular reporting requirements may be amended. Such arrangements will be considered on a case-by-case basis and will be appropriately notified on the Agency website.

VI.C.2.2.10. Reports from Class Action Lawsuits

Stimulated reports arising from class action lawsuits should be managed as spontaneous reports. Valid ICSRs should describe adverse reactions related to the concerned medicinal product. They should be reported in accordance with the time frames and modalities described in VI.C.3., and VI.C.6.

Where large batches of potential ICSRs are received, marketing authorisation holders may request, in exceptional circumstances, for an exemption in order to submit serious cases of suspected adverse reactions within 30 days from their date of receipt instead of 15 days. The 90 days reporting time frame for non-serious ICSRs remains unchanged. It will be possible to apply for this exemption only once the functionalities of the EudraVigilance database specified in Article 24(2) of Regulation (EC) No 726/2004 are established.

---

32. *See* also chapter 1, section 5.1.1 of Volume 2A (Notice to Applicants) of The Rules Governing Medicinal Products in theEuropean Union. http://ec.europa.eu/health/documents/eudralex/vol-2/index_en.htm.

The request should be made to the Agency's pharmacovigilance department.

VI.C.2.2.11. Reports from Patient Support Programmes and Market Research Programmes

A patient support programme is an organised system where a marketing authorisation holder receives and collects information relating to the use of its medicinal products. Examples are post-authorisation patient support and disease management programmes, surveys of patients and healthcare providers, information gathering on patient compliance, or compensation/reimbursement schemes.

A market research programme refers to the systematic collection, recording and analysis by a marketing authorisation holder of data and findings about its medicinal products, relevant for marketing and business development.

Safety reports originating from those programmes should be considered as solicited reports. Marketing authorisation holders should have the same mechanisms in place as for all other solicited reports (*see* VI.C.2.2.2.) to manage that information and report valid cases of adverse reactions, which are suspected to be related to the concerned medicinal product.

Valid ICSRs should be reported as solicited in accordance with the electronic reporting requirements provided in VI.C.6.2.3.7.

VI.C.3. Reporting Time Frames

The general rules in relation to the reporting of initial and follow-up reports, including those for defining the clock start are detailed in VI.B.7.

According to Articles 107(3) and 107a(4) of Directive 2001/83/EC:
- Serious valid ICSRs shall be reported by competent authorities in Member States or by marketing authorisation holders within 15 days from the date of receipt of the reports;
- Non-serious valid ICSRs shall be reported by competent authorities in Member States or by marketing authorisation holders within 90 days from the date of receipt of the reports.

This should be done in accordance with the reporting modalities detailed in VI.C.4.

VI.C.4. Reporting Modalities

In addition to the recommendations provided in VI.B.8., competent authorities in Member States and marketing authorisation holders shall use the formats, standards and terminologies for the electronic transmission of suspected adverse reactions as referred to in chapter IV of the Commission Implementing Regulation (EU) No 520/2012. ICSRs shall be used for reporting to the EudraVigilance database suspected adverse reactions to a medicinal product that occur in a single patient at a specific point in time [IR Art 27]. Competent authorities in Member States and marketing authorisation holders shall also ensure that all reported electronic ICSRs are well documented and as complete as possible in accordance with the requirements provided in [IR Art 28].

The time frames for reporting serious and non-serious valid ICSRs are provided in VI.C.3. The recommendations provided in VI.C.6. should be adhered to as regards the electronic exchange of pharmacovigilance information between competent authorities in Member States, marketing authorisation holders and the Agency.

ICSRs reported electronically to the EudraVigilance database will be made accessible to stakeholders such as competent authorities, healthcare professionals, consumers, as well as marketing authorisation holders and research organisations in accordance with Article 24(2) of Regulation (EC) No 726/2004 and the EudraVigilance Access Policy for Medicines for Human Use.[33] This policy defines the overall principles of the provision of access to EudraVigilance data in line with the current legal framework, while guaranteeing personal data protection. As detailed in the EudraVigilance access policy, a selection of ICSRs could be downloaded by marketing authorisation holders in ICH E2B format and in accordance with the ICH M2 message specifications, to facilitate their pharmacovigilance activities.

VI.C.4.1. Interim Arrangements

In accordance with the provisions set out in Article 2(4), Article 2(5) and Article 2(6) of Directive 2010/84/EU, until the Agency can ensure the

---

33. http://www.ema.europa.eu

functionalities of the EudraVigilance database as specified in Article 24(2) of Regulation (EC) No 726/2004, the following reporting requirements shall apply to valid unsolicited and solicited ICSRs reported by healthcare professionals and non-healthcare professionals. This is independently of the condition of use of the suspected medicinal product and of the expectedness of the adverse reaction.

a. Serious ICSRs

- Marketing authorisation holders shall report all serious ICSRs that occur in the EU to the competent authority of the Member State on whose territory the suspected adverse reactions occurred.
- Marketing authorisation holders shall report to the EudraVigilance database all serious ICSRs that occur outside the EU, including those received from competent authorities. If required by Member States, those reports shall also be submitted to the competent authorities in the Member States in which the medicinal product is authorised.
- Competent authorities in Member States shall ensure that all serious ICSRs that occur in their territory and that are reported to them, including those received from marketing authorisation holders, are made available to the EudraVigilance database. Competent authorities in Member States should also make available, to the marketing authorisation holders of the suspected medicinal products, all serious ICSRs reported directly to them.

b. Non-Serious ICSRs

- If required by Member States, marketing authorisation holders shall report all non-serious ICSRs that occur in the EU to the competent authority of the Member State on whose territory the suspected adverse reactions occurred.

Overviews of the reporting requirements of serious and non-serious reports during the interim period, applicable to marketing authorisation holders or competent authorities in Member States, are presented in VI.App3.1., together with a detailed business process map.

Member States reporting requirements for serious non-EU ICSRs and for non-serious EU ICSRs are also included in this Appendix.

VI.C.4.2. Final Arrangements

Once the functionalities of the EudraVigilance database specified in Article 24(2) of Regulation (EC) No 726/2004 are established, the following requirements, detailed in Articles 107(3) and 107a(4) of Directive 2001/83/EC, shall apply within 6 months of the announcement by the Agency to valid unsolicited and solicited ICSRs reported by healthcare professionals and non-healthcare professionals. This is independently of the condition of use of the suspected medicinal product and of the expectedness of the adverse reaction.

a. Serious ICSRs

- Marketing authorisation holders shall submit all serious ICSRs that occur within or outside the EU, including those received from competent authorities outside the EU, to the EudraVigilance database only.
- Competent authorities in Member States shall submit to the EudraVigilance database all serious ICSRs that occur in their territory and that are directly reported to them.

b. Non-Serious ICSRs

- Marketing authorisation holders shall submit all non-serious ICSRs that occur in the EU to the EudraVigilance database only.
- Competent authorities in Member States shall submit all non-serious ICSRs that occur in their territory to the EudraVigilance database.

Overviews of the reporting requirements of serious and non-serious reports, applicable to marketing authorisation holders or competent authorities in Member States once the final arrangements are implemented, are presented in VI. App3.2., together with a detailed business process map.

In accordance with the requirement detailed in Article 24(4) of Regulation (EC) No 726/2004 for the final arrangements, the ICSRs submitted to the EudraVigilance database by marketing authorisation holders shall be automatically transmitted upon receipt, to the competent authority of the Member State where the reaction occurred. A detailed business process map is included in VI.App3.3.

VI.C.5. Collaboration with the World Health Organization and the European Monitoring Centre for Drugs and Drug Addiction

The Agency shall make available to the WHO (in practice the WHO Collaborating Centre for International Drug Monitoring) all suspected adverse reaction reports occurring in the EU [REG Art 28c(1)]. This will take place on a weekly basis after their transmission to the EudraVigilance database by competent authorities in Member States or marketing authorisation holders. It will replace the requirements of Member States participating in the WHO Programme for International Drug Monitoring to directly report to WHO suspected adverse reactions reports occurring in their territory. This will be implemented once the functionalities of the EudraVigilance database specified in Article 24(2) of Regulation (EC) No 726/2004 are established.

A detailed business process map for the reporting of ICSRs, from the EudraVigilance database to the WHO Collaborating Centre for International Drug Monitoring, is presented in VI. Appendix 4.

The Agency and the European Monitoring Centre for Drugs and Drug Addiction shall also exchange information that they receive on the abuse of medicinal products including information related to illicit drugs [REG Art 28c(2)].

VI.C.6. Electronic Exchange of Safety Information in the EU

VI.C.6. highlights the requirements, as defined in Articles 24(1) and 24(3) of Regulation (EC) No 726/2004, for the establishment and maintenance of the European database and data processing network (the EudraVigilance database) in order to collate and share pharmacovigilance information electronically between competent authorities in Member States, marketing authorisation holders and the Agency, in ways which ensure the quality and integrity of the data collected.

The information provided here is relevant for the electronic exchange of ICSRs in the EU between all stakeholders and for the electronic submission of information on medicinal products to the Agency.

VI.C.6.1. Applicable Guidelines, Definitions, International Formats, Standards and Terminologies

For the classification, retrieval, presentation, risk-benefit evaluation and assessment, electronic exchange and communication of pharmacovigilance and medicinal product information, Member States, marketing authorisation holders and the Agency shall adhere to the legal requirements provided in chapter IV of the Commission Implementing Regulation (EU) No 520/2012.

In addition the following guidelines should be applied:
- Note for guidance - EudraVigilance Human - Processing of Safety Messages and Individual Case Safety Reports (ICSRs)(EMA/H/20665/04/Final ReVI. 2) (EudraVigilance Business Rules);
- Note for Guidance on the Electronic Data Interchange (EDI) of Individual Case Safety Reports (ICSRs) and Medicinal Products (MPRS) in Pharmacovigilance during the pre- and post- authorisation phase in the European economic area (EEA)(EMEA/115735/2004);
- The ICH guidelines detailed in VI.B.8.;
- The ICH-M5 guideline 'Routes of Administration Controlled Vocabulary'(CHMP/ICH/175860/2005), which provides standard terms for routes of administration;

The latest version of these documents should always be considered.

VI.C.6.2. Electronic Reporting of Individual Case Safety Reports

The reporting of valid ICSRs electronically, by competent authorities in Member States and marketing authorisation holders, is mandatory for all medicinal products authorised in the EU [DIR Art 107(3), Art 107a(4)]. Non-adherence to this requirement constitutes a non-compliance with EU legislation. Responsibilities in case of communication failure (including adherence to compliance for reporting) are detailed in chapter

IV of the Note for Guidance on the Electronic Data Interchange (EDI) of Individual Case Safety Reports (ICSRs) and Medicinal Product Reports (MPRs) in Pharmacovigilance during the Pre- and Post-authorisation Phase in the European Economic Area (EEA)(EMEA/115735/2004).

Technical tools (EVWEB) have been made available by the Agency to interested electronic data interchange partners, including small and medium-sized enterprises, to facilitate compliance with the electronic reporting requirements as defined in EU legislation. Information is available on EudraVigilance website.[34]

VI.C.6.2.1. EudraVigilance Database Modules

Two modules are available in the EudraVigilance database to address the collection of reports of suspected adverse reactions related to medicinal products for human use, in accordance with EU legislation:
- EudraVigilance Post-Authorisation Module (EVPM), implemented based on the requirements defined in Regulation (EC) No 726/2004 and Directive 2001/83/EC;and
- EudraVigilance Clinical Trial Module (EVCTM), implemented based on the requirements defined in Directive2001/20/EC.

VI.C.6.2.1.1. Adverse Reaction Data Collected in the Eudravigilance Post-authorisation Module

The adverse reaction reports collected in the EudraVigilance Post-Authorisation Module (EVPM) refer to unsolicited reports and solicited reports which do not fall under the scope of the Clinical Trials Directive 2001/20/EC (see VI.C.1.). The ICSRs should be submitted with the value 'EVHUMAN' in the data element 'Message receiver identifier' (ICH M2 M.1.6).

Depending on their type, these ICSRs should be classified with one of the following options, in accordance with the EudraVigilance Business Rules:[35]
- Data element 'Type of report' (ICH-E2B(R2) A.1.4):
  - spontaneous report;
  - other;
  - not available to sender (unknown);or
  - report from study.

- In addition, when the value in the data element ICH-E2B(R2) A.1.4 is 'Report from study', the data element 'Study type in which the reaction(s)/event(s) were observed' (ICH-E2B(R2) A.2.3.3) should be populated with:
  - Individual patient use, e.g. compassionate use or named-patient basis;or
  - Other studies, e.g. pharmacoepidemiology, pharmacoeconomics, intensive monitoring, PMS.

VI.C.6.2.1.2. Adverse Reaction Data Collected in the EudraVigilance Clinical Trial Module

Only cases of suspected unexpected serious adverse reactions (SUSARs), related to investigational medicinal products studied in clinical trials which fall under the scope of Directive 2001/20/EC (see VI.C.1.), should be reported by the sponsor to the EudraVigilance Clinical Trial Module (EVCTM). The requirements provided in chapter II of EudraLex Volume 10 of The Rules Governing Medicinal Productsin the European Union should be applied. The ICSRs should be submitted with the value 'EVCTMPROD' in the data element 'Message receiver identifier' (ICH M2 M.1.6) and should be classified as followed, in accordance with the EudraVigilance Business Rules:[36]
- Data element 'Type of report' (ICH-E2B(R2) A.1.4):
  - Report from study; and
- Data element 'Study type in which the reaction(s)/event(s) were observed' (ICH-E2B(R2)A.2.3.3):
  - Clinical trials.

VI.C.6.2.2. Preparation of Individual Case Safety Reports

VI.C.6.2.2.1. General Principles

The content of each valid ICSR transmitted electronically between all stakeholders should comply with the legal requirements and guidelines detailed in the Commission Implementing Regulation (EU) No 520/2012 and in VI.C.6.1., particularly:
- The requirements provided in chapters IV and V of the Commission Implementing Regulation (EU) No 520/2012;
- The latest version of the ICH-Endorsed Guide for MedDRA Users - MedDRA Term Selection:

---

34. http://eudravigilance.ema.europa.eu
35. Note for guidance - EudraVigilance Human - Processing of Safety Messages and Individual Case Safety Reports (ICSRs)(EMA/H/20665/04/Final ReVI.2).
36. *See* Footnote 38.

Points to Consider Document (*see* GVP Annex IV);
- The EudraVigilance business rules for the electronic transmission of ICSRs detailed in the Note for Guidance - EudraVigilance Human - Processing of Safety Messages and Individual Case Safety Reports (ICSRs)(EMA/H/20665/04/Final ReVI.2).

It is recognised that it is often difficult to obtain all the details on a specific case. However, the complete information (medical and administrative data) for a valid ICSR that is available to the sender should be reported in a structured manner in the relevant ICH-E2B(R2) data elements (*see* GVP Annex IV) (which should be repeated as necessary when multiple information is available) and in the narrative section (*see* VI.C.6.2.2.4.). This applies to all types of ICSRs, such as reports with initial information on the case, follow-up information and cases highlighted for nullification.[37]

In the situation where it is evident that the sender has not transmitted the complete information available on the case, the receiver may request the sender to re-transmit the ICSR within 24 hours with the complete case information in electronic format in accordance with the requirements applicable for the electronic reporting of ICSRs. This should be seen in the light of the qualitative signal detection and evaluation activity, where it is important for the receiver to have all the available information on a case to perform the medical assessment (*see* VI.C.6.2.4.).

Where the suspected adverse reactions reported in a single ICSR impact on the known risk-benefit balance of a medicinal product, this should be considered as an emerging safety issue (*see* VI.C.2.2.6.), which should be immediately notified in writing to the competent authorities of the Member States where the medicinal product is authorised and to the Agency. This is in addition to the reporting requirements detailed in VI.C.4. A summary of the points of concerns and the action proposed should be recorded in the ICSR in data element 'Sender's comments' (ICH-E2B(R2) B.5.4).

VI.C.6.2.2.2. Information on Suspect, interacting and concomitant medicinal products
The suspect, interacting and/or concomitant active substances/invented names of the reported medicinal products should be provided in accordance with IR Art 28 (3) (g) to (i), ICH-E2B(R2) (*see* GVP Annex IV) and the EudraVigilance Business Rules.

The characterisation of medicinal products as suspect, interacting or concomitant is based on the information provided by primary source.

For combination medicinal products, which contain more than one active substance, each active substance needs to be reflected individually in the data element 'Active substance name(s)' (ICH E2B(R2) B.4.k.2.2), which needs to be repeated for each active substance contained in the combination medicinal product.

When the primary source reports a suspect or interacting branded/proprietary medicinal product name without indicating the active substance(s) of the medicinal product and where the proprietary medicinal product can be one of two or more possible generics, which have a different composition depending on the country where the medicinal product is marketed, the ICSR should be populated as follows:
- Data element 'Proprietary medicinal product name' (ICH-E2B(R2) B.4.k.2.1) should be populated with the proprietary/branded medicinal product name as reported by the primary source;
- Data element 'Active substance name(s)' (ICH-E2B(R2) B.4.k.2.2) should be completed with the active substance(s) that correspond(s) to the composition of the proprietary/branded medicinal product of the country where the reaction/event occurred.

However if the information is available on:
- The 'Identification of the country where the drug was obtained' (data element ICH E2B(R2) B.4.k.2.3),
- The 'Authorization/application number' (data element ICH-E2B(R2)B.4.k.4.1),
- The 'Country of authorization/application' (data element ICH-E2B(R2) B.4.k.4.2),and/or
- The 'Batch/lot number' (data element ICH-E2B(R2) B.4.k.3), the composition with regard the active substance(s) of the proprietary medicinal product should be provided accordingly.

Where the primary source reports a suspect or interacting branded/proprietary medicinal product

---

37. *See* also VI.C.6.2.2.10.on nullification of individual cases.

name without indicating the pharmaceutical form/presentation of the product and where the proprietary/branded medicinal product can be one of two or more possible pharmaceutical forms/presentations, which have different compositions in a country, the ICSR should be populated as follows:
- Data element 'Proprietary medicinal product name' (ICH-E2B(R2) B.4.k.2.1) should be populated with the medicinal product name as reported by the primary source;
- Data element 'Active substance name(s)' (ICH-E2B(R2) B.4.k.2.2) should be completed with those active substances which are in common to all pharmaceutical forms/presentations in the country of authorisation.

Where medicinal products cannot be described on the basis of the active substances or the invented names, for example, when only the therapeutic class is reported by the primary source, or in case of other administered therapies that cannot be structured, this information should only be reflected in the case narrative (data element ICH-E2B(R2) B.5.1). The data elements 'Proprietary medicinal product name' (ICH-E2B(R2) B.4.k.2.1) and 'Active substance name(s)' (ICH-E2B(R2) B.4.k.2.2) should not be populated. The same applies if a suspected food interaction is reported (e.g. to grapefruit juice).

Where a case of adverse reactions is reported to be related only to a therapeutic class, it is considered incomplete and does not qualify for reporting (*see* VI.B.2.). Efforts should be made to follow-up the case in order to collect the missing information regarding the suspected medicinal product (*see* VI.B.3.).

As regards the reporting of drug interactions, which concerns drug/drug (including biological products), drug/food, drug/device, and drug/alcohol interactions, the coding of the interaction should be performed in section 'Reactions/Events' (ICH-E2B(R2) B.2) in line with the latest version of the ICH-Endorsed Guide for MedDRA Users-MedDRA Term Selection: Points to Consider Document (*see* GVP Annex IV). In addition, for drug/drug interactions, information on the active substances/proprietary medicinal product names should be provided in the section 'Drug information' (ICH-E2B(R2) B.4), which should be characterised as interacting in the data element 'Characterisation of drug role' (ICH- E2B(R2)B.4.k.1).

If the primary source suspects a possible causal role of one of the ingredients (e.g., excipient or adjuvant) of the suspected medicinal product, this information should be provided in the section 'Drug information' (ICH-E2B(R2) B.4) as a separate entry in addition to the information given regarding the suspected medicinal product. This should also be specified in the case narrative (data element ICH-E2B(R2) B.5.1). If available, tests results (positive or negative) in relation to the causal role of the suspected ingredient should be included in the section 'Results of tests and procedures relevant to the investigation of the patient' (ICH E2B(R2) B.3).

VI.C.6.2.2.3. Suspected adverse reactions
All available information as described in [IR Art 28 (3) (j)] shall be provided for each individual case. The coding of diagnoses and provisional diagnoses with signs and symptoms in the data element 'Reaction/event in MedDRA terminology (Lowest Level Term)' (ICH-E2B(R2) B.2.i.1) should be performed in line with the latest version of the ICH-Endorsed Guide for MedDRA Users, MedDRA Term Selection: Points to Consider (*see* GVP Annex IV).

In practice, if a diagnosis is reported with characteristic signs and symptoms, the preferred option is to select a term for the diagnosis only and to MedDRA code it in the ICH-E2B(R2) section B.2 'Reaction(s)/event(s)'. If no diagnosis is provided, all reported signs and symptoms should be listed and MedDRA coded in the ICH-E2B(R2) section B.2 'Reaction(s)/event(s)'. If these signs and symptoms are typically part of a diagnosis, the diagnosis can be MedDRA coded in addition by competent authorities in Member States or marketing authorisation holders in the ICH-E2B(R2) data element B.5.3 'Sender's diagnosis/syndrome and/or reclassification of reaction/event'.

If in the narrative other events have been reported, which are not typically signs or symptoms of the primary source's diagnosis or provisional diagnosis, and those events are suspected to be adverse reactions, they should also be listed and MedDRA coded in the ICH-E2B(R2) section B.2 'Reaction(s)/event(s)'.

In case a competent authority in a Member State or a marketing authorisation holder disagrees with the diagnosis reported by the primary source, an alternative diagnosis can be provided in the ICH-E2B(R2) data element B.5.3 'Sender's diagnosis/

syndrome and/or reclassification of reaction/event' in addition to the reported diagnosis provided in the ICH-E2B(R2) section B.2 'Reaction(s)/event(s)'. In this situation, a reasoning should be included in the data element 'Sender's comments' (ICH-E2B(R2) B.5.4) (see VI.C.6.2.2.4.).

In the event of death of the patient, the date, cause of death including autopsy-determined causes shall be provided as available [IR 28 (3) (l)]. If the death is unrelated to the reported suspected adverse reaction(s) and is linked for example, to disease progression, the seriousness criterion of the ICSR should not be considered as fatal; the recommendation provided in the EudraVigilance Business Rules should be followed.

VI.C.6.1.1.4. Case narrative, causality assessment and comments

In accordance with [IR Art 28 (3) (m)], a case narrative (data element ICH-E2B(R2) B.5.1) shall be provided, where possible,[38] for all cases with the exception of non-serious cases. The information shall be presented in a logical time sequence, in the chronology of the patient's experience including clinical course, therapeutic measures, outcome and follow-up information obtained. Any relevant autopsy or post-mortem findings shall also be summarised.

The narrative should be presented in line with the recommendations described in chapter 5.2 of ICH- E2D (*see* GVP Annex IV). In this aspect, it should serve as a comprehensive, stand-alone "medical report" containing all known relevant clinical and related information, including patient characteristics, therapy details, medical history, clinical course of the event(s), diagnosis, adverse reactions and their outcomes, relevant laboratory evidence (including normal ranges) and any other information that supports or refutes the suspected adverse reactions. An example of a standard narrative template is available in the Report of the CIOMS Working Group V.[39]

The information provided in the narrative should be consistent with the data appropriately reflected in all the other relevant ICH-E2B(R2) data elements of the ICSR (*see* GVP Annex IV).

During the interim arrangements (*see* VI.C.4.1.), the case narratives included in the ICSRs submitted to the competent authorities in Member States by marketing authorisation holders, should not be modified or deleted when the ICSRs are forwarded to the EudraVigilance database by the competent authorities.

Where available, comments from the primary source on the diagnosis, causality assessment or other relevant issue, should be provided in the data element 'Reporter's comments' (ICH-E2B(R2) B.5.2). Competent authorities in Member States and marketing authorisation holders may provide an assessment of the case and describe a disagreement with, and/or alternatives to the diagnoses given by the primary source (*see* VI.C.6.2.2.3.). This should be done in the data element 'Sender's comments' (ICH-E2B(R2) B.5.4), where discrepancies or confusions in the information notified by the primary source may also be highlighted. Where applicable, a summary of the points of concerns and actions proposed should also be included in the data element 'Sender's comments' (ICH-E2B(R2) B.5.4), if the ICSR leads to notification of an emerging safety issue (*see* VI.C.2.2.6.). The degree of suspected relatedness of each medicinal product to the adverse reaction(s) may be indicated in the data element 'Relatedness of drug to reaction(s)/event(s)' (ICH-E2B(R2) B.4.k.18), which should be repeated as necessary. This also allows presenting the degree of relatedness from different sources or with different methods of assessment.

VI.C.6.2.2.5. Test results

Results of tests and procedures relevant to the investigation of the patient shall be provided [IR Art 28 (3) (k)].

As described in ICH-E2B(R2) (*see* GVP Annex IV), the section B.3 'Results of tests and procedures relevant to the investigation of the patient' should capture the tests and procedures performed to diagnose or confirm the reaction/event, including those tests done to investigate (exclude) a non-drug cause, (e.g. serologic tests for infectious hepatitis in suspected drug-induced hepatitis). Both positive and negative results should be reported.

---

38. 'Where possible' should be interpreted as having received sufficient information from the primary source to prepare a concise clinical summary of the individual case.
39. Council for International Organizations of Medical Sciences (CIOMS). Current Challenges in Pharmacovigilance: Pragmatic Approaches (CIOMS V). Geneva: CIOMS; 2001. http://www.cioms.ch/.

The coding of investigations should be performed in line with the latest version of the ICH-Endorsed Guide for MedDRA Users, MedDRA Term Selection: Points to Consider (*see* GVP Annex IV). If it is not possible to provide information on tests and test results in a structured manner, provisions have been made to allow for the transmission of the information as free text in the data element ICH-E2B(R2) B.3.2. 'Results of tests and procedures relevant to the investigation'.

VI.C.6.2.2.6. Supplementary information
Key information from supplementary records should be provided in the relevant section of the ICSR, and their availability should be mentioned in the data element 'List of documents held by sender' (ICH- E2B(R2) A.1.8.2).

Other known case identifiers relevant for the detection of duplicates should be presented systematically in the data element 'Other case identifiers in previous transmissions' (ICH-E2B(R2) A.1.11).

VI.C.6.2.2.7. Follow-up information
ICSRs are sent at different times to multiple receivers. Therefore the initial/follow-up status is dependent upon the receiver. For this reason an item to capture follow-up status is not included in the ICH-E2B(R2) data elements. However, the data element 'Date of receipt of the most recent information for this report' (ICH-E2B(R2) A.1.7) taken together with the data element 'Sender identifier' (ICH E2B(R2) A.3.1.2) and the data element 'Sender's (case) report unique identifier' (ICH-E2B(R2) A.1.0.1) provide a mechanism for each receiver to identify whether the report being transmitted is an initial or a follow-up report. For this reason these items are considered critical for each transmission and a precise date should always be used (i.e. day, month, year). The data element 'Date of receipt of the most recent information for this report' (ICH-E2B(R2) A.1.7) should therefore always be updated each time a follow-up information is received by a competent authority or a marketing authorisation holder, independently whether the follow-up information received is significant enough to be reported. The data element 'Date report was first received from the source' (ICH-E2B(R2) A.1.6) should remain unchanged to the date the competent authority or the marketing authorisation holder became aware of the initial report.

New information should be clearly identifiable in the case narrative (data element ICH-E2B(R2) B.5.1) and provided in a structured format in the applicable ICH-E2B(R2) data elements.

Competent authorities in Member States or marketing authorisation holders should report follow-up information if significant new medical information has been received. Significant new information relates to for example new suspected adverse reaction(s), a change in the causality assessment and any new or updated information on the case that impacts on its medical interpretation. Therefore, the identification of significant new information requiring to be reported always necessitates medical judgement.

Situations where the seriousness criteria and/or the causality assessment are downgraded (e.g. follow- up information leads to a change of the seriousness criteria from serious to non-serious; causality assessment is changed from related to non-related) should also be considered as significant changes and thus reported (*see* VI.B.7.1. for reporting time frames).

In addition, competent authorities in Member States or marketing authorisation holders should also report follow-up information, where new administrative information is available, that could impact on the case management; for example, if new case identifiers have become known to the sender, which may have been used in previous transmissions (data element 'Other case identifiers in previous transmissions' (ICH-E2B(R2) A.1.11). This information may be specifically relevant to manage potential duplicates. Another example refers to data element 'Additional available documents held by sender' (ICH-E2B(R2) A.1.8), whereby new documents that have become available to the sender may be relevant for the medical assessment of the case.

In contrast, a follow-up report which contains non-significant information does not require to be reported. This may refer, for example, to minor changes to some dates in the case with no implication for the evaluation or transmission of the case, or corrections of typographical errors in the previous case version. Medical judgement should be applied since a change to the birth date may constitute a significant modification (e.g. with implications on the age information of the patient). Similarly, a change of the status of a MedDRA code/term from current to non-current, due to a version change of MedDRA, can be considered as a non-significant change as long as this change has no impact on the medical content of a case. However, an amendment of the MedDRA coding due to a change in the interpretation of a previously reported suspected adverse reaction may constitute a significant change and therefore should be reported.

In situations where the case is modified without impacting on its medical evaluation, while no new follow-up is received (e.g. for correcting a mistake or typographical error), the date of receipt of the most recent information reported in the data element 'Date of receipt of the most recent information for this report' (ICH-E2B(R2) A.1.7) should not be changed. This data element should however be updated in any other situations, to the date when new follow-up information is received (independently whether it is significant or not) or to the date when changes are made which impact on the interpretation of the case.

Where follow-up information of a case initially reported by a marketing authorisation holder is received directly by a competent authority, the 'Worldwide unique case identification number' (ICH-E2B(R2) A.1.10) of the initial report should be maintained, in adherence with ICH-E2B(R2) (see GVP Annex IV). The same principle should be applied if a follow-up is received by a marketing authorisation holder of a case initially reported by a competent authority.

VI.C.6.2.2.8. What to take into account for data privacy laws

To detect, assess, understand and prevent adverse reactions and to identify, and take actions to reduce the risks of, and increase the benefits from medicinal products for the purpose of safeguarding public health, the processing of personal data within the EudraVigilance database is possible while respecting EU legislation in relation to data protection (Directive 95/46/EC, Regulation (EC) No 45/2001).

Where in accordance with applicable national legislation, information related to personal data cannot be transferred to the EudraVigilance database, pseudonymisation may be applied by competent authorities in Member States and by marketing authorisation holders, thereby replacing identifiable personal data such as name and address with pseudonyms or key codes, for example, in accordance with the ISO Technical Specification DD ISO/TS 25237:2008, Health informatics – Pseudonymization [IR Recital 17]. The application of pseudonymisation will facilitate the ability of the EudraVigilance system to adequately support case processing and detect duplicates. This should however be done without impairing the information flow in the EudraVigilance database and the interpretation and evaluation of safety data relevant for the protection of public health; given the high-level nature of the information, data elements such as patient's age, age group and gender should in principle be kept un-redacted/visible.

VI.C.6.2.2.9. Handling of languages

The ICH-E2B(R2) (see GVP Annex IV) concept for the electronic reporting of ICSRs is based on the fact that structured and coded information is used for data outputs of pharmacovigilance systems (e.g. listings) and for signal detection. However, for scientific case assessment and signal evaluation, the medical summary provided in the data element 'Case narrative including clinical course, therapeutic measures, outcome and additional relevant information' (ICH-E2B(R2) B.5.1) is normally required (see VI.6.2.2.4.).

Where suspected adverse reactions are reported by the primary source in narrative and textual descriptions in an official language of the Union other than English, the original verbatim text and the summary thereof in English shall be provided by the marketing authorisation holder.[40] Member States may report case narratives in their official language(s). For those reports, case translations shall be provided when requested by the Agency or other Member States for the evaluation of potential signals. For suspected adverse reactions originating outside the EU, English shall be used in the ICSR [IR 28 (4)].

---

40. In practice, the original verbatim text reported by the primary source in an official language of the Union other than English should be included in the ICSR, if it is requested by the Member State where the reaction occurred or by the Agency.

Additional documents held by the sender, which may be only available in a local language, should only be translated if requested by the receiver.

VI.C.6.2.2.10. Nullification of cases
In line with ICH-E2B(R2) (*see* GVP Annex IV), the nullification of individual cases should be used to indicate that a previously transmitted report should be considered completely void (nullified), for example when the whole case was found to be erroneous or in case of duplicate reports. It is essential to use the same case report numbers previously submitted in the data element 'Sender's (case) safety report unique identifier' (ICH-E2B(R2) A.1.0.1) and in the data element 'Worldwide unique case identification number' (ICH-E2B(R2) A.1.10).

A nullified case is one that should no longer be considered for scientific evaluation. The process of the nullification of a case is by means of a notification by the sender to the receiver that this is no longer a valid case. However, the case should be retained in the sender's pharmacovigilance database for auditing purposes.

The principles to be considered when nullifying a case are detailed in VI. Appendix 5.

VI.C.6.2.3. Special Situations

VI.C.6.1.3.1. Use of a medicinal product during pregnancy or breastfeeding
General recommendations are provided in VI.B.6.1.

With regard to the electronic reporting of parent-child/foetus cases, the following should be adhered to:

- In the situation where a foetus or nursing infant is exposed to one or several medicinal products through the parent and experiences one or more suspected adverse reactions (other than early spontaneous abortion/foetal demise), information on both the parent and the child/foetus should be provided in the same report. These cases are referred to as parent-child/foetus reports. The information provided in the section 'Patients characteristics' (ICH-E2B(R2) B.1) applies only to the child/foetus. The characteristics concerning the parent (mother or father), who was the source of exposure to the suspect medicinal product should be provided in the data element 'For a parent-child/fetus report, information concerning the parent' (ICH-E2B(R2) B.1.10). If both parents are the source of the suspect drug(s) then the case should reflect the mother's information in the data element 'For a parent-child/fetus report, information concerning the parent' (ICH E2B(R2) B.1.10). The data element 'Case narrative including clinical course, therapeutic measures, outcome and additional relevant information' (ICH-E2B(R2) B.5.1) should describe the entire case, including the father's information.
- If both the parent and the child/foetus experience suspected adverse reactions, two separate reports, i.e. one for the parent (mother or father) and one for the child/foetus, should be created but they should be linked by using the data element 'Identification number of the report which is linked to this report' (ICH-E2B(R2) A.1.12) in each report.
- If there has been no reaction affecting the child, the parent-child/foetus report does not apply; i.e. the section 'Patients characteristics' (ICH-E2B(R2) B.1) applies only to the parent (mother or father) who experienced the suspected adverse reaction.
- For those cases describing miscarriage or early spontaneous abortion, only a parent report is applicable, i.e. the section 'Patients characteristics' (ICH-E2B(R2) B.1) apply to the mother. However, if the suspect medicinal product was taken by the father, the data element 'Additional information on drug' (ICH-E2B(R2) B.4.k.19) should specify that the medication was taken by the father.

VI.C.6.1.3.2. Suspected adverse reaction reports published in the scientific literature
EU requirements in relation to the monitoring of suspected drug reactions reported in the scientific and medical literature are provided in VI.C.2.2.3. With regard to the electronic reporting of ICSRs published in the scientific and medical literature, the following applies:

- The literature references shall be included in the data element 'Literature reference(s)' (ICH-E2B (R2) A.2.2) in the Vancouver Convention (known as "Vancouver style"), developed by the International Committee of Medical Journal Editors [IR Art 28 (3) (b)]. The standard format as well as those for special situations can be found in the following reference: International Committee of Medical Journal Editors. Uniform requirements for manuscripts submitted to biomedical journals. NEngl J Med. 1997; 336: 309-16, which is in the Vancouverstyle.[41]

- A comprehensive English summary of the article shall be provided in the data element 'Case narrative including clinical course, therapeutic measures, outcome and additional relevant information' (ICH-E2B(R2) B.5.1) [IR Art 28 (3)(b)].
- Upon request of the Agency, for specific safety review, a full translation in English and a copy of the relevant literature article shall be provided by the marketing authorisation holder that transmitted the initial report, taking into account copyright restrictions [IR 28 (3)]. The recommendations detailed in VI.App2.10, regarding the mailing of the literature article, should be adhered to.
- Recommendations presented in VI.App2.10, for the reporting of several cases when they are published in the same literature article, should be followed.

VI.C.6.2.3.3. Suspected adverse reactions related to overdose, abuse, off-label use, misuse, medication error or occupational exposure

General principles are provided in VI.B.6.3.

If a case of overdose, abuse, off-label use, misuse, medication error or occupational exposure is reported with clinical consequences, the MedDRA Lowest Level Term code, corresponding to the term closest to the description of the reported overdose, abuse, off-label use, misuse, medication error or occupational exposure should be added to the observed suspected adverse reaction(s) in the data element 'Reaction/event in MedDRA terminology (Lowest Level Term)' (ICH-E2B(R2) B.2.i.1), in line with recommendations included in the latest version of the ICH-Endorsed Guide for MedDRA Users'MedDRA Term Selection: Points to Consider'(*see* GVP Annex IV).

VI.C.6.2.3.4. Lack of therapeutic efficacy

General principles are provided in VI.B.6.4.

If the primary source suspects a lack of therapeutic efficacy, the MedDRA Lowest Level Term code, corresponding to the term closest to the description of the reported lack of therapeutic efficacy, should be provided in the data element 'Reaction/event in MedDRA terminology (Lowest Level Term)' (ICH- E2B(R2) B.2.i.1), in line with recommendations included in the latest version of the ICH-EndorsedGuide for MedDRA Users 'MedDRA Term Selection: Points to Consider'(*see* GVP Annex IV).

Unless aggravation of the medical condition occurs, the indication for which the suspected medicinal product was administered should not be included in the data element 'Reaction/event in MedDRA terminology (Lowest Level Term).

The same reporting modalities as for serious ICSRs (*see* VI.C.4.) should be applied for those cases related to classes of medicinal products where, as described in VI.B.6.4., reports of lack of therapeutic efficacy should be reported within a 15-day time frame. If no seriousness criterion is available, it is acceptable to submit the ICSR within 15 days as non-serious.

VI.C.6.2.3.5. Suspected adverse reactions related to quality defect or falsified medicinal products

EU requirements are provided in VI.C.2.2.4. In order to be able to clearly identify cases related to quality defect or falsified medicinal products when they are exchanged between stakeholders, the following recommendations should be applied:

a. Quality defect

Where a report of suspected adverse reactions is associated with a suspected or confirmed quality defect of a medicinal product, the MedDRA Lowest Level Term code of the term corresponding most closely to the product quality issue, should be added to the observed suspected adverse reaction(s) in the data element 'Reaction/event in MedDRA terminology (Lowest Level Term)' (ICH-E2B(R2) B.2.i.1).

b. Falsified medicinal products

Where a report of suspected adverse reactions is associated with a suspected or confirmed falsified[42] ingredient, active substance or medicinal product, the MedDRA Lowest Level Term code of the term corresponding most closely to the reported information should be added to the observed suspected adverse reaction(s) in the data element 'Reaction/event in MedDRA terminology (Lowest Level Term)' (ICH-E2B(R2) B.2.i.1). Information on the suspected medicinal product, active substance(s) or excipient(s) should be provided in the data elements 'Proprietary medicinal product

---

41. The Vancouver recommendations are also available on the International Committee of Medical Journal Editors website http://www.icmje.org.
42. As presented in EU legislation (Directive 2011/62/EU).

name' (ICH- E2B(R2) B.4.k.2.1) and/or 'Active substance name(s)' (ICH-E2B(R2) B.4.k.2.2) as reported by the primary source.

VI.C.6.2.3.6. Suspected transmission via a medicinal product of an infectious agent

EU requirements are provided in VI.C.2.2.5.

The coding of a suspected transmission of an infectious agent via a medicinal product in the data element 'Reaction/event in MedDRA terminology (Lowest Level Term)' (ICH-E2B(R2) B.2.i.1) should be performed in line with the latest version of the ICH-Endorsed Guide for MedDRA Users 'MedDRA Term Selection: Points to Consider'(*see* GVP Annex IV).

In addition, if the infectious agent is specified, the MedDRA Lowest Level Term code corresponding to the infectious agent should also be included in the data element 'Reaction/event in MedDRA terminology (Lowest Level Term)' (ICH-E2B(R2) B.2.i.1).

VI.C.6.2.3.7. Reports of suspected adverse reactions originating from organised data collection systems and other systems

General safety reporting requirements in the EU for post-authorisation studies are provided in VI.C.1. and VI.C.2.2.2. Individual case safety reports originating from those studies shall contain information on study type, study name and the sponsor's study number or study registration number [IR Art 28 (3)(c)]. This should be provided in ICH E2B(R2) section A.2.3 'Study identification'.

Safety reporting requirements regarding patient support programmes or market research programmes are provided in VI.C.2.2.11.

The following reporting rules should be applied based on (i) the type of data collection system and (ii) whether the suspected medicinal product is part of the scope of the data collection system.

1. For cases of suspected adverse reactions (i) in relation to those adverse events for which the protocol of non-interventional post-authorisation studies does not provide differently and requires their systematic collection (*see* VI.C.1.2.1.), (ii) originating from compassionate use or named patient use conducted in Member States where the active collection of adverse events occurring in these programmes is required (*see* VI.C.1.2.2.), or (iii) originating from patient support programmes, or market research programmes (*see* VI.C.2.2.11.):

   a. Where the adverse reaction is suspected to be related at least to the studied (or supplied) medicinal product:
      - The report should be considered as solicited;
      - The ICH E2B(R2) data element A.1.4 'Type of report' should be populated with the value 'Report from study';
      - The ICH E2B(R2) data element A.2.3.3 'Study type in which the reaction(s)/event(s) were observed' should be populated with the value 'Other studies' or 'Individual patient use'.
   b. Where the adverse reaction is only suspected to be related to a medicinal product which is not subject to the scope of the organised data collection system and there is no interaction with the studied (or supplied) medicinal product:
      - The report should be considered as spontaneous report; as such it conveys the suspicion of the primary source;
      - The ICH E2B(R2) data element A.1.4 'Type of report' should be populated with the value 'Spontaneous'.

2. For suspected adverse reactions (i) in relation to those adverse events for which the protocol of non-interventional post-authorisation studies provides differently and does not require their systematic collection (*see* VI.C.1.2.1.) or (ii) originating from compassionate use or named patient use conducted in Member States where the active collection of adverse events occurring in these programmes is not required (*see* VI.C.1.2.2.):
   - The report should be considered as spontaneous report; as such it conveys the suspicion of the primary source;
   - The ICH E2B(R2) data element A.1.4 'Type of report' should be populated with the value 'Spontaneous'.

3. For clinical trial conducted in accordance with Directive 2001/20/EC and where the adverse reaction is only suspected to be related to a non-investigational medicinal product (or another medicinal product which is not subject to the scope of the clinical trial) and there is no interaction with the investigational medicinal product:
   - The report should be considered as spontaneous report; as such it conveys the suspicion of the primary source;

- The ICH E2B(R2) data element A.1.4 'Type of report' should be populated with the value 'Spontaneous'.

All ICSRs which are reportable to the EudraVigilance database and which originate from post-authorisation studies which do not fall under the scope of the clinical trials Directive 2001/20/EC, should be submitted to EVPM (see VI.C.6.2.1.). The same applies to cases of adverse reactions originating in clinical trials if they are not suspected to be related to the investigational medicinal product.

VI.C.6.2.3.8. Receipt of missing minimum information
When missing minimum information (see VI.B.2.) has been obtained about a non-valid ICSR, the following rules should be applied:
- The data element 'Date report was first received from source' (ICH-E2B(R2) A.1.6) should contain the date of receipt of the initial non-valid ICSR;
- The data element 'Date of receipt of the most recent information for this report' (ICH-E2B(R2) A.1.7) should contain the date when all the four elements of the minimum information required for reporting have become available;
- Clarification should be provided in the case narrative (data element ICH-E2B(R2) B.5.1) that some of the four elements were missing in the initial report.;
- As for any reported cases, compliance monitoring is performed against the data element 'Date of receipt of the most recent information for this report' (ICH-E2B(R2)A.1.7).

VI.C.6.2.4. Data Quality of Individual Case Safety Reports Transmitted Electronically and Duplicate Management

The EudraVigilance database should contain all cases of suspected adverse reactions that are reportable according to Directive 2001/83/EC and Regulation (EC) No 726/2004 to support pharmacovigilance activities. This applies to all medicinal products authorised in the EU independent of their authorisation procedure.

The EudraVigilance database should also be based on the highest internationally recognised data quality standards.

To achieve these objectives, all competent authorities in Member States and marketing authorisation holders should adhere to:
- The electronic reporting requirements as defined in EU legislation;
- The concepts of data structuring, coding and reporting in line with the EU legislation, guidelines, standards and principles referred to in VI.C.6.2.2.1.

This is a pre-requisite to maintain a properly functioning EudraVigilance database intended to fully support the protection of public health.

The Agency shall, in collaboration with the stakeholder that submitted an ICSR to the EudraVigilance database, be responsible for operating procedures that ensure the highest quality and full integrity of the information collected in the EudraVigilance database [REG Art 24(3)]. This includes as well the monitoring of use of the terminologies referred to in chapter IV of the Commission Implementing Regulation (EU) No 520/2012 [IR Art 25(3)].

Specific quality system procedures and processes shall be in place in order to ensure:
- The submission of accurate and verifiable data on serious and non-serious suspected adverse reactions to the Eudravigilance data base within the 15 or 90-day time frame [IR Art 11(1)(c)];
- The quality, integrity and completeness of the information submitted on the risks of medicinal products, including processes to avoid duplicate submissions [IR Art 11 (1)(d)].

In this regard, marketing authorisation holders and competent authorities in Member States should have in place an audit system, which ensures the highest quality of the ICSRs transmitted electronically to the EudraVigilance database within the correct time frames, and which enables the detection and management of duplicate ICSRs in their system. Those transmitted ICSRs should be complete, entire and undiminished in their structure, format and content.

High level business process maps and process descriptions in relation to the quality review of ICSRs and the detection and management of duplicate ICSRs are provided in VI. Appendix 6 and VI. Appendix 7. Further guidance on the detection of duplicate ICSRs is available in the Guideline on the Detection and Management of Duplicate Individual Cases and Individual Case Safety Reports (ICSRs)(EMA/13432/2009).

A review of the ICSRs quality, integrity and compliance with the reporting time frames will be performed by the Agency at regular intervals for all organisations reporting to the EudraVigilance database. Feedback from these reviews will be provided to those organisations.

VI.C.6.2.5. Electronic Re-transmission of ICSRS between Multiple Senders and Receivers

The electronic re-transmission of cases refers to the electronic exchange of ICSRs between multiple senders and receivers, for example, where in case of contractual agreement, a third country ICSR is first reported by a marketing authorisation holder outside the EU to another marketing authorisation holder in the EU and from there to the Agency. This applies as well for the interim arrangements period, where based on the reporting requirements detailed in VI.C.4.1., ICSRs originating in the EU are submitted by marketing authorisation holders to the competent authorities in the Member State where the reaction occurred and then re-transmitted to the EudraVigilance database.

During this re-transmission process, information on the case should not in principle be omitted or changed if no new information on the case is available to the re-transmitting sender.

Exceptions apply to the following data elements or sections:
- 'Sender's (case) safety report unique identifier' (ICH-E2B(R2)A.1.0.1);
- 'Date of this transmission' (ICH-E2B(R2)A.1.3);
- 'Date report was first received from source' (ICH-E2B(R2) A.1.6), for initial reports;
- 'Date of receipt of the most recent information for this report' (ICH-E2B(R2)A.1.7);
- 'Information on sender and receiver of case safety report' (ICH-E2B(R2)A.3);
- 'Relatedness of drug to reaction(s)/event(s)' (ICH-E2B(R2)B.4.k.18);
- 'Sender's diagnosis/syndrome and/or reclassification of reaction/event' (ICH-E2B(R2)B.5.3);
- 'Sender's comments' (ICH-E2B(R2)B.5.4).

In the interest of improving data quality, in case of errors or inconsistencies in the report, the re- transmitters should go back to the originator of the report to correct the case accordingly. However, if this cannot be done within normal reporting time frame, the re-transmitter can correct information that has been incorrectly structured.

In addition, any electronic data interchange partner should adhere to the ICH-E2B(R2) rules regarding the provision of follow-up information, whereby the 'Worldwide unique case identification number' (ICH-E2B(R2) A.1.10) should be maintained in accordance with the ICH-E2B(R2) guideline (*see* GVP Annex IV). Non-adherence to these administrative requirements endangers the electronic case management and leads to the potential for unnecessary duplication of reports in the receiver's database.

VI.C.6.2.6. Electronic reporting through company's headquarters

If a pharmaceutical company decides to centralise the electronic reporting of ICSRs (e.g. by reporting through the company's global or EU headquarter), the following should be taken into account:
- The central reporting arrangement should be clearly specified in the marketing authorisation holder's pharmacovigilance system master file and in the internal standard operating procedures;
- The company's headquarter designated for reporting the ICSRs should be registered with EudraVigilance;
- The same principles may be applied for reporting ICSRs from the competent authorities in Member States to the marketing authorisation holders during the interim arrangements period, that is the competent authorities in Member States report electronically to the company's headquarter instead of to the local affiliates.

VI.C.6.3. Electronic Submission of Information on Medicinal Products

To support the objectives of Directive 2001/83/EC and Regulation (EC) No 726/2004, the provisions provided in second sub-paragraph of Article 57(2) of Regulation (EC) No 726/2004, regarding the electronic submission and update of information on medicinal products for human use authorised or registered in the EU, shall be followed by marketing authorisation holders. In this aspect marketing authorisation holders shall apply the internationally agreed formats and terminologies described in chapter IV of the Commission Implementing Regulation (EU) No 520/2012. Recommendations related to the electronic submission of information on medicines are provided on the Agency's website.[43]

---

43. *See* EMA documents for electronic submission of information on medicines: http://www.ema.europa.eu/ema/index.jsp?curl=pages/regulation/document_listing/document_listing_000336.jsp&murl=menus/regulations/regulations.jsp&mid=WC0b01ac0580410138&jsenabled=true

… Textbook of Pharmacovigilance

VI. APPENDIX 1 IDENTIFICATION OF BIOLOGICAL MEDICINAL PRODUCTS[44]

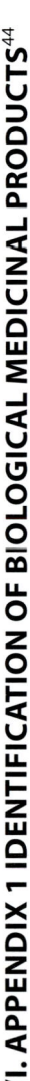

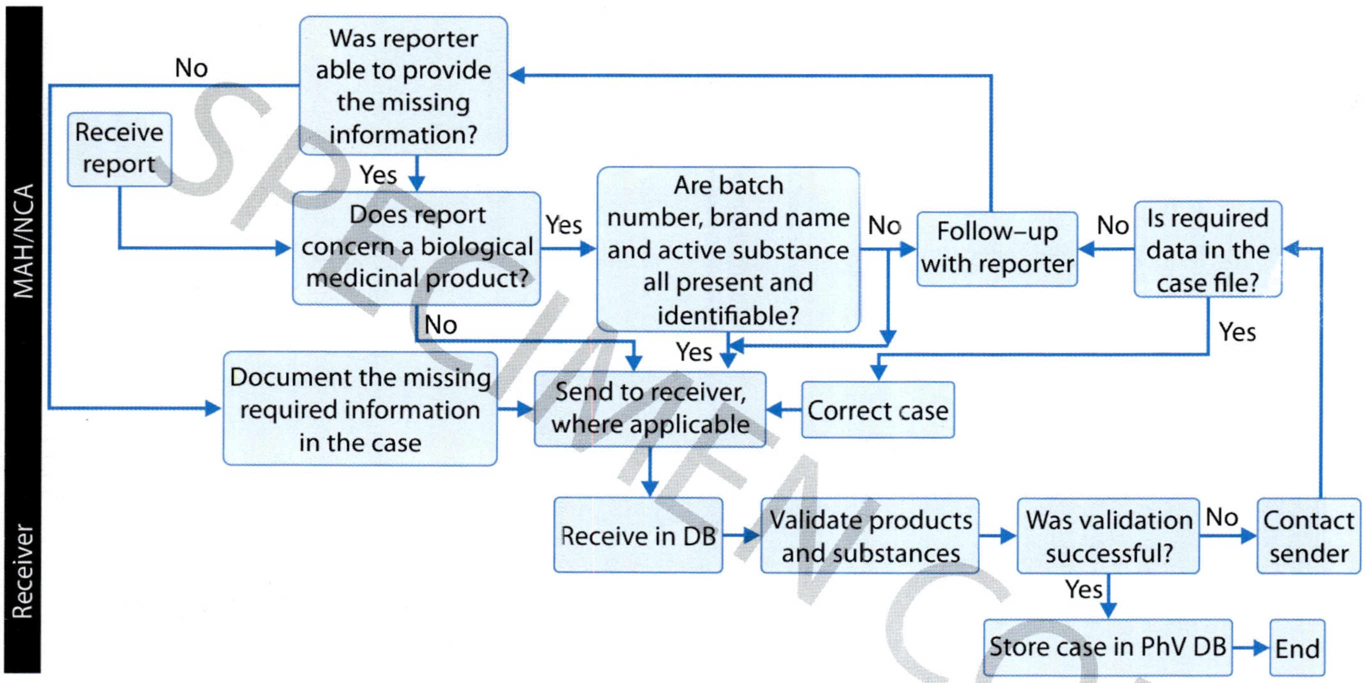

Fig VI.2: Business process map - Identification of biological medicinal products.

44. Mandatory when they are the subject of reports of suspected adverse reactions [DIR Art 102(e) and IR Art 28 (3)].

Annexure 8: Guideline on Good Pharmacovigilance Practices (GVP)

Table VI.2: Process description - Identification of biological medicinal products.

Sl. No.	Step	Description	Responsible Organisation
1	**Start. Receive report.**	Day 0. Receipt of the information for the case that indicates that one of the suspect drugs is of biological origin.	MAH/NCA
2	Does report concern a biological medicinal product?	If Yes, go to step 3. If No, go to step 4	
3	Are batch number, brand name and active substance all present and identifiable?	If Yes, create the case and send it to the correct receiver (step 3). If there is more than one batch number, structure the batch number that coincided with the adverse reaction in the Drug section (ICH-E2B(R2) B.4) and enter the other batch numbers in the case narrative. If No, create the case and send it to the correct receiver (step 3) and follow-up with the reporter (step 3.1).	MAH/NCA
3.1	Follow-up with reporter.	Follow-up with the reporter to attempt to identify the missing information.	MAH/NCA
3.2	Was reporter able to provide the missing information?	If Yes, return to step 1 – the information should be treated as follow-up and a new version created and transmitted. If No, document this (step 3.3).	MAH/NCA
3.3	Document the required missing information in the case.	Document in the case that the missing required information has been sought but the reporter was not able or willing to provide it.	MAH/NCA
4	Send to receiver, where applicable.	If the case requires transmission to a receiver, transmit the case electronically, in E2B(R2) format within the relevant timelines (15 or 90 days), to the relevant receiver.	MAH/NCA
5	**Receive in PharmacoVigilance DataBase (PhV DB).**	Receive the case electronically and load it into the PharmacoVigilance DataBase.	**Receiver**
6	Validate products and substances	Validate the products and substances to ensure that the brand name, active substance and batch number are all present and identifiable. This validation should be complementary to the usual business rules validations.	Receiver
7	Was validation successful?	If Yes, store the case in the PharmacoVigilance DataBase (step 8). If No, contact the sender (step 7.1).	Receiver
7.1	Contact sender.	Contact the sender regarding the missing or not identifiable information.	Receiver
7.2	*Is required data in the case file?*	Upon receipt of communication from the receiver, check in the case file to *see* if the missing or unidentifiable information is already on file. If it is on file, correct the case (step 7.3). If the information is not on file, contact the reporter to request the missing information (step 3.1).	MAH/NCA
7.3	Correct case.	Correct the case to include the missing information and send updated version to receiver (step 4).	MAH/NCA
8	*Store case in PharmacoVigilance DataBase (PhV DB).*	The case should now be stored in the pharmacovigilance database.	*Receiver*
9	End.	*The case is now available for signal detection and data quality analyses.*	

VI. APPENDIX 2 DETAILED GUIDANCE ON THE MONITORING OF SCIENTIFIC LITERATURE

VI. App2.1. When to Start and Stop Searching in the Scientific Literature

EU specific requirements, as regards the monitoring of scientific and medical literature are provided in VI.C.2.2.3.

In addition to the reporting of serious and non-serious ICSRs or their presentation in periodic safety update reports, the marketing authorisation holder has an obligation to review the worldwide experience with medicinal product in the period between the submission of the marketing authorisation application and the granting of the marketing authorisation. The worldwide experience includes published scientific and medical literature. For the period between submission and granting of a marketing authorisation, literature searching should be conducted to identify published articles that provide information that could impact on the risk-benefit assessment of the product under evaluation. For the purpose of the preparation of periodic safety update reports (see Module VII) and the notification of emerging safety issues (see VI.C.2.2.6.), the requirement for literature searching is not dependent on a product being marketed. Literature searches should be conducted for all products with a marketing authorisation, irrespective of commercial status. It would therefore be expected that literature searching would start on submission of a marketing authorisation application and continue while the authorisation is active.

VI. App2.2. Where to Look

Articles relevant to the safety of medicinal products are usually published in well-recognised scientific and medical journals, however, new and important information may be first presented at international symposia or in local journals. Although the most well-known databases (e.g. Medline) cover the majority of scientific and medical journals, the most relevant publications may be collated elsewhere in very specialised medical fields, for certain types of product (e.g. herbal medicinal products) or where safety concerns are subject to non-clinical research.

A marketing authorisation holder should establish the most relevant source of published literature for each product.

Medline, Embase and Excerpta Medica are often used for the purpose of identifying ICSRs. These databases have broad medical subject coverage. Other recognised appropriate systems may be used. The database providers can advise on the sources of records, the currency of the data, and the nature of database inclusions. It is best practice to have selected one or more databases appropriate to a specific product. For example, in risk-benefit assessment, safety issues arising during non-clinical safety studies may necessitate regular review of a database that has a less clinical focus and includes more laboratory-based publications.

Relevant published abstracts from meetings and draft manuscripts should be reviewed for reportable ICSRs and for inclusion in periodic safety update reports. Although it is not a requirement for marketing authorisation holders to attend all such meetings, if there are company personnel at such a meeting, or it is sponsored by a marketing authorisation holder, it is expected that articles of relevance would be available to the marketing authorisation holder's pharmacovigilance system. In addition, literature that is produced or sponsored by a marketing authorisation holder should be reviewed, so that any reportable ICSRs can be reported as required in advance of publication.

If ICSRs are brought to the attention of a marketing authorisation holder from this source, they should be processed in the same way as ICSRs found on searching a database or reviewing a journal.

Abstracts from major scientific meetings are indexed and available in some databases, but posters and communications are rarely available from this source.

VI.App2.3. Database Searches

A search is more than a collection of terms used to interrogate a database. Decisions about the database selection, approach to records retrieval, term or text selection and the application of limits need to be relevant to the purpose of the search. For searches in pharmacovigilance, some of the considerations for database searching are described below.

VI.App 2.3.1. Precision and Recall

Medical and scientific databases are a collection of records relating to a set of publications. For any given record, each database has a structure that facilitates the organisation of records and searching by various means, from simple text to complex indexing terms with associated subheadings. Search terms (text or indexed) can be linked using Boolean operators and proximity codes to combine concepts, increasing or decreasing the specificity of a search. In addition, limits to the output can be set. When searching, the application of search terms means that the output is less than the entire database of the records held. The success of a search can be measured according to precision and recall (also called sensitivity). Recall is the proportion of records retrieved ("hits") when considering the total number of relevant records that are present in the database. Precision is the proportion of "hits" that are relevant when considering the number of records that were retrieved. In general, the higher recall searches would result in low precision.

VI.App 2.3.2. Search Construction

Databases vary in structure, lag time in indexing and indexing policy for new terms. While some database providers give information about the history of a particular indexing term or the application of synonyms, other databases are less sophisticated. In addition, author abstracts are not always consistent in the choice of words relating to pharmacovigilance concepts or medicinal products/active substances names.

When constructing a search for pharmacovigilance, the highest recall for a search would be to enter the medicinal product name and active substance name (in all their variants) only. In practice, additional indexing terms and text are added to increase precision and to reduce the search result to return records that are of relevance to pharmacovigilance. There is a balance to be achieved. It is, therefore, expected that complicated searches are accompanied by initial testing to check that relevant records are not omitted, however, there is no defined acceptable loss of recall when searching for pharmacovigilance purposes. Term selection should be relevant to the database used and the subject of the search.

VI.App2.3.3. Selection of Product Terms

Searches should be performed to find records for active substances and not for brand names only. This can also include excipients or adjuvants that may have a pharmacological effect. When choosing search terms for medicinal products, there are a number of considerations.
- Is the active substance an indexed term?
- What spellings might be used by authors (particularly if the active substance is not indexed)?
- What alternative names might apply (numbers or codes used for products newly developed, chemical names, brand names, activemetabolites)?
- Is it medically relevant to search only for a particular salt or specific compound for an active substance?

During searches for ICSRs, it may be possible to construct a search that excludes records for pharmaceutical forms or routes of administration different to that of the subject product, however, restrictions should allow for the inclusion of articles where this is not specified. Search construction should also allow for the retrieval of overdose, medication error, abuse, misuse, off-label use or occupational exposure information, which could be poorly indexed. Searches should also not routinely exclude records of unbranded products or records for other company brands.

VI.App2.3.4. Selection of Search Terms

As described previously, there is no acceptable loss of recall when searching published literature for pharmacovigilance. The use of search terms (free text or use of indexing) to construct more precise searches may assist in managing the output. Deficiencies that have been found frequently during Competent Authority inspections include:
- The omission of outcome terms, for example "death" as an outcome may be the only indexed term in a case of sudden death;
- The omission of pregnancy terms to find adverse outcomes in pregnancy for ICSR reporting;
- The omission of terms to include special types of reports which needs to be addressed as well in periodic safety update reports, for example,
  - Reports of asymptomatic overdose, medication error, off-label use, misuse, abuse, occupational exposure;
  - Reports of uneventful pregnancy.

VI.App2.3.5. Limits to a Search

Some databases apply indexing that allows the application of limits to a search, for example, by subject age, sex, publication type. The limits applied to a search are not always shown in the "search strategy" or search string.

If limits are applied, they should be relevant to the purpose of the search. When searching a worldwide scientific and medical literature database, titles and abstracts are usually in English language. The use of limits that reduce the search result to only those published in the English language is generally not acceptable. Limits applied to patient types, or other aspects of an article, for example human, would need to be justified in the context of the purpose of a search.

Limits can be applied to produce results for date ranges, for example, weekly searches can be obtained by specifying the start and end date for the records to be retrieved. Care should be taken to ensure that the search is inclusive for an entire time period, for example, records that may have been added later in the day for the day of the search should be covered in the next search period. The search should also retrieve all records added in that period, and not just those initially entered or published during the specified period (so that records that have been updated or retrospectively added are retrieved). This should be checked with the database provider if it is not clear.

Although one of the purposes of searching is to identify ICSRs for reporting, the use of publication type limits is not robust. ICSRs may be presented within review or study publications, and such records may not be indexed as "case-reports", resulting in their omission for preparation of periodic safety update reports from search results limited by publication type.

VI.App2.4. Record Keeping

Records of literature searches should be maintained in accordance with the requirements described in [IR Art 12]. Marketing authorisation holders should demonstrate due diligence in searching published scientific and medical literature. It is always good practice to retain a record of the search construction, the database used and the date the search was run. In addition, it may be useful to retain results of the search for an appropriate period of time, particularly in the event of zero results. If decision making is documented on the results, it is particularly important to retain this information.

VI.App2.5. Outputs

Databases can show search results in different ways, for example, titles only or title and abstract with or without indexing terms. Some publications are of obvious relevance at first glance, whereas others may be more difficult to identify. Consistent with the requirement to provide the full citation for an article and to identify relevant publications, the title, citation and abstract (if available) should always be retrieved and reviewed.

VI.App2.6. Review and Selection of Articles

It is recognised that literature search results are a surrogate for the actual article. Therefore, it is expected that the person reviewing the results of a search is trained to identify the articles of relevance. This may be an information professional trained in pharmacovigilance or a pharmacovigilance professional with knowledge of the database used. Recorded confirmation that the search results have been reviewed will assist in demonstrating that there is a systematic approach to collecting information about suspected adverse reactions from literature sources. It is recommended that quality control checks are performed on a sample of literature reviews/selection of articles to check the primary reviewer is identifying the relevant articles.

A common issue in selecting relevant articles from the results of a search is that often this process is conducted for the purposes of identification of ICSRs only. Whereas the review should also be used as the basis for collating articles for the periodic safety update report production, therefore relevant studies with no ICSRs should also be identified, as well as those reports of events that do not qualify for reporting.

Outputs from searches may contain enough information to be a valid ICSR, in which case the article should be ordered. All articles for search results that are likely to be relevant to pharmacovigilance requirements should be obtained, as they may contain valid ICSRs or relevant safety information. The urgency with which this occurs should be proportionate to the content of the material reviewed and the resulting requirement for action as applicable for the marketing authorisation holder.

Articles can be excluded from reporting by the marketing authorisation holder if another company's branded medicinal product is the suspected medicinal product. In the absence of a specified medicinal product source and/or invented name, ownership of the medicinal product should be assumed for articles about an active substance. Alternative reasons for the exclusion of a published article for the reporting of ICSRs are detailed in VI.C.2.2.3.

VI.App2.7. Day Zero

As described in VI.B.7., day zero is the date on which an organisation becomes aware of a publication containing the minimum information for an ICSR to be reportable. Awareness of a publication includes any personnel of that organisation, or third parties with contractual arrangements with the organisation. It is sometimes possible to identify the date on which a record was available on a database, although with weekly literature searching, day zero for a reportable adverse reaction present in an abstract is taken to be the date on which the search was conducted. For articles that have been ordered as a result of literature search results, day zero is the date when the minimum information for an ICSR to be valid is available. Organisations should take appropriate measures to obtain articles promptly in order to confirm the validity of a case.

VI.App2.8. Duplicates

Consistent with the requirements for reporting ICSRs, literature cases should be checked to prevent reporting of duplicates, and previously reported cases should be identified as such when reported. It is, therefore, expected that ICSRs are checked in the organisation database to identify literature articles that have already been reported.

VI.App2.9. Contracting Out Literature Search Services

It is possible to use the services of another party to conduct searches of the published scientific and medical literature. In this event, the responsibility for the performance of the search and subsequent reporting still remains. The transfer of a pharmacovigilance task or function should be detailed in a contract between the organisation and the service provider. The nature of third party arrangements for literature searching can range from access to a particular database interface only (access to a technology) to full literature searching, review and reporting (using the professional pharmacovigilance services of another organisation). It is recognised that more than one organisation may share services of a third party to conduct searches for generic active substances. In this instance, each organisation should satisfy itself that the search and service is appropriate to their needs and obligations.

Where an organisation is dependent on a particular service provider for literature searching, it is expected that an assessment of the service(s) is undertaken to determine whether it meets the needs and obligations of the organisation. In any case, the arrangement should be clearly documented.

The clock start for the reporting of ICSRs begins with awareness of the minimum information by either the organisation or the contractual partner (whichever is the earliest). This also applies where a third party provides a review or a collated report from the published scientific and medical literature, in order to ensure that published literature cases are reported as required within the correct time frames. That is, day zero is the date the search was run if the minimum criteria are available in the abstract and not the date the information was supplied to the organisation.

VI.App2.10. Electronic Submission of Copies of Articles Published in the Scientific Literature

Until standards for the electronic transmission of attachments (e.g. copies of literature articles) are developed in the framework of ICH, the sender should follow the rules outlined below for the submission of a copy of the literature article as detailed in VI.C.6.2.3.2.:

1. Mailing address and format of literature articles: Literature articles reportable to the Agency should be provided in PDF format and sent via

e-mail to the following e-mail address: EVLIT@ema.europa.eu.

In relation to copies of articles from the published scientific and medical literature, marketing authorisation holders are recommended to consider potential copyright issues specifically as regards the electronic transmission and handling of electronic copies in the frame of regulatory activities.

2. File name of literature articles sent in electronic format to the Agency:

The file name of a literature article sent in PDF format should match exactly the 'World-Wide Unique Case Identification Number' (ICH-E2B(R2) A.1.10.1 or A.1.10.2 as applicable) assigned to the individual case, which is described in the article and which is reported in the E2B(R2) ICSR format.

If there is a follow-up article to the individual case published in the literature, the file name with the World-Wide Unique Case Identification Number must be maintained but should include a sequence number separated with a dash.

Examples:
- Initial ICSR published in the literature: FR-ORGABC-23232321 (data element 'World-Wide Unique Case Identification Number' (ICH-E2B(R2)A.1.10.1));
  – File name of the literature article: FR-ORGABC-23232321.pdf.
- Follow-up information published in the literature in a separate article:
  – ICSR: FR-ORGABC-23232321 (data element World-Wide Unique Case Identification Number remains unchanged (ICH-E2B(R2) A.1.10.1);
  – File name: FR-ORGABC-23232321-1.pdf.

3. Reporting of cases reported in the scientific and medical literature referring to more than one patient:

When the literature article refers to the description of more than one patient, the copy of the literature article should be sent only once.

The file name of a literature article sent in PDF format should match exactly the 'World-Wide Unique Case Identification Number' (data element ICH-E2B(R2) A.1.10.1 or A.1.10.2 as applicable) assigned to the first reportable individual case described in the article.

In addition, all ICSRs which relate to the same literature article should be cross referenced in the data element 'Identification number of the report which is linked to this report' (ICH-E2B(R2) A.1.12). The data element should be repeated as necessary to cross refer all related cases (*see* Table VI.2.).

Table VI.3: Examples for the reporting of ICSRs described in the scientific and medical literature and referring to more than one patient.

Ex.	Scenario	Action
1	A literature article describes suspected adverse reactions that have been experienced by up to 3 single patients. 3 ICSRs should be created and reported for each individual identifiable patient described in the literature article. Each ICSR should contain all the available information on the case.	For Case 1 described in the literature article: • ICH-E2B(R2) A.1.10.1 'World-Wide Unique Case Identification Number': UK-ORGABC-0001 • ICH-E2B(R2) A.1.12 'Identification number of the report which is linked to this report': UK-ORGABC-0002 • ICH-E2B(R2) A.1.12 'Identification number of the report which is linked to this report': UK-ORGABC-0003 • ICH-E2B(R2) A.2.2 'Literature reference(s): Literature reference in line with uniform requirements for manuscripts submitted to biomedical journals: N Engl J Med. 1997;336:309-15. • File name for the copy of literature article to be sent via e-mail to EVLIT@ema.europa.eu: UK-ORGABC-0001.pdf

Contd..

Annexure 8: Guideline on Good Pharmacovigilance Practices (GVP)

Contd..

Ex.	Scenario	Action
		For Case 2 described in the literature article: • ICH-E2B(R2) A.1.10.1 'World-Wide Unique Case Identification Number': UK-ORGABC-0002 • ICH-E2B(R2) A.1.12 'Identification number of the report which is linked to this report': UK-ORGABC-0001 • ICH-E2B(R2) A.1.12 'Identification number of the report which is linked to this report': UK-ORGABC-0003 • ICH-E2B(R2) A.2.2 'Literature reference(s): Literature reference in line with uniform requirements for manuscripts submitted to biomedical journals: N Engl J Med. 1997;336:309-15. • No copy of the literature article required since the copy was already submitted for case 1. For Case 3 described in the literature article: • ICH-E2B(R2) A.1.10.1 'World-Wide Unique Case Identification Number': UK-ORGABC-0003 • ICH-E2B(R2) A.1.12 'Identification number of the report which is linked to this report': UK-ORGABC-0001 • ICH-E2B(R2) A.1.12 'Identification number of the report which is linked to this report': UK-ORGABC-0002 • ICH-E2B(R2) A.2.2 'Literature reference(s): Literature reference in line with uniform requirements for manuscripts submitted to biomedical journals: N Engl J Med. 1997;336:309-15. • No copy of the literature article required since the copy was already submitted for case 1.
2.	A literature article describes suspected adverse reactions that have been experienced by more than 3 single patients. ICSRs should be created and reported for each individual identifiable patient described in the literature article. Each ICSR should contain all the available information on the case. The cross reference with all the linked ICSRs from this literature article should only be provided in the first case, in the data element ICH-E2B(R2) A.1.12 'Identification number of the report which is linked to this report'. There is no need to repeat all the cross references in the other ICSRs.	For the IC7SRs which relate to the same literature article, the cross reference in the data element 'Identification number of the report which is linked to this report' ICH (E2B(R2) field A.1.12) should be conducted as follows: • The first case should be linked to all other cases related to the same article; • All the other cases should be only linked to the first one, as in the example below. *Example for the reporting of cases originally reported in the scientific and medical literature referring to a large number of patients:* For Case 1 described in the literature article: • ICH E2B(R2) A.1.10.1 'Worldwide Unique Case Identification Number': UK-ORGABC-0001 • ICH-E2B(R2) A.1.12 'Identification number of the report which is linked to this report': UK-ORGABC-0002 • ICH-E2B(R2) A.1.12 'Identification number of the report which is linked to this report': UK-ORGABC-0003

Contd..

Contd..

Ex.	Scenario	Action
		• ICH-E2B(R2) A.1.12 'Identification number of the report which is linked to this report': UK-ORGABC-0004
• ICH-E2B(R2) A.1.12 'Identification number of the report which is linked to this report': UK-ORGABC-000N
• ICH-E2B(R2) A.2.2 'Literature reference(s)': N Engl J Med.1997;336:309-15.
• File name for the copy of literature article to be sent via e-mail to EVLIT@ema.europa.eu: UK-ORGABC-0001.pdf.
For Case 2 described in the literature article:
• ICH E2B(R2) A.1.10.1 'Worldwide Unique Case Identification Number': UK-ORGABC-0002
• ICH-E2B(R2) A.1.12 'Identification number of the report which is linked to this report':
• UK-ORGABC-0001
• ICH-E2B(R2) A.2.2 'Literature reference(s)':
• N Engl J Med. 1997;336:309-15.
• No copy of the literature article required since the copy was already submitted for case1.
For Case N described in the literature article:
• ICH-E2B(R2) A.1.10.1 'Worldwide Unique Case Identification Number': UK-ORGABC-000N
• ICH-E2B(R2) A.1.12 'Identification number of the report which is linked to this report': UK-ORGABC-0001
• ICH-E2B(R2) A.2.2 'Literature reference(s)': N Engl J Med.1997;336:309-15.
• No copy of the literature article required since the copy was already submitted for case 1.

Annexure 8: Guideline on Good Pharmacovigilance Practices (GVP)

VI. APPENDIX 3 MODALITIES FOR REPORTING

VI. App3.1. Interim Arrangements

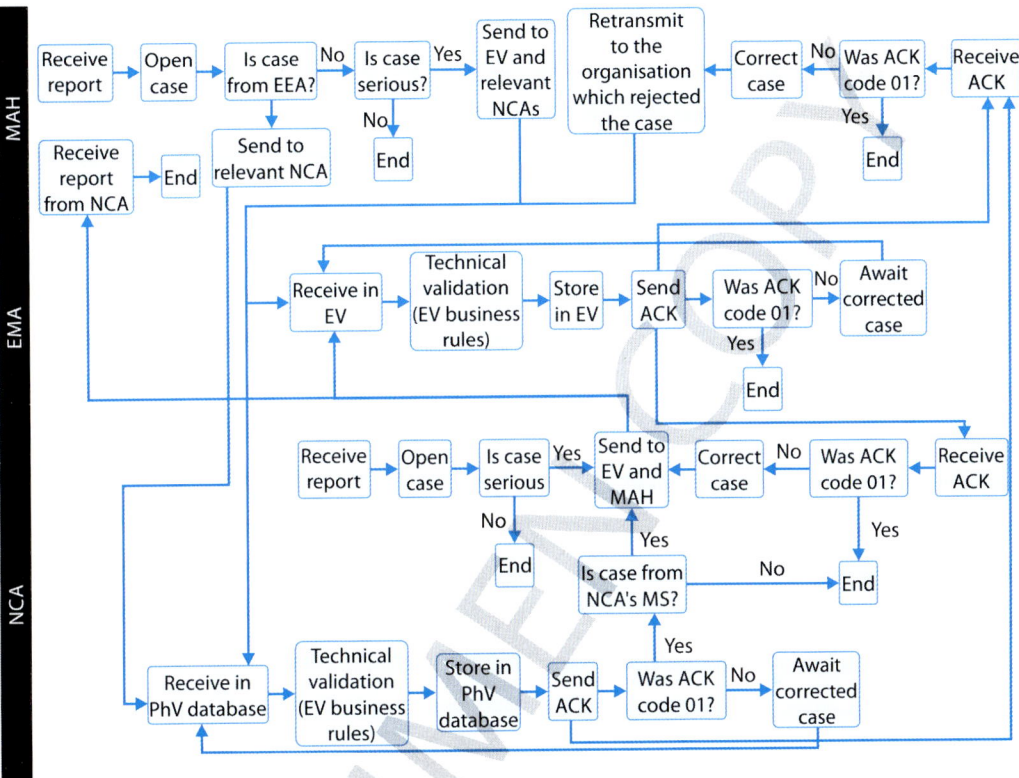

FIG. VI.3: Business process map—Suspected adverse reaction reporting in EU—Interim arrangements.

Table VI.4: Process description—Suspected adverse reaction reporting in EU—Interim arrangements

No.	Step	Description	Responsible Organisation
1	Start. Receive report.	Marketing Authorisation Holder (MAH) receives information on a suspected adverse reaction from a patient, healthcare professional or other valid reporter. If the case has been received from an EU NCA, do not retransmit it to Eudra Vigilance (EV).	MAH
2	Open case.	Open and create an individual case safety report.	MAH
3	Is case from EEA?	Did the adverse reactions occur in the EU? If No, go to step 3.1. If Yes, got so step 5.	MAH
3.1	Is case serious?	If No, go to step 3.2. If Yes, got to step 4.	MAH
3.2	End.	The case is now stored in the MAHs pharmacovigilance database. Normal follow-up activities should continue and if any follow-up is received, return to step 1.	MAH
4	Send to EV & relevant NCAs.	Transmit the serious case electronically, in ICH E2B(R2) format as an xml message within the 15-day time frame to EV and to the relevant NCAs, where required. The case goes to step 4.1 and step 6.	MAH
4.1	Receive in EV.	Receive the message in EV database from MAH or NCA.	EMA
4.2	Technical Validation (EV Business Rules).	Every message that is received in EV is validated against the EudraVigilance Business Rules and an Acknowledgement message (ACK) is created specifying whether or not the message and the case(s) therein are valid. A valid message will have an ACK code 01. A non-valid message will have an ACK code 02 (if a case contained therein is non-valid) or 03 (if the message itself is not correctly formatted).	EMA
4.3	Store in EV.	Once the case has been validated, it is stored in EV.	EMA
4.4	Send ACK.	The acknowledgement message created in step 4.2 is transmitted to the case sender, no later than 2 business days following receipt of the case. Go to step 16 for MAHs receiving the ACK. Go to step 20 for NCAs receiving the ACK. Go to step 4.5 for the EMA's next step.	EMA
4.5	Was ACK code 01?	If No, go to step 4.6. If Yes, go to step 4.7.	EMA
4.6	Await corrected case.	The sender should correct every case with an error ACK and retransmit within the regulatory reporting timelines. Periodically the EMA should assess all cases with an error ACK for which a corrected case has not been transmitted and contact the Qualified Person responsible for PharmacoVigilance (QPPV) to inform of these missing corrected cases. If a sender fails to correct cases, then this information should be incorporated into data quality assessments and the appropriate committees should be informed. Go back to step 4.1 upon receipt of the corrected case.	EMA

Contd..

Annexure 8: Guideline on Good Pharmacovigilance Practices (GVP)

Contd..

No.	Step	Description	Responsible Organisation
4.7	End.	The case is now stored in EV and, following duplicate detection and recoding will be available for signal detection and data quality analyses.	EMA
5	Send to relevant NCA.	Transmit the case (serious, and if required non-serious) electronically, in ICH E2B(R2) format as an xml message within the relevant time frames (15 or 90 days, as applicable), to the relevant NCA for the Member State where the reaction occurred. If country of occurrence has not been specified, then country of primary source should normally be taken to be the occurrence country.	MAH
6	Receive in PharmacoVigilance DataBase (PhV DB).	Receive the message from MAH in the NCA's PhV DB.	NCA
7	Technical Validation (EV Business Rules).	Every message that is received in the NCA's PhV DB should be validated against the EudraVigilance Business Rules and an Acknowledgement message (ACK) is created specifying wheather or not the message & the case(s) therein are valid. A valid message will have an ACKcode 01. A non-valid message will have an ACK code 02 (if a case contained therein is non-valid) or 03 (if the message itself is not correctly formatted).	NCA
8	Store in EV.	Once the case has been validated, it is stored in the NCA's PhV DB.	NCA
9	Send ACK.	The acknowledgement message created in step 7 is transmitted to the case sender no later than 2 business days following receipt of the case. Go to step 16 for MAHs receiving the ACK. Go to step 10 for the NCA's next step.	NCA
10	Was ACK code 01?	If No, go to step 10.1. If Yes, go to step 11.	NCA
10.1	Await corrected case.	The MAH should correct every case with an error ACK and retransmit it within the regulatory reporting timelines. Periodically the NCA should assess all cases with an error ACK for which a corrected case has not been transmitted and contact the QPPV to inform them of these missing corrected cases. If a sender fails to correct cases, then this information should be incorporated into any data quality assessments performed and the appropriate action can be taken. Go back to step 6 upon receipt of the corrected case.	NCA
11	Was case from NCA's MS?	Did the case occur in the territory of the receiving NCA? If No, go to step 11.1. If Yes, go to step 12.	NCA
11.1	End.	The case is now stored in the NCA's PharmacoVigilance Data Base and, following duplicate detection and recoding will be available for signal detection and data quality analyses.	NCA

Contd..

Contd..

No.	Step	Description	Responsible Organisation
12	Send to EV & MAH.	Transmit the serious case electronically, in ICH E2B(R2) format as an xml message within the 15-day time frame to EV and to the relevant MAH(s). Go to step 4.1 for reception of the case in EV Go to step 24 for reception of the case by the relevant MAH(s)	NCA
13	**Start.** **Receive report.**	**NCA receives information on a suspected adverse reaction from a patient, healthcare professional or other valid reporter concerning a suspected adverse reaction occurring in the territory of the receiving competent authority.**	NCA
14	Open case.	Open and create an individual case safety report.	NCA
15	Is case serious?	If No, go to step 15.1 If Yes, go to step 12	NCA
15.1	**End**	**The case is now stored in the NCA's PharmacoVigilance Data Base and, following duplicate detection and recoding will be available for signal detection and data quality analyses.**	NCA
16	**Receive ACK.**	Receive the ACK message, associate it with the relevant case(s) and check to ensure that the case was considered valid.	MAH
17	Was ACK code 01?	If yes, go to step 17.1. If no, then the regulatory timeline clock has not stopped and the case should be corrected and re-transmitted to EV within the relevant regulatory reporting timelines. Day 0 remains as the day that the first information was received. A 02 or 03 ACK does not constitute new information. Go to step 18 (Correct case).	MAH
17.1	**End.**	**End the process of transmitting this version of the case to EV or NCA. Normal follow-up activities should continue and if any follow-up is received, return to step 1.**	MAH
18	Correct case.	Correct the case to remove the errors identified in the ACK.	MAH
19	Retransmit to the organisation which rejected the case.	Retransmit the corrected case to the organisation which rejected the case with ACK code 02 or 03. Got to step 4.1 &/or step 6 as appropriate.	MAH
20	**Receive ACK.**	Receive the ACK message, associate it with the relevant case(s) and check to ensure that the case was considered valid.	NCA
21	Was ACK code 01?	If yes, go to step 23. If no, then the regulatory timeline clock has not stopped and the case should be corrected and re-transmitted to EV within the relevant regulatory reporting timelines. Day 0 remains as the day that the first information was received. A 02 or 03 ACK does not constitute new information. Go to step 22 (Correct case).	NCA

Contd..

Contd..

No.	Step	Description	Responsible Organisation
22	Correct case.	Correct the case to remove the errors identified in the ACK and retransmit the case to EV and to the relevant MAH(s) (go back to step 12).	NCA
23	End.	End the process of transmitting this version of the case to EV and to the relevant MAH(s). Normal follow-up activities should continue and if any follow-up is received, return to step 6 or 13.	NCA
24	Receive report from NCA	MAH receives information on a suspected adverse reaction from an NCA. This case should not be retransmitted to EV and to the NCA which transmitted it to the MAH	MAH
25	End	The case is now stored in the MAH's PharmacoVigilance DataBase and, following duplicate detection and recoding will be available for signal detection and data quality analyses.	MAH

VI. App3.1.1. Interim Arrangements Applicable to Marketing Authorisation Holders

Reporting requirements of individual case safety reports applicable to marketing authorisation holders during the interim period are detailed in the latest version of Doc. EMA/321386/2012 available on EMA website.

VI. App3.1.2. Interim Arrangements Applicable to Competent Authorities in Member States

Table VI.5: Reporting requirements applicable to competent authorities in Member States—Interim arrangements.

Marketing authorisation procedure	Origin	Adverse reaction type	Destination	Time frame
• Centralised • Mutual recognition, decentralised or subject to referral • Purely national	EU	All serious	• EudraVigilance database • Marketing authorisation holder of the suspected medicinal product	15 days

VI. App3.2. Final Arrangements

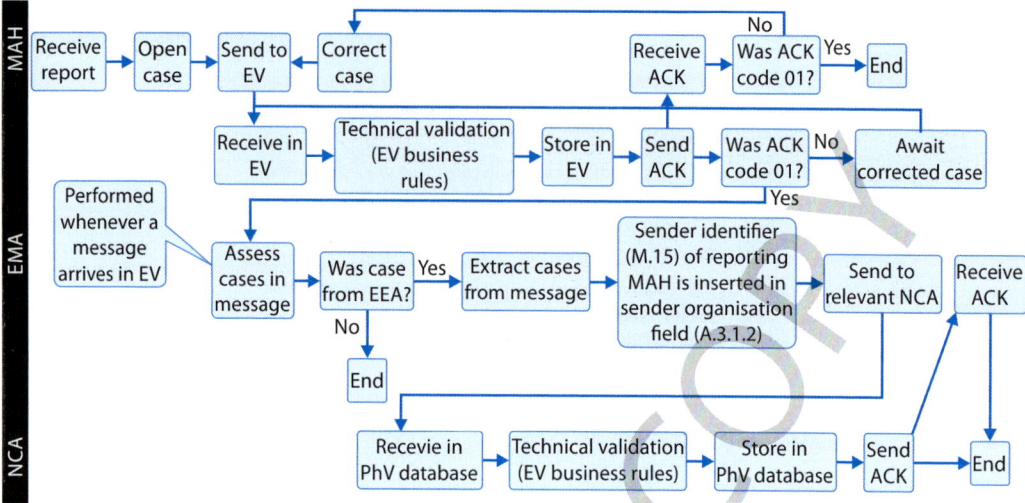

Fig. VI.4: Business process map—Suspected adverse reaction reporting in EU—Final arrangements

No.	Step	Description	Responsible Organisation
		Table VI.6: Process description—Suspected adverse reaction reporting in EU—Final arrangements	
1	Start. Receive report.	National Competent Authority (NCA) or Marketing Authorisation Holder (MAH) receives information on a suspected adverse reaction from a patient, healthcare professional or other valid reporter. If the case has been received from an EU NCA, do not retransmit it to EudraVigilance (EV).	MAH/NCA
2	Open case.	Open and create an individual case safety report.	MAH/NCA
3	Is case serious?	If No go to step 3.1. If Yes, go to step 4.	
3.1	Is case from EEA?	If No go to step 11.1. If Yes, go to step 4.	
4	Send to EV.	Transmit the case (all serious and EU non-serious) electronically, in ICH E2B(R2) format as an xml message within the relevant time frame (15 or 90 days, as applicable), to EV.	MAH/NCA
5	**Receive in EV.**	Receive the message in the EV.	EMA
6	Technical Validation (EV Business Rules).	Every message that is received in EV is validated against the EudraVigilance Business Rules and an Acknowledgement message (ACK) is created specifying whether or not the message and the case(s) therein are valid.	EMA

Contd..

Contd..

No.	Step	Description	Responsible Organisation
		A valid message will have an ACK code 01. A non-valid message will have an ACK code 02 (if a case contained therein is non-valid) or 03 (if the message itself is not correctly formatted).	
7	Store in EV.	Once the case has been validated, it is stored in the EV.	EMA
8	Send ACK.	The acknowledgement message created in step 6 is transmitted to the case sender no later than 2 business days following receipt of the case. Go to step 9 for the EMA's next step. Go to step 10 for MAH/NCA's next step.	EMA
9	Was ACK code 01?	If no, go to step 9.1. If yes, go to step 9.2.	EMA
9.1	Await corrected case.	The sender should correct every case with an error ACK and retransmit it within the regulatory reporting timelines. Periodically the EMA should assess all cases with an error ACK for which a corrected case has not been transmitted and contact the Qualified Person responsible for PharmacoVigilance (QPPV) to inform these missing corrected cases. If a sender fails to correct cases, this information should be incorporated into data quality assessments and the appropriate committees should be informed. Go back to step 5 upon receipt of the corrected case.	EMA
9.2	End.	**The case is now stored in EV &, following duplicate detection & recoding will be available for signal detection and data quality analyses. If the case occurred in the EU and was transmitted to EV by a MAH, it will be rerouted to the relevant NCA** (see **VI. Appendix 3.3**)	EMA
10	Receive ACK.	Receive the ACK message, associate it with the relevant case(s) and check to ensure that the case was considered valid.	**MAH/NCA**
11	Was ACK code 01?	If yes, go to step 11.1. If no, then the regulatory timeline clock has not stopped and the case should be corrected and re-transmitted to EV within the relevant regulatory reporting timelines. Day 0 remains as the day that the first information was received. A 02 or 03 ACK does not constitute new information. Go to step 12 (Correct case)	MAH/NCA
11.1	End.	**End the process for this version of the case. Normal follow-up activities should continue and if any follow-up is received, return to step 1.**	MAH/NCA
12	Correct case.	Correct the case to remove the errors identified in the ACK and re-transmit the case to EV (go back to step 4).	MAH/NCA

VI. App3.2.1. Final Arrangements Applicable to Marketing Authorisation Holders

Table VI.7: Reporting requirements applicable to marketing authorisation holders—Final arrangements

Marketing authorisation procedure	Origin	Adverse reaction type	Destination	Time frame
• Centralised	EU	All serious	• EudraVigilance database	15 days
• Mutual recognition, decentralised or subject to referral		All non-serious	• EudraVigilance database	90 days
• Purely national	Non-EU	All serious	• EudraVigilance database	15 days

VI. App3.2.2. Final Arrangements Applicable to Competent Authorities in Member States

Table VI.8: Reporting requirements applicable to competent authorities in Member States—Final arrangements

Marketing authorisation procedure	Origin	Adverse reaction type	Destination	Time frame
• Centralised	EU	All serious	• EudraVigilance database	15 days
• Mutual recognition, decentralised or subject to referral		All non-serious	• EudraVigilance database	90 days
• Purely national				

VI. App3.3. Transmission and Rerouting of ICSRs to Competent Authorities in Member States[45]

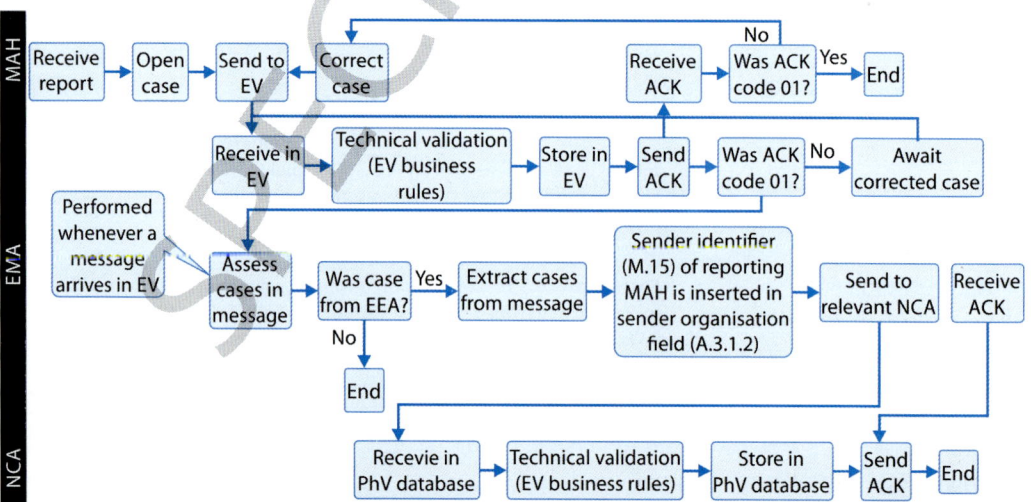

Fig. VI.5: Business process map: Transmission and rerouting of ICSRs to competent authorities in Member States.

Annexure 8: Guideline on Good Pharmacovigilance Practices (GVP)

Table VI.9: Process description: Transmission and rerouting of ICSRs to competent authorities in Member States[46]

No.	Name	Description	Responsible Organisation
1	Start. Receive report.	Marketing Authorisation Holder (MAH) receives information on a suspected adverse reaction from a patient, healthcare professional or other valid reporter.	MAH
2	Open case.	Open and create an individual case safety report.	MAH
3	Send to EudraVigilance (EV).	Transmit the case electronically, in ICH E2B(R2) format as an xml message within the relevant time frames (15 or 90 days, as applicable), to EVI.	MAH
4	Receive in EV.	Receive the message in the EV.	EMA
5	Technical Validation (EV Business Rules).	Every message that is received in EV is validated against the EudraVigilance Business Rules and an Acknowledgement message (ACK) is created specifying whether or not the message & the case(s) therein are valid. A valid message will have an ACK code 01. A non-valid message will have an ACK code 02 (if a case contained therein is non-valid) or 03 (if the message itself is not correctly formatted).	EMA
6	Store in EV.	Once the case has been validated, it is stored in EV.	EMA
7	Send ACK.	The acknowledgement message created in step 5 is transmitted to the case sender no later than 2 business days following receipt of the case.	EMA
7.1	Receive ACK.	Receive the ACK message, associate it with the relevant case(s) and check to ensure that the case was considered valid.	MAH
7.2	Was ACK code 01?	If yes, go to step 7.2.1. If no, then the regulatory timeline clock has not stopped and the case should be corrected and re-transmitted to EV within the relevant regulatory reporting timelines. Day 0 remains as the day that the first information was received. A 02 or 03 ACK does not constitute new information. Go to step 7.2.2 (Correct case).	MAH
7.2.1	End.	End the process of transmitting this version of the case to EVI. Normal follow-up activities should continue and if any follow-up is received, return to step 1.	MAH
7.2.2	Correct case.	Correct the case to remove the errors identified in the ACK and re-transmit the case to EV (go back to step 3).	MAH
8	Was ACK code 01?	If yes, go to step 9. If no, perform no further processing on this version of the case and go to step 8.1	EMA

Contd..

---

46. Once the functionalities of the EudraVigilance database specified in [REG Art 24(2)] are established.

Contd..

No.	Name	Description	Responsible Organisation
8.1	Await corrected case.	The sender should correct every case with an error ACK and re-transmit it within the regulatory reporting timelines. Periodically the EMA should assess all cases with an error ACK for which a corrected case has not been transmitted and contact the Qualified Person responsible for PharmacoVigilance (QPPV) to inform of these missing corrected cases. If a sender fails to correct cases, his information should be incorporated into data quality assessments and the appropriate committees should be informed.	EMA
9	Assess cases in message.	Whenever a message has passed the technical validation, the cases therein should be immediately assessed to determine the country where the reaction occurred for regulatory reporting purposes.	EMA
10	Was case from EU?	For every case, assess whether the country of occurrence is in the EU. If Yes, go to step 11. If No, go to step 10.1	EMA
10.1	**End.**	**The case is now stored in EV &, following duplicate detection & recoding will be available for signal detection and data quality analyses.**	EMA
11	Extract cases from message.	The cases occurring in the EU will be extracted from the message for processing prior to re-transmission.	EMA
12	Technical Validation.	Message sender identifier (ICH M2 M.1.5) of reporting MAH is inserted in Sender organisation field (ICH-E2B(R2) A.3.1.2) prior to re-transmission. This is to permit the receiving National Competent Authority (NCA) to unambiguously identify the MAH responsible for transmitting the case to EV.	EMA
13	Send to relevant NCA	The case is transmitted to the relevant NCA of the Member State where the reaction occurred with no other changes. Where a Member State has more than one NCA responsible for post-marketing reports, the cases occurring in that Member State are sent to all relevant NCAs.	EMA
14	**Receive in PharmacoVigilance DataBase (PhV DB).**	**The relevant NCA receives the message in its PhV DB**	**NCA**
15	Technical Validation (EV Business Rules).	Every message should be validated against the EudraVigilance Business Rules (the same business rules as in Step 5 and an Acknowledgement message (ACK) is created specifying whether or not the message & the case(s) therein are valid. A valid message will have an ACK code 01. A non-valid message will have an ACK code 02 (if a case contained therein is non-valid) or 03 (if the message itself is not correctly formatted).	NCA
16	Store in PharmacoVigilance DataBase (PhV DB).	Once the case has been validated, it is stored in the PhV DB.	NCA

Contd..

Annexure 8: Guideline on Good Pharmacovigilance Practices (GVP)

Contd..

No.	Name	Description	Responsible Organisation
17	Send ACK.	The acknowledgement message created in step 15 is transmitted to EV no later than 2 business days following receipt of the case.	NCA
17.1	End	The case is now stored in the NCA's PharmacoVigilance DataBase &, following duplicate detection & recoding will be available for signal detection and data quality analyses.	NCA
18	Receive ACK	The acknowledgement message sent in step 17 is received & stored in EV.	EMA
19	End	The case has now been successfully retransmitted to the relevant NCA.	EMA

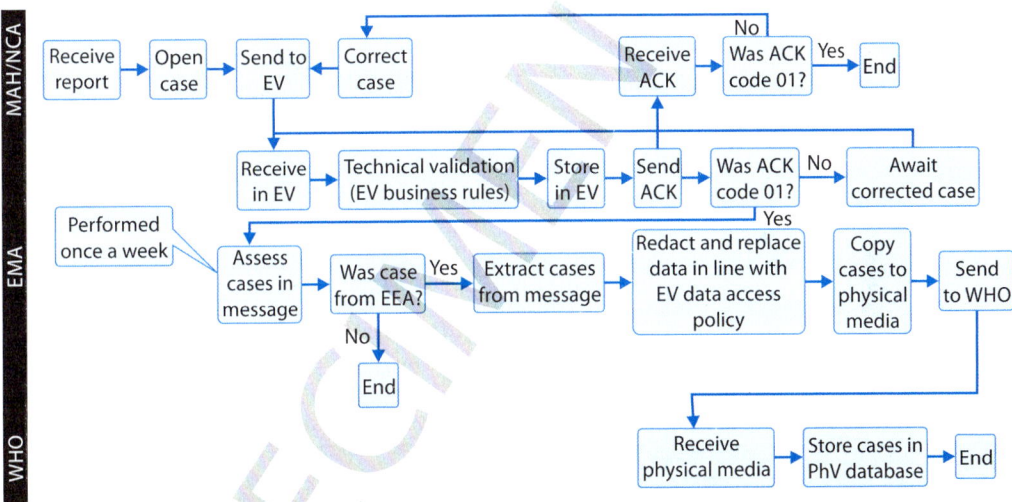

Fig. VI.6: Business process map: Transmission of ICSRs to World Health Organization (WHO) Collaborating Centre for International Drug Monitoring

---

47. Once the functionalities of the EudraVigilance database specified in [REG Art 24(2)] are established.

VI. APP 4 TRANSMISSION OF ICSRS TO WORLD HEALTH ORGANIZATION (WHO)[47]

Table VI.10: Process description: Transmission of ICSRs to World Health Organisation (WHO) Collaborating Centre for International Drug Monitoring[48]

No.	Step	Description	Responsible Organisation
1	**Start. Receive report.**	National Competent Authority (NCA) or Marketing Authorisation Holder (MAH) receives information on a suspected adverse reaction from a patient, healthcare professional or other valid reporter.	MAH/NCA
2	Open case.	Open and create an individual case safety report.	MAH/NCA
3	Send to EV.	Transmit the case electronically, in ICH E2B(R2) format as an xml message within the relevant time frames (15 or 90 days, as applicable), to EudraVigilance (EV).	MAH/NCA
4	**Receive in EV.**	**Receive the message in EV.**	EMA
5	Technical Validation (EV Business Rules).	Every message that is received in EV is validated against the EudraVigilance Business Rules and an Acknowledgement message (ACK) is created specifying whether or not the message & the case(s) therein are valid. A valid message will have an ACK code 01. A non-valid message will have an ACK code 02 (if a case contained therein is non-valid) or 03 (if the message itself is not correctly formatted).	EMA
6	Store in EV.	Once the case has been validated, it is stored in EV.	EMA
7	Send ACK.	The acknowledgement message created in step 5 is transmitted to the case sender no later than 2 business days following receipt of the case.	EMA
7.1	**Receive ACK.**	Receive the ACK message, associate it with the relevant case(s) and check to ensure that the case was considered valid.	**MAH/NCA**
7.2	Was ACK code 01?	If Yes, go to step 7.2.1. If no, then the regulatory timeline clock has not stopped and the case should be corrected and re-transmitted to EV within the relevant regulatory reporting timelines. Day 0 remains as the day that the first information was received. A 02 or 03 ACK does not constitute new information. Go to step 7.2.2 (Correct case).	MAH/NCA
7.2.1	End	End the process of transmitting this version of the case to EV. Normal follow-up activities should continue and if any follow-up is received, return to step 1.	**MAH/NCA**
7.2.2	Correct case	Correct the case to remove the errors identified in the ACK and retransmit the case to EV (go back to step 3).	MAH/NCA
8	**Was ACK code 01?**	If yes, go to step 9. If no, perform no further processing on this version of the case and go to step 8.1	EMA

Contd..

---

48. Once the functionalities of the EudraVigilance database specified in [REG Art 24(2)] are established.

Annexure 8: Guideline on Good Pharmacovigilance Practices (GVP)

Contd..

No.	Step	Description	Responsible Organisation
8.1	Await corrected case.	The sender should correct every case with an error ACK and re-transmit within the regulatory reporting timelines. Periodically the EMA should assess all cases with an error ACK for which a corrected case has not been transmitted and contact the Qualified Person responsible for PharmacoVigilance (QPPV) to inform of these missing corrected cases. If a sender fails to correct cases, this information should be incorporated into data quality assessments and the appropriate committees should be informed.	EMA
9	Assess cases in message.	Once a week, for every message that has passed the technical validation, the cases therein should be assessed to determine the country where the reaction occurred for regulatory reporting purposes.	EMA
10	Was case from EU?	For every case, assess whether the country of occurrence is in the EU. If yes, go to step 11. If no, go to step 10.1.	EMA
10.1	**End.**	**The case is now stored in EV &, following duplicate detection & recoding will be available for signal detection and data quality analyses.**	EMA
11	Extract cases from message	The cases occurring in the EU is extracted from the message for processing prior to retransmission.	EMA
12	Redact & replace data in line with EV Data Access policy.	Prior to sending the cases to the World Health Organization (WHO) Collaborating Centre for International Drug Monitoring, the extracted copies of the cases have some data elements redacted and replaced in line with the EV Data Access Policy in order to ensure personal data protection.	EMA
13	Copy cases to physical media.	The cases are copied to physical media.	EMA
14	Send to WHO.	The physical media is sent to WHO Collaborating Centre.	EMA
15	**Receive physical media**	**WHO Collaborating Centre receives the physical media.**	**WHO**
16	Store cases in PharmacoVigilance DataBase (PhV DB).	Once the cases have been validated, they are stored in the PhV DB.	WHO
17	**End.**	**Cases are stored in the WHO Collaborating Centre's PharmacoVigilance DataBase &, following duplicate detection & recoding will be available for signal detection and data quality analyses.**	**WHO**

VI. APPENDIX 5 NULLIFICATION OF CASES

General principles regarding the nullification of cases are provided in VI.C.6.2.2.10. The following recommendations should also be applied:

- The value in the data element 'Report nullification' (ICH-E2B(R2) A.1.13) should be set to 'Yes' and the nullification reason should be provided in the data element 'Reason for nullification' (ICH- EB(R2) A.1.13.1). The nullification reason should be clear and concise to explain why this case is no longer considered to be a valid report. For example, a nullification reason stating, 'the report no longer meets the reporting criteria' or 'report sent previously in error' are not detailed enough explanations.
- An individual case can only be nullified by the sending organisation.
- Once an individual case has been nullified, the case cannot be reactivated.
- If it becomes necessary to resubmit the case that has been previously nullified, a new 'Sender's (case) safety report unique identifier' (ICH-E2B(R2) A.1.0.1) and 'Worldwide unique case identification number' (ICH-E2B(R2) A.1.10) should be assigned.
- Individual versions (i.e. follow-up reports) of a case cannot be nullified, only the entire individual case to which they refer.
- Individual cases that have been nullified should not be used for scientific evaluation, however, they should remain in the database for auditing purposes.
- In addition, in case of duplicate reports where one report needs to be nullified, the update of the remaining case should be performed in the form of a follow up report.[49] Information on the identification of the nullified case(s) should be provided in the data element 'Source(s) of the case identifier (e.g. name of the company, name of regulatory agency)' (ICH-E2B(R2) A.1.11.1) and in the data element 'Case identifier(s)' (ICH-E2B(R2)A.1.11.2).

Table VI.11: Examples of scenarios for which ICSRs should be nullified

Ex.	Scenario	Action
1	An individual case has been identified as a duplicate of another individual case previously submitted.	One of the individual cases should be nullified. The remaining valid case should be updated with any additional relevant information from the nullified case.
2	A wrong 'Worldwide unique case identification number' (ICH-E2B(R2) A.1.10) was accidentally used and does not refer to an existing case.	The case with the wrong 'Worldwide unique case identification number' (ICH-E2B(R2) A.1.10) should be nullified. A new case should be created with a correct 'Worldwide unique case identification number'.
3	On receipt of further information it is confirmed that that the adverse reaction occurred before the suspect drug(s) was taken.	The case should be nullified.
4	On receipt of further information on an individual case, it is confirmed that the patient did not receive the suspect drug. Minimum reporting criteria for an ICSR as outlined in VI.B.2 are no longer met.	The case should be nullified.
5	On receipt of further information it is confirmed by the same reporter that the reported adverse reaction(s) did not occur to the patient. Minimum reporting criteria for an ICSR as outlined in VI.B.2 are no longer met.	The case should be nullified.
6	On receipt of further information it is confirmed that there was no valid patient for the individual case. Minimum reporting criteria for an ICSR as outlined in VI.B.2 are no longer met.	If it is not possible to obtain confirmation of the patient's existence, then the case should be nullified.

---

49. As presented in the Guideline on the Detection and Management of Duplicate Individual Cases and Individual Case Safety Reports (ICSRs), EMA/13432/2009.

Annexure 8: Guideline on Good Pharmacovigilance Practices (GVP) **463**

Table VI.12: Examples of scenarios for which ICSRs should NOT be nullified

Ex.	Scenario	Action
7	A wrong 'Worldwide unique case identification number' (ICH E2B(R2) A.1.10) was accidentally used. This wrong ICH-E2B(R2) A.1.10 'Worldwide unique case identification number' referred to an existing case.	The report with the wrong 'Worldwide unique case identification number' (ICH-E2B(R2) A.1.10) should not be nullified. A follow-up report should be submitted to correct the information previously submitted. A new ICSR should be created and submitted with the correct 'Worldwide unique case identification number'.
8	On receipt of further information on an individual case, it is confirmed that the patient did not receive the marketing authorisation holder's suspect drug. However, the patient received other suspect drugs and the minimum reporting criteria for an ICSR are still met.	The case should not be nullified.
9	On receipt of further information the reporter has confirmed that the reported adverse reaction is no longer considered to be related to the suspect medicinal product(s).	The case should not be nullified. A follow-up report should be submitted within the appropriate time frame with the updated information on the case.
10	Change of the individual case from serious to non-serious (downgrading).	The case should not be nullified. A follow-up report should be submitted with the data element 'Seriousness' (ICH-E2B(R2) A.1.5.1) populated with the value 'No' without selection of a value for the data element 'Seriousness criteria' (ICH-E2B(R2) A.1.5.2). The data element 'Does this case fulfil the local criteria for an expedited report?' (ICH-E2B(R2) field A.1.9) should remain populated with the value 'Yes'.
11	The primary source country has changed, which has an impact on the ICH-E2B(R2) convention regarding the creation of the 'Worldwide unique case identification number' (ICH-E2B(R2) A.1.10).	The case should not be nullified. The 'Sender's (case) safety report unique identifier' (ICH-E2B(R2) A.1.0.1) can be updated on the basis of the new primary source country code. However, the 'Worldwide unique case identification number' (ICH-E2B(R2) A.1.10) should remain unchanged. If, for some technical reason, the sender's local system is not fully ICH-E2B(R2) compliant and cannot follow this policy, then the sender should nullify the original case. A new case should be created with a new 'Worldwide unique case identification number' (ICH-E2B(R2) A.1.10) reflecting the changed primary source country code. The 'Worldwide unique case identification number' (ICH-E2B(R2) A.1.10) of the case that was nullified should be reflected in the data elements 'Other case identifiers in previous transmissions' (ICH-E2B(R2) A.1.11).

Contd..

Contd..

Ex	Scenario	Action
12	The suspected medicinal product belongs to another marketing authorisation holder (e.g. a product with the same active substance but marketed under a different invented name).	The case should not be nullified. It is recommended that the initial sender informs the other marketing authorisation holder about this case (including the 'Worldwide unique case identification number' (ICH-E2B(R2) A.1.10) used). The original organisation should also submit a follow-up report to provide this new information. The other concerned marketing authorisation holder should create a new case and specify the reference case number and the name of the initial sending marketing authorisation holder in the data elements 'Source(s) of the case identifier (e.g. name of the company name of regulatory agency)' (ICH-E2B(R2) A.1.11.1) and 'Case identifier(s)' (ICH-E2B(R2) A.1.11.2). This will allow grouping the cases in the EudraVigilance database.
13	The suspected medicinal product taken does not belong to the marketing authorisation holder (same active substance, the invented name is unknown and the report originates from a country, where the marketing authorisation holder has no marketing authorisation for the medicinal product in question).	The case should not be nullified. The marketing authorisation holder should submit a follow-up report with this information within the appropriate time frame.
14	The case is mistakenly reported by the marketing authorisation holder A although the marketing authorisation holder B as co-marketer is responsible for reporting the case.	The case should not be nullified. An explanation should be sent by the marketing authorisation holder A to the co-marketer marketing authorisation holder B that the case has already been reported. The marketing authorisation holder B should provide any additional information on the case as a follow-up report with the same 'Worldwide unique case identification number' (ICH-E2B(R2) A.1.10).

VI. APPENDIX 6 DATA QUALITY MONITORING OF ICSRs TRANSMITTED ELECTRONICALLY

The business map and process description describe a system where there is a separation between a PharmacoVigilance DataBase (PhV DB) holder, the PhV DB holder's data Quality Assessors (QA) and the PhV DB holder's auditors; however this is not mandatory and these functions may be performed by the same people or groups.

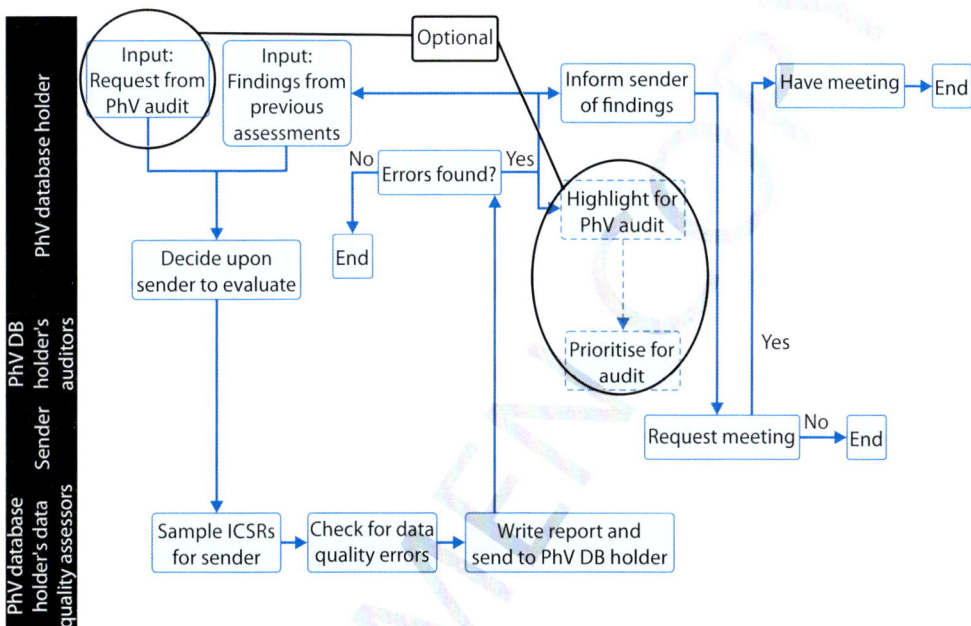

Fig VI.7: Business process map: Data quality monitoring of ICSRs transmitted electronically

Table VI.13: Process description—Data quality monitoring of ICSRs transmitted electronically.

No.	Step	Description	Responsible Organisation
1	Start. Decide upon Sender to evaluate.	Select one of the organisations that has transmitted ICSRs to your database. Inputs into this decision can include, but need not be limited to findings from previous assessments and requests from pharmacovigilance audits.	PhV DB holder
2	Sample ICSRs from Sender.	Take a sample of ICSRs that were transmitted by the selected sender	QA
3	Check for data quality errors.	Check the cases for data quality errors. The cases should be assessed against appropriate published standards and similar documents, for example the MedDRA Term Selection Points to Consider document.	QA
4	Write report and send to PhV DB holder.	The findings from the data quality assessment should be collated into a single report. These can include related checks, such as 15-day reporting compliance, whether error reports are corrected and similar statistical information.	QA
5	Errors found?	Were any errors found during the analysis of the cases? If no, go to step 5.1. If yes go to steps 5.2, 5.3 and 6.	PhV DB holder
5.1	End.	If there were no errors found, then no further action needs to be taken. The process can end until the next time the sender is assessed. The PhV DB holder may choose to share this information with the assessed sender and their auditors who may wish to factor this in to determinations of which sender to assess.	PhV DB holder
5.2	Highlight for PhV audit.	If the PhV DB holder's organisation has an audit department, any significant findings should always be shared with them.	PhV DB holder
5.2.1	Prioritise for Audit.	The audit or inspections department should use the information provided to them to feed into decisions about prioritising organisations for audit or inspection.	PhV DB holder's auditors
5.3	INPUT: Findings from previous assessments.	Any errors found (or even lack thereof) should be incorporated into decisions about which senders to evaluate & should also inform the performance of the assessments (e.g. targeting particular types of case) and the report (documenting whether previously identified issues have been addressed).	PhV DB holder
6	Inform sender of findings.	Inform the sender of the findings, including requested remedial actions (e.g. re-transmitting certain cases) and time frames for those actions	PhV DB holder
7	Request meeting?	The sender should have the option to choose to request a meeting to discuss the findings and appropriate remedial action and time frames. If no, meeting is requested, go to step 7.1. If a meeting is requested go to step 8.	Sender
7.1	Address the findings and retransmit any required cases.	Address all findings, take necessary steps to prevent recurrence of such findings and re-transmit any required cases.	Sender

Contd..

Contd..

No.	Step	Description	Responsible Organisation
7.2	End.	Once all findings have been addressed, the necessary steps taken to prevent recurrence of such findings and any required cases have been retransmitted, the process can end until the next time the sender is assessed.	Sender
8	Have meeting.	Upon request from one party, a meeting should be held to discuss the findings of quality assessments and appropriate remedial and preventive actions to ensure that the cases in the database are correct and shall be so in the future.	PhV DB holder & Sender
9	End.	Unless further action has been specified (e.g. future meetings or assessments), the process can end until the next time the sender is assessed.	PhV DB holder

VI. APPENDIX 7 DUPLICATE DETECTION AND MANAGEMENT OF ICSRs

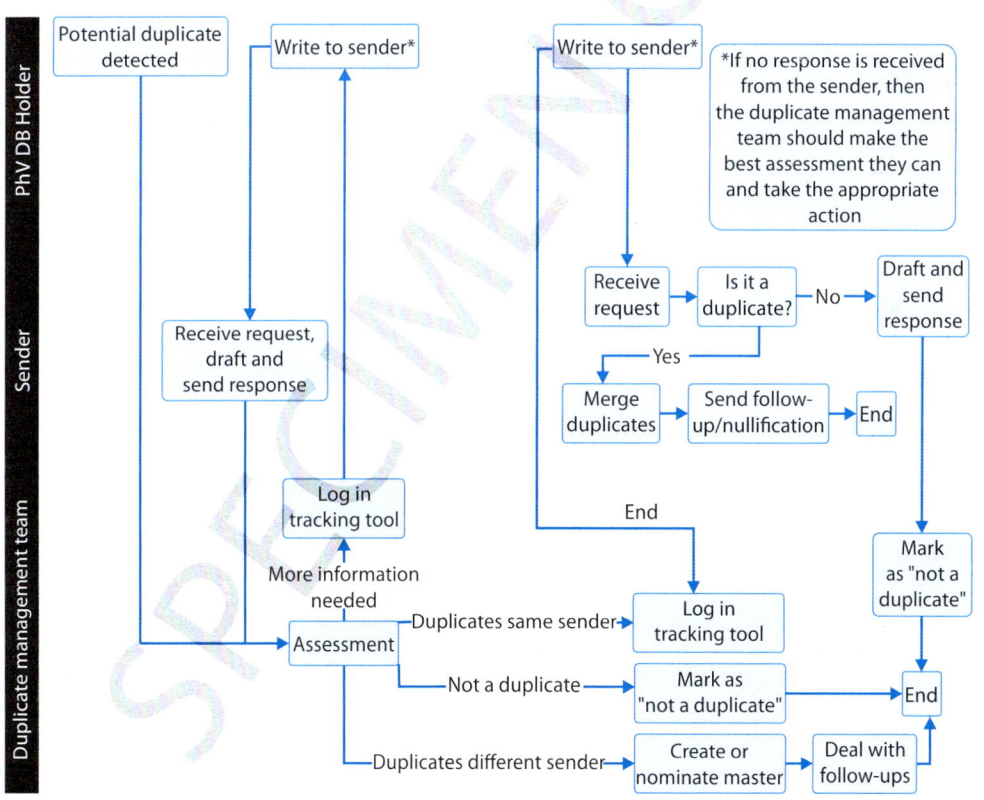

FIG. VI.8: Business process map: Duplicate detection and management of ICSRs.

Table VI.14: Process description—Duplicate detection and management of ICSRs

No.	Step	Description	Responsible Organisation
1	Start. Potential duplicate detected.	Potential duplicates have been detected by the PharmacoVigilance DataBase (PhV DB) holder organisation or the PhV DB holder organisation is notified of potential duplicates by a receiver of the cases.	PhV DB holder
2	Assessment.	All potential duplicates need assessment by the organisation Duplicate Management Team (DMT) to confirm or deny their duplicate status. Following assessment there are 4 possible outcomes: • Not a duplicate (go to step 2.1), • More information needed (go to step 2.2), • Duplicates from different sender (go to step 2.3), • Duplicates from same sender (go to step 2.4). The outcome of all assessments should be recorded to avoid continually reassessing the same cases when further versions arrive. These recorded outcomes can also be used to refine the duplicate detection methods during future development.	DMT
2.1	Not a Duplicate: Mark as not a duplicate.	If the cases are assessed as not being duplicates of one another, then mark both cases as such. Go to step 3 (End).	DMT
2.2	More information needed: Log in tracking tool.	There should be some form of tool for tracking when more information is needed, when correspondence has been sent, whether an answer was received and, if so, when.	DMT
2.2.1	Write to sender.	More information is required in order to be able to make a definite assessment. The sender (who transmitted the case(s) in question to the PhVDB holder's organisation) should be contacted to request specific information necessary to confirm or deny duplication. Personal data protection must remain paramount, so unsecured communications should not include sufficient data to identify an individual.	PhV DB holder
2.2.2	Receive request, draft and send response.	Once a request for more information has been received, the Sender of the case should respond promptly, either as a follow-up version of the case or by responding to the requester. The DMT should then reassess the case based on the new information (Go back to step 2).	Sender
2.3	Duplicates different senders: Create or nominate master.	Once cases have been determined to be duplicates of one another and have been transmitted to the PhV DB holder by different senders or reporters, then they should be merged under a master case, following the process described in chapter 2.3 "Management of duplicate cases" of the Guideline on the Detection and Management of Duplicate Individual Cases and Individual Case Safety Reports (ICSRs), EMA/13432/2009.	DMT
2.3.1	Deal with follow-ups.	If any follow-ups arrive for any of the cases, this information may require a reassessment of the master case. Reassess and, if necessary, amend the master case as with any received follow-up information. Go to step 3 (End).	DMT

Contd..

Contd..

No.	Step	Description	Responsible Organisation
2.4	**Duplicates same sender: Log in tracking tool.**	Once cases have been determined to be duplicates of one another, and have been transmitted to the PhV DB holder by the same sender, then this decision and the correspondence referred to in step 2.4.1 should be logged in the tracking tool referred to in step 2.2.	DMT
2.4.1	**Write to sender.**	The sender organisation, as the source of the duplicates, should be contacted in accordance with chapter 2.3.3 of the Guideline on the Detection and Management of Duplicate Individual Cases and Individual Case Safety Reports (ICSRs), EMA/13432/2009. The sender should be asked to confirm or deny duplication and take appropriate steps in accordance with chapter 2.3.1 of the aforementioned Guideline.	**PhV DB holder**
2.4.2	**Receive request.**	Receive and log the communication containing information on suspected duplicates in the Sender's PhV DB.	**Sender**
2.4.3	Is it a duplicate?	Assess the potential duplicates. Are the cases duplicates of one another? If yes, go to step 2.4.3.1. If no, go to step 2.4.3.2.	Sender
2.4.3.1	Merge duplicates.	Merge the duplicates, taking into account Flowchart 1 of chapter 2.3.1.3 of the Guideline on the Detection and Management of Duplicate Individual Cases and Individual Case Safety Reports (ICSRs), EMA/13432/2009.	Sender
2.4.3.1.1	Send follow-up/ nullification.	For the cases that are merged under the master, send a nullification message to the PhV DB holder. For the case that is master, send the updated case to the PhV DB holder as follow-up information. The merging and transmission should be completed promptly and in any case within 15 days of the date of receipt of the information from the PhV DB holder that the cases were considered to be possible duplicates. This date should be treated as the date of receipt of most recent information for regulatory reporting purposes.	Sender
2.4.3.1.2	End.	**The duplicates have now been removed from both the Sender's system and that of the PhV DB holder and only the master should be available for signal detection and data quality analyses. Unless follow-up information is received, then no further steps need be taken.**	**Sender**
2.4.3.2	Draft and send a response.	Reply to the PhV DB holder who sent the communication informing that the cases are not duplicates.	Sender
2.4.3.2.1	**Mark as "Not a duplicate".**	Upon receipt of confirmation from the Sender organisation that the cases are not duplicates, mark the cases as "Not a duplicate" and go to step 3 (End).	DMT
3	End.	No further action is required for this couple.	DMT

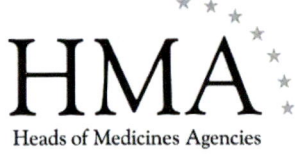
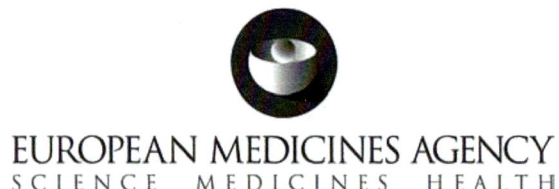

9 December 2013
EMA/816292/2011 Rev 1*

GUIDELINE ON GOOD PHARMACOVIGILANCE PRACTICES (GVP)

Module VII Periodic safety update report (Rev 1)

Date for coming into effect of first version	2 July 2012
Draft Revision 1* finalised by the Agency in collaboration with Member States	21 March 2013
Draft Revision 1 agreed by ERMS FG	27 March 2013
Draft Revision 1 adopted by Executive Director	19 April 2013
Release for consultation	25 April 2013
End of consultation (deadline for comments)	25 June 2013
Revised draft Revision 1 finalised by the Agency in collaboration with Member States	23 October 2013
Revised draft Revision 1 agreed by ERMS FG	11 November 2013
Revised draft Revision 1 adopted by Executive Director as final	9 December 2013
Date for coming into effect of Revision 1* (for PSURs with data lock point after 12 December 2013)	13 December 2013

*Note: Revision 1 contains the following:
- Updates in VII.B and VII.C.5. following finalisation of the ICH-E2C(R2) guideline on "Periodic Benefit-Risk Evaluation Report (PBRER)", which reached Step 4 of the ICH process in November 2012, in order to harmonise the principles and agreements reached by the ICH Expert Working Group;
- Further guidance regarding technical aspects on the implementation of Regulation (EU) No 1235/2010 and Directive 2010/84/EU based on the experience gained since July 2012;
- Practical instructions for the application, description and maintenance of the EU reference date list in VII.C.3.2., VII.C.3.3. and VII.C.3.4. and amendments to the marketing authorisation in VII.C.3.7.;
- Further instructions regarding the PSUR assessment process, product information and transitional arrangements within the EU regulatory network in VII.C.

VII.A. INTRODUCTION

Periodic safety update reports (PSURs) are pharmacovigilance documents intended to provide an evaluation of the risk-benefit balance of a medicinal product for submission by marketing authorisation holders at defined time points during the post-authorisation phase.

The legal requirements for submission of PSURs are established in Regulation (EC) No 726/2004, Directive 2001/83/EC and in the Commission Implementing Regulation (EU) No 520/2012 on the performance of pharmacovigilance activities provided for in Regulation (EC) No 726/2004 and Directive 2001/83/EC (hereinafter referred to as IR). All applicable legal requirements in this Module are referenced in the way explained in the GVP Introductory Cover Note and are usually identifiable by the modal verb "shall". Guidance for the implementation of legal requirements is provided using the modal verb "should".

The format of PSURs shall follow the structure described in the IR Article 35. This Module provides guidance on the preparation, submission and assessment of PSURs.

The scope, objectives, format and content of the PSUR are described in VII.B. The required format and content of PSURs in the EU are based on those for the Periodic Benefit Risk Evaluation Report (PBRER) described in the ICH-E2C(R2) guideline (see Annex IV ICH-E2C(R2)). The PBRER format replaces the PSUR format previously described in the ICH-E2C(R1). In line with the EU legislation, the report is described as PSUR in the GVP Modules.

Further details and guidance for the submission of PSURs in the EU, including the list of Union references dates and frequency of submission are provided in VII.C., which also covers the single EU assessment of PSURs in VII.C.4. Details related to the quality system are provided in VII.C.6. and the publication of PSUR-related documents in VII.C.7. as transparency provisions.

Each marketing authorisation holder shall be responsible for submitting PSURs for its own products [DIR Art 107b] [REG Art 28 (2)] and should submit PSURs to the Agency (see VII.C.9. for transitional arrangements) according to the following timelines:

- Within 70 calendar days of the data lock point (day 0) for PSURs covering intervals up to 12 months (including intervals of exactly 12 months); and
- Within 90 calendar days of the data lock point (day 0) for PSURs covering intervals in excess of 12 months;
- The timeline for the submission of ad hoc PSURs requested by competent authorities will normally be specified in the request, otherwise the ad hoc PSURs should be submitted within 90 calendar days of the data lock point.

It should be noted that detailed listings of individual cases shall not be included systematically [IR Art 34(4)]. The PSUR should focus on summary information, scientific safety assessment and integrated benefit-risk evaluation.

Recital 23 of Directive 2010/84/EU states that the obligations imposed in respect of PSURs should be proportionate to the risks posed by medicinal products. PSUR reporting should therefore be linked to the risk management systems of a medicinal product (see Module V). The "modular approach" of the PSUR described in VII.B.5. aims to minimise duplication and improve efficiency during the preparation and review of PSURs along with other regulatory documents such as the development safety update report (DSUR)[1] or the safety specification in the Risk Management Plan (RMP), by enabling the common content of particular sections where appropriate to be utilised interchangeably across different PSURs, DSURs and RMPs.

The amended Directive 2001/83/EC also waives the obligation to submit PSURs routinely for generic medicinal products (authorised under DIR Art 10(1)), well-established use medicinal products (authorised under DIR Art 10a), homeopathic medicinal products (authorised under DIR Art 14) and traditional herbal medicinal products (authorised under DIR Art 16a), [DIR Art 107b(3)]. For such products, PSURs shall be submitted where there is a condition in the marketing authorisation or when requested by a competent authority in a Member State on the basis of concerns relating to pharmacovigilance data or due to the lack of PSURs for an active substance after its authorisation [DIR Art 107b(3)(a) and (3)(b)].

---

1. *See* Detailed Guidance on the Collection, Verification and Presentation of Adverse Event/Reaction Reports Arising from Clinical Trials on Medicinal Products for Human Use; available on http://ec.europa.eu/health/documents/eudralex/vol-10/

Competent authorities in the Member States shall assess PSURs to determine whether there are new risks or whether risks have changed or whether there are changes to the risk-benefit balance of medicinal products [DIR Art 107d].

In order to increase the shared use of resources between competent authorities in Member States, a single assessment of PSURs should be performed in the EU for different medicinal products containing the same active substance or the same combination of active substances authorised in more than one Member State for which a Union reference date and frequency of submission of PSURs has been established. The EU single assessment can include joint assessment for medicinal products authorised through either national or centralised procedures for marketing authorisation. The Agency shall make available a list of Union reference dates and frequency of submission [REG Art 26(g)] which will be legally binding.

As part of the assessment, it should be considered whether further investigations need to be carried out and whether any action concerning the marketing authorisations of products containing the same active substance or the same combination of active substances, and their product information is necessary.

The Agency shall make the PSURs available to the competent authorities in Member States, members of the Pharmacovigilance Risk Assessment Committee (PRAC), of the Committee for Medicinal Products for Human use (CHMP) and of the Coordination Group for Mutual Recognition and Decentralised Procedures - Human (CMDh) and the European Commission by means of a PSUR repository [DIR Art 107b(2)].

VII.B. STRUCTURES AND PROCESSES

VII.B.1. Objectives of the Periodic Safety Update Report (PSUR)

The main objective of a PSUR is to present a comprehensive, concise and critical analysis of the risk-benefit balance of the medicinal product taking into account new or emerging information in the context of cumulative information on risks and benefits. The PSUR is therefore a tool for post-authorisation evaluation at defined time points in the lifecycle of a product.

For the purposes of lifecycle benefit-risk management, it is necessary to continue evaluating the risks and benefits of a medicine in everyday medical practice and long term use in the post-authorisation phase. This may extend to evaluation of populations and endpoints that could not be investigated in the pre-authorisation clinical trials. A different risk-benefit balance may emerge as pharmacovigilance reveals further information about safety. The marketing authorisation holder should therefore re-evaluate the risk-benefit balance of its own medicinal products in populations exposed. This structured evaluation should be undertaken in the context of ongoing pharmacovigilance (*see* Module XII) and risk management (*see* Module V) to facilitate optimisation of the risk-benefit balance through effective risk minimisation.

Urgent safety information should be reported through the appropriate mechanism. A PSUR is not intended, in the first instance, for notification of significant new safety or efficacy information or to provide the means by which new safety issues are detected, (*see* Module IX and XII). It is acknowledged that the review of the data in the PSUR may lead to new safety issues being identified.

VII.B.2. Principles for the Evaluation of the Risk-benefit Balance within PSURs and Scope of the Information to be Included

Benefit-risk evaluation should be carried out throughout the lifecycle of the medicinal product to promote and protect public health and to enhance patient safety through effective risk minimisation.

After a marketing authorisation is granted, it is necessary to continue evaluating the benefits and risks of medicinal products in actual use and/or long term use, to confirm that the risk-benefit balance remains favourable.

The analysis of the risk-benefit balance should incorporate an evaluation of the safety, efficacy and effectiveness information that becomes available,[2]

---

2. The ICH-E2C(R2) guideline should not serve to limit the scope of the information to be provided in the benefit-risk evaluation of a medicinal product. Please refer to the applicable laws and regulations in the countries and regions. For EU specific requirements, *see* VII.C.5.

with reasonable and appropriate effort, during the reporting interval for the medicinal product in the context of what was known previously.

The risk evaluation should be based on all uses of the medicinal product. The scope includes evaluation of safety in real medical practice including use in unauthorised indications and use which is not in line with the product information. If use of the medicinal product is identified where there are critical gaps in knowledge for specific safety issues or populations, such use should be reported in the PSUR (e.g. use in paediatric population or in pregnant women). Sources of information on use outside authorisation may include drug utilisation data, information from spontaneous reports and publications in the literature.

The scope of the benefit information should include both clinical trial and real world data in authorised indications.

The integrated benefit-risk evaluation should be performed for all authorised indications and should incorporate the evaluation of risks in all use of the medicinal product (including use in unauthorised indications).

The evaluation should involve:

1. Critically examining the information which has emerged during the reporting interval to determine whether it has generated new signals, led to the identification of new potential or identified risks or contributed to knowledge of previously identified risks.
2. Critically summarising relevant new safety, efficacy and effectiveness information that could have an impact on the risk-benefit balance of the medicinal product.
3. Conducting an integrated benefit-risk analysis for all authorised indications based on the cumulative information available since the development international birth date (DIBD), the date of first authorisation for the conduct of an interventional clinical trial in any country. For the cases where the DIBD is unknown or the marketing authorisation holder does not have access to data from the clinical development period, the earliest possible applicable date should be used as starting point for the inclusion and evaluation of the cumulative information.
4. Summarising any risk minimisation actions that may have been taken or implemented during the reporting interval, as well as risk minimisation actions that are planned to be implemented.
5. Outlining plans for signal or risk evaluations including timelines and/or proposals for additional pharmacovigilance activities.

VII.B.3. Principles for the Preparation of PSURs

Unless otherwise specified by competent authorities, the marketing authorisation holder shall prepare a single PSUR for all its medicinal products containing the same active substance with information covering all the authorised indications, route of administration, dosage forms and dosing regiments, irrespective of whether authorised under different names and through separate procedures. Where relevant, data relating to a particular indication, dosage form, route of administration or dosing regimen, shall be presented in a separate section of the PSUR and any safety concerns shall be addressed accordingly [IR Art 34(6)]. There might be exceptional scenarios where the preparation of separate PSURs might be appropriate, for instance, in the event of different formulations for entirely different indications. In this case, agreement should be obtained from the relevant competent authorities preferably at the time of authorisation.

Case narratives shall be provided in the relevant risk evaluation section of the PSUR where integral to the scientific analysis of a signal or safety concern [IR Art 34(4)]. In this context, the term "case narratives" refers to clinical evaluations of individual cases rather than the CIOMS narratives. It should not be necessary to provide the actual CIOMS narrative text included in the individual case safety report (ICSR) but rather a clinical evaluation of important or illustrative cases in the context of the evaluation of the safety concern/signal.

When data received at the marketing authorisation holder from a partner might contribute meaningfully to the safety, benefit and/or benefit-risk analyses and influence the reporting marketing authorisation holder's product information, these data should be included and discussed in the PSUR.

The format and table of contents of all PSURs shall be as described in the IR Art 35 and each report should include interval as well as cumulative data. As the PSUR should be a single stand–alone document for the reporting interval, based on cumulative data, summary bridging reports and addendum reports, introduced in ICH-E2C(R1) guideline, will not be accepted.

The GVP Modules on Product- or Population-Specific Considerations[3] should be consulted as applicable when preparing a PSUR.

VII.B.4. Reference Information

Risk minimisation activities evaluated in the PSUR include updates to the product information.

The reference product information for the PSUR should include "core safety" and "authorised indications" components. In order to facilitate the assessment of benefit and risk-benefit balance by indication in the evaluation sections of the PSUR, the reference product information document should list all authorised indications in ICH countries[4] or regions. When the PSUR is also submitted to other countries in which there are additional locally authorised indications, these indications may be either added to the reference product information or handled as a regional appendix as considered most appropriate by the marketing authorization holder. The basis for the benefit evaluation should be the baseline important efficacy and effectiveness information summarised in the PSUR section 17.1 ("Important baseline efficacy and effectiveness information").

Information related to a specific indication, formulation or route of administration should be clearly identified in the reference product information.

The following possible options can be considered by the marketing authorisation holders when selecting the most appropriate reference product information for a PSUR:

- Company core data sheet (CCDS)
  - It is common practice for marketing authorisation holders to prepare their own company core data sheet which covers data relating to safety, indications, dosing, pharmacology, and other information concerning the product. The core safety information contained within the CCDS is referred to as the company core safety information (CCSI). A practical option for the purpose of the PSUR is for each marketing authorisation holder to use the CCDS in effect at the end of the reporting interval, as reference product information for both the risk sections of the PSUR as well as the main authorised indications for which benefit is evaluated.
  - When the CCDS does not contain information on authorised indications, the marketing authorisation holder should clearly specify which document is used as reference information for the authorised indications in the PSUR.
- Other options for the reference product information
  - When no CCDS or CCSI exist for a product (e.g. where the product is authorised in only one country or region, or for established/generics products on the market for many years), the marketing authorisation holder should clearly specify the reference information being used. This may comprise national or regional product information such as the EU summary of product characteristics (SmPC).
  - Where the reference information for the authorised indications is a separate document to the reference safety information (the core safety information contained within the reference product information), the version in effect at the end of the reporting interval should be included as an appendix to the PSUR (see VII.B.5.20.).

The marketing authorisation holder should continuously evaluate whether any revision of the reference product information/reference safety information is needed whenever new safety information is obtained during the reporting interval and ensure that significant changes made over the interval are described in PSUR section 4 ("Changes to the reference safety information") and where relevant, discussed in PSUR section 16 ("Signal and risk evaluation"). These changes may include:

- Changes to contraindications, warnings/precautions sections;
- Addition to adverse reactions and interactions;
- Addition of important new information on use in overdose; and

---

3. http://www.ema.europa.eu
4. http://www.ich.org/

- Removal of an indication or other restrictions for safety or lack of efficacy reasons.

The marketing authorisation holder should provide a clean copy of all versions of the reference product information in effect at the end of the reporting interval (e.g. different formulations included in the same PSUR) as an appendix to the PSUR (see VII.B.5.20.). The reference product information should be dated and version controlled.

Where new information on safety that could warrant changes to the authorised product information (e.g. new adverse drug reaction, warning or contraindication) has been added to the reference safety information during the period from the data lock point to the submission of the PSUR, this information should be included in the PSUR section 14 ("Late-breaking information"), if feasible.

If stipulated by applicable regional requirements, the marketing authorisation holder should provide, in the regional appendix, information on any final, ongoing and proposed changes to the national or local authorised product information (see VII.C.5.).

VII.B.5. Format and Contents of the PSUR

The PSUR shall be based on all available data and shall focus on new information which has emerged since the data lock point of the last PSUR [IR Art 34(1)]. Cumulative information should be taken into account when performing the overall safety evaluation and integrated benefit-risk assessment.

Because clinical development of a medicinal product frequently continues following marketing authorisation, relevant information from post-authorisation studies or clinical trials in unauthorised indications or populations should also be included in the PSUR. Similarly, as knowledge of the safety of a medicinal product may be derived from evaluation of other data associated with off-label use, such knowledge should be reflected in the risk evaluation where relevant and appropriate.

The PSUR shall provide summaries of data relevant to the benefits and risks of the medicinal product, including results of all studies with a consideration of their potential impact on the marketing authorisation [DIR Art 107b(1)(a)].

Examples of sources of efficacy, effectiveness and safety information that may be used in the preparation of PSURs include the following:
- Non-clinical studies;
- Spontaneous reports (e.g. on the marketing authorisation holder's safety database);
- Active surveillance systems (e.g. sentinel sites);
- Investigations of product quality;
- Product usage data and drug utilisation information;
- Clinical trials, including research in unauthorised indications or populations;
- Observational studies, including registries;
- Patient support programs;
- Systematic reviews and meta-analysis;
- Marketing authorisation holders sponsored websites;[5]
- Published scientific literature or reports from abstracts, including information presented at scientific meetings;
- Unpublished manuscripts;
- Licensing partners, other sponsors or academic institutions and research networks;
- Competent authorities (worldwide).

The above list is not intended to be all inclusive, and additional data sources may be used by the marketing authorisation holder to present safety, efficacy and effectiveness information in the PSUR and to evaluate the risk-benefit balance, as appropriate to the product and its known and emerging important benefits and risks. When desired by the marketing authorisation holder, a list of the sources of information used to prepare the PSUR can be provided as an appendix to the PSUR.

A PSUR shall be prepared following the full modular structure set out in Annex II of the IR [IR Art 35].

For the purposes of this Module, sources of information include data regarding the active substance(s) included in the medicinal product, or the medicinal product that the marketing authorisation holder may reasonably be expected to have access to and that are relevant to the evaluation of the safety, and/or risk-benefit balance. It is therefore recognised that while the same format (as defined in the IR) shall be followed for all products, the extent of the information provided may vary where justified according to what is accessible to the marketing authorisation holder. For example, for a marketing authorisation holder sponsored

---

5. ICH-E2D Post-Approval Safety Data Management: Definitions and Standards for Expedited Reporting.

clinical trial, there should be access to patient level data while for a clinical trial not sponsored by the marketing authorisation holder, only the published report may be accessible.

The level of detail provided in certain sections of the PSUR should depend on known or emerging important information on the medicinal product's benefits and risks. This approach is applicable to those sections of the PSUR in which there is evaluation of information about safety, efficacy, effectiveness, safety signals and risk-benefit balance.

When preparing the PSUR, the ICH-E2C(R2) guideline (see Annex IV ICH-E2C(R2)) on PBRER should also be applied. Guidance on the titles, order and content of the PSUR sections is provided in VII.B.5.1. to VII.B.5.21. When no relevant information is available for any of the sections, this should be stated.

- Part I: Title page including signature[6]
- Part II: Executive Summary
- Part III: Table of Contents

1. Introduction
2. Worldwide marketing authorisation status
3. Actions taken in the reporting interval for safety reasons
4. Changes to reference safety information
5. Estimated exposure and use patterns
   5.1. Cumulative subject exposure in clinical trials
   5.2. Cumulative and interval patient exposure from marketing experience
6. Data in summary tabulations
   6.1. Reference information
   6.2. Cumulative summary tabulations of serious adverse events from clinical trials
   6.3. Cumulative and interval summary tabulations from post-marketing data sources
7. Summaries of significant findings from clinical trials during the reporting interval
   7.1. Completed clinical trials
   7.2. Ongoing clinical trials
   7.3. Long-term follow-up
   7.4. Other therapeutic use of medicinal product
   7.5. New safety data related to fixed combination therapies
8. Findings from non-interventional studies
9. Information from other clinical trials and sources
   9.1. Other clinical trials
   9.2. Medication errors
10. Non-clinical data
11. Literature
12. Other periodic reports
13. Lack of efficacy in controlled clinical trials
14. Late-breaking information
15. Overview of signals: new, ongoing or closed
16. Signal and risk evaluation
    16.1. Summaries of safety concerns
    16.2. Signal evaluation
    16.3. Evaluation of risks and new information
    16.4. Characterisation of risks
    16.5. Effectiveness of risk minimisation (if applicable)
17. Benefit evaluation
    17.1. Important baseline efficacy and effectiveness information
    17.2. Newly identified information on efficacy and effectiveness
    17.3. Characterisation of benefits
18. Integrated benefit-risk analysis for authorised indications
    18.1. Benefit-risk context – Medical need and important alternatives
    18.2. Benefit-risk analysis evaluation
19. Conclusions and actions
20. Appendices to the PSUR

PSUR title page

The title page should include the name of the medicinal product(s)[7] and substance, international birth date (IBD) (the date of the first marketing authorisation for any product containing the active substance granted to any company in any country in the world), reporting interval, date of

---

6. For PSURs submission in the EU, it is at the discretion of the QPPV to determine the most appropriate person to sign the document according to the marketing authorisation holder structure and responsibilities. A statement confirming the designation by the QPPV should be included. No delegation letters should be submitted.
7. For PSURs covering multiple products, for practical reasons, this information may be provided in the PSUR Cover Page (See Annex II)

the report, marketing authorisation holder details and statement of confidentiality of the information included in the PSUR.

The title page shall also contain the signature.

PSUR executive summary

An executive summary should be placed immediately after the title page and before the table of contents. The purpose of the executive summary is to provide a concise summary of the content and the most important information in the PSUR and should contain the following information:
- Introduction and reporting interval;
- Medicinal product(s), therapeutic class(es), mechanism(s) of action, indication(s), pharmaceutical formulation(s), dose(s) and route(s) of administration;
- Estimated cumulative clinical trials exposure;
- Estimated interval and cumulative exposure from marketing experience;
- Number of countries in which the medicinal product is authorised;
- Summary of the overall benefit-risk analysis evaluation (based on sub-section 18.2 "benefit-risk analysis evaluation" of the PSUR);
- Actions taken and proposed for safety reasons, (e.g. significant changes to the reference product information, or other risk minimisation activities);
- Conclusions.

PSUR table of contents

The executive summary should be followed by the table of contents.

VII.B.5.1. PSUR Section "Introduction"

The marketing authorisation holder should briefly introduce the product(s) so that the PSUR "stands alone" but it is also placed in perspective relative to previous PSURs and circumstances. The introduction should contain the following information:
- IBD, and reporting interval;
- Medicinal product(s), therapeutic class(es), mechanism(s) of action, authorised indication(s), pharmaceutical form(s), dose(s) and route(s) of administration;
- A brief description of the population(s) being treated and studied;

VII.B.5.2. PSUR Section "Worldwide Marketing Authorisation Status"

This section of the PSUR should contain a brief narrative overview including: date of the first authorisation worldwide, indications(s), authorised dose(s), and where authorised.

VII.B.5.3. PSUR Section "Actions Taken in the Reporting Interval for Safety Reasons"

This section of the PSUR should include a description of significant actions related to safety that have been taken worldwide during the reporting interval, related to either investigational uses or marketing experience by the marketing authorisation holder, sponsors of clinical trial(s), data monitoring committees, ethics committees or competent authorities that had either:
- A significant influence on the risk-benefit balance of the authorised medicinal product; and/or
- An impact on the conduct of a specific clinical trial(s) or on the overall clinical development programme.

If known, the reason for each action should be provided and any additional relevant information should be included as appropriate. Relevant updates to previous actions should also be summarised in this section.

Examples of significant actions taken for safety reasons include:

Actions related to investigational uses:
- Refusal to authorise a clinical trial for ethical or safety reasons;
- Partial[8] or complete clinical trial suspension or early termination of an ongoing clinical trial because of safety findings or lack of efficacy;
- Recall of investigational drug or comparator;
- Failure to obtain marketing authorisation for a tested indication including voluntary withdrawal of a marketing authorisation application;
- Risk management activities, including:
  - Protocol modifications due to safety or efficacy concerns (e.g. dosage changes, changes in study inclusion/exclusion criteria, intensification of subject monitoring, limitation in trial duration);

- Restrictions in study population or indications;
- Changes to the informed consent document relating to safety concerns;
- Formulation changes;
- Addition by regulators of a special safety-related reporting requirement;
- Issuance of a communication to investigators or healthcare professionals; and
- Plans for new studies to address safety concerns.

Actions related to marketing experience:
- Failure to obtain or apply for a marketing authorisation renewal;
- Withdrawal or suspension of a marketing authorisation;
- Actions taken due to product defects and quality issues;
- Suspension of supply by the marketing authorisation holder;
- Risk management activities including:
  - Significant restrictions on distribution or introduction of other risk minimisation measures;
  - Significant safety-related changes in labelling documents including restrictions on use or population treated;
  - Communications to health care professionals; and
  - New post-marketing study requirement(s) imposed by competent authorities.

VII.B.5.4. PSUR Section "Changes to Reference Safety Information"

This PSUR section should list any significant changes made to the reference safety information within the reporting interval. Such changes might include information relating to contraindications, warnings, precautions, serious adverse drug reactions, interactions, important findings from ongoing or completed clinical trials and significant non-clinical findings (e.g. carcinogenicity studies). Specific information relevant to these changes should be provided in the appropriate sections of the PSUR.

VII.B.5.5. PSUR Section "Estimated Exposure and Use Patterns"

PSURs shall provide an accurate estimate of the population exposed to the medicinal product, including all data relating to the volume of sales and volume of prescriptions. This estimate of exposure shall be accompanied by a qualitative and quantitative analysis of actual use, which shall indicate, where appropriate, how actual use differs from the indicated use based on all data available to the marketing authorisation holder, including the results of observational or drug utilisation studies [IR Art 34 (2)].

This PSUR section should provide estimates of the size and nature of the population exposed to the medicinal product including a brief description of the method(s) used to estimate the subject/patient exposure and the limitations of that method.

Consistent methods for calculating subject/patient exposure should be used across PSURs for the same medicinal product. If a change in the method is appropriate, both methods and calculations should be provided in the PSUR introducing the change and any important difference between the results using the two methods should be highlighted.

VII.B.5.5.1. PSUR Sub-section "Cumulative Subject Exposure in Clinical Trials"

This section of the PSUR should contain the following information on the patients studied in clinical trials sponsored by the marketing authorisation holder, if applicable presented in tabular formats:
- Cumulative numbers of subjects from ongoing and completed clinical trials exposed to the investigational medicinal product, placebo, and/or active comparator(s) since the DIBD. It is recognised that for "old products", detailed data might not be available;
- More detailed cumulative subject exposure in clinical trials should be presented if available (e.g. sub-grouped by age, sex, and racial/ethnic group for the entire development programme);
- Important differences among trials in dose, routes of administration, or patient populations can be noted in the tables, if applicable, or separate tables can be considered;

---

8. "Partial suspension" might include several actions (e.g. suspension of repeat dose studies, but continuation of single dose studies; suspension of trials in one indication, but continuation in another, and/or suspension of a particular dosing regimen in a trial but continuation of other doses). ICH-E2C(R2) guideline (*see* Annex IV).

- If clinical trials have been or are being performed in special populations (e.g. pregnant women; patients with renal, hepatic, or cardiac impairment; or patients with relevant genetic polymorphisms), exposure data should be provided as appropriate;
- When there are substantial differences in time of exposure between subjects randomised to the investigational medicinal product or comparator(s), or disparities in length of exposure between clinical trials, it can be useful to express exposure in subject-time (subject-days, -months, or -years);
- Investigational drug exposure in healthy volunteers might be less relevant to the overall safety profile, depending on the type of adverse reaction, particularly when subjects are exposed to a single dose. Such data can be presented separately with an explanation as appropriate;
- If the serious adverse events from clinical trials are presented by indication in the summary tabulations, the patient exposure should also be presented by indication, where available;
- For individual trials of particular importance, demographic characteristics should be provided separately.

Examples of tabular format for the estimated exposure in clinical trials are presented in VII. Appendix 1, Tables VII.2, VII.3 and VII.4.

VII.B.5.5.2. PSUR Sub-section "Cumulative and Interval Patient Exposure from Marketing Experience"

Separate estimates should be provided for cumulative exposure (since the IBD), when possible, and interval exposure (since the data lock point of the previous PSUR). Although it is recognised that it is often difficult to obtain and validate exposure data, the number of patients exposed should be provided whenever possible, along with the method(s) used to determine the estimate. Justification should be provided if it is not possible to estimate the number of patients exposed. In this case, alternative estimates of exposure, if available, should be presented along with the method(s) used to derive them. Examples of alternative measures of exposure include patient-days of exposure and number of prescriptions. Only if such measures are not available, measures of drug sales, such as tonnage or dosage units, may be used. The concept of a defined daily dose may also be used to arrive at patient exposure estimates.

The data should be presented according to the following categories:

1. Post-authorisation (non-clinical trial) exposure: An overall estimation of patient exposure should be provided. In addition, the data should be routinely presented by sex, age, indication, dose, formulation and region, where applicable. Depending upon the product, other variables may be relevant, such as number of vaccination courses, route(s) of administration, and duration of treatment.

   When there are patterns of reports indicating a safety signal, exposure data within relevant subgroups should be presented, if possible.

2. Post-authorisation use in special populations: Where post-authorisation use has occurred in special populations, available information regarding cumulative patient numbers exposed and the method of calculation should be provided. Sources of such data may include for instance non-interventional studies designed to obtain this information, including registries. Other sources of information may include data collection outside a study environment including information collected through spontaneous reporting systems (e.g. information on reports of pregnancy exposure without an associated adverse event may be summarised in this section). Populations to be considered for discussion include, but might not be limited to:
   - Paediatric population;
   - Elderly population;
   - Pregnant or lactating women;
   - Patients with hepatic and/or renal impairment;
   - Patients with other relevant co-morbidity;
   - Patients with disease severity different from that studied in clinical trials;
   - Sub-populations carrying relevant genetic polymorphism(s);
   - Populations with specific racial and/or ethnic origins.

3. Other post-authorisation use:
   If the marketing authorisation holder becomes aware of a pattern of use of the medicinal product, which may be regional, considered relevant for the interpretation of safety data,

provide a brief description thereof. Examples of such patterns of use may include evidence of overdose, abuse, misuse and use beyond the recommendation(s) in the reference product information (e.g. an anti-epileptic drug used for neuropathic pain and/or prophylaxis of migraine headaches). Where relevant to the evaluation of safety and/or benefit-risk, information reported on patterns of use without reference to adverse reactions should be summarised in this section as applicable. Such information may be received via spontaneous reporting systems, medical information queries, customer's complaints, screening of digital media or via other information sources available to the marketing authorisation holder. If quantitative information on use is available, it should be provided.

If known, the marketing authorisation holder may briefly comment on whether other use beyond the recommendation(s) in the reference product information may be linked to clinical guidelines, clinical trial evidence, or an absence of authorised alternative treatments. For purposes of identifying patterns of use outside the terms of the reference product information, the marketing authorisation holder should use the appropriate sections of the reference product information that was in effect at the end of the reporting interval of the PSUR (e.g. authorised indication, route of administration, contraindications).

Signals or risks identified from any data or information source should be presented and evaluated in the relevant sections of the PSUR.

Examples of tabular format for the estimated exposure from marketing experience are presented in VII. Appendix 1, Tables VII.5 and VII.6.

VII.B.5.6. PSUR section "Data in Summary Tabulations"

The objective of this PSUR section is to present safety data through summary tabulations of serious adverse events from clinical trials, spontaneous serious and non-serious reactions from marketing experience (including reports from healthcare professionals, consumers, scientific literature, competent authorities (worldwide)) and serious reactions from non-interventional studies and other non-interventional solicited source. At the discretion of the marketing authorisation holder graphical displays can be used to illustrate specific aspects of the data when useful to enhance understanding.

When the Medical Dictionary for Regulatory Activities (MedDRA) terminology is used for coding the adverse event/reaction terms, the preferred term (PT) level and system organ class (SOC) should be presented in the summary tabulations.

The seriousness of the adverse events/reactions in the summary tabulations should correspond to the seriousness assigned to events/reactions included in the ICSRs using the criteria established in ICH-E2A[9] (see Annex IV). When serious and non-serious events/reactions are included in the same ICSR, the individual seriousness per reaction should be reflected in the summary tabulations. Seriousness should not be changed specifically for the preparation of the PSURs.

VII.B.5.6.1. PSUR Sub-section "Reference Information"

This sub-section of the PSUR should specify the version(s) of the coding dictionary used for presentation of adverse events/reactions.

VII.B.5.6.2. PSUR Sub-section "Cumulative Summary Tabulations of Serious Adverse Events from Clinical Trials"

This PSUR sub-section should provide background for the appendix that provides a cumulative summary tabulation of serious adverse events reported in the marketing authorisation holder's clinical trials, from the DIBD to the data lock point of the current PSUR. The marketing authorisation holder should explain any omission of data (e.g. clinical trial data might not be available for products marketed for many years). The tabulation(s) should be organised by MedDRA SOC (listed in the internationally agreed order), for the investigational drug, as well as for the comparator arm(s) (active comparators, placebo) used in the clinical development programme. Data can be integrated across the programme. Alternatively, when useful and feasible, data can be presented by

---

9 ICH Topic E2A. Clinical safety data management: Definitions and standards for expedited reporting.

trial, indication, route of administration or other variables.

This sub-section should not serve to provide analyses or conclusions based on the serious adverse events.

The following points should be considered:
- Causality assessment is generally useful for the evaluation of individual rare adverse drug reactions. Individual case causality assessment has less value in the analysis of aggregate data, where group comparisons of rates are possible. Therefore, the summary tabulations should include all serious adverse events and not just serious adverse reactions for the investigational drug, comparators and placebo. It may be useful to give rates by dose.
- In general, the tabulation(s) of serious adverse events from clinical trials should include only those terms that were used in defining the case as serious and non-serious events should be included in the study reports.
- The tabulations should include blinded and unblinded clinical trial data. Unblinded serious adverse events might originate from completed trials and individual cases that have been unblinded for safety-related reasons (e.g. expedited reporting), if applicable. Sponsors of clinical trials and marketing authorisation holders should not unblind data for the specific purpose of preparing the PSUR.
- Certain adverse events can be excluded from the clinical trials summary tabulations, but such exclusions should be explained in the report. For example, adverse events that have been defined in the protocol as "exempt" from special collection and entry into the safety database because they are anticipated in the patient population, and those that represent study endpoints, can be excluded (e.g. deaths reported in a trial of a drug for congestive heart failure where all-cause mortality is the primary efficacy endpoint, disease progression in cancer trials).

An example of summary tabulation of serious adverse events from clinical trials can be found in VII. Appendix 1 Table VII.7.

VII.B.5.6.3. PSUR Sub-section "Cumulative and Interval Summary Tabulations from Post-Marketing Data Sources"

This sub-section of the PSUR should provide background for the appendix that provides cumulative and interval summary tabulations of adverse reactions, from the IBD to the data lock point of the current PSUR. These adverse reactions are derived from spontaneous ICSRs including reports from healthcare professionals, consumers, scientific literature, competent authorities (worldwide) and from solicited non-interventional ICSRs including those from non-interventional studies.[10] Serious and non-serious reactions from spontaneous sources, as well as serious adverse reactions from non-interventional studies and other non-interventional solicited sources should be presented in a single table, with interval and cumulative data presented side-by-side. The table should be organised by MedDRA SOC (listed in the internationally agreed order). For special issues or concerns, additional tabulations of adverse reactions can be presented by indication, route of administration, or other variables.

As described in ICH-E2D[11] (see Annex IV) guideline, for marketed medicinal products, spontaneously reported adverse events usually imply at least a suspicion of causality by the reporter and should be considered to be suspected adverse reactions for regulatory reporting purposes.

Analysis or conclusions based on the summary tabulations should not be provided in this PSUR sub-section.

An example of summary tabulations of adverse drug reactions from post-marketing data sources can be found in VII. Appendix 1 Table VII.8.

VII.B.5.7. PSUR Section "Summaries of Significant Findings from Clinical Trials During the Reporting Interval"

This PSUR section should provide a summary of the clinically important emerging efficacy and safety findings obtained from the marketing authorisation holder's sponsored clinical trials during the reporting interval, from the sources specified in the sub-sections listed below. When possible

---

10. ICH-E2D Post-Approval Safety Data Management: Definitions and Standards for Expedited Reporting.
11. ICH-E2D Post-Approval Safety Data Management: Definitions and Standards for Expedited Reporting.

and relevant, data categorised by sex and age (particularly paediatrics versus adults), indication, dose, and region should be presented.

Signals arising from clinical trial sources should be tabulated in PSUR section 15 ("Overview on signals: new, ongoing or closed"). Evaluation of the signals, whether or not categorised as refuted signals or either potential or identified risk, that were closed during the reporting interval should be presented in PSUR section 16.2 ("Signal evaluation"). New information in relation to any previously known potential or identified risks and not considered to constitute a newly identified signal should be evaluated and characterised in PSUR sections 16.3 ("Evaluation of risks and new information") and 16.4 ("Characterisation of risks") respectively.

Findings from clinical trials not sponsored by the marketing authorisation holder should be described in the relevant sections of the PSUR.

When relevant to the benefit-risk evaluation, information on lack of efficacy from clinical trials for treatments of non-life-threatening diseases in authorised indications should also be summarised in this section. Information on lack of efficacy from clinical trials with products intended to treat or prevent serious or life-threatening illness should be summarised in section 13 ("Lack of efficacy in controlled clinical trials") (VII.B.5.13).

Information from other clinical trials/study sources should be included in the PSUR sub-section 9.1 ("other clinical trials") (VII.B.5.9.1).

In addition, the marketing authorisation holder should include an appendix listing the sponsored post-authorisation interventional trials with the primary aim of identifying, characterising, or quantifying a safety hazard or confirming the safety profile of the medicinal product that were completed or ongoing during the reporting interval. The listing should include the following information for each trial:
- Study ID (e.g. protocol number or other identifier);
- Study title (abbreviated study title, if applicable);
- Study type (e.g. randomised clinical trial, cohort study, case-control study);
- Population studied, including country and other relevant population descriptors (e.g. paediatric population or trial subjects with impaired renal function);
- Study start (as defined by the marketing authorisation holder) and projected completion dates;
- Status: ongoing (clinical trial has begun) or completed (clinical study report is finalised).

VII.B.5.7.1. PSUR sub-section "Completed Clinical Trials"

This sub-section of the PSUR should provide a brief summary of clinically important emerging efficacy and safety findings obtained from clinical trials completed during the reporting interval. This information can be presented in narrative format or as a synopsis.[12] It could include information that supports or refutes previously identified safety concerns as well as evidence of new safety signals.

VII.B.5.7.2. PSUR Sub-section "Ongoing Clinical trials"

If the marketing authorisation holder is aware of clinically important information that has arisen from ongoing clinical trials (e.g. learned through interim safety analyses or as a result of unblinding of subjects with adverse events), this sub-section should briefly summarise the concern(s). It could include information that supports or refutes previously identified safety concerns, as well as evidence of new safety signals.

VII.B.5.7.3. PSUR Sub-section "Long-term follow-up"

Where applicable, this sub-section should provide information from long-term follow-up of subjects from clinical trials of investigational drugs, particularly advanced therapy products (e.g. gene therapy, cell therapy products and tissue engineered products).

VII.B.5.7.4. PSUR Sub-section "Other Therapeutic Use of Medicinal Product"

This sub-section of the PSUR should include clinically important safety information from other programmes conducted by the marketing authorisation holder that follow a specific protocol,

---

12. Examples of synopses can be found in ICH-E3: Structure and Content of Clinical Study Reports and CIOMS VII (Council for International Organizations of Medical Sciences (CIOMS). Development Safety Update Report (DSUR): Harmonizing the Format and Content for Periodic Safety Reporting During Clinical Trials - Report of CIOMS Working Group VII). Geneva: CIOMS; 2006. http://www.cioms.ch/.
13. ICH-E2D Post-Approval Safety Data Management: Definitions and Standards for Expedited Reporting.

with solicited reporting as per ICH-E2D[13] (e.g. expanded access programmes, compassionate use programmes, particular patient use, and other organised data collection).

VII.B.5.7.5. PSUR Sub-section "New Safety Data Related to Fixed Combination Therapies"

Unless otherwise specified by national or regional regulatory requirements, the following options can be used to present data from combination therapies:
- If the active substance that is the subject of the PSURs is also authorised or under development as a component of a fixed combination product or a multi-drug regimen, this sub-section should summarise important safety findings from use of the combination therapy.
- If the product itself is a fixed combination product, this PSUR sub-section should summarise important safety information arising from the individual components whether authorised or under development.

The information specific to the combination can be incorporated into a separate section(s) of the PSUR for one or all of the individual components of the combination.

VII.B.5.8. PSUR Section "Findings from Non-interventional Studies"

This section should also summarise relevant safety information or information with potential impact in the benefit-risk assessment from marketing authorisation holder-sponsored non-interventional studies that became available during the reporting interval (e.g. observational studies, epidemiological studies, registries, and active surveillance programmes). This should include relevant information from drug utilisation studies when relevant to multiple regions.

The marketing authorisation holder should include an appendix listing marketing authorisation holder-sponsored non-interventional studies conducted with the primary aim of identifying, characterising or quantifying a safety hazard, confirming the safety profile of the medicinal product, or of measuring the effectiveness of risk management measures which were completed or ongoing during the reporting interval. (*see* VII.B.5.7. for the information that should be included in the listing).

Final study reports completed during the reporting interval for the studies mentioned in the paragraph above should also be included in the regional appendix of the PSUR (*see* VII.B.5.20. and VII.C.5.4.).

Summary information based on aggregate evaluation of data generated from patient support programs may be included in this section when not presented elsewhere in the PSUR. As for other information sources, the marketing authorisation holder should present signals or risks identified from such information in the relevant sections of the PSUR.

VII.B.5.9. PSUR Section "Information from other Clinical Trials and Sources"

VII.B.5.9.1. PSUR Sub-section "Other Clinical Trials"

This PSUR sub-section should summarise information relevant to the benefit-risk assessment of the medicinal product from other clinical trial/study sources which are accessible by the marketing authorisation holder during the reporting interval (e.g. results from pool analysis or meta-analysis of randomised clinical trials, safety information provided by co-development partners or from investigator-initiated trials).

VII.B.5.9.2. PSUR Sub-section "Medication Errors"

This sub-section should summarise relevant information on patterns of medication errors and potential medication errors, even when not associated with adverse outcomes. A potential medication error is the recognition of circumstances that could lead to a medication error, and may or may not involve a patient. Such information may be relevant to the interpretation of safety data or the overall benefit-risk evaluation of the medicinal product. A medication error may arise at any stage in the medication use process and may involve patients, consumers, or healthcare professionals.

VII.B.5.10. PSUR Section "Non-clinical Data"

This PSUR section should summarise major safety findings from non-clinical in vivo and in vitro studies (e.g. carcinogenicity, reproduction or immunotoxicity studies) ongoing or completed during the reporting interval. Results from studies designated to address specific safety concerns should be included in the PSUR, regardless of the outcome. Implications of these findings should be discussed in the relevant evaluation sections of the PSUR.

VII.B.5.11. PSUR Section "Literature"

This PSUR section should include a summary of new and significant safety findings, either published in the peer-reviewed scientific literature or made available as unpublished manuscripts that the marketing authorisation holder became aware of during the reporting interval, when relevant to the medicinal product.

Literature searches for PSURs should be wider than those for individual adverse reaction cases as they should also include studies reporting safety outcomes in groups of subjects and other products containing the same active substance.

The special types of safety information that should be included, but which may not be found by a search constructed specifically to identify individual cases, include:
- Pregnancy outcomes (including termination) with no adverse outcomes;
- Use in paediatric populations;
- Compassionate supply, named patient use;
- Lack of efficacy;
- Asymptomatic overdose, abuse or misuse;
- Medication error where no adverse events occurred;
- Important non-clinical safety results.

If relevant and applicable, information on other active substances of the same class should be considered.

The publication reference should be provided in the style of the Vancouver Convention[14,15].

VII.B.5.12. PSUR Section "Other Periodic Reports"

This PSUR section will only apply in certain circumstances concerning fixed combination products or products with multiple indications and/or formulations where multiple PSURs are prepared in agreement with the competent authority. In general, the marketing authorisation holder should prepare a single PSUR for a single active substance (unless otherwise specified by the competent authority); however if multiple PSURs are prepared for a single medicinal product, this section should also summarise significant findings from other PSURs if they are not presented elsewhere within the report.

When available, based on the contractual agreements, the marketing authorisation holder should summarise significant findings from periodic reports provided during the reporting interval by other parties (e.g. sponsors, other marketing authorisation holders or other contractual partners).

VII.B.5.13. PSUR Section "Lack of Efficacy in Controlled Clinical Trials"

This section should summarise data from clinical trials indicating lack of efficacy, or lack of efficacy relative to established therapy(ies), for products intended to treat or prevent serious or life-threatening illnesses (e.g. excess cardiovascular adverse events in a trial of a new anti-platelet medicine for acute coronary syndromes) that could reflect a significant risk to the treated population.

VII.B.5.14. PSUR Section "Late-breaking Information"

The marketing authorisation holder should summarise in this PSUR section the potentially important safety, efficacy and effectiveness findings that arise after the data lock point but during the period of preparation of the PSUR. Examples include clinically significant new publications, important follow-up data, clinically relevant toxicological findings and any action that the marketing authorisation holder, a data monitoring committee, or a competent authority (worldwide) has taken for safety reasons. New individual case

---

14. Uniform requirements for manuscripts submitted to biomedical journals. International Committee of Medical Journal Editors. N Engl J Med. 1997 Jan 23;336(4):309-15. Available online: http://www.nejm.org/doi/full/10.1056/NEJM199701233360422
15. Uniform Requirements for Manuscripts Submitted to Biomedical Journals: Writing and Editing for Biomedical Publication [Updated April 2010] Publication Ethics: Sponsorship, Authorship, and Accountability, International Committee of Medical Journal Editors. http://www.icmje.org/urm_full.pdf

reports should not be routinely included unless they are considered to constitute an important index case (i.e. the first instance of an important event) or an important safety signal or where they may add information to the evaluation of safety concerns already presented in the PSUR (e.g. a well documented case of aplastic anaemia in a medicinal product known to be associated with adverse effects on the bone marrow in the absence of possible alternative causes).

Any significant change proposed to the reference product information (e.g. new adverse reaction, warning or contraindication) which has occurred during this period, should also be included in this section of the PSUR (see VII.B.4.), where feasible.

The data presented in this section should also be taken into account in the evaluation of risks and new information (see VII.B.5.16.3.).

VII.B.5.15. PSUR Section "Overview of Signals: New, Ongoing, or Closed"

The general location for presentation of information on signals and risks within the PSUR is shown in figure VII.1 (see VII.B.5.21.). The purpose of this section is to provide a high level overview of signals[16] that were closed (i.e. evaluation was completed) during the reporting interval as well as ongoing signals that were undergoing evaluation at the end of the reporting interval. For the purposes of the PSUR, a signal should be included once it has undergone the initial screening or clarification step, and a determination made to conduct further evaluation by the marketing authorisation holder[17]. It should be noted that a safety signal is not synonymous with a statistic of disproportionate reporting for a specific medicine/event combination as a validation step is required. Signals may be qualitative (e.g., a pivotal individual case safety report, case series) or quantitative (e.g. a disproportionality score, findings of a clinical trial or epidemiological study). Signals may arise in the form of an information request or inquiry on a safety issue from a competent authority (worldwide) (see Module IX).

Decisions regarding the subsequent classification of these signals and the conclusions of the evaluation, involve medical judgement and scientific interpretation of available data, which is presented in section 16 ("Signal and risk evaluation") of the PSUR.

A new signal refers to a signal that has been identified during the reporting interval. Where new clinically significant information on a previously closed signal becomes available during the reporting interval of the PSUR, this would also be considered a new signal on the basis that a new aspect of a previously refuted signal or recognised risk warrants further action to verify. New signals may be classified as closed or ongoing, depending on the status of signal evaluation at the end of the reporting interval of the PSUR.

Examples of new signals would therefore include new information on a previously:

- Close and refuted signal, which would result in the signal being re-opened.
- Identified risk where the new information suggests a clinically significant difference in the severity or frequency of the risk (e.g. transient liver enzyme increases are identified risks and new information indicative of a more severe outcome such as hepatic failure is received, or neutropenia is an identified risk and a well documented case report of agranulocytosis with no presence of possible alternative causes is received).
- Identified risk for which a higher frequency or severity of the risk is newly found (e.g. in an indicated subpopulation).
- Potential risk which, if confirmed, would warrant a new warning, precaution, a new contraindication or restriction in indication(s) or population or other risk minimisation activities.

Within this section, or as an appendix the marketing authorisation holder should provide a tabulation of all signals ongoing or closed at the end of the reporting interval. This tabulation should include the following information:

- A brief description of the signal;
- Date when the marketing authorisation holder became aware of the signal;

---

16 "Signal" means information arising from one or multiple sources, including observations and experiments, which suggests a new potentially causal association, or a new aspect of a known association between an intervention and an event or set of related events, either adverse or beneficial, that is judged to be of sufficient likelihood to justify verificatory action [IR Art 19(1)].

17 In the EU-regulatory network and for the purpose of the PSUR, the term "signal" in this section corresponds with the term "validated signal" described in GVP Module IX.

- Status of the signal at the end of the reporting interval (close or ongoing);
- Date when the signal was closed, if applicable;
- Source of the signal;
- A brief summary of the key data;
- Plans for further evaluation; and
- Actions taken or planned.

An example of tabulation of signals can be found in VII. Appendix 2.

The detailed signal assessments for closed signals are not to be included in this section but instead should be presented in sub-section 16.2 ("Signal evaluation") of the PSUR.

Evaluation of new information in relation to any previously known identified and potential risks and not considered to constitute a new signal should be provided in PSUR sub-section 16.3 ("Evaluation of risks and new information").

When a competent authority (worldwide) has requested that a specific topic (not considered a signal) be monitored and reported in a PSUR, the marketing authorisation holder should summarise the result of the analysis in this section if it is negative. If the specific topic becomes a signal, it should be included in the signal tabulation and discussed in sub-section 16.2 ("Signal evaluation").

VII.B.5.16. PSUR Section "Signal and Risk Evaluation"

The purpose of this section of the PSUR is to provide:
- A succinct summary of what is known about important identified and potential risks and missing information at the beginning of the reporting interval covered by the report (VII.B.5.16.1.).
- An evaluation of all signals closed during the reporting interval (VII.B.5.16.2.).
- An evaluation of new information with respect to previously recognised identified and potential risks (VII.B.5.16.3).
- An updated characterisation of important potential and identified risks, where applicable (VII.B.5.16.4.).
- A summary of the effectiveness of risk minimisation activities in any country or region which may have utility in other countries or regions (VII.B.5.16.5.).

A flowchart illustrating the mapping of signals and risks to specific sections/sub-sections of the PSUR can be found in VII.B.5.21.

These evaluation sub-sections should not summarise or duplicate information presented in previous sections of the PSUR but should rather provide interpretation and critical appraisal of the information, with a view towards characterising the profile of those risks assessed as important. In addition, as a general rule, it is not necessary to include individual case narratives in the evaluation sections of the PSUR but where integral to the scientific analysis of a signal or risk, a clinical evaluation of pivotal or illustrative cases (e.g. the first case of suspected agranulocytosis with an active substance belonging to a class known to be associated with this adverse reaction) should be provided (*see* VII.B.3.).

VII.B.5.16.1. PSUR Sub-section "Summary of Safety Concerns"

The purpose of this sub-section is to provide a summary of important safety concerns at the beginning of the reporting interval, against which new information and evaluations can be made. For products with an existing safety specification, this section can be either the same as, or derived from the safety specification summary[18] that is current at the start of the reporting interval of the PSUR. It should provide the following safety information:
- Important identified risks;
- Important potential risks; and
- Missing information.

The following factors should be considered when determining the importance of each risk:
- Medical seriousness of the risk, including the impact on individual patients;
- Its frequency, predictability, preventability, and reversibility;
- Potential impact on public health (frequency; size of treated population); and
- Potential for avoidance of the use of a medicinal product with a preventive benefit due to a disproportionate public perception of risk (e.g. vaccines).

For products without an existing safety specification, this section should provide information on the important identified and

---

18 ICH-E2E – Pharmacovigilance planning (*see* Annex IV).

potential risks and missing information associated with use of the product, based on pre- and post-authorisation experience. Important identified and potential risks may include, for example:
- Important adverse reactions;
- Interactions with other medicinal products;
- Interactions with foods and other substances;
- Medication errors;
- Effects of occupational exposure; and
- Pharmacological class effects.

The summary on missing information should take into account whether there are critical gaps in knowledge for specific safety issues or populations that use the medicinal product.

VII.B.5.16.2. PSUR Sub-section "Signal Evaluation"

This sub-section of the PSUR should summarise the results of evaluations of all safety signals (whether or not classified as important) that were closed during the reporting interval. A safety signal can be closed either because it is refuted or because it is determined to be a potential or identified risk, following evaluation. The two main categories to be included in this sub-section are:
1. Those signals that, following evaluation, have been refuted as "false" signals based on medical judgement and scientific evaluation of the currently available information.
2. Those signals that, following evaluation, have been categorised as either a potential or identified risk, including lack of efficacy.

For both categories of closed signals, a concise description of each signal evaluation should be included in order to clearly describe the basis upon which the signal was either refuted or considered to be a potential or identified risk by the marketing authorisation holder.

It is recommended that the level of detail provided in the description of the signal evaluation should reflect the medical significance of the signal (e.g. severe, irreversible, lead to increased morbidity or mortality) and potential public health importance (e.g. wide usage, frequency, significant use outside the recommendations of the product information) and the extent of the available evidence. Where multiple evaluations will be included under both categories of closed signals, they can be presented in the following order:
- Closed and refuted signals.
- Closed signals that are categorised as important potential risks.
- Closed signals that are categorised as important identified risks.
- Closed signals that are potential risks not categorised as important.
- Closed signals that are identified risks not categorised as important.

Where applicable the evaluations of closed signals can be presented by indication or population.

The description(s) of the signal evaluations can be included in this sub-section of the PSUR or in an appendix. Each evaluation should include the following information as appropriate:
- Source or trigger of the signal;
- Background relevant to the evaluation;
- Method(s) of evaluation, including data sources, search criteria (where applicable, the specific MedDRA terms (e.g. PTs, HLTs, SOCs, etc.) or Standardised MedDRA Queries (SMQs) that were reviewed), and analytical approaches;
- Results - a summary and critical analysis of the data considered in the signal evaluation; where integral to the assessment, this may include a description of a case series or an individual case (e.g. an index case of well documented agranulocytosis or Stevens Johnson Syndrome);
- Discussion;
- Conclusion.

Marketing authorisation holder's evaluations and conclusions for refuted signals should be supported by data and clearly presented.

VII.B.5.16.3. PSUR Sub-section "Evaluation of Risks and New Information"

This sub-section should provide a critical appraisal of new information relevant to previously recognised risks that is not already included in sub-section 16.2 ("Signal evaluation").

New information that constitutes a signal with respect to a previously recognised risk or previously refuted signal should be presented in the signals tabulation (*see* VII.B.5.15.) and evaluated in sub-section 16.2 ("Signal evaluation"), if the signal is also closed during the reporting interval of the PSUR.

Updated information on a previously recognised risk that does not constitute a signal should be included in this sub-section. Examples includes information that confirms a potential risk as an identified risk, or information which allows any other further characterisation of a previously recognised risk.

New information can be organised as follows:
1. New information on important potential risks.
2. New information on important identified risks.
3. New information on other potential risks not categorised as important.
4. New information on other identified risks not categorised as important.
5. Update on missing information.

The focus of the evaluation(s) is on new information which has emerged during the reporting interval of the PSUR. This should be concise and interpret the impact, if any, on the understanding and characterisation of the risk. Where applicable, the evaluation will form the basis for an updated characterisation of important potential and identified risks in sub-section 16.4 ("Characterisation of risks") of the report. It is recommended that the level of detail of the evaluation included in this sub-section should be proportional to the available evidence on the risk and its medical significance and public health relevance.

The evaluation(s) of the new information and missing information update(s) can be included in this sub-section of the PSUR, or in an appendix. Each evaluation should include the following information as appropriate:
- Source of the new information;
- Background relevant to the evaluation;
- Method(s) of evaluation, including data sources, search criteria, and analytical approaches;
- Results – a summary and critical analysis of the data considered in the risk evaluation;
- Discussion;
- Conclusion, including whether or not the evaluation supports an update of the characterisation of any of the important potential and identified risks in sub-section 16.4 ("Characterisation of risks")

Any new information on populations exposed or data generated to address previously missing information should be critically assessed in this sub-section. Unresolved concerns and uncertainties should be acknowledged.

VII.B.5.16.4. PSUR Sub-section "Characterisation of Risks"

This sub-section should characterise important identified and potential risks based on cumulative data (i.e. not restricted to the reporting interval), and describe missing information.

Depending on the nature of the data source, the characterisation of risk may include, where applicable:
- Frequency;
- Numbers of cases (numerator) and precision of estimate, taking into account the source of the data;
- Extent of use (denominator) expressed as numbers of patients, patient-time, etc., and precision of estimate;
- Estimate of relative risk and precision of estimate;
- Estimate of absolute risk and precision of estimate;
- Impact on the individual patient (effects on symptoms, quality or quantity of life);
- Public health impact;
- Patient characteristics relevant to risk (e.g. patient factors (age, pregnancy/lactation, hepatic/renal impairment, relevant co-morbidity, disease severity, genetic polymorphism);
- Dose, route of administration;
- Duration of treatment, risk period;
- Preventability (i.e. predictability, ability to monitor for a "sentinel" adverse reaction or laboratory marker);
- Reversibility;
- Potential mechanism; and
- Strength of evidence and its uncertainties, including analysis of conflicting evidence, if applicable.

When missing information could constitute an important risk, it should be included as a safety concern. The limitations of the safety database (in terms of number of patients studied, cumulative exposure or long term use, etc.) should be discussed.

For PSURs for products with several indications, formulations, or routes of administration, where there may be significant differences in the identified and potential risks, it may be appropriate to present risks by indication, formulation, or route of

administration. Headings that could be considered include:
- Risks relating to the active substance;
- Risks related to a specific formulation or route of administration (including occupational exposure);
- Risks relating to a specific population; and
- Risks associated with non-prescription use (for compounds that are available as both prescription and non-prescription products).

VII.B.5.16.5. PSUR Sub-section: "Effectiveness of Risk Minimisation (if applicable)"

Risk minimisation activities are public health interventions intended to prevent the occurrence of an adverse drug reaction(s) associated with the exposure to a medicinal product or to reduce its severity should it occur. The aim of a risk minimisation activity is to reduce the probability or severity of an adverse drug reaction. Risk minimisation activities may consist of routine risk minimisation (e.g. product labelling) or additional risk minimisation activities (e.g. Direct Healthcare Professional Communication/Educational materials).

The PSUR shall contain the results of assessments of the effectiveness of risk minimisation activities relevant to the risk-benefit assessment [IR Art 34(3)].

Relevant information on the effectiveness and/or limitations of specific risk minimisation activities for important identified risks that has become available during the reporting interval should be summarised in this sub-section of the PSUR.

Insights into the effectiveness of risk minimisation activities in any country or region that may have utility in other countries or regions are of particular interest. Information may be summarised by region, if applicable and relevant.

When required for reporting in a PSUR, results of evaluations that became available during the reporting interval, which refer to an individual region should be provided in the PSUR regional appendix (*see* VII.B.5.20. and VII.C.5.5.).

VII.B.5.17. PSUR Section "Benefit Evaluation"

PSUR sub-sections 17.1 ("Important baseline efficacy and effectiveness information") and 17.2 ("Newly identified information on efficacy and effectiveness") provide the baseline and newly identified benefit information that support the characterisation of benefit described in sub-section 17.3 ("Characterisation of benefits") that in turn supports the benefit-risk evaluation in section 18 ("Integrated benefit-risk analysis for authorised indications").

VII.B.5.17.1. PSUR Sub-section "Important Baseline Efficacy and Effectiveness Information"

This sub-section of the PSUR summarises information on both efficacy and effectiveness of the medicinal product at the beginning of the reporting interval and provides the basis for the benefit evaluation. This information should relate to authorised indication(s) of the medicinal product listed in the reference product information (*See* VII.B.4.).

For medicinal products with multiple indications, populations, and/or routes of administration, the benefit should be characterised separately by these factors when relevant.

The level of detail provided in this sub-section should be sufficient to support the characterisation of benefit in the PSUR sub-section 17.3 ("Characterisation of benefits") and the benefit-risk assessment in section 18 ("Integrated benefit-risk analysis for authorised indications").

VII.B.5.17.2. PSUR Sub-section "Newly Identified Information on Efficacy and Effectiveness"

For some products, additional information on efficacy or effectiveness in authorised indications may have become available during the reporting interval. Such information should be presented in this sub-section of the PSUR. For authorised indications, new information on efficacy and effectiveness under conditions of actual use should also be described in this sub-section, if available. New information on efficacy and effectiveness in uses other than the authorised indications should not be included unless relevant for the benefit-risk evaluation in the authorised indications.

Information on indications newly authorised during the reporting interval should also be included in this sub-section. The level of detail provided in this section should be sufficient to support the characterisation of benefit in sub-section 17.3 ("Characterisation of benefits") and the benefit-risk assessment in section 18 ("Integrated benefit-risk analysis for authorised indications").

In this sub-section, particular attention should be given to vaccines, anti-infective agents or other medicinal products where changes in the therapeutic environment may impact on efficacy/effectiveness over time.

VII.B.5.17.3. PSUR Sub-section "Characterisation of Benefits"

This sub-section provides an integration of the baseline benefit information and the new benefit information that has become available during the reporting interval, for authorised indications.

The level of detail provided in this sub-section should be sufficient to support the analysis of benefit-risk in section 18 ("Integrated benefit-risk analysis for authorised indications").

When there are no new relevant benefit data, this sub-section should provide a characterisation of the information in sub-section 17.1 ("Important baseline efficacy and effectiveness information").

When there is new positive benefit information and no significant change in the risk profile in this reporting interval, the integration of baseline and new information in this sub-section should be succinct.

This sub-section should provide a concise but critical evaluation of the strengths and limitations of the evidence on efficacy and effectiveness, considering the following when available:

- A brief description of the strength of evidence of benefit, considering comparator(s), effect size, statistical rigor, methodological strengths and deficiencies, and consistency of findings across trials/studies;
- New information that challenges the validity of a surrogate endpoint, if used;
- Clinical relevance of the effect size;
- Generalisability of treatment response across the indicated patient population (e.g. information that demonstrates lack of treatment effect in a sub-population);
- Adequacy of characterization of dose-response;
- Duration of effect;
- Comparative efficacy; and
- A determination of the extent to which efficacy findings from clinical trials are generalisable to patient populations treated in medical practice.

VII.B.5.18. PSUR Section "Integrated Benefit-Risk Analysis for Authorised Indications"

The marketing authorisation holder should provide in this PSUR section an overall appraisal of the benefit and risk of the medicinal product as used in clinical practice. Whereas sub-sections 16.4 ("Characterisation of risks") and 17.3 ("Characterisation of benefits") present the risks and benefits, this section should provide a critical analysis and integration of the key information in the previous sections and should not simply duplicate the benefit and risk characterisation presented in the sub-sections mentioned above.

VII.B.5.18.1. PSUR Sub-section "Benefit-risk Context - Medical Need and Important Alternatives"

This sub-section of the PSUR should provide a brief description of the medical need for the medicinal product in the authorised indications and summarised alternatives (medical, surgical or other; including no treatment).

VII.B.5.18.2. PSUR Sub-section "Benefit-risk Analysis Evaluation"

A risk-benefit balance is specific to an indication and population. Therefore, for products authorised for more than one indication, risk-benefit balances should be evaluated and presented by each indication individually. If there are important differences in the risk-benefit balance among populations within an indication, the benefit-risk evaluation should be presented by population, if possible.

The benefit-risk evaluation should be presented and discussed in a way that facilitates the comparison of benefits and risks and should take into account the following points:

- Whereas previous sections/sub-sections should include all important benefit and risk information, not all benefits and risks contribute importantly to the overall benefit-risk evaluation, therefore, the key benefits and risks considered in the evaluation should be specified. The key information presented in the previous benefit and risk section/sub-sections should be carried forward for integration in the benefit-risk evaluation.

- Consider the context of use of the medicinal product: the condition to be treated, prevented, or diagnosed; its severity and seriousness; and the population to be treated (relatively healthy; chronic illness, rare conditions).
- With respect to the key benefit(s), consider its nature, clinical importance, duration, and generalisability, as well as evidence of efficacy in non-responders to other therapies and alternative treatments. Consider the effect size. If there are individual elements of benefit, consider all (e.g. for therapies for rheumatoid arthritis: reduction of symptoms and inhibition of radiographic progression of joint damage).
- With respect to risk, consider its clinical importance, (e.g. nature of toxicity, seriousness, frequency, predictability, preventability, reversibility, impact on patients), and whether it arose from clinical trials in unauthorised indications or populations, off-label use, or misuse.
- The strengths, weaknesses, and uncertainties of the evidence should be considered when formulating the benefit-risk evaluation. Describe how uncertainties in the benefits and risks impact the evaluation. Limitations of the assessment should be discussed.

Provide a clear explanation of the methodology and reasoning used to develop the benefit-risk evaluation:

- The assumptions, considerations, and judgement or weighting that support the conclusions of the benefit-risk evaluation should be clear.
- If a formal quantitative or semi-quantitative assessment of benefit-risk is provided, a summary of the methods should be included.
- Economic considerations (e.g. cost-effectiveness) should not be considered in the benefit-risk evaluation.

When there is important new information or an ad hoc PSUR has been requested, a detailed benefit-risk analysis should be presented based on cumulative data. Conversely, where little new information has become available during the reporting interval, the primary focus of the benefit-risk evaluation might consist of an evaluation of updated interval safety data.

VII.B.5.19. PSUR Section "Conclusions and Actions"

A PSUR should conclude with the implications of any new information that arose during the reporting interval in terms of the overall evaluation of benefit-risk for each authorised indication, as well as for relevant subgroups, if appropriate.

Based on the evaluation of the cumulative safety data and the benefit-risk analysis, the marketing authorisation holder should assess the need for changes to the reference product information and propose changes as appropriate.

In addition and as applicable, the conclusions should include preliminary proposal(s) to optimise or further evaluate the risk-benefit balance for further discussion with the relevant competent authority(ies). This may include proposals for additional risk minimisation activities.

For products with a pharmacovigilance or risk management plan, the proposals should also be considered for incorporation into the pharmacovigilance plan and/or risk minimisation plan, as appropriate (*see* Module V).

Based on the evaluation of the cumulative safety data and the risk-benefit analysis, the marketing authorisation holder shall draw conclusions in the PSUR as to the need for changes and/or actions, including implications for the approved summary of product characteristics (SmPC) for the product(s) for which the PSUR is submitted [IR Art 34(5)].

Proposed changes to the reference product information should be described in this section of the PSUR. The regional appendix should include proposals for product information (SmPC and package leaflet) together with information on ongoing changes when applicable.

VII.B.5.20. Appendices to the PSUR

A PSUR should contain the following appendices as appropriate, numbered as follows:
1. Reference information (*see* VII.B.4.).
2. Cumulative summary tabulations of serious adverse events from clinical trials; and cumulative and interval summary tabulations of serious and non-serious adverse reactions from post-marketing data sources.

3. Tabular summary of safety signals (if not included in the body of the report)[19].
4. Listing of all the marketing authorisation holder-sponsored interventional and non-interventional studies with the primary aim of identifying, characterising, or quantifying a safety hazard or confirming the safety profile of the medicinal product, or of measuring the effectiveness of risk management measures, in case of non-interventional studies.
5. List of the sources of information used to prepare the PSUR (when desired by the marketing authorisation holder).
6. Regional appendix:

The requirements for the regional appendix in the EU are provided in section VII.C.5.

VII.B.5.21. Mapping Signals and Risks to PSUR Sections/Sub-sections

The following flowchart (Figure VII.1) reflects the general location for the presentation of information on signals and risks within the PSUR.

VII.B.6. Quality Systems for PSURs at the Level of Marketing Authorisation Holders

Marketing authorisation holders should have in place structures and processes for the preparation, quality control, review and submission of PSURs including follow-up during and after their assessment. These structures and processes should be described by means of written policies and procedures in the marketing authorisation holder's quality system (*see* Module I).

There are a number of areas in the pharmacovigilance process that can directly impact the quality of PSURs, some examples are case management of spontaneous and study reports, literature screening, signal management, additional pharmacovigilance and post-marketing research activities, procedures for integration of information on benefits and risks from all available data sources and maintenance of product information. The quality system should describe the links between the processes, the communication channels and the responsibilities with the aim of gathering all the relevant information for the production of PSURs. There should be documented procedures including quality control checks in place to check the accuracy and completeness of the data presented in the PSURs. In ensuring completeness of data, a documented template or plan for drawing data from various data sources could be developed. The importance of an integrated approach to benefit-risk evaluation should underpin processes and cross departmental input to PSUR preparation.

The PSUR should also contain the assessment of specific safety issues requested by competent authorities in accordance with agreed timelines and procedures. The marketing authorisation holder should have mechanisms in place to ensure that the requests made by competent authorities during the time of their PSUR assessment are properly addressed.

The provision of the data included in the summary tabulations (*see* VII.B.5.6.) should undergo source data verification against the marketing authorisation holder's safety database to ensure accuracy of the number of events/reactions provided. The process for querying the safety database, the parameters used for the retrieval of the data and the quality control performed should be properly documented.

An appropriate quality system should be in place in order to avoid failure to comply with PSUR requirements such as:
- Non-submission: complete non-submission of PSURs, submission outside the correct submission schedule or outside the correct time frames (without previous agreement with the competent authorities);
- Unjustified omission of information required by VII.B.5.;
- Poor quality reports: poor documentation or insufficient information or evaluation provided to perform a thorough assessment of the new safety information, signals, risk evaluation, benefit evaluation and integrated benefit-risk analysis, misuse not highlighted, absence of use of standardised medical terminology (e.g. MedDRA) and inappropriate dismissal of cases with no reported risk factors in cumulative reviews;

---

19. It is preferred to include the tabulation of signals in the body of the PSUR, if feasible.

Annexure 8: Guideline on Good Pharmacovigilance Practices (GVP)

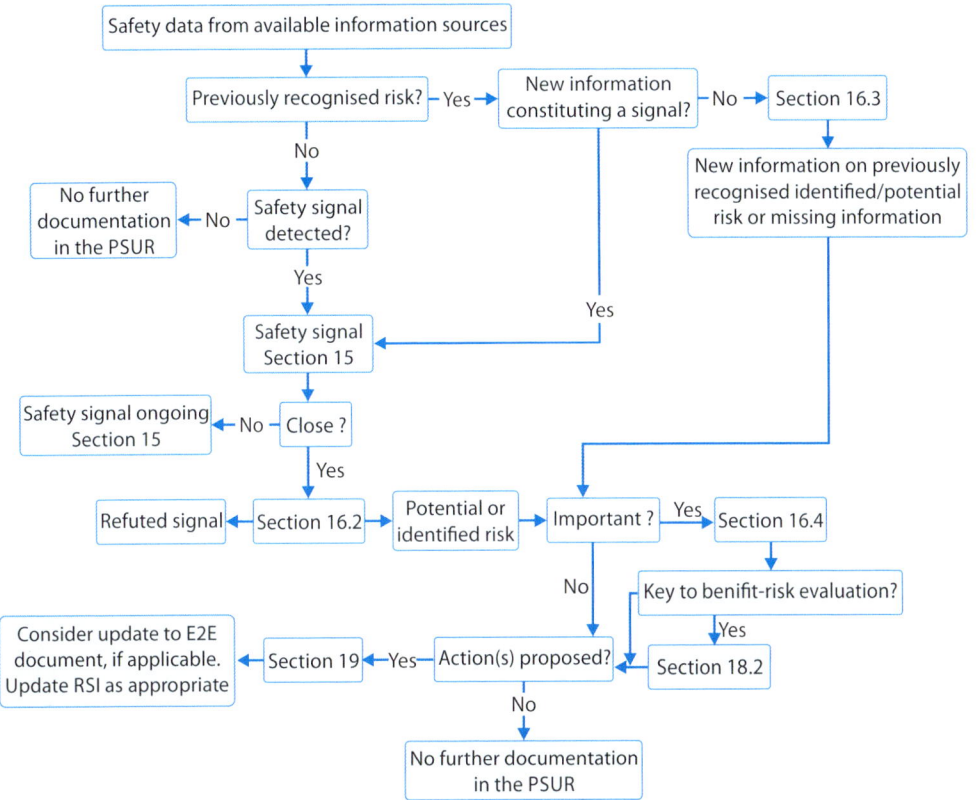

FIG. VII.1: PSUR sections/subsections – signals and risks.

- Submission of a PSUR where previous requests from competent authorities have not been addressed;
- Failure to provide an explicit evaluation of the risk-benefit balance of the medicinal product;
- Failure to provide adequate proposals for the local authorised product information.

Any significant deviation from the procedures relating to the preparation or submission of PSURs should be documented and the appropriate corrective and preventive action should be taken. This documentation should be available at all times.

When marketing authorisation holders are involved in contractual arrangements (e.g. licensor-licensee), respective responsibilities for preparation and submission of the PSUR to the competent authorities should be clearly specified in the written agreement.

When the preparation of the PSUR is delegated to third parties, the marketing authorisation holder should ensure that they are subject to a quality system compliant with the current legislation. Explicit procedures and detailed agreements should exist between the marketing authorisation holder and third parties. The agreements may specifically detail the options to audit the PSUR preparation process.

VII.B.7. Training of Staff Members Related to the PSUR Process

For all organisations, it is the responsibility of the person responsible for the pharmacovigilance system to ensure that the personnel, including pharmacovigilance, medical and quality personnel involved in the preparation, review, quality control, submission and assessment of PSURs are adequately qualified, experienced and trained according to the applicable guidelines (e.g. ICH E2C(R2) and this GVP Module VII). When appropriate, specific training for the different processes, tasks and responsibilities relating to the PSUR should be in place.

Training to update knowledge and skills should also take place as necessary.

Training should cover legislation, guidelines, scientific evaluation and written procedures related to the PSUR process. Training records should demonstrate that the relevant training was delivered prior to performing PSUR-related activities.

VII.C. OPERATION OF THE EU NETWORK

VII.C.1. PSUR Process in the EU - General Process

The following flowchart (Figure VII.2.) reflects the general process cycle for the PSUR procedure at the EU level when recommendations by the PRAC are issued. This represents a high level cycle to outline the entire process, from the preparation of the report to the implementation of the European Commission decision/national actions when applicable. Different single steps in this flowchart are formed by intermediate steps further explained and developed in different sections in this Module.

VII.C.2. Standard Submission Schedule of PSURs

Marketing authorisation holders for products authorised before 02 July 2012 (centrally authorised products) and 21 July 2012 (nationally authorised products) and for which the frequency and dates of submission of PSURs are not laid down as a condition to the marketing authorisation or determined otherwise in the list of Union reference dates, shall submit PSURs according to the following submission schedule [REG 28(2), DIR Art 107c(2)].
- At 6 months intervals once the product is authorised, even if it is not marketed;
- Once a product is marketed, 6 monthly PSUR submission should be continued following initial placing on the market in the EU for 2 years, then once a year for the following 2 years and thereafter at 3-yearly intervals.

VII.C.3. List of European Union Reference Dates and Frequency of Submission of PSURs[20]

VII.C.3.1. Objectives of the EU Reference Dates List

The Agency shall make public a list of Union reference dates (hereinafter referred to as list of EU reference dates) and frequency of submission of PSURs by means of the European medicines web-portal [DIR Art 107c(7), REG Art 26(1)(g)].

The objectives of the list of EU reference dates and frequency of submission of PSURs are:
- Harmonisation of data lock point and frequency of submission of PSURs for the same active substance and combination of active substances:
For medicinal products containing the same active substance or combination of active substances subject to different marketing authorisations, an EU reference date should be set up and the frequency and date of submission of PSURs harmonised in order to allow the preparation of a single assessment established in DIR Art 107e(1). Such information should be included in the list published by the Agency.
- Optimisation of the management of PSURs and PSURs assessments within the EU:
The list overrules the submission schedule described in DIR Art 107c(2)(b).
For active substances or combinations of active substances included in the list, marketing authorisation holders shall vary, if applicable, the condition laid down in their marketing authorisations in order to allow the submission of PSURs in accordance to the frequency and submission date as indicated in the list [DIR 107c(4) to (7)].
The periodicity is defined on the basis of a risk-based approach in order to prioritise the periodic re-evaluation of the risk-benefit balance of active substances in a way that best

---

20 The initial EU reference dates list was adopted by the CHMP/CMDh following consultation of the PRAC in September 2012 and was published on 01 October 2012.

Annexure 8: Guideline on Good Pharmacovigilance Practices (GVP)

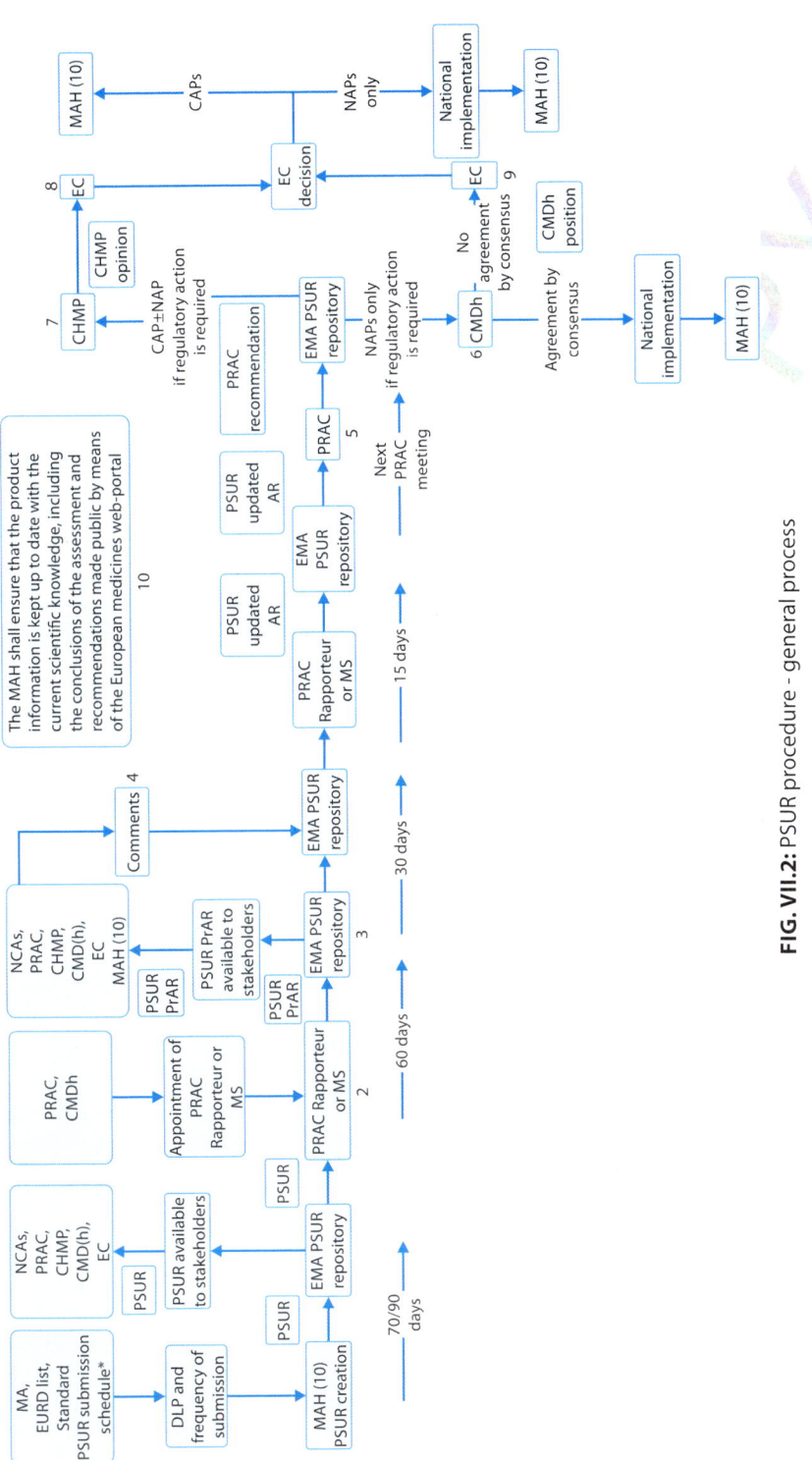

FIG. VII.2: PSUR procedure - general process

protects public health [Directive 2010/84/EU Preamble Recital 23].
- Single EU assessment and reassessment of the risk-benefit balance of an active substance based on all available safety data:

The list enables the harmonisation of PSUR submissions for medicinal products containing the same active substance or the same combination of active substances.

A single EU PSUR assessment provides a mechanism for evaluating the totality of available data on the benefits and risks of an active substance or combination of active substances. The effective application of work sharing principles is important in avoiding duplication of efforts and in prioritising the use of limited resources in the best interests of European citizens.

VII.C.3.2. Description of the EU Reference Dates List

The Union reference date of medicinal products containing the same active substance or the same combination of active substances shall be [DIR Art 107c(5)]:
- The date of the first marketing authorisation in the EU of a medicinal product containing that active substance or that combination of active substances; or
- If the date of first marketing authorisation cannot be ascertained, the earliest of the known dates of the marketing authorisations for a medicinal product containing that active substance or that combination of active substances.

The list of EU reference dates and frequency of submission of PSURs consists of a comprehensive list of substances and combinations of active substances in alphabetical order, for which PSURs, where required, shall be submitted in accordance with the EU reference date and the frequency as determined by the Committee for Medicinal Products for Human Use (CHMP) and the Coordination Group for Mutual Recognition and Decentralised Procedures - Human (CMDh) following consultation with the Pharmacovigilance Risk Assessment Committee (PRAC) [DIR Art 107c(4) and (6)]. The list should be updated in line with the "list of all medicinal products for human use authorised in the Union" as referred to in REG Art 57(1)(b).

The EU reference dates list should contain the following information:
- The EU reference dates;
- The frequencies of submission of PSURs;
- The data lock points of the next submissions of PSURs;
- The date of publication (on the European Medicines web-portal) of the frequency for PSURs submission and data lock point for each active substance and combination of active substances. Any change to the dates of submission and frequency on PSURs specified in the marketing authorisation shall take effect 6 months after the date of such publication [DIR Art 107c(7)].

Where specificity is deemed necessary, the list should include the scope of the PSUR and related EU single assessment procedure (*see* VII.C.3.3.) such as:
- Whether or not it should cover all the indications of the substance or combination of active substances;
- Whether or not it should cover all the formulations/routes of administration of the products containing a substance or combination of active substances;
- Whether generic, well-established use, traditional herbal and homeopathic medicinal products shall submit a PSUR due to a request from a competent authority or due to concerns relating to pharmacovigilance data or due to the lack of PSURs relating to an active substance after the marketing authorisation has been granted [DIR Art 107c(2) second subparagraph] (*see* VII.C.3.3.2.).

VII.C.3.3. Application of the List of EU Reference Dates to Submission of PSURs

Figure VII.3 presents the various potential scenarios for the submission of a PSUR as a general requirement.

VII.C.3.3.1. Submission of PSURs for Medicinal Products: General Requirement
The data lock points included in the list of EU references dates enable the synchronisation of PSURs submission for products subject to different

marketing authorisations and permit the EU single assessment. These data lock points are fixed on a certain date of the month, and should be used to determine the submission date (which has legal status) of the PSUR. Marketing authorisation holders can request to amend those dates in accordance with section VII.C.3.5.2.

Unless otherwise specified in the list of EU reference dates and frequency of submission, or agreed with competent authorities in Member States or the Agency, as appropriate, a single PSUR shall be prepared for all medicinal products containing the same active substance and authorised for one marketing authorisation holder. The PSUR shall cover all indications, routes of administration, dosage forms and dosing regimens, irrespective of whether authorised under different names and through separate procedures. Where relevant, data relating to a particular indication, dosage form, route of administration or dosing regimen shall be presented in a separate section of the PSUR and any safety concerns shall be addressed accordingly [IR Art 34(6)].

For medicinal products containing an active substance or a combination of active substances not included in the EU reference dates list, PSURs shall be submitted according to the PSUR frequency defined in the marketing authorisation or if not specified, in accordance with the submission schedule specified in DIR Art 107c(2) and REG Art 28(2).

VII.C.3.3.2. Submission of PSURs for Generic, Well-established Use, Traditional Herbal and Homeopathic Medicinal Products

By way of derogation, generics (authorised under DIR Art 10(1)), well-established use (authorised under DIR Art 10a), homeopathic (authorised under DIR Art 14) and traditional herbal (authorised under DIR Art 16a) medicinal products are exempted from submitting PSURs except in the following circumstances [DIR Art 107b(3)]:

- The marketing authorisation provides for the submission of PSURs as a condition;
- PSURs is (are) requested by a competent authority in a Member State on the basis of concerns relating to pharmacovigilance data or due to the lack of PSURs relating to an active substance after the marketing authorisation has been granted (e.g. when the "reference" medicinal product is no longer marketed). The assessment reports of the requested PSURs shall be communicated to the PRAC, which shall consider whether there is a need for a single assessment report for all marketing authorisations for medicinal products containing the same active substance and

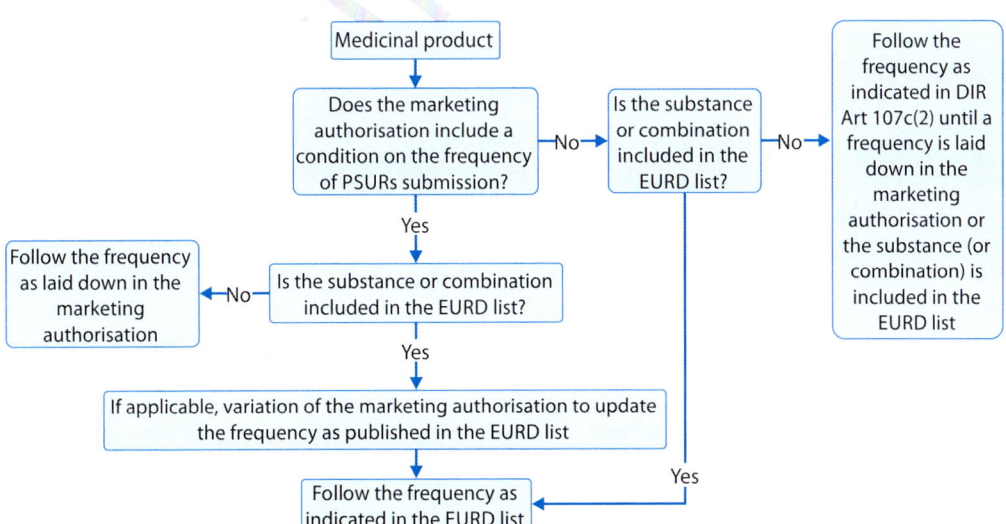

FIG. VII.3: Conditions for PSURs submission as general requirement.

inform the CMDh or CHMP accordingly, in order to apply the procedures laid down in DIR Art 107c(4) and 107e.

In order to facilitate and optimise the PSUR EU single assessment process, to avoid duplications of requests for PSURs and to provide transparency and predictability for the marketing authorisation holders, the legislative provision laid down in DIR 107b(3)(b) is applied by specifying in the list of EU reference dates, the substances for which PSURs for generic, well-established use, traditional herbal and homeopathic medicinal products are required. This specification is based on the request made by a competent authority in a Member State during the creation or maintenance of the list of EU reference dates and on the basis of concerns relating to pharmacovigilance data or due to the lack of PSURs relating to an active substance.

The harmonised frequency for the submission of the reports and the EU reference dates are determined by the CHMP and/or CMDh after consultation of the PRAC.

The application of the list of EU reference dates for the submission of PSURs for generic, well-established use, traditional herbal and homeopathic medicinal products does not undermine the right of a competent authority in a Member State to request the submission of PSURs at any time under the provision laid down in [DIR Art 107c(2) second subparagraph].

For products where PSURs are no longer required to be submitted routinely, it is expected that marketing authorisation holders will continue to evaluate the safety of their products on a regular basis and report any new safety information that impacts on the risk-benefit balance or the product information (*See* Module VI and Module IX).

Figure VII.4 presents the various potential scenarios as regard the submission of a PSUR for generic, well-established use, traditional herbal and homeopathic medicinal products.

VII.C.3.3.3. Submission of PSURs for Fixed Dose Combination Products

Unless otherwise specified in the list of EU reference dates and frequency of submission, if the substance that is the subject of the PSUR is also authorised as a component of a fixed combination medicinal product, the marketing authorisation holder shall either submit a separate PSUR for the combination of active substances authorised for the same marketing authorisation holder with cross-references to the single-substance PSUR(s), or provide the combination data within one of the single-substance PSURs [IR Art 34(7)].

VII.C.3.3.4. Submission of PSURs on Demand of a Competent Authority in a Member State

Marketing authorisation holders shall submit PSURs immediately upon request from a competent authority in a Member State [DIR Art 107c(2)]. To facilitate the EU assessment and avoid duplication of requests, the competent authorities in the Member States should normally make use of the list of EU reference dates to request the submission of PSURs, however in especial circumstances competent authorities in Member States can directly request the submission of a PSUR. When the timeline for submission has not been specified in the request, marketing authorisation holders should submit the PSUR within 90 calendar days of the data lock point.

VII.C.3.4. Criteria Used for Defining the Frequency of Submission of PSURs

When deviating from the PSUR submission schedule defined in DIR Art 107c(2)(b), the frequencies of submission of PSURs and the corresponding data lock points should be defined on a risk-based approach by the CHMP where at least one of the marketing authorisations concerned has been granted in accordance with the centralised procedure or by the CMDh otherwise, after consultation with the PRAC.

The following prioritisation criteria should be taken into account when defining the frequency of submission for a given active substance or combination of active substances:
- Information on risks or benefits that may have an impact on the public health;
- New product for which there is limited safety information available to date (includes pre- and post-authorisation experiences);
- Significant changes to the product (e.g. new indication has been authorised, new pharmaceutical form or route of administration broadening the exposed patient population);
- Vulnerable patient populations/poorly studied patient populations, missing information

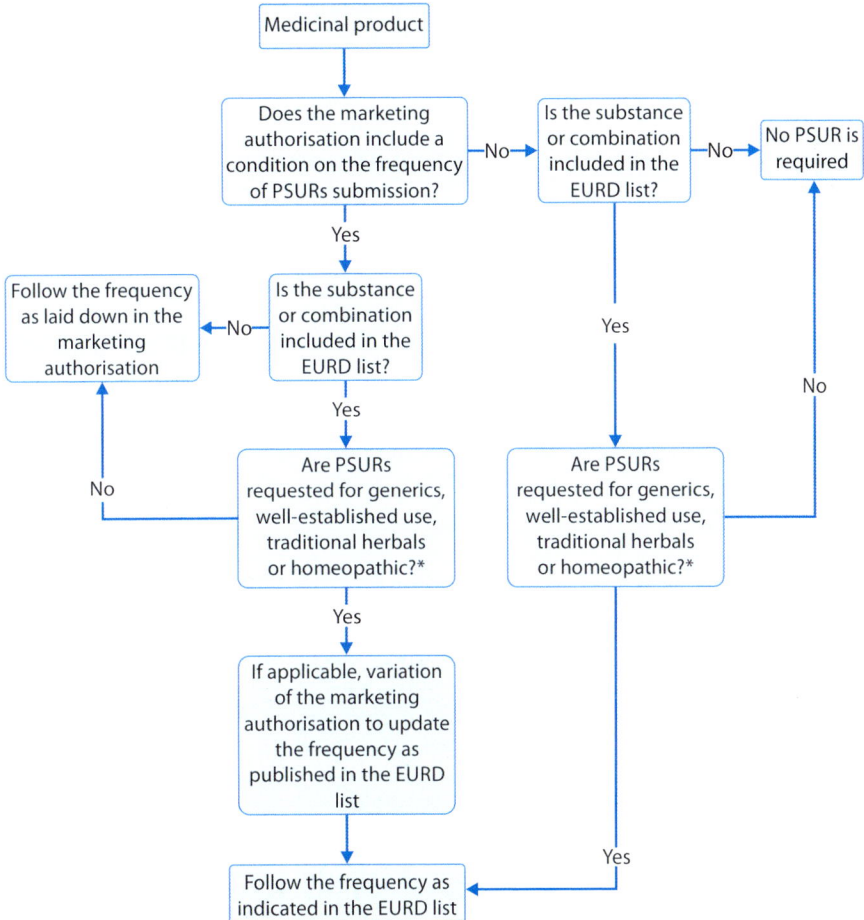

*Whether marketing authorisation holders for generics, well-established use, traditional herbal and homeopathic medicinal products are requested to submit PSURs following a request of a competent authority in a Member State due to concerns relating to pharmacovigilance data or lack of PSUR submission.

FIG. VII.4: Conditions for PSURs submission for generic, well-established use, traditional herbal and homeopathic medicinal products.

(e.g. children, pregnant women) while these populations are likely to be exposed in the post-authorisation setting;
- Signal of/potential for misuse, medication error, risk of overdose or dependency;
- The size of the safety database and exposure to the medicinal product;
- Medicinal products subjected to additional monitoring.

Any change in the criteria listed above for a given active substance or combination of active substances may lead to an amendment of the list of EU reference dates (e.g. increase of the frequency for PSUR submission).

VII.C.3.5. Maintenance of the List of EU Reference Dates

VII.C.3.5.1. General Principles
The maintenance of the list of EU reference dates should facilitate regulatory responsiveness to public health concerns identified within the EU

and therefore the list will be subject to changes to reflect the decisions taken (e.g. by the Agency's committees following signal detection).

The information included in the list such as the active substances and combinations of active substances, the frequencies of submission of PSURs and data lock points may need to be updated when considered necessary by the CHMP or CMDh after consultation with the PRAC. Changes to the list may be applied on one of the following grounds:

- Emergence of new information that might have an impact on the risk-benefit balance of the active substances or combinations of active substances, and potentially on public health;
- Any change in the criteria used for the allocation of frequency for PSUR submission and defined under VII.C.3.4.;
- A request from the marketing authorisation holders as defined under DIR Art 107c(6);
- Active substance newly authorised.

Figure VII.5. provides a general overview of the maintenance of the list of EU reference dates and frequency of submission of PSURs:

VII.C.3.5.2. Requests from Marketing Authorisation Holders to Amend the List of EU Reference Dates

Marketing authorisation holders shall be allowed to submit a request to the CHMP or the CMDh, as appropriate, to determine the Union reference dates or to change the frequency of submission of PSURs on one of the following grounds [DIR Art 107c(6)]:

- For reasons relating to public health;
- In order to avoid a duplication of the assessment;
- In order to achieve international harmonisation.

The request and its grounds should be considered by the PRAC and the CHMP if it concerns at least one marketing authorisation granted in accordance with the centralised procedure or the CMDh otherwise, which will either approve or deny the request.

The list will then be amended accordingly when appropriate and published on the European medicines web-portal (*see* section VII.C.3.6.).

For details about how to submit requests for amendments to the list, refer to the EU reference dates cover note and the related template published on the European medicines web-portal.[21]

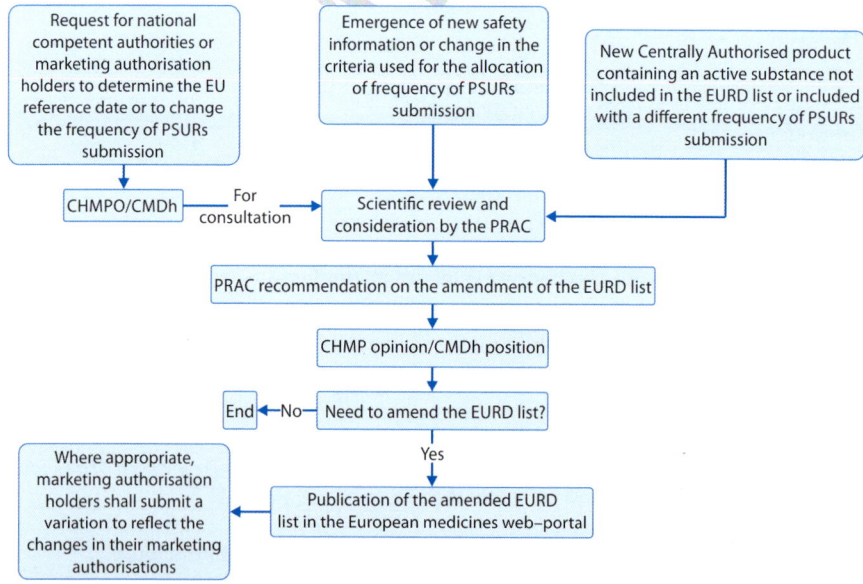

FIG. VII.5: Maintenance of the list of EU reference dates and frequency of submission of PSURs.

---

21. http://www.emea.europa.eu

VII.C.3.6. Publication of the List

Upon its establishment and adoption by the CHMP and CMDh following PRAC consultation, the list of EU reference dates and frequency of submission of PSURs is published on the European medicines web-portal.

In case of amendments, the updated list should be published following its adoption by the CHMP or the CMDh. It is expected to be updated monthly.

VII.C.3.7. Amendment of the Marketing Authorisation According to the List of EU Reference Dates

Any changes to the dates and frequencies of submission of PSURs specified in the list take effect six months after the date of the publication on the European medicines web-portal. Where appropriate, marketing authorisation holders shall submit the relevant variation in order to reflect the changes in their marketing authorisation [DIR 107c(6)], unless the marketing authorisation contains a direct cross reference to the list of EU references dates.

VII.C.4. Processes for PSUR Assessment in the EU Network

The competent authorities in the Member States shall assess PSURs to determine whether there are new risks or whether risks have changed or whether there are changes to the risk-benefit balance of the medicinal product [DIR Art 107d].

For purely nationally authorised medicinal products authorised in one Member State, the assessment of PSURs is conducted by the competent authority in the Member State where the product is authorised (*see* VII.C.4.1.).

For medicinal products authorised in more than one Member State, containing the same active substance or the same combination of active substances whether or not held by the same marketing authorisation holders and for which the frequency and dates of submission of PSURs have been harmonised in the list of EU reference dates, an EU single assessment of all PSURs is conducted with recommendation from the PRAC in accordance with the procedure described in VII.C.4.2.1. and VII.C.4.2.2.

Further to assessment of the PSUR and opinion from the CHMP or position from the CMDh, as applicable, following the recommendation from the PRAC, the competent authorities in Member States, or the European Commission for centrally authorised products, shall take the necessary measures to vary, suspend or revoke the marketing authorisation(s), in accordance with outcome of the assessment [DIR Art 107g(2)] [REG Art 28(4) and (5)] (*see* VII.C.4.2.3. and VII.C.4.2.4.).

The outcome of the PSUR assessment results in a legally binding decision or position in case of any action to vary, suspend, revoke the marketing authorisations of the medicinal products containing the concerned active substance or combination of active substances, on the basis of the position of the CMDh or the opinion of the CHMP following the recommendations from the PRAC. Furthermore, marketing authorisation holders are reminded of their obligation to keep their marketing authorisation up to date in accordance with REG Art 16(3) and DIR Art 23(3). The recommendations are therefore implemented in a harmonised and timely manner for all products within the scope of the procedure across the EU.

Amendments to the SmPC, package leaflet and labelling as a result of the PSUR assessment should be implemented without subsequent variation submission for centrally authorised products and through the appropriate variation for nationally authorised products, including those authorised through the mutual recognition and decentralised procedures.

When the proposals for the product information include new adverse reactions in section 4.8 ("Undesirable effects") of the SmPC, or modifications in the description, frequency and severity of the existing reactions, marketing authorisation holders should provide in the relevant sections of the PSUR appropriate information to allow the adequate description and classification of the frequency of the adverse reactions. If other sections of the SmPC (e.g. SmPC section 4.4 "Special warnings and precautions for use") are considered to be updated, clear proposals should be provided for the competent authorities in the Member States to consider during the PSUR assessment.[22] The proposals should be included in the PSUR regional appendix (VII.C.5.).

Harmonisation of the entire product information in all the Member States where the product is authorised is not one of the objectives of the PSUR assessment procedure. Instead, the outcome of the assessment should incorporate the new safety warnings and key risk minimisation recommendations, arising from the assessment of the data in the PSUR, to be included in the relevant sections of the product information.

VII.C.4.1. PSURs for Purely Nationally Authorised Medicinal Products

It is the responsibility of the competent authority in the Member State where the product is authorised to evaluate the PSURs for these medicinal products and the assessment is conducted in accordance with the national legislation.

Listings of individual cases may be requested in the context of the PSUR assessment procedure for adverse reactions of special interest and should be provided by the marketing authorisation holder within an established timeframe to be included in the request. This may be accompanied by a request for an analysis of individual case safety reports, (including information on numbers of cases, details of fatal cases and as necessary, analysis of non-serious cases), where necessary for the scientific evaluation. Information on the context or rationale for the request should generally be provided.

Following the assessment of PSURs, the competent authority in the Member State should consider whether any action concerning the marketing authorisation for the medicinal product concerned is necessary. They should vary, suspend or revoke the marketing authorisation when applicable according to the appropriate procedure at national level.

The assessment report and conclusions of the competent authority in the Member State should be provided to the marketing authorisation holder.

VII.C.4.2. Medicinal Products Authorised in More than One Member State

VII.C.4.2.1. Assessment of PSURs for a Single Centrally Authorised Medicinal Product

This section describes the assessment of PSURs where only one centrally authorised medicinal product is involved according to the procedure set up in Article 28 of Regulation (EC) No 726/2004 (*see* Figure VII.6.).

The assessment of PSURs for a single centrally authorised medicinal product is coordinated by the Agency and shall be conducted by a Rapporteur appointed by the PRAC [REG Art 28(3)] (hereinafter referred to as "PRAC Rapporteur").

Upon receipt, the Agency should perform a technical validation of the report to ensure that the PSUR application is in a suitable format.

Listings of individual cases from EudraVigilance database may be retrieved to support the PSUR assessment.

Further to the above verifications, the procedure starts in accordance with the official starting dates published on the Agency's website. The detailed procedural timetables are published as a generic calendar on the Agency's website.

The published timetables identify the submission, start and finish dates of the procedures as well as other interim dates/milestones that occur during the procedure.

During the assessment, additional listings of individual cases may be requested by the PRAC Rapporteur through the Agency for adverse reactions of special interest and should be provided by the marketing authorisation holder(s) within an established timeframe to be included in the request. This may be accompanied by a request for an analysis of individual cases safety reports, (including information on numbers of cases, details of fatal cases and as necessary, analysis of non-serious cases), where necessary for the scientific evaluation. Information on the context or rationale for the request should generally be provided.

During the drafting of the assessment report, the PRAC Rapporteur shall closely collaborate with the CHMP Rapporteur [REG Art 28(3)].

---

22. *See* "Guideline on Summary of Product Characteristics" as published on the Website of the European Commission in the Notice to Applicants, Volume 2C: http://ec.europa.eu/health/files/eudralex

Annexure 8: Guideline on Good Pharmacovigilance Practices (GVP)

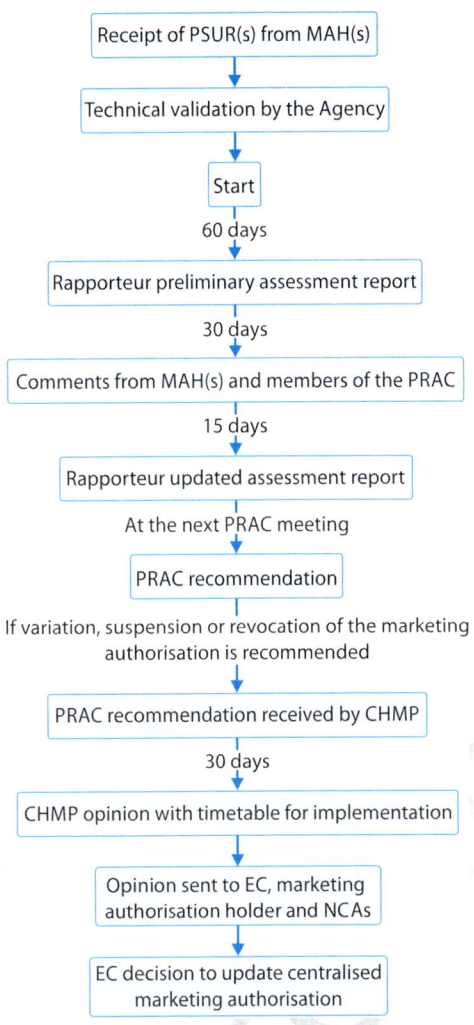

FIG. VII.6: PSUR assessment procedure for a single centrally authorised medicinal product.

The PRAC Rapporteur shall prepare an assessment report and send it to the Agency and to the members of the PRAC [REG Art 28(3)] within 60 days of the start of the procedure.

The Agency shall send the PRAC Rapporteur's preliminary assessment report to the marketing authorisation holder [REG Art 28(3)].

By Day 90, the marketing authorisation holder and members of the PRAC may send comments on the PRAC Rapporteur's preliminary assessment report to the Agency and the PRAC Rapporteur. Those comments should also include responses to outstanding issues or questions raised by the PRAC Rapporteur in the preliminary assessment report and which can be addressed within the timeframe of the comments phase.

Following receipt of comments, the PRAC Rapporteur shall prepare an updated assessment report [REG Art 28(3)] within 15 days (i.e. by Day 105). The updated assessment report is made available to the members of the PRAC and should be forwarded to the marketing authorisation holder by the Agency.

An oral explanation to the PRAC can be held at the request of the PRAC or the marketing authorisation holder in case of recommendation for a revocation or suspension of the marketing authorisation, a new contraindication, a restriction of the indication or a reduction of the recommended dose.

The PRAC shall adopt the updated assessment report with or without further changes at its next meeting [REG Art 28(3)], together with a recommendation on the maintenance of the marketing authorisation or the need to vary, suspend or revoke the marketing authorisation. The PRAC recommendation may also highlight the need to conduct a post-authorisation safety study, request an update of the RMP, review of safety issues and/or close monitoring of events of interest.

Divergent positions of PRAC members and the grounds on which they are based shall be reflected in the recommendation issued by the PRAC [REG Art 28(3)].

The Agency shall include the PRAC recommendation and adopted assessment report in the repository, and forward both to the marketing authorisation holder [REG Art 28(3)].

Further to adoption at the PRAC meeting, in case of any regulatory action is recommended, the assessment report and PRAC recommendation are sent to the CHMP for adoption of an opinion for the centrally authorised product concerned as described in VII.C.4.2.3.

VII.C.4.2.2. Assessment of PSURs for Medicinal Products Subject to Different Marketing Authorisations Containing the Same Active Substance (EU Single Assessment)

This section describes the assessment of PSURs for medicinal products subject to different marketing authorisations, authorised in more than one Member State, containing the same active substance or the same combination of active substances whether or not held by the same marketing authorisation holder and for which the frequency and dates of submission of PSURs have been harmonised in the list of EU reference dates. This could include a mixture of centrally authorised products, products authorised through the mutual recognition, decentralised and national procedures. [DIR Art 107e to 107g] (so-called PSUR "EU single assessment" procedure).

The assessment of PSURs for medicinal products, also called "EU single assessment", shall be conducted by [DIR Art 107e(1)]:
- A "Member State" appointed by the CMDh where none of the marketing authorisations concerned has been granted in accordance with the centralised procedure;
- A "Rapporteur" appointed by the PRAC, where at least one of the marketing authorisations concerned has been granted in accordance with the centralised procedure (hereinafter referred to as "PRAC Rapporteur").

The PSUR EU single assessment procedure is coordinated by the Agency. Upon receipt, the Agency should perform a technical validation of the reports to ensure that the PSURs applications are in a suitable format.

Upon establishment of the list of all medicinal products for human use authorised in the EU referred to in REG Art 57, the Agency should ensure that all marketing authorisation holder(s) of the given substance have submitted PSUR(s), as required. In the event where a PSUR has not been submitted, the Agency should contact the concerned marketing authorisation holder(s). However, this will not preclude the start of the single assessment procedure for other PSUR(s) of the same active substance.

Listings of individual cases from EudraVigilance database may be retrieved to support the PSURs assessment.

Further to the above verifications, the procedure starts in accordance with the official starting dates published on the Agency's website. The detailed procedural timetables are published as a generic calendar on the Agency's website.

The published timetables identify the submission, start and finish dates of the procedures as well as other interim dates/milestones that occur during the procedure.

Further to the start of procedure, the PRAC Rapporteur or Member State conducts the single assessment of all PSURs submitted for the given active substance.

During the assessment, additional listings of individual cases may be requested by the PRAC Rapporteur or Member State through the Agency for adverse drug reactions of special interest and should be provided by the marketing authorisation holder(s) within an established timeframe to be included in the request. This may be accompanied by a request for an analysis of individual cases safety reports, (including information on numbers of cases, details of fatal cases and as necessary, analysis of non-serious cases), where necessary for the scientific evaluation. Information on the context or rationale for the request should generally be provided.

The PRAC Rapporteur or Member State shall prepare an assessment report and send it to the Agency and to the Member States concerned [DIR Art 107e(2)] within 60 days of the start of the procedure. This preliminary assessment report should be circulated to the members of the PRAC.

The Agency shall send the PRAC Rapporteur's/Member State preliminary assessment report to the concerned marketing authorisation holder(s) [DIR Art 107e(2)]. This assessment report should be

Annexure 8: Guideline on Good Pharmacovigilance Practices (GVP)

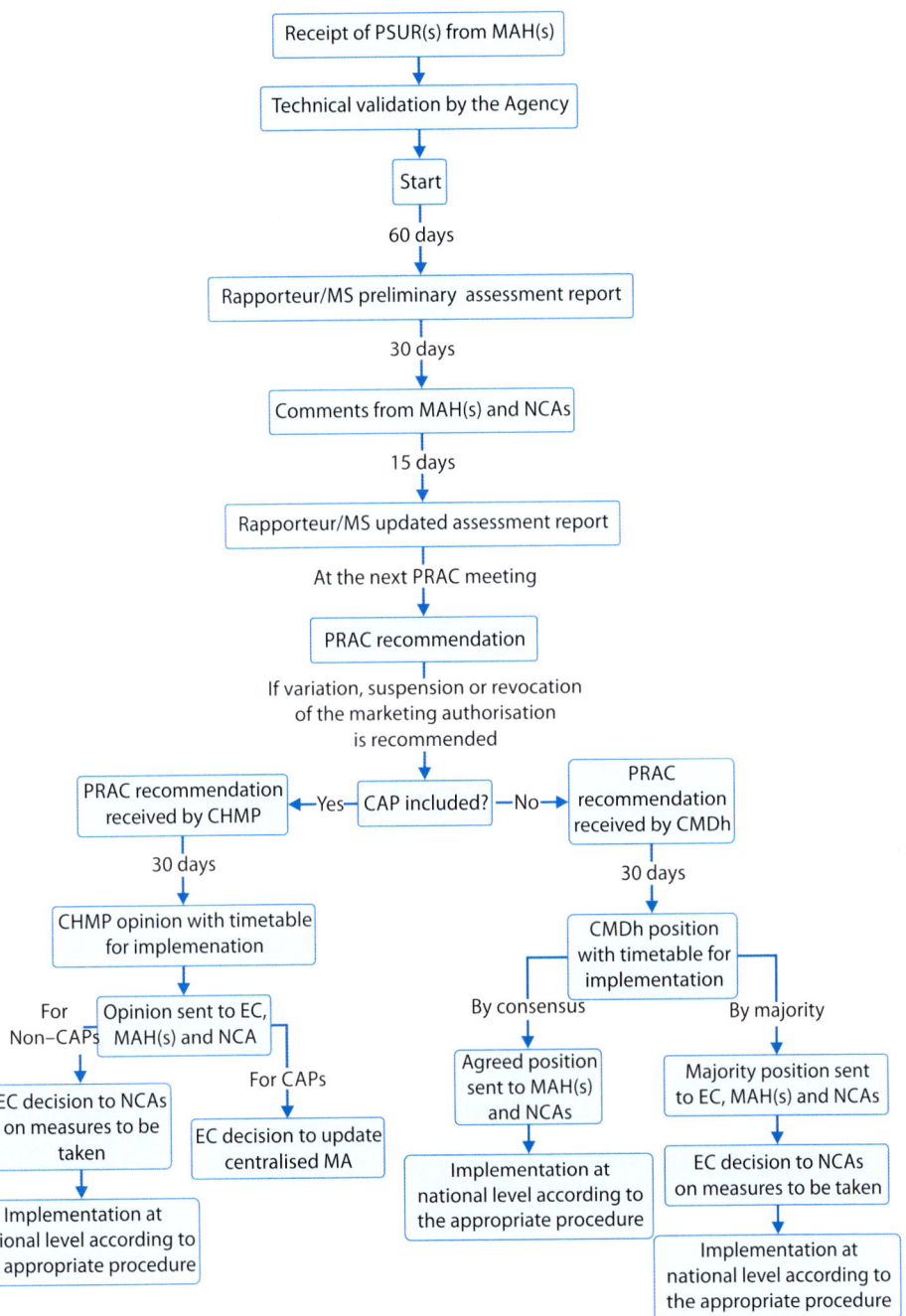

FIG. VII.7: PSUR assessment procedure for "EU single assessment".

circulated amongst all the marketing authorisation holders whose medicinal product(s) are part of the EU single assessment.

By Day 90, the marketing authorisation holder(s), Member States and members of the PRAC as applicable may send comments on the PRAC Rapporteur's/Member State's preliminary assessment report to the Agency and the PRAC Rapporteur/Member State, as applicable. Those comments should also include responses to outstanding issues or questions raised by the PRAC Rapporteur/Member State in the preliminary assessment report and which can be addressed within the timeframe of the comments phase.

Following receipt of comments, the PRAC Rapporteur/Member State shall prepare an updated assessment report [DIR Art 107e (3)] within 15 days (i.e. by Day 105). The updated assessment report is forwarded to the members of the PRAC and should be circulated by the Agency amongst all the marketing authorisation holders whose medicinal product(s) are part of the EU single assessment.

An oral explanation to the PRAC can be held at the request of the PRAC or the marketing authorisation holder in case of recommendation for a revocation or suspension of the marketing authorisation, a new contraindication, a restriction of the indication or a reduction of the recommended dose.

The PRAC shall adopt the updated assessment report with or without further changes at its next meeting [DIR Art 107e(3)], together with a recommendation on maintenance of the marketing authorisation or the need to vary, suspend or revoke the marketing authorisation. The PRAC recommendation may also highlight the need to conduct a post-authorisation safety study (*see* Module VIII), request an update of the RMP (*see* Module V), review of safety issue and/or close monitoring of events of interest.

Divergent positions of PRAC members and the grounds on which they are based shall be reflected in the recommendation issued by the PRAC [DIR Art 107e(3)].

The Agency shall include the PRAC recommendation and adopted assessment report in the repository, and forward both to the marketing authorisation holder(s) [DIR Art 107e(3)].

Further to adoption at the PRAC meeting, in case of any regulatory action is recommended, the assessment report and PRAC recommendation are sent to:

- The CHMP where at least one centrally authorised product is included in the single assessment, for adoption of an opinion as described in VII.C.4.2.3.;
- The CMDh where no centrally authorised product is included in the single assessment, for agreement of a position as described in VII.C.4.2.4.

VII.C.4.2.3. Single Assessment Including at least One Centrally Authorised Product Leading to a CHMP Opinion

The CHMP acknowledges receipt of the PRAC recommendation and assessment report, in case of any regulatory action, at their next meeting following the PRAC adoption. Within 30 days from receipt, the CHMP shall consider the PRAC assessment report and recommendation and adopt an opinion on the maintenance, variation, suspension, revocation of the marketing authorisation(s) concerned [DIR 107g(3)].

An oral explanation to the CHMP can be held at the request of the CHMP or the marketing authorisation holder(s) only in case of differences with the PRAC recommendation where CHMP considers the possibility of adopting an opinion on the suspension or revocation of the marketing authorisation(s), a new contraindication, a restriction of the indication or a reduction of the recommended dose.

The opinion will contain the following:

- The final assessment report and recommendation adopted by the PRAC;
- Detailed explanation of the scientific grounds for differences with the PRAC recommendation, if applicable [DIR Art 107g(3)];
- In the case of a CHMP opinion to vary the marketing authorisation(s):
    - The scientific conclusions and grounds recommending the variation to the terms of the marketing authorisation;
    - For centrally authorised products, revised product information and if applicable, conditions imposed to the marketing authorisation holder and where appropriate, the conditions or restrictions imposed to the Member States for the safe and effective used of the medicinal

product, in accordance with the provision provided in DIR Art 127a;
- For nationally authorised products, including those authorised through the mutual recognition and decentralised procedures, an annex indicating the new safety warnings and key risk minimisation recommendations to be included in the relevant sections of the product information as applicable.
- In the case of a CHMP opinion to suspend the marketing authorisation(s), the scientific conclusions together with the grounds for suspension and conditions for lifting the suspension;
- In the case of a CHMP opinion to revoke the marketing authorisation(s), the scientific conclusions together with the grounds for revocation;
- Divergent positions of CHMP members, where applicable.

Further to adoption, the Agency should send the CHMP opinion together with its annexes and appendices to the European Commission, marketing authorisation holder(s) and competent authorities in Member States.

The final assessment conclusions and recommendations are published in the European medicines web-portal (VII.C.7.).

a. Post CHMP opinion - Centrally authorised products

Where the CHMP opinion states that the terms of the marketing authorisation(s) needs to be varied, the marketing authorisation holder(s) of centrally authorised products should provide the translations of the product information and the scientific conclusions and grounds recommending the variation to the terms of the marketing authorisation, in all EU official languages, in accordance with the translation timetable adopted by the CHMP.

Further to receipt of a CHMP opinion stating that regulatory action to the concerned marketing authorisation is necessary, the European Commission shall adopt a decision addressed to marketing authorisation holders to vary, suspend or revoke the marketing authorisation(s) of centrally authorised product(s) [DIR Art 107g(4b)].

Further to adoption, the European Commission should notify the decisions amending the terms of the marketing authorisation of centrally authorised products to the marketing authorisation holder(s).

b. Post CHMP opinion - Nationally authorised products, including those authorised through the mutual recognition and decentralised procedures

Further to receipt of a CHMP opinion stating that regulatory action to the concerned marketing authorisations is necessary, the European Commission shall adopt a decision addressed to the competent authorities in Member States concerning the measures to be taken [DIR Art 107g(a)] in respect of nationally authorised products, including those authorised through the mutual recognition and decentralised procedures.

Further to the receipt of the decision from the European Commission, the competent authorities in Member States shall take the necessary measures to vary, suspend or revoke the marketing authorisation(s) within 30 days [DIR Art 107g(4)].

VII.C.4.2.4. Single Assessment not Including Centrally Authorised Product Leading to a CMDh Position

The CMDh acknowledges receipt of the PRAC recommendation and assessment report, in case of any regulatory action, at their next meeting following the PRAC adoption.

Within 30 days from receipt, the CMDh shall consider the PRAC assessment report and recommendation and reach a position on the maintenance, variation, suspension, revocation of the marketing authorisation(s) concerned [DIR Art 107g(1)].

An oral explanation to the CMDh can be held at the request of the CMDh or the marketing authorisation holder(s), only in case of differences with the PRAC recommendation where the CMDh considers the possibility to reach a position on the suspension or revocation of the marketing authorisation(s), a new contraindication, a restriction of the indication or a reduction of the recommended dose.

The position will contain the following:
- The final assessment report and recommendation adopted by the PRAC;

- Detailed explanation of the scientific grounds for differences with the PRAC recommendation, if applicable [DIR Art 107g(2)];
- In the case of a CMDh position to vary the marketing authorisation(s), the scientific conclusions and grounds recommending the variation to the terms of the marketing authorisation and an annex indicating the new safety warnings and key risk minimisation recommendations to be included in the relevant sections of the product information, as applicable;
- In the case of a CMDh position to suspend the marketing authorisation(s), the scientific conclusions together with the grounds for suspension and conditions for lifting the suspension;
- In the case of a CMDh position to revoke the marketing authorisation(s), the scientific conclusions together with the grounds for revocation;
- Divergent position(s) for the CMDh members, where applicable.

The final assessment conclusions and recommendations shall be published by the Agency in the European medicines web-portal [DIR Art 107l] (VII.C.7.).

If the CMDh position is reached by consensus:
The position agreed including the action to be taken is recorded by the chairperson in the minutes of the CMDh meeting where agreed.

The chairman shall send the agreed CMDh position [DIR Art 107g(2)] and its appendices to the marketing authorisation holder(s) and competent authorities in Member States.

Further to receipt of the CMDh position stating that regulatory action to the concerned marketing authorisation is necessary, the competent authorities in Member States shall adopt necessary measures to vary, suspend or revoke the marketing authorisation(s) concerned in accordance with the timetable for implementation determined in the agreed position [DIR Art 107g(2)].

In case the position of the CMDh agreed that variation to the terms of marketing authorisation is required, the marketing authorisation holder(s) shall submit the relevant variation to that effect within the timetable for implementation [DIR Art 107g(2)] as appended to the agreed position.

If the CMDh position is reached by majority vote:
The majority position on the action to be taken is recorded by the chairman in the minutes of the CMDh meeting where agreed.

The majority position of the CMDh together with its annexes and its appendices, including translations in all EU official languages where applicable, shall be forwarded to the European Commission [DIR Art 107g(2)]. The position of the CMDh should also be forwarded to the competent authorities in Member States.

Further to receipt of a CMDh position stating that regulatory action to the concerned marketing authorisation is necessary, the European Commission shall adopt decision(s) [DIR Art 107g(2)] addressed to the competent authorities in Member States in order for them to vary, suspend or revoke the marketing authorisation(s) of nationally authorised product(s) which is addressed to marketing authorisation holders.

Further to receipt of the decision from the European Commission, the competent authorities in Member States shall take the necessary measures to maintain, vary, suspend or revoke the marketing authorisation(s) within 30 days [DIR Art 107g(2)].

VII.C.4.3. Relationship between PSUR and Risk Management Plan

The general relationship between the risk management plan (RMP) and the PSUR is described in Module V, while an overview of the common RMP/PSUR modules is provided in VII.C.4.3.1.

During the preparation of a PSUR, the marketing authorisation holder should consider whether any identified or potential risks discussed within the PSUR is important and requires an update of the RMP. In these circumstances, updated revised RMP including the new important safety concern should be submitted with the PSUR and assessed in parallel, following the timetable for the assessment of PSUR as described above.

If important safety concerns are identified by the national competent authorities in the Member States during the assessment of a PSUR and no updated RMP or no RMP has been submitted, recommendations should be made to submit an update or a new RMP within a defined timeline.

VII.C.4.3.1. PSUR and Risk Management Plan – Common Modules

The proposed modular formats for the PSUR and the RMP aim to address duplication and facilitate flexibility by enabling common PSUR/RMP sections to be utilised interchangeably across both reports. Common sections with the above mentioned reports are identified in Table VII.1.:

VII.C.5. EU-specific Requirements for Periodic Safety Update Reports

The scientific evaluation of the risk-benefit balance of the medicinal product included in the PSUR detailed in VII.B.5. shall be based on all available data, including data from clinical trials in unauthorised indications and populations according to the provisions of DIR Art 107b and IR Art 34(1).

The EU-specific requirements should be included in the PSUR EU regional appendix.

Table VII.1: Common sections between PSUR and RMP

PSUR section	RMP section
Section 3 – "Actions taken in the reporting interval for safety reasons"	Part II, module SV – "Post-authorisation experience", section "Regulatory and marketing authorisation holder action for safety reason"
Sub-section 5.2 – "Cumulative and interval patient exposure from marketing experience"	Part II, module SV – "Post-authorisation experience", section "Non-study post-authorisation exposure"
Sub-section 16.1 – "Summary of safety concerns"	Part II, module SVIII – "Summary of the safety concerns" (as included in the version of the RMP which was current at the beginning of the PSUR reporting interval)
Sub-section 16.4 – "Characterisation of risks"	Part II, Module SVII – "Identified and potential risks"
Sub-section 16.5 – "Effectiveness of risk minimisation (if applicable)"	Part V – "Risk minimisation measures", section "Evaluation of the effectiveness of risk minimisation activities"

VII.C.5.1. PSUR EU Regional Appendix, Sub-section "Proposed Product Information"

The assessment of the need for amendments to the product information is incorporated within the PSUR assessment procedure in the EU. The regulatory opinion/position should include recommendations for updates to product information where needed. Marketing authorisation holders should provide the necessary supportive documentation and references within the PSUR or in this appendix to facilitate this.

Within the PSUR, the marketing authorisation holder is required to consider the impact of the data and evaluations presented within the report, on the marketing authorisation. Based on the evaluation of the cumulative safety data and the risk-benefit analysis, the marketing authorisation holder shall draw conclusions in the PSUR as to the need for changes and/or actions, including implications for the approved SmPC(s) for the product(s) for which the PSUR is submitted [IR Art 34 (5)].

In this sub-section, the marketing authorisation holder should provide the proposals for product information (SmPC and package leaflet) based on the above mentioned evaluation. These should be based on all EU authorised indications.

A track change version of the proposed SmPCs and package leaflets based on the assessment and conclusions of the PSUR should be provided. For centrally authorised medicinal products, the proposed product information should also be submitted to Module 1.3.1 of the Electronic Common Technical Document (eCTD).

All the SmPCs and packages leaflets covered by the PSUR and in effect at the data lock point, should be reviewed to ensure that they reflect the appropriate information according to the cumulative data included and analysed in the PSUR.

Amendments to the product information should not be postponed or delayed until the PSUR submission and amendments not related to the information presented in the PSUR, should not be proposed within the PSUR procedure. It is the obligation of the marketing authorisation holder to submit a variation in accordance with the Regulation (EC) No 1234/2008 on variations to the terms of a marketing authorisation.

A brief description of ongoing procedures (e.g. variations) to update the product information should be provided in this section.

VII.C.5.2. PSUR EU Regional Appendix, Sub-section "Proposed Additional Pharmacovigilance and Risk Minimisation Activities"

Considering the provision established in IR Art 34 (5), this sub-section should include proposals for additional pharmacovigilance and additional risk minimisation activities based on the conclusions and actions of the PSUR, including a statement of the intention to submit a RMP or an updated RMP when applicable.

VII.C.5.3. PSUR EU Regional Appendix, Sub-section "Summary of Ongoing Safety Concerns"

In order to support the information provided in the PSUR section 16.1 "Summary of safety concerns" (*see* VII.B.5.16.1.), Table 1.10 (according to the current RMP template) "Summary – Ongoing safety concerns" should be included in this PSUR sub-section. This table should be extracted from the version of RMP available at the beginning of the PSUR reporting interval (*see* Module V).

VII.C.5.4. PSUR EU Regional Appendix, Sub-section "Reporting of Results from Post-authorisation Safety Studies"

Findings from both interventional and non-interventional (for further guidance *see* Module VIII) post-authorisation safety studies (PASS) should be reported in the PSUR. While the marketing authorisation holder should inform competent authorities in Member States and the Agency as applicable about any new information that may impact on the risk-benefit balance immediately, the PSUR should provide comprehensive information on the findings of all PASS, both interventional and non-interventional, in PSUR sections 7 and 8 respectively.

Final study reports for studies conducted with the primary aim of identifying, characterising or quantifying a safety hazard, confirming the safety profile of the medicinal product, or of measuring the effectiveness of risk management measures which were completed during the reporting interval should also be included as an annex to the PSUR.

For such studies discontinued during the reporting interval, the reasons for stopping the study should also be explained.

If an important safety concern has been identified in the course of a study, regardless of whether it has been detected through pre-specified methods and whether the study is considered a PASS, the marketing authorisation holder and specifically the qualified person responsible for pharmacovigilance (QPPV) will have informed the relevant competent authorities in Member States immediately.

PSURs should not be used as the initial communication method either for the submission of final study reports to the competent authorities in Member States or for the notification of any new information that might influence the evaluation of the risk-benefit balance.

VII.C.5.5. PSUR EU Regional Appendix, Sub-section "Effectiveness of Risk Minimisation"

Risk minimisation activities are public health interventions intended to prevent the occurrence of an adverse drug reaction(s) associated with the exposure to a medicinal product or to reduce its severity should it occur. The success of risk minimisation activities in delivering these objectives needs to be evaluated throughout the lifecycle of a product to ensure that the burden of adverse reactions is minimised and hence the overall risk-benefit balance is optimised. In accordance with section VII.B.5.16.5., evaluation of broad global experience should be reflected in the body of the report, when provides insights into the effectiveness of risk minimisation activities in any country or region that may have utility in other countries or regions are of particular interest.

This sub-section should additionally provide an evaluation of the effectiveness of routine and/or additional risk minimisation activities specifically relevant to an EU context. This should take account of regulatory imposed obligations for implementation of risk minimisation measures in addition to the overall requirement for monitoring of safety and benefit-risk. Results of any studies to assess the impact or other formal assessment(s) of risk minimisation activities in the EU should be included when available. As part of this critical evaluation, the marketing authorisation holder should make observations on factors contributing to the success or weakness of risk minimisation activities. If a particular risk minimisation strategy proves ineffective, then alternative activities need to be put in place. In certain cases, it may be judged that risk minimisation cannot control the risks to the extent possible to ensure a positive risk-benefit balance and that the medicinal product needs to be withdrawn either from the market or restricted to those patients in whom the benefits outweigh the risks. More extensive guidance on monitoring the effectiveness of risk minimisation activities is included in Module XVI. As a principle, the marketing authorisation holder should distinguish in their evaluation between implementation success and attainment of the intended outcome.

VII.C.6. Quality Systems and Record Management Systems for PSURs in the EU Network

VII.C.6.1. Quality Systems and Record Management Systems at the Level of the Marketing Authorisation Holder

Specific quality system procedures and processes shall be in place in order to ensure the update of product information by the marketing authorisation holder in the light of scientific knowledge, including the assessments and recommendations made public via the European medicines web-portal, and on the basis of a continuous monitoring by the marketing authorisation holder of information published on the European medicines web-portal [IR Art 11(1)(f)].

It is the responsibility of the marketing authorisation holder to check regularly the list of EU reference dates and frequency of submission published in the European medicines web-portal to ensure compliance with the PSUR reporting requirements for their medicinal products (*see* VII.C.3.).

Systems should be in place to schedule the production of PSURs according to:
- The list of EU reference dates and frequency of PSURs submission; or
- The conditions laid down in the marketing authorisation; or
- The standard PSUR submission schedule established according to DIR Art 107c(2) for products authorised before 2 July 2012 (for centrally authorised products) and 21 July 2012 (for nationally authorised products) as applicable (without any conditions in their marketing authorisation or not included in the list of EU references dates and frequency of submission or not affected by the derogation established in [DIR Art 107b(3)]); or
- Ad hoc requests for PSURs by a competent authority in a Member State or the Agency.

For those medicinal products where the submission of an RMP is not required, the marketing authorisation holder should maintain on file a specification of important identified risks, important potential risks and missing information in order to support the preparation of the PSURs.

The marketing authorisation holder should have procedures in place to follow the requirements established by the Agency for the submission of PSURs.

The QPPV shall be responsible for the establishment and maintenance of the pharmacovigilance system [DIR Art 104(e)] and therefore should ensure that the pharmacovigilance system in place enables the compliance with the requirements established for the production and submission of PSURs. In relation to the medicinal products covered by the pharmacovigilance system, specific additional responsibilities of the QPPV in relation to PSURs should include:
- Ensuring the necessary quality, including the correctness and completeness, of the data submitted in the PSURs;
- Ensuring full response according to the timelines and within the procedure agreed (e.g. next PSUR) to any request from the competent authorities in Member States and the Agency related to PSURs;
- Awareness of the PSUR and assessment report conclusions, PRAC recommendations, CHMP opinions, CMDh positions and European Commission decisions in order to ensure that appropriate action takes place.

The record retention times for product-related documents in Module I also apply to PSURs and source documents related to the creation of PSURs, including documents related to actions taken for safety reasons, clinical trials and post-authorisation studies, relevant benefit information and documents utilised for the calculation of patient exposure.

VII.C.6.2. Quality Systems and Record Management Systems at the Level of the European Medicines Agency

The application of the Agency's quality system (*see* Module I) should support compliance by the Agency when fulfilling its tasks and responsibilities for the management of PSUR procedures and EU single assessments.

The Agency should have in place a process to technically validate the completeness of PSUR submissions.

Line listings and summary tabulations from the EudraVigilance database utilised to support the PSUR assessment should be created using reports by means of the EudraVigilance data analysis system.

Effective communication and circulation of PSURs and related documents is crucial for the successful completeness of the procedure; therefore processes have to be in place for the circulation of documents between the Agency, marketing authorisation holders, the Commission and the competent authorities in Member States. Where applicable, the procedures should establish the necessity for quality checks with the aim to remove any information of a personal or commercially confidential nature.

Written procedures should reflect the different steps to follow for the maintenance of the list of EU references dates and frequency of submission of PSURs published by the Agency in the European medicines web-portal (*see* VII.C.3.).

Prior to the publication of summaries of PSUR assessment reports in the European medicines web-portal (*see* VII.C.7.) the appropriate personnel at the Agency should adhere to the procedures established for web publication of documents produced by the Agency or competent authorities in the Member States.

All records related to PSURs created by the Agency's staff members, experts or consultants are the property of the Agency and all PSURs and related documents received are in the custody of the Agency. Both types of PSURs records (created or received by the Agency) are subject to the Agency's overall control via the PSUR repository set up according to the provisions laid down in REG Art 25a.

The Agency's policy on records management (EMEA/590678/2007)[23], provides the basis for a consistent, sustainable and efficient records management program and it has been developed in accordance with the commonly recognised international standard for records management, "ISO 15489-1:2001 Information and documentation – Records management[24]". According to the records classification stated by the Agency's policy, PSURs would be considered business, legal, evidential and research/historical value records.

The record retention times for product-related documents in Module I also apply to PSUR-system related documents (e.g. standard operating procedures) and PSUR-related documents (e.g. PSURs, assessment reports, the data retrieved from the EudraVigilance database or other data used to support the PSUR assessment).

VII.C.6.3. Quality Systems and Record Management Systems at the Level of the Competent Authorities in Member States

Each competent authority in the Member States shall have in place a pharmacovigilance system [DIR Art 101] for the surveillance of medicinal products and for receipt and evaluation of all pharmacovigilance data including PSURs. For the purpose of operating its tasks relating to PSURs in addition to the pharmacovigilance system the national competent authorities in Member States should implement a quality system (*see* Module I).

Competent authorities in the Member States should monitor marketing authorisation holders for compliance with regulatory obligations for PSURs. Additionally, competent authorities should

---

23. www.ema.europa.eu
24. www.ISO.org

exchange information in cases of non-compliance and take appropriate regulatory actions as required.

No PSUR assessment at EU level is foreseen for purely nationally authorised products authorised in only one Member State; therefore the national competent authority in the Member State where the medicinal product is authorised should have procedures in place for the assessment of PSURs related to those medicinal products.

The procedures established by the national competent authorities in Member States for the performance of the EU single assessment of PSURs, should be in line with the procedures established by the Agency for the coordination of PSUR assessment in the EU regulatory network (see VII.C.4.). These procedures should establish effective communication across the EU regulatory network and the actions to be taken regarding the variation, suspension or revocation of the marketing authorisation following the PRAC recommendations, CHMP opinion, CMDh position and European Commission decision as applicable.

The procedures established by the Agency for the use of the PSUR repository to support the single assessment, should be followed by the national competent authorities in Member States.

Where tasks related to PSUR procedures are delegated to third parties, the national competent authorities in Member States should ensure that they are subject to a quality system in compliance with the obligations provided by the European legislation.

The record retention times for product-related documents in Module I also apply to PSUR-system related documents (e.g. standard operating procedures) and PSUR -related documents (e.g. PSURs, assessment reports, the data retrieved from the EudraVigilance database or other data used to support the PSUR assessment).

VII.C.7. Transparency

VII.C.7.1. Publication of PSUR-related Documents on the European Medicines and National Medicines Web-Portals

The following documents shall be made publicly available by means of the European medicines web-portal [DIR Art 107l, REG Art 26(g)]:

- List of EU reference dates and frequency of submission of PSURs (see VII C.3.);
- Final assessment conclusions of the adopted assessment reports;
- PRAC recommendations including relevant annexes;
- CMDh position including relevant annexes and where applicable, detailed explanation on scientific grounds for any differences with the PRAC recommendations;
- CHMP opinion including relevant annexes and where applicable, detailed explanation on scientific grounds for any differences with the PRAC recommendations;
- European Commission decision.

The version and date of publication are reflected in each document as they define the issue of the PRAC recommendations, CHMP opinions, CMDh positions and European Commission decisions at a certain point of time.

Links between the European medicines web-portal and the National medicines web-portals should be made whenever possible and relevant.

Any personal or confidential data made public by the Agency or the competent authorities in Member States as referred to in paragraphs 2 and 3 of Article 106a of Directive 2001/83/EC shall be deleted unless considered necessary in terms of protection of the public health [DIR Art 106a(4)].

VII.C.8. Renewal of Marketing Authorisations

Marketing authorisations need to be renewed after 5 years on the basis of a re-evaluation of the risk-benefit balance in order to continue to be valid to place the product on the market. This renewal is irrespective of whether the marketing authorisation is suspended. Further details on the procedure and the documentation requirements can be found in the current versions of the "Guideline on Processing of Renewals in the Centralised Procedure" (EMEA/CHMP/2990/00) for Centralised products and the "CMDh Best Practice Guide on the processing of renewals in the MRP/DCP" (CMDh/004/2005) for other products.

No PSURs, addendum reports and summary bridging reports should be submitted within the renewal application. The clinical overview should include an addendum containing the relevant sections for the re-assessment of the risk-benefit balance of the medicinal product. These sections are identified in the above-mentioned guidelines for renewal. Marketing authorisation holders are advised to consider this GVP Module VII as guidance for the preparation of the addendum to the clinical overview.

Following the submission of a renewal application, the PRAC may be consulted for medicinal products authorised through the centralised procedure as regards safety issues. For nationally authorised products, including those authorised through the mutual recognition or decentralised procedure, the PRAC may also be consulted upon request by a competent authority in a Member State on the basis of safety concerns.

Conditional marketing authorisations should be renewed annually [REG Art 14(7)]. Further details on the procedure and the documentation to be submitted can be found in the "Guideline on the scientific application and the practical arrangements necessary to implement Commission Regulation (EC) No 507/2006 on the conditional marketing authorisation for medicinal products for human use falling within the scope of regulation (EC) no 726/2004" (EMEA/509951/2006).

VII.C.9. Transition and Interim Arrangements

VII.C.9.1. Submission and Availability of Documents before the Agency's Repository is in Place

The Agency shall, in collaboration with the competent authorities in Member States and the European Commission set up and maintain a repository for PSURs and the corresponding assessment reports so that they are fully and permanently accessible to European Commission, the competent authorities in Member States, the PRAC, the CHMP and the CMDh [REG Art 25a].

The repository shall undergo an independent audit before the functionalities are announced by the Agency's management board [REG Art 25a].

As established in the transitional provisions introduced in Directive 2010/84/EU Art 2(7), until the Agency can ensure the functionalities agreed for the repository, marketing authorisation holders under the obligation to submit PSURs irrespective of whether the medicinal product is authorised in one or more Member States and irrespective of whether the active substance or combination of active substances is on the EU reference date list shall submit the PSURs to all competent authorities in Member States in which the medicinal products are authorised. For the substances or combination of active substances subject to the EU single assessment, and for which an EU reference date has been established, the PSURs should be also sent to the Agency.

The competent authorities in Member States requirements for the submission of PSURs during this transitional period are published in the Agency web-site[25].

From 12 months after the functionalities of the repository have been established and have been announced by the Agency, the marketing authorisation holders shall submit the PSURs electronically to the Agency regardless of the authorisation procedure of the medicinal product [DIR Art 107b(1)]. The competent authorities in Member States shall ensure that this obligation applies as required [DIR Art 2(7)].

Once the structured electronic format "ePSUR", based on content agreed in the ICH-E2C(R2), becomes available, marketing authorisation holders will have the possibility to submit PSURs and related documents automatically via an electronic gateway.

Until the repository is in place, the relevant documents should be circulated as follows:
- The preliminary assessment report created by the PRAC Rapporteur/Member State within 60 days of the start of the procedure should be circulated to the Agency and the members of the PRAC through a dedicated mailbox. The Agency should send the report to the concerned marketing authorisation holder(s);
- Members of the PRAC should circulate their comments through a dedicated mailbox by

---
25. www.ema.europa.eu

Day 90 on the PRAC Rapporteur/Member State preliminary assessment report;
- Comments by the marketing authorisation holder(s) by Day 90 on the PRAC Rapporteur/Member State preliminary assessment report, should be submitted to the Agency, PRAC Rapporteur and all members of the PRAC, according to the instructions for submission published by the Agency;
- Updated PRAC Rapporteur/Member State assessment report created within 15 days (i.e. by Day 105) should be circulated to the Agency and members of the PRAC through a dedicated mailbox. The Agency should forward the updated PRAC Rapporteur/Member State assessment report to the marketing authorisation holders concerned.

Further to adoption, the Agency should send the CHMP opinion together with its annexes and appendices to the European Commission, marketing authorisation holder(s) and competent authorities in Member States, through secure email until the repository is in place.

VII.C.9.2. Quality Systems and Record Management Systems at the Level of the Competent Authorities in Member States

Special considerations should be taken for the management of the PSURs submitted to the concerned competent authorities in Member States until the Agency can ensure the functionalities agreed for the PSUR repository and 12 months after the establishment of the repository according to the transitional provisions.

VII.C.9.3. Publication of the EU List of Union References Dates and Start of the EU- PSUR Single Assessment Procedure

As stated in VII.C.3.6., the list of EU reference dates and frequency of submission should be published in the European medicines web-portal, nevertheless, the EU single assessment procedure for substances included only in nationally authorised products, detailed in VII.C.4.2.2., and VII.C.4.2.4. will be delayed until funds are available.

Table VII.2: Estimated cumulative subject exposure from clinical trials.

Treatment	Number of Subjects
Medicinal product	
Comparator	
Placebo	

Table VII.3: Cumulative subject exposure to investigational drug from completed clinical trials by age and sex.

Number of subjects			
Age range	Male	Female	Total

Data from completed trials as of [date]

Table VII.4: Cumulative subject exposure to investigational drug from completed clinical trials by racial/ethnic group.

Racial/ethnic group	Number of subjects
Asian	
Black	
Caucasian	
Other	
Unknown	
Total	

Data from completed trials as of [date]

VII. APPENDICES

VII. Appendix 1. Examples of Tabulations for Estimated Exposure and Adverse Events/Reactions Data

Marketing authorisation holders can modify these examples tabulations to suit specific situations, as appropriate.

Estimates of cumulative subject exposure, based upon actual exposure data from completed clinical trials and the enrolment/randomisation schemes for ongoing trials.

Table VII.5: Cumulative exposure from marketing experience.

Indication	Sex		Age (years)			Dose			Formulation				Region			
	Male	Female	2 to ≤16	>16 to 65	>65	Unknown	<40	≥40	Unknown	Intravenous	Oral	EU	Japan	Colombia	US/Canada	Other
Overall																
Depression																
Migraine																

Table VII.5 includes cumulative data obtained from day/month/year throughout day/month/year, where available

Table VII.6: Interval exposure from marketing experience.

Indication	Sex		Age (years)			Dose			Formulation				Region			
	Male	Female	2 to ≤16	>16 to 65	>65	Unknown	<40	≥40	Unknown	Intravenous	Oral	EU	Japan	Colombia	US/Canada	Other
Depression																
Migraine																

Table VII.6 includes interval data obtained from day/month/year throughout day/month/year

Table VII.7: Cumulative tabulation of serious adverse events from clinical trials.

System Organ Class	Preferred term	Investigational medicinal product	Blinded	Active comparator	Placebo
Blood and lymphatic system disorders					
	Anaemia				
	Bone marrow necrosis				
Cardiac disorders					
	Tachycardia				
	Ischaemic cardiomyopathy				

Annexure 8: Guideline on Good Pharmacovigilance Practices (GVP)

Table VII.8: Numbers of adverse reactions by preferred term from post-authorisation sources.*

SOC MedDRA PT	Spontaneous, including competent authorities (worldwide) and literature					Non-interventional post-marketing study and reports from other solicited sources **	
	Serious		Non-serious		Total Spontaneous	Serious	
	Interval	Cumulative	Interval	Cumulative	Cumulative	Interval	Cumulative
<SOC 1>							
<PT>							
<PT>							
<PT>							
<SOC 2>							
<PT>							
<PT>							
<PT>							
<PT>							

*Non-interventional post-authorisation studies, reports from other solicited sources and spontaneous ICSRs (i.e., reports from healthcare professionals, consumers, competent authorities (worldwide), and scientific literature)
** This does not include interventional clinical trials.

VII. Appendix 2. Example of Tabular Summary of Safety Signals that Were Ongoing or Closed During the Reporting Interval

Reporting interval: DD-MMM-YYYY to DD-MMM-YYYY

Table VII.9: The tabular summary below is a fictitious example of tabular summary of safety signals ongoing or closed during the reporting interval

Signal term	Date detected	Status (ongoing or closed)	Date closed (for closed signals)	Source of signal	Reason for evaluation and summary of key data	Method of signal evaluation	Pending
Stroke	MMM/ YYYY	Ongoing	MMM/ YYYY	meta-analysis (published trials)	Statistically significant increase in frequency	Review meta-analysis and available data	Pending
SJS	MMM/ YYYY	Closed	MMM/ YYYY	Spontaneous case reports	Rash already an identified risk SJS not reported in pre-authorisation CTs. 4 reports within 6 months of authorisation; plausible time to onset and no possible alternative causes.	Targeted follow up of reports with site visit to one hospital. Full review of cases by MAH dermatologist and literature searches.	RSI updated with a warning and precaution DHPC sent Effectiveness survey planned 6 months post DHPC. RMP updated.

Explanatory notes:

Signal term:
- A brief descriptive name of a medical concept for the signal. This may evolve and be refined as the signal is evaluated. The concept and scope may or may not be limited to specific MedDRA term(s), depending on the source of signal.

Date detected:
- Month and year the marketing authorisation holder became aware of the signal.

Status:
- *Ongoing:* Signal under evaluation at the data lock point of the PSUR. Anticipated completion date, if known, should be provided.
- *Closed:* Signal for which evaluation was completed before the data lock point of the PSUR.

Note: A new signal of which the marketing authorisation holder became aware during the reporting interval may be classified as closed or ongoing, depending on the status of the signal evaluation at the end of the reporting interval of the PSUR.

Date closed:
- Month and year when the signal evaluation was completed.

Source of signal:
- Data or information source from which a signal arose. Examples include, but may not be limited to, spontaneous reports, clinical trial data, scientific literature, and non-clinical study results, or information request or inquiries from a competent authority (worldwide).

Reason for evaluation and summary of key data:
- A brief summary of key data and rationale for further evaluation.

Action(s) taken or planned:

State whether or not a specific action has been taken or is planned for all closed signals that have been classified as potential or identified risks. If any further actions are planned for newly or previously identified signals under evaluation at the data lock point, these should be listed, otherwise leave blank for ongoing signals.

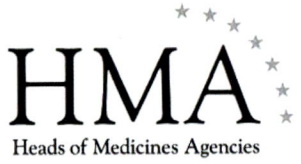
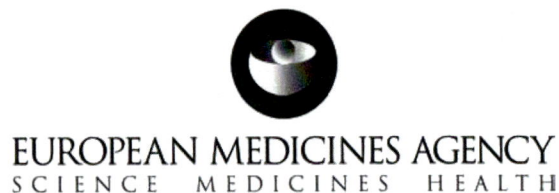

4 August 2016
EMA/813938/2011 Rev 2* Corr**

GUIDELINE ON GOOD PHARMACOVIGILANCE PRACTICES (GVP)

Module VIII   Post-Authorisation Safety Studies (Rev 2)

Date for coming into effect of first version	2 July 2012
Date for coming into effect of Revision 1	25 April 2013
Draft Revision 2 finalised by the Agency in collaboration with Member States	23 June 2015
Draft Revision 2 agreed by the European Risk Management Facilitation Group (ERMS FG)	16 July 2015
Draft Revision 2 adopted by Executive Director	3 August 2015
Release for public consultation	11 August 2015
End of consultation (deadline for comments)	9 October 2015
Revised draft Revision 2 finalised by the Agency in collaboration with Member States	14 April 2016
Revised draft Revision 2 agreed by ERMS FG	15 July 2016
Revised draft Revision 2 adopted by Executive Director as final	4 August 2016
Date for coming into effect of Revision 2*	9 August 2016

** The correction relates to adding 'holder' after 'marketing authorisation' in the 4th bullet point on page 4.
Note: Revision 2 contains the following:
- Changes to VIII.A., clarifying the link between the legislation on non-interventional PASS and categories 1-3 of non-interventional PASS described in GVP Module V;
- Changes to VIII.B., amending and re-organising the text of several sections to provide a better distinction between legal obligations and recommendations to marketing authorisation holders;
- Changes to VIII.B.3.1, adding text in line with GVP Module VI Rev 1 to provide a recommendation on adverse events that will not be collected or reported;
- Changes to VIII.B.3. and VIII.B.4 with the sentences referring to the notification of study information to the Agency (substantial amendments to PASS protocols, progress reports and final reports) moved to GVP Module VIII Addendum I Rev 2;
- Change to VIII.B.4.3.2. (Format of study report) to add a section "Conclusion";
- Changes to VIII.B.8. (Impact on the risk management system) to only refer to GVP Module V;
- Changes to previous VIII.C.1.d./now VIII.C.1.4., revising the text on joint studies to emphasise the role of the Agency and national competent authority to systematically encourage submission of joint protocols;
- Updating of the structure to bring the Module in line with other GVP Modules as structuring has consolidated over time (previous B.1. and C.1. on scope moved to A and previous B.2. moved to A.1);
- Editorial amendments throughout the Module;
- Revision of nearly all sections of VIII. Appendix 1 in order to:
  - Provide updated and more detailed information on some study designs;
  - Revise the terminology where needed.

VIII.A. INTRODUCTION

Regulation (EC) No 726/2004, Directive 2001/83/EC and Commission Implementing Regulation (EU) No 520/2012 (hereinafter referred to as REG, DIR and IR) include provisions for post-authorisation safety studies applicable in the European Union (EU).

A post-authorisation safety study (PASS) is defined in DIR Art 1(15) as any study relating to an authorised medicinal product conducted with the aim of identifying, characterising or quantifying a safety hazard, confirming the safety profile of the medicinal product, or of measuring the effectiveness of risk management measures.

A PASS may be interventional or non-interventional. This Module concerns both interventional and non-interventional PASS, with a main focus on non-interventional ones. It does not concern pre-clinical safety studies.

Non-interventional PASS concerned by this guidance are those initiated, managed or financed by a marketing authorisation holder voluntarily or pursuant to an obligation imposed by an EU competent authority [DIR Art 107m(1), REG Art 28b].

Non-interventional PASS concerned can be:
- Imposed as an obligation in accordance with REG Art 9(4)(cb) and Art 10a(1)(a) and with DIR Art 21a(b) and Art 22a(1)(a) (category 1 of studies in GVP Module V);
- Imposed as a specific obligation in the framework of a marketing authorisation granted under exceptional circumstances (category 2 of studies in GVP Module V);
- Required in the risk management plan (RMP) to investigate a safety concern or to evaluate the effectiveness of risk minimisation activities (category 3 of studies in GVP Module V); or
- Conducted voluntarily by a marketing authorisation holder.

Non-interventional PASS shall be conducted in accordance with the following provisions:
- DIR Art 107m for non-interventional PASS initiated, managed or financed by a marketing authorisation holder voluntarily or pursuant to imposed obligations,
- DIR Art 107n-q, REG Art 28b and IR Art 36-38 for non-interventional PASS conducted pursuant to an obligation imposed by an EU competent authority (categories 1 and 2 of studies in GVP Module V).

A PASS is non-interventional if the following requirements are cumulatively fulfilled (see Volume 10 of The Rules Governing Medicinal Products in the European Union, Questions and Answers, Version 11.0, 15 May 2013, Question 1.10)[1]:
- The medicinal product is prescribed in the usual manner in accordance with the terms of the marketing authorisation;
- The assignment of the patient to a particular therapeutic strategy is not decided in advance by a trial protocol but falls within current practice and the prescription of the medicine is clearly separated from the decision to include the patient in the study; and
- No additional diagnostic or monitoring procedures are applied to the patients and epidemiological methods are used for the analysis of collected data.

Non-interventional studies are defined by the methodological approach used and not by its scientific objectives. Non-interventional studies include database research or review of records where all the events of interest have already happened (this may include case-control, cross-sectional, cohort or other study designs making secondary use of data). Non-interventional studies also include those involving primary data collection (e.g. prospective observational studies and registries in which the data collected derive from routine clinical care), provided that the conditions set out above are met. In these studies, interviews, questionnaires, blood samples and patient follow-up may be performed as part of normal clinical practice.

If a PASS is interventional, the provisions of Directive 2001/20/EC and of Volume 10 of The Rules Governing Medicinal Products in the European Union[2] shall apply.

The purposes of this Module are to:
- Provide general guidance for the transparency, scientific standards and quality standards of non-interventional PASS conducted voluntarily

---

1. http://ec.europa.eu/health/files/eudralex/vol-10/ctqa_v11.pdf
2. http://ec.europa.eu/health/documents/eudralex/vol-10/

or pursuant to an obligation imposed by an EU competent authority (VIII.B.);
- Describe procedures whereby an EU competent authority may impose on a marketing authorisation holder an obligation to conduct a PASS (VIII.C.1.);
- Describe procedures that apply to non-interventional PASS pursuant to an obligation imposed by an EU competent authority for the protocol oversight and reporting of results (VIII.C.2.) and for subsequent changes to the marketing authorisation (VIII.C.3.).

Legal requirements are identifiable by the modal verb "shall". Recommendations that are not legal requirements are provided using the modal verb "should". National and Union requirements for ensuring the well-being and rights of participants in non-interventional PASS shall also apply [DIR Art 107m(2)].

In VIII.B., some legal requirements which are mandatory to non-interventional PASS conducted pursuant to an obligation imposed by an EU competent authority are recommended for non-interventional PASS conducted voluntarily in order to support the same level of transparency, scientific standards and quality standards. This applies, for example, to the format and content of the study protocol and of the final study report and its abstract.

For non-interventional PASS, this guidance applies to studies that involve primary collection of safety data directly from patients and healthcare professionals as well as those that make secondary use of data previously collected from patients and healthcare professionals for another purpose.

VIII.A.1. Terminology

Date at which a study commences: date of the start of data collection.

Start of data collection: the date from which information on the first study subject is first recorded in the study dataset or, in the case of secondary use of data, the date from which data extraction starts [IR Art 37(1)]. Simple counts in a database to support the development of the study protocol, for example, to inform the sample size and statistical precision of the study, are not part of this definition.

End of data collection: the date from which the analytical dataset is completely available [IR Art 37(2)].

Analytical dataset: the minimum set of data required to perform the statistical analyses leading to the results for the primary objective(s) of the study.

Substantial amendment to the study protocol: amendment to the protocol likely to have an impact on the safety, physical or mental well-being of the study participants or that may affect the study results and their interpretation, such as changes to the primary or secondary objectives of the study, the study population, the sample size, the study design, the data sources, the method of data collection, the definitions of the main exposure, outcome and confounding variables or the statistical analytical plan as described in the study protocol.

VIII.B. STRUCTURES AND PROCESSES

VIII.B.1. Principles

In the light of DIR Art 1(15), a post-authorisation study should be classified as a post-authorisation safety study when the main aim for initiating the study includes any of the following objectives:
- To quantify potential or identified risks, e.g. to characterise the incidence rate, estimate the rate ratio or rate difference in comparison to a non-exposed population or a population exposed to another medicinal product or class of medicinal products as appropriate, and investigate risk factors, including effect modifiers;
- To evaluate the risks of a medicinal product used in a patient population for which safety information is limited or missing (e.g. pregnant women, specific age groups, patients with renal or hepatic impairment or other relevant comorbidity or co-medication);
- To evaluate the risks of a medicinal product after long-term use;
- To provide evidence about the absence of risks;
- To assess patterns of drug utilisation that add knowledge regarding the safety of the medicinal product or the effectiveness of a risk management measure (e.g. collection of information on indication, off-label use,

dosage, co-medication or medication errors in clinical practice that may influence safety, as well as studies that provide an estimate of the public health impact of any safety concern);
- To measure the effectiveness of a risk management measures.

Whereas the PASS design should be appropriate to address the study objective(s), the classification of a post-authorisation study as a PASS is not constrained by the type of design chosen if it fulfils the criteria as set in DIR Art 1(15). For example, a systematic literature review or a meta-analysis may be considered as PASS depending on its aim.

Relevant scientific guidance should be considered by marketing authorisation holders and investigators for the development of study protocols, the conduct of studies and the writing of study reports, and by the Pharmacovigilance Risk Assessment Committee (PRAC) and national competent authorities for the evaluation of study protocols and study reports. Relevant scientific guidance includes, amongst others, the ENCePP Guide on Methodological Standards in Pharmacoepidemiology[3], the ENCePP Checklist for Study Protocols[4], the Guideline on Conduct of Pharmacovigilance for Medicines Used by the Paediatric Population[5], and the Guidelines for Good Pharmacoepidemiology Practices of the International Society of Pharmacoepidemiology (ISPE GPP)[6].

For studies that are funded by a marketing authorisation holder, including studies developed, conducted or analysed fully or partially by investigators who are not employees of the marketing authorisation holder, the marketing authorisation holder should ensure that the investigators are qualified by education, training and experience to perform their tasks. The research contract between the marketing authorisation holder and investigators should ensure that the study meets its regulatory obligations while permitting their scientific expertise to be exercised throughout the research process. In the research contract, the marketing authorisation holder should consider the provisions of the ENCePP Code of Conduct[7], and address the following aspects:
- Rationale, main objectives and brief description of the intended methods of the research to be carried out by the investigator(s);
- Rights and obligations of the investigator(s) and marketing authorisation holder;
- Clear assignment of tasks and responsibilities;
- Procedure for achieving agreement on the study protocol;
- Provisions for meeting the marketing authorisation holder's pharmacovigilance obligations, including the reporting of adverse reactions and other safety data by investigators, where applicable;
- Intellectual property rights arising from the study and access to study data;
- Storage and availability of analytical dataset and statistical programmes for audit and inspection;
- Communication strategy for the scheduled progress and final reports;
- Publication strategy of interim and final results.

Non-interventional post-authorisation safety studies shall not be performed where the act of conducting the study promotes the use of a medicinal product [DIR Art 107m(3)]. This requirement applies to all studies and to all activities performed in the study, including for studies conducted by the personnel of the marketing authorisation holder and by third parties on behalf of the marketing authorisation holder.

Payments to healthcare professionals for participating shall be restricted to compensation for time and expenses incurred [DIR Art 107m(4)].

VIII.B.2. Study Registration

For non-interventional PASS conducted pursuant to an obligation imposed by an EU competent authority, the date of study registration in the electronic study register shall be included as a milestone in the final study report [IR Annex III]. For this purpose, the EU PAS Register maintained by the Agency and accessible through the European

---

3. http://www.encepp.eu/standards_and_guidances/methodologicalGuide.shtml
4. http://www.encepp.eu/standards_and_guidances/checkListProtocols.shtml
5. http://www.ema.europa.eu
6. http://www.pharmacoepi.org/resources/.guidelines_08027.cfm
7. http://www.encepp.eu/code_of_conduct/documents/ENCePPCodeofConduct_Rev3.pdf
8. http://www.encepp.eu/encepp_studies/indexRegister.shtml

medicines web-portal serves as the electronic study register[8].

In order to support transparency on all non-interventional PASS and to facilitate exchange of pharmacovigilance information between the Agency, national competent authorities and marketing authorisation holders, the marketing authorisation holders should also enter in the EU PAS Register all non-interventional PASS required in the risk management plan agreed in the EU or conducted voluntarily in the EU.

Non-interventional PASS should be registered in the EU PAS Register before the study commences or at the earliest possible date, for example if data collection had already started for a study included in the risk management plan. The study protocol should be uploaded as soon as possible after its finalisation and prior to the start of data collection. Updated study protocols in case of substantial amendments, progress reports and the final study report should also be entered in the register (as soon as possible and preferably within two weeks after their finalisation). Study information should normally be submitted in English. If the study protocol or the study report is written in another language, the marketing authorisation should facilitate access to study information by including an English translation of the title, the abstract of the study protocol and the abstract of the final study report.

Where prior publication of the protocol could threaten the validity of the study (for example, in studies with primary data collection where prior knowledge of the study objective could lead to information bias) or the protection of intellectual rights, a study protocol with redactions made by the marketing authorisation holder may be entered into the register prior to the start of data collection. These redactions should be justified and kept to the minimum necessary for the objective aimed by the redaction process. Whenever a redacted study protocol is published prior to the start of data collection, the title page of the protocol should include the mention "Redacted protocol" and the complete study protocol should be made available to the Agency and national competent authorities upon request. The complete study protocol should be entered in the register as soon as possible and preferably within two weeks after the end of data collection.

VIII.B.3. Study Protocol

Non-interventional PASS conducted pursuant to an obligation imposed by an EU competent authority or conducted voluntarily shall have a written study protocol. The study protocol should be developed by individuals with appropriate scientific background and experience. An overview of study designs and databases frequently used in post-authorisation safety studies is provided in VIII.App.1.

For non-interventional PASS imposed as an obligation, the draft study protocol shall be submitted by the marketing authorisation holder to the PRAC or to the national competent authority of the Member State that requested the study if the study is conducted in only one Member State [DIR Art 107n(1)] (see VIII. C.2.).

The marketing authorisation holder may be required by the national competent authority to submit the protocol to the competent authorities of the Member States in which the study is conducted [DIR Art 107m(5)]. Requirements and recommendations for submission of the study protocol to the Agency and national competent authorities are specified in GVP Module VIII Addendum I.

In order to ensure compliance of the marketing authorisation holder with its pharmacovigilance obligations, the qualified person responsible for pharmacovigilance (QPPV) or his/her delegate should be involved in the review and sign-off of study protocols required in the risk management plan agreed in the EU or conducted voluntarily in the EU (see GVP Module I).

Where applicable, the marketing authorisation holder's pharmacovigilance contact person at national level should be informed of any study sponsored or conducted by the marketing authorisation holder in that Member State and have access to the protocol.

VIII.B.3.1. Format and content of the study protocol

For non-interventional PASS conducted pursuant to an obligation imposed by an EU competent authority, the study protocol shall follow the format described in this section [IR Annex III]. This format should also be followed for non-interventional

PASS required in the risk management plan agreed in the EU or conducted voluntarily in the EU.
1. **Title:** informative title including a commonly used term indicating the study design and the medicinal product, substance or medicinal product class concerned, and a sub-title with a version identifier and the date of the last version. If the study protocol has been registered in the EU PAS Register, subsequent versions of the protocol should mention on the title page "EU PAS Register No:" with the registration number.
2. **Marketing authorisation holder:** name and address of the marketing authorisation holder.
3. **Responsible parties:** names, titles, qualifications, addresses, and affiliations of all main responsible parties, including the main author(s) of the protocol, the principal investigator, a coordinating investigator for each country in which the study is to be performed and other relevant study sites. A list of all collaborating institutions and investigators should be made available to the Agency and national competent authorities upon request.
4. **Abstract:** stand-alone summary of the study protocol including the following sub-sections:
   – Title with subtitles including version and date of the protocol and name and affiliation of main author
   – Rationale and background
   – Research question and objectives
   – Study design
   – Population
   – Variables
   – Data sources
   – Study size
   – Data analysis
   – Milestones.
5. **Amendments and updates:** any substantial amendment and update to the study protocol after the start of data collection, including a justification for each amendment or update, dates of each change and a reference to the section of the protocol where the change has been made.
6. **Milestones:** table with planned dates for the following milestones:
   – Start of data collection
   – End of data collection
   – Study progress report(s) as referred to in Article 107m(5) of Directive 2001/83/EC (see VIII.B.4.3.1.)
   – Interim report(s) of study results, where applicable, in line with phases of data analyses (see VIII.B.4.3.1.)
   – Final report of study results (see VIII.B.4.3.2.).
   Any other important timelines in the conduct of the study should be presented.
7. **Rationale and background:** short description of the safety hazard(s), the safety profile or the risk management measures that led to the initiation or imposition of the study, and short critical review of relevant published and unpublished data to explain gaps in knowledge that the study is intended to fill. The review may encompass relevant animal and human experiments, clinical studies, vital statistics and previous epidemiologic studies. The review should cite the findings of similar studies, and the expected contribution of the current study.
8. **Research question and objectives:** research question that explains how the study will address the issue which led to the study being initiated or imposed, and research objectives, including any pre-specified hypotheses and main summary measures.
9. **Research methods:** description of the research methods, including:
9.1. **Study design:** overall research design and rationale for this choice.
9.2. **Setting:** study population defined in terms of persons, place, time period, and selection criteria, including the rationale for any inclusion and exclusion criteria. Where any sampling from a source population is undertaken, description of the source population and details of sampling methods should be provided. Where the study design is a systematic review or a meta-analysis, the criteria for the selection and eligibility of studies should be explained.
9.3. **Variables:** outcomes, exposures and other variables including measured risk factors should be addressed separately, including operational definitions; potential confounding variables and effect modifiers should be specified.
9.4. **Data sources:** strategies and data sources for determining exposures, outcomes and all other variables relevant to the study objectives, such as potential confounding variables and effect modifiers. Where the study will use an existing data source,

such as electronic health records, any information on the validity of the recording and coding of the data should be reported. In case of a systematic review or meta-analysis, the search strategy and processes and any methods for confirming data from investigators should be described. If data collection methods or instruments are tested in a pilot study, plans for the pilot study should be presented. If a pilot study has already been performed, a summary of the results should be reported. Involvement of any expert committees to validate diagnoses should be stated.

9.5. **Study size:** any projected study size, precision sought for study estimates and any calculation of the sample size that can minimally detect a pre-specified risk with a pre-specified statistical precision.

9.6. **Data management:** data management and statistical programmes to be used in the study, including procedures for data collection, retrieval and preparation.

9.7. **Data analysis:** the major steps that lead from raw data to a final result, including methods used to correct inconsistencies or errors, impute values, modify raw data, categorise, analyse and present results, and procedures to control sources of bias and their influence on results; statistical procedures to be applied to the data to obtain point estimates and confidence intervals of measures of occurrence or association, and sensitivity analyses. The primary analyses should be clearly identified from sub-group analyses and secondary analyses.

9.8. **Quality control:** description of any mechanisms and procedures to ensure data quality and integrity, including accuracy and legibility of collected data and original documents, extent of source data verification and validation of endpoints, storage of records and archiving of statistical programmes. As appropriate, certification and/or qualifications of any supporting laboratory or research groups should be included.

9.9. **Limitations of the research methods:** any potential limitations of the study design, data sources, and analytic methods, including issues relating to confounding, bias, generalisability, and random error. The likely success of efforts taken to reduce errors should be discussed.

10. **Protection of human subjects:** safeguards in order to comply with national and European Union requirements for ensuring the well-being and rights of participants in non-interventional post-authorisation safety studies.

11. **Management and reporting of adverse events/adverse reactions:** procedures for the collection, management and reporting of individual cases of suspected adverse reactions and of and other medically important events while the study is being conducted that might influence the evaluation of the risk-benefit balance of the product while the study is being conducted.

For studies with primary data collection where information on certain adverse events will not be collected (see GVP Module VI), the marketing authorisation holder should provide in the protocol a justification for the overall approach to the collection of safety data. Any reference to adverse events that will not be collected should be made using the appropriate level of the MedDRA classification. If information on certain adverse events will not be collected, the channels and documents to be used to inform the healthcare professionals and consumers of the possibility to report adverse reactions to the marketing authorisation holder or to the national spontaneous reporting system should be included in this section (see GVP Module VI). In certain circumstances where suspected adverse reactions with fatal outcome will not be subject to expedited reporting as individual case safety reports (see GVP Module VI), each of these adverse reactions should be listed in a table using the appropriate level of the MedDRA classification with a rationale for not reporting them.

A statement should indicate if the study is only based on secondary use of data for which all adverse events must be collected but the reporting of suspected adverse reactions in the form of individual case safety reports is not required (see GVP Module VI).

For combined study designs with primary and secondary data collection, the same requirements as for studies with primary data collection should be followed (see GVP Module VI).

12. **Plans for disseminating and communicating study results**, including any plans for submission of progress reports and final reports.
13. **References.**

The format of the study protocol should follow the Guidance for the Format and Content of the Protocol of Non-Interventional Post-Authorisation Safety Studies[9].

Feasibility or pilot studies that were carried out to support the development of the protocol, for example, the testing of a questionnaire or simple counts of medical events or prescriptions in a database to determine the statistical precision of the study, should be reported in the appropriate section of the study protocol with a summary of their methods and results. The full report should be made available to the Agency and national competent authorities upon request. Feasibility or pilot studies that are part of the research process should be described in the protocol, for example, a pilot evaluation of the study questionnaire(s) used for the first set of patients recruited into the study.

An annex should list all separate documents and list or include any additional or complementary information on specific aspects not previously addressed (e.g. questionnaires, case report forms), with clear document references.

VIII.B.3.2. Substantial Amendments to the Study Protocol

The study protocol should be amended and updated as needed throughout the course of the study. Any substantial amendments to the protocol after the study start should be documented in the protocol in a traceable and auditable way including the dates of the changes. If changes to the protocol lead to the study being considered an interventional clinical trial, the national competent authorities and the Agency should be informed immediately. The study shall subsequently be conducted in accordance with Directive 2001/20/EC and Volume 10 of The Rules Governing Medicinal Products in the European Union.

For non-interventional PASS conducted pursuant to an obligation imposed by an EU competent authority, see VIII.C.2. for the submission of substantial amendments to the study protocol.

Requirements and recommendations for the submission of substantial amendments to the study protocol are specified in GVP Module VIII Addendum I.

VIII.B.4. Reporting of Pharmacovigilance Data to Competent Authorities

VIII.B.4.1. Data Relevant to the Risk-Benefit Balance of the Product

The marketing authorisation holder shall monitor the data generated while the study is being conducted and consider their implications for the risk-benefit balance of the medicinal product concerned [DIR Art. 107m(7)]. Any new information that may affect the risk-benefit balance of the medicinal product should be communicated immediately in writing as an emerging safety issue to competent authorities of the Member States in which the product is authorised and to the Agency via email (P-PV-emerging-safety-issue@ema.europa.eu). Information affecting the risk-benefit balance of the medicinal product may include an analysis of adverse reactions and aggregated data.

This communication is without prejudice of the information on the findings of studies which should be provided by means of periodic safety update reports (PSURs) (see GVP Module VII) and in the RMP updates (see GVP Module V), where applicable.

VIII.B.4.2. Reporting of Adverse Reactions/Adverse Events

Adverse reactions/adverse events should be reported to competent authorities in accordance with the provisions of GVP Module VI. Procedures for the collection, management (including a review by the marketing authorisation holder if appropriate) and reporting of suspected adverse reactions/adverse events should be put in place and summarised in the study protocol. If appropriate, reference can be made to the pharmacovigilance system master file (see GVP Module II) but details

---
9. www.ema.europa.eu

specific to the study should be described in the study protocol.

VIII.B.4.3. Study Reports

VIII.B.4.3.1. Progress Report and Interim Report of Study Results

The progress report is meant to include relevant information to document the progress of the study, for example, the number of patients who have entered the study, the number of exposed patients or the number of patients presenting the outcome, problems encountered and deviations from the expected plan. The progress report may include an interim report of study results.

The interim report of study results is meant to include results of any planned interim analysis of study data before or after the end of data collection.

Upon request from a national competent authority, progress reports for PASS imposed as an obligation or conducted voluntarily shall be submitted to the competent authorities of the Member States in which the study is conducted [DIR Art 107m(5)]. They may also be requested by the Agency for PASS concerning centrally-authorised products. Requests for progress reports may be made before the study commences or any time during the study conduct. They may be guided by the communication of risk-benefit information arising from the study or the need for information about the study progress in the context of regulatory procedures or important safety communication about the product. Requirements and recommendations for submission of progress reports are specified in GVP Module VIII Addendum I.

The timing of the submission of progress reports should be agreed with the relevant competent authorities and specified in the study protocol when they have been agreed before the study commences.

VIII.B.4.3.2. Final Study Report

For non-interventional PASS conducted pursuant to an obligation imposed by an EU competent authority, the final study report shall follow the format described in this section [IR Annex III] and shall be submitted within 12 months of the end of data collection [DIR Art 107p(1)] (see VIII.C.2.). This format and timeline should also be followed for PASS required in the risk management plan agreed in the EU or conducted voluntarily in the EU.

Requirements and recommendations for submission of the final study report are specified in Module VIII Addendum I.

If a study is discontinued, a final report should be submitted and the reasons for terminating the study should be provided.

The final study report should include the following information:

1. **Title:** title including a commonly used term indicating the study design; sub-titles with date of final report and name and affiliation of main author. If the study has been registered in the EU PAS Register, the final study report should mention on the title page "EU PAS Register No:" with the registration number and the web link to the study record.
2. **Abstract:** stand-alone summary in the format presented below [IR Annex III].
3. **Marketing authorisation holder:** name and address of the marketing authorisation holder.
4. **Investigators:** names, titles, degrees, addresses and affiliations of the principal investigator and all co-investigators, and list of all collaborating primary institutions and other relevant study sites. Such information should be provided for each country in which the study is to be performed and other relevant study sites. A list of all collaborating institutions and investigators should be made available to the Agency and national competent authorities upon request.
5. **Milestones:** dates for the following milestones:
   - Start of data collection (planned and actual dates)
   - End of data collection (planned and actual dates) or date of early termination, if applicable, with reasons for termination
   - Study progress report(s) (see VIII.B.4.3.1.)
   - Interim report(s) of study results, where applicable (see VIII.B.4.3.1.)
   - Final report of study results (planned and actual date)
   - Any other important milestone applicable to the study, including date of study registration in the EU PAS Register and date of protocol approval by an Institutional Review Board/Independent Ethics Committee if applicable.
6. **Rationale and background:** description of the safety concerns that led to the study being

initiated or imposed, and critical review of relevant published and unpublished data evaluating pertinent information and gaps in knowledge that the study is intended to fill.

7. **Research question and objectives:** research question and research objectives, including any pre-specified hypotheses, as stated in the study protocol.
8. **Amendments and updates to the protocol:** list of any substantial amendments and updates to the initial study protocol after the start of data collection, including a justification for each amendment or update.
9. **Research methods:**
   9.1. **Study design:** key elements of the study design and the rationale for this choice.
   9.2. **Setting:** setting, locations, and relevant dates for the study, including periods of recruitment, follow-up, and data collection. In case of a systematic review or meta-analysis, study characteristics used as criteria for eligibility, with rationale.
   9.3. **Subjects:** any source population and eligibility criteria of study subjects. Sources and methods of selection of participants should be provided, including, where relevant methods for case ascertainment, as well as number of and reasons for dropouts.
   9.4. **Variables:** all outcomes, exposures, predictors, potential confounders, and effect modifiers, including operational definitions and diagnostic criteria, if applicable.
   9.5. **Data sources and measurement:** for each variable of interest, sources of data and details of methods of assessment and measurement. If the study has used an existing data source, such as electronic health records, any information on the validity of the recording and coding of the data should be reported. In case of a systematic review or meta-analysis, description of all information sources, search strategy, methods for selecting studies, methods of data extraction and any processes for obtaining or confirming data from investigators.
   9.6. **Bias:** any efforts to assess and address potential sources of bias at the design stage.
   9.7. **Study size:** study size, rationale for any study size calculation and any method for attaining projected study size.
   9.8. **Data transformation:** transformations, calculations or operations on the data, including how quantitative data were handled in the analyses and which groupings were chosen and why.
   9.9. **Statistical methods:** description of the following items:
   - Main summary measures
   - All statistical methods applied to the study, including those used to control for confounding and, for meta-analyses, methods for combining results of studies
   - Any methods used to examine subgroups and interactions
   - How missing data were addressed
   - Any sensitivity analyses
   - Any amendment to the plan of data analysis included in the study protocol, with rationale for the change.
   9.10. **Quality control:** mechanisms to ensure data quality and integrity.
10. **Results:** presentation of tables, graphs, and illustrations to present the pertinent data and reflect the analyses performed. Both unadjusted and adjusted results should be presented. Precision of estimates should be quantified using confidence intervals. This section should include the following sub-sections:
    10.1. **Participants:** numbers of study subjects at each stage of study, e.g. numbers potentially eligible, examined for eligibility, confirmed eligible, included in the study, completing follow-up, and analysed, and reasons for non-participation at any stage. In the case of a systematic review or meta-analysis, number of studies screened, assessed for eligibility and included in the review with reasons for exclusion at each stage.
    10.2. **Descriptive data:** characteristics of study participants, information on

exposures and potential confounders and number of participants with missing data for each variable of interest. In case of a systematic review or meta-analysis, characteristics of each study from which data were extracted (e.g. study size, follow-up).
10.3. **Outcome data:** numbers of participants across categories of main outcomes.
10.4. **Main results:** unadjusted estimates and, if applicable, confounder-adjusted estimates and their precision (e.g. 95% confidence interval). If relevant, estimates of relative risk should be translated into absolute risk for a meaningful time period.
10.5. **Other analyses:** other analyses done, e.g. analyses of subgroups and interactions, and sensitivity analyses.
10.6. **Adverse events and adverse reactions:** summary of all adverse events/adverse reactions reported in the study, in line with requirements described in GVP Module VI.
11. **Discussion:**
11.1. **Key results:** key results with reference to the study objectives, prior research in support of and conflicting with the findings of the completed post-authorisation safety study, and, where relevant, impact of the results on the risk-benefit balance of the product.
11.2. **Limitations:** limitations of the study taking into account circumstances that may have affected the quality or integrity of the data, limitations of the study approach and methods used to address them (e.g. response rates, missing or incomplete data, imputations applied), sources of potential bias and imprecision and validation of the events. Both direction and magnitude of potential biases should be discussed.
11.3. **Interpretation:** interpretation of results considering objectives, limitations, multiplicity of analyses, results from similar studies and other relevant evidence.
11.4. **Generalisability:** the generalisability (external validity) of the study results.
12. **Other information:** any additional or complementary information on specific aspects not previously addressed.
13. **Conclusions:** main conclusions of the study deriving from the analysis of the data.
14. **References.**

The format of the final study report should follow the Guidance for the Format and Content of the Final Study Report of Non-Interventional Post-Authorisation Safety Studies[10].

The abstract of the final study report should include a summary of the study methods and findings presented in the following format:
1. Title, with subtitles including date of the abstract and name and affiliation of main author
2. Keywords (not more than five keywords indicating the main study characteristics)
3. Rationale and background
4. Research question and objectives
5. Study design
6. Setting
7. Subjects and study size (including dropouts)
8. Variables and data sources
9. Results
10. Discussion (including, where relevant, an evaluation of the impact of study results on the risk-benefit balance of the product)
11. Conclusion
12. Marketing authorisation holder
13. Names and affiliations of principal investigators.

VIII.B.5. Publication of Study Results

For studies that are fully or partially conducted by investigators who are not employees of the marketing authorisation holder, the marketing authorisation holder and the investigator should agree in advance on a publication policy allowing the principal investigator to independently prepare publications based on the study results irrespective of data ownership. The marketing authorisation holder should be entitled to view the results and interpretations included in the manuscript and provide comments prior to submission of the manuscript for publication.

---

10. www.ema.europa.eu

VIII.B.5.1. Submission of Manuscripts Accepted for Publication

In order to allow competent authorities to review in advance the results and interpretations to be published, the marketing authorisation holder initiating, managing or financing a non-interventional PASS should communicate to the Agency and the competent authorities of the Member States in which the product is authorised the final manuscript of the article within two weeks after first acceptance for publication.

VIII.B.6. Data Protection

Marketing authorisation holders and investigators shall follow relevant national legislation and guidance of those Member States where the study is being conducted [DIR Art 107m(2)]. The legislation on data protection must be followed in accordance with Directive 95/46/EC of the European Parliament and of the Council on the protection of individuals with regard to the processing of personal data and on the free movement of such data.

For non-interventional PASS imposed as an obligation, the marketing authorisation holder shall ensure that all study information is handled and stored so as to allow for accurate reporting, interpretation and verification of that information and shall ensure that the confidentiality of the records of the study subjects remains protected [IR Art 36]. This provision should be also followed for PASS required in the risk management plan agreed in the EU or conducted voluntarily in the EU.

VIII.B.7. Quality Systems, Audits and Inspections

The marketing authorisation holder shall ensure the fulfilment of its pharmacovigilance obligations in relation to the study and that this can be audited, inspected and verified. For PASS imposed as an obligation, the marketing authorisation holder shall ensure that the analytical dataset and statistical programmes used for generating the data included in the final study report are kept in electronic format and are available for auditing and inspection [IR 12, IR Art 36].

For PASS required in the risk management plan agreed in the EU or conducted voluntarily in the EU, record management and data retention shall follow the provisions of IR Art 12.

VIII.B.8. Impact on the Risk Management System

Information on non-interventional PASS conducted pursuant to an obligation imposed by an EU competent authority or required in the risk management plan should be included in the risk management plan as described in GVP Module V.

VIII.C. OPERATION OF THE EU NETWORK

VIII.C.1. Procedure for Imposing Post-Authorisation Safety Studies

In the EU, the conduct of any post-authorisation safety study (PASS) can be imposed by the Agency or the national competent authority as applicable during the evaluation of the initial marketing authorisation application [REG Art 9(4)(cb), DIR Art 21a(b)] or during the post-authorisation phase [REG Art 10a(1)(a), DIR Art 22a(1)(a)], whenever there are concerns about the risks of an authorised medicinal product for which PASS results would significantly impact on the risk-benefit of the product. This obligation shall be duly justified, shall be notified in writing and shall include the objectives and timeframe for the submission and conduct of the study. The request may also include recommendations on key elements of the study (e.g. study design, setting, exposure(s), outcome(s), study population).

VIII.C.1.1. Request for a Post-authorisation Safety Study As Part of the Initial Marketing Authorisation Application

A marketing authorisation may be granted subject to the conduct of a PASS. If, during the evaluation of a marketing authorisation application, the need for a PASS is identified, the PRAC may adopt an advice with an assessment report to the Committee for Medicinal Products for Human Use (CHMP) or to the Member State that requested such advice as applicable.

VIII.C.1.2. Request for a Post-authorisation Safety Study during a Post-authorisation Regulatory Procedure

The need for a PASS could be identified by the Agency or a national competent authority during a post-authorisation regulatory procedure, for example, an extension or a variation to a marketing authorisation, a renewal procedure or a PSUR procedure. If, during the evaluation of a post-authorisation procedure, the need for a PASS is identified, the PRAC may adopt an advice or a recommendation with an assessment report to the CHMP or the Member States as applicable.

VIII.C.1.3. Request for a Post-authorisation Safety Study due to an Emerging Safety Concern

After the granting of the marketing authorisation, the Agency or a national competent authority, as applicable, may impose on the marketing authorisation holder an obligation to conduct a post-authorisation safety study if there are concerns about the risk of the authorised medicinal product. If the need for a PASS is identified, the PRAC may adopt an advice or a recommendation with an assessment report to the CHMP or the Member States as applicable.

VIII.C.1.4. Joint Post-authorisation Safety Studies

If safety concerns apply to more than one medicinal product, the Agency or the national competent authority shall, following consultation with the PRAC, encourage the marketing authorisation holders concerned to conduct a joint PASS [REG Art 10a(1)(a), DIR Art 22a(1)(a)]. Requests to the marketing authorisation holders should contain the justification for the request of a joint study and may include core elements for the study protocol. The national competent authority or the Agency should support interactions between the concerned marketing authorisation holders and providing suggestions for the joint study proposal.

VIII.C.1.5. Written Observations in Response to the Imposition of an Obligation

Within 30 days of receipt of the written notification of an obligation imposed, the marketing authorisation holder may request to present written observations in response to the imposition of the obligation [REG Art 10a(2), DIR Art 22a(2)]. The national competent authority or the Agency shall specify a time limit for the provision of these observations. On the basis of the written observations submitted by the marketing authorisation holder, the national competent authority or the European Commission shall withdraw or confirm the obligation. When the obligation is confirmed, the marketing authorisation shall be varied to include the obligation as a condition of the marketing authorisation and the risk management plan, where applicable, shall be updated accordingly [REG Art 10a(3), DIR Art 22a(3)] (see GVP Module V).

VIII.C.2. Supervision of Non-interventional Post-authorisation Safety Studies Conducted Pursuant to an Obligation

Non-interventional PASS conducted pursuant to obligations imposed by a competent authority in the EU (categories 1 and 2 of studies in GVP Module V) are supervised and assessed by the PRAC, unless for PASS requested by a national competent authority of a single Member State according to DIR Art 22a and conducted only in that Member State, where national oversight procedures will apply [DIR Art 107n(1)].

VIII.C.2.1. Roles and Responsibilities of the Marketing Authorisation Holder

If the study is a non-interventional study (see VIII.A.), the marketing authorisation holder shall ensure that the study meets the requirements applicable to non-interventional PASS set out in DIR Art 107m-q, REG Art 28b, IR Art 36-38 and this Module. The marketing authorisation holder shall ensure the fulfilment of its pharmacovigilance

---

11. http://ec.europa.eu/health/documents/eudralex/vol-10/

obligations in relation to the study and that this fulfilment can be audited, inspected and verified (see VIII.B.6. and VIII.B.7.).

Following the imposing as a condition to the marketing authorisation to conduct a non-interventional PASS, the marketing authorisation holder shall develop a study protocol and submit it to the national competent authority or the PRAC for review [DIR Art 107n(1)] as appropriate. The marketing authorisation holder has the responsibility to ensure that the study is not a clinical trial, in which case Directive 2001/20/EC and Volume 10 of The Rules Governing Medicinal Products in the European Union[11] shall apply.

The study may commence only when the written endorsement from the national competent authority or the PRAC, as appropriate, has been issued. When a letter of endorsement has been issued by the PRAC, the marketing authorisation holder shall forward the protocol to the national competent authority of the Member State(s) in which the study is to be conducted and may thereafter commence the study according to the endorsed protocol [DIR Art 107n(3)]. EU and national requirements shall be followed to ensure the well-being and rights of participants in the study [DIR Art 107m(2)].

Prior to submission of the protocol, the marketing authorisation holder may submit a request to the national competent authority or the Agency, as appropriate, for a pre-submission meeting (with the Agency and the PRAC rapporteur in case the request is submitted to the Agency) in order to clarify specific aspects of the requested study (such as study objectives, study population, definition of exposure and outcomes) and to facilitate the development of the protocol in accordance with the objectives determined by the national competent authority or the PRAC.

After a non-interventional imposed PASS has been commenced, the marketing authorisation holder shall submit any substantial amendments to the protocol, before their implementation, to the national competent authority or to the PRAC, as appropriate [DIR Art 107o] (see VIII.A.1. for the definition of a substantial amendment).

Upon completion of the study, the marketing authorisation holder shall submit a final study report, including a public abstract, to the national competent authority or to the PRAC as soon as possible and not later than 12 months after the end of data collection, unless a written waiver has been granted by the national competent authority or the PRAC, as appropriate [DIR Art 107p(1)].

When the PRAC is responsible for supervision of the PASS, the marketing authorisation holder should request the waiver in writing to the Agency at least three months before the due date for the submission of the report. The request should include a justification for the waiver. The request should be assessed by the PRAC rapporteur and granted or rejected by the PRAC on the basis of the justification and timeline submitted by the marketing authorisation holder.

The marketing authorisation holder shall submit the study protocol, the abstract of the final study report and the final study report in English except for studies to be conducted in only one Member State that requests the study according to DIR Art 22a. For the latter studies, the marketing authorisation holder shall provide an English translation of the title and abstract of the study protocol as well as an English translation of the abstract of the final study report [IR Art 36].

VIII.C.2.2. Roles and Responsibilities of the PRAC and the National Competent Authority

Within 60 days from submission of the draft protocol, the national competent authority or the PRAC, as appropriate, shall issue a letter endorsing the draft protocol, a letter of objection or a letter notifying the marketing authorisation holder that the study is a clinical trial falling under the scope of Directive 2001/20/EC. The letter of objection shall set out in detail the grounds for the objection in any of the following cases:

- It is considered that the conduct of the study promotes the use of a medicinal product;
- It is considered that the design of the study does not fulfil the study objectives [DIR Art 107n(2)].

If the study proves to be interventional, the PRAC or the national competent authority as applicable should issue an explanatory statement to the marketing authorisation holder that the study is a clinical trial falling under the scope of Directive 2001/20/EC.

When the PRAC is involved in the oversight of the study, the PRAC will nominate a PRAC rapporteur responsible for the supervision of the

PASS. The PRAC rapporteur should draft a protocol assessment report and submit it for review and approval by the PRAC.

In case of submission of an amended study protocol, the national competent authority or the PRAC, as appropriate, shall assess the amendments and inform the marketing authorisation holder of its endorsement or objection [DIR Art 107o]. The national competent authority or the PRAC will provide the marketing authorisation holder with a letter of endorsement or objection to the protocol amendment within 60 days of submission. The letter of objection will provide a timeline by which the marketing authorisation holder should resubmit an amended version of the protocol.

Where the study protocol is assessed by a national competent authority, this national competent authority should share its assessment with the other concerned Member States where the product is authorised.

Concerning the assessment of study results, in cases where the PRAC is involved in the oversight of the study, the PRAC will produce an assessment report and issue a recommendation that will be addressed to the CHMP or CMDh, as applicable.

VIII.C.2.3. Roles and Responsibilities of the Agency

The Agency shall provide scientific secretariat to the PRAC.

The Agency will inform the marketing authorisation holder in writing and within the appropriate timelines of the decisions of the PRAC with respect to the assessment of the following:
- Study protocol;
- Study protocol amendments;
- Final study report;
- Waiver request for the submission of the final study report.

When the marketing authorisation holder submits a request to the Agency for a pre-submission meeting, the Agency will be responsible for a timely set up of the meeting with the Agency and the PRAC rapporteur.

The Agency shall make public on the European medicines web-portal protocols and public abstracts of results of the post-authorisation safety studies referred to in DIR Art 107n and 107p.

VIII.C.3. Changes to the Marketing Authorisation Following Results from a Non-Interventional Post-Authorisation Safety Study

The marketing authorisation holder shall submit a final study report to the national competent authority or the PRAC as applicable within 12 months of the end of data collection unless a written waiver has been granted [DIR Art 107p(1)].

The marketing authorisation holder shall evaluate whether the study results have an impact on the marketing authorisation and shall, if necessary, submit to the national competent authorities or the Agency an application to vary the marketing authorisation [DIR Art 107p(2)]. In such case, the variation should be submitted to the national competent authority or the Agency.

Following the review of the final study report, the PRAC or a national competent authority in a Member State may recommend variation, suspension or revocation of the marketing authorisation [REG Art 28b(2), DIR Art 107q(2)]. The recommendation by the PRAC shall mention any divergent positions and the grounds on which they are based [DIR Art 107q(1)].

Where at least one centrally-authorised product is concerned by the final study results, the recommendation made by the PRAC shall be transmitted to the CHMP which shall adopt an opinion taking into account the recommendation. When the opinion of the CHMP differs from the recommendation of the PRAC, the CHMP shall attach to its opinion a detailed explanation of the scientific grounds for the differences [REG Art 28b(2)].

Where nationally authorised products are concerned by the final study results, the Member States represented within the CMDh shall agree a position taking into account the PRAC recommendation and include a timetable for the implementation of this agreed position. When a consensus agreement is reached, the agreed position shall be sent by the CMDh to the marketing authorisation holder and Member States which should adopt necessary measures to vary, suspend or revoke the marketing authorisation in line with the implementation timetable of the CMDh. In case a variation is agreed upon, the marketing authorisation holder shall submit to the national competent authorities an appropriate application for a variation, including an updated summary of product characteristics (SmPC) and package leaflet within the determined timetable for implementation [DIR Art 107q(2)]. In case an agreement by consensus cannot be reached, the position of the majority of the Member States represented within the CMDh should be forwarded to the Commission who shall apply the procedure laid down in DIR Art 33 and 34 [DIR Art 107q(2)].

Where the agreement or position of the CMDh differs from the recommendation of the PRAC, the CMDh shall attach to the agreement or majority position a detailed explanation of the scientific grounds for differences together with the recommendation [DIR Art 107q(2)].

More urgent action may be required in certain circumstances, for example, based on interim results included in progress reports (see also VIII.B.4.3.1.). In such case, an appropriate procedure will be initiated (see GVP Module VI).

VIII. APPENDIX 1. METHODS FOR POST-AUTHORISATION SAFETY STUDIES

VIII. App1.1. Study Designs

Post-authorisation safety studies may adopt different designs depending on their objectives. A brief description of the main types of studies, as well as the types of data resources available, is provided hereafter. This Appendix is not intended to be exhaustive and should be complemented with other information sources, such as the ENCePP Guide for Methodological Standards in Pharmacoepidemiology.

VIII.App1.1.1. Active Surveillance

Active surveillance, in contrast to passive surveillance, seeks to ascertain more completely the number of adverse events in a given population via a continuous organised process. An example of active surveillance is the follow-up of patients treated with a particular medicinal product through a risk management system. Patients who fill a prescription for this product may be asked to complete a brief survey and give permission to be contacted at a later stage. In general, it is more feasible to get comprehensive data on individual adverse event reports through an active surveillance system than through a passive reporting system. However, some of the limitations of spontaneous reporting systems still apply, especially when evaluating delayed effects. For example, adverse events that occur a long time after the exposure (e.g. cancer, birth defects) may not be readily detected via spontaneous reporting systems. Automatic detection of abnormal laboratory values from computerised laboratory reports in certain clinical settings may also provide an efficient active surveillance system.

VIII.App1.1.1.1. Intensive Monitoring Schemes

Intensive monitoring is a system of record collection in designated areas, e.g. hospital units or by specific healthcare professionals in community practice. In such case, the data collection may be undertaken by monitors who attend ward rounds, where they gather information concerning undesirable or unintended events thought by the attending physician to be (potentially) causally related to the medication. Monitoring may also be focused on certain major events that tend to be medicine-related such as hepatic disorders, renal failure, haematological disorders or bleeding. The major strength of such systems is that the monitors may document important information about the events and exposure to medicinal products. The major limitation is the need to maintain a trained monitoring team over time.

Intensive monitoring may be achieved by reviewing medical records or interviewing patients and/or physicians/pharmacists in a sample of sentinel sites to ensure complete and accurate data on reported adverse events. The selected sites may provide information, such as data from specific patient subgroups that would not be available in a passive spontaneous reporting system. Further, collection of information on the use of a medicinal product, such as the potential for abuse, may be targeted at selected sentinel sites. Some of the major weaknesses of sentinel sites are problems with selection bias, small numbers of patients and increased costs. Intensive monitoring with sentinel sites is most efficient for those medicinal products used mainly in institutional settings such as hospitals, nursing homes and haemodialysis centres. Institutional settings may have a greater frequency of use for certain products and may provide an infrastructure for dedicated reporting.

In addition, automatic detection of abnormal laboratory values from computerised laboratory reports in certain clinical settings may provide an efficient intensive monitoring scheme.

VIII.App1.1.1.2. Prescription Event Monitoring

In prescription event monitoring (PEM), patients may be identified from electronic prescription data or automated health insurance claims. A follow-up questionnaire can then be sent to each prescribing physician or patient at pre-specified intervals to obtain outcome information. Information on patient demographics, indication for treatment, duration of therapy (including start date), dosage, clinical events and reasons for discontinuation can be included in the questionnaire. PEM tends to be used as a method to study safety just after product launch. Limitations of prescription event monitoring include substantial loss to follow-up, relatively short duration of follow-up, selective sampling, selective reporting and limited scope to study products which are used exclusively in hospitals. However, in PEM, there is the opportunity to collect more detailed information on adverse events from a large number of physicians and/or patients.

VIII.App1.1.1.3. Registries

A registry is an organised system that uses observational methods to collect uniform data on specified outcomes in a population defined by a particular disease, condition or exposure. A registry can be used as a data source within which studies can be performed.

Entry in a registry is generally defined either by diagnosis of a disease, prescription of a medicinal product, or both (patients with a certain disease treated with a defined medicinal product, defined active substance or any medicine of a defined class of medicinal products). The choice of the registry population and the design of the registry should be driven by its objective(s) in terms of outcomes to be measured and analyses and comparisons to be performed.

Registries are particularly useful when dealing with a rare disease, rare exposure or special population. In many cases, registries can be enriched with data on outcomes, confounding variables and effect modifiers obtained from a linkage to an existing database such as national cancer registries, prescription databases or mortality records.

Depending on their objective, registries may provide data on patient, disease and treatment outcomes, and of their determinants. Data on outcomes may include data on patient-reported outcomes, clinical conditions, medicines utilisation patterns and safety and effectiveness. It is acknowledged that on occasion, registries may be the only opportunity to provide insight into efficacy aspects of a medicinal product. However, observational registries should not normally be used to demonstrate efficacy. Rather, once efficacy has been demonstrated in randomised clinical trials (RCTs), patient registries may be useful to study effectiveness in heterogeneous populations, effect modifiers, such as doses that have been prescribed by physicians and that may differ from those used in RCTs, patient sub-groups defined by variables such as age, co-morbidities, use of concomitant medication or genetic factors, or factors related to a defined country or healthcare system.

Where adequate data are already available or can be collected, patient registries may be used to compare risks of outcomes between different groups. For example, a case-control study may be performed to compare the exposure to the medicinal product of cases of severe adverse reactions identified from the registry and of controls selected from either patients within the registry or from outside the registry. Likewise, a cohort study may be embedded in a registry. Case-only designs may also be applied (see VIII.App 1.1.2.4.).

Patient registries may address exposure to medicinal products in specific populations, such as pregnant women. Patients may be followed over time and included in a cohort study to collect data on adverse events using standardised questionnaires. Simple cohort studies may measure incidence, but, without a comparison group, cannot evaluate any association between exposures and outcomes. Nonetheless, they may be useful for signal amplification particularly for rare outcomes. This type of registry may be very valuable when examining the safety of an orphan medicinal product authorised for a specific condition.

VIII.App1.1.2. Observational Studies

Traditional epidemiological methods are a key component in the evaluation of adverse events. There are a number of observational study designs that are useful in validating signals from spontaneous reports, active surveillance programmes or case series. Major types of these designs are cross-sectional studies, case-control studies, and cohort studies, based on primary data collection or secondary use of existing data.

VIII.App1.1.2.1. Cross-sectional Study

Data collected on a population of patients at a single point in time (or interval of time) regardless of exposure or disease status constitute a cross-sectional study. These types of studies are primarily used to gather data for surveys or for ecological analyses. A drawback of cross-sectional studies is that the temporal relationship between exposure and outcome cannot be directly addressed, which limits its use for etiologic research unless the exposure does change over time. These studies are best used to examine the prevalence of a disease at one point in time or to examine trends over time where data for serial time-points can be captured. These studies may also be used to examine the crude association between exposure and outcome in ecological analyses.

VIII.App1.1.2.2. Cohort Study

In a cohort study, a population-at-risk for an event of interest is followed over time for the occurrence of that event. Information on exposure status is known throughout the follow-up period for each study participant. A study participant might be exposed to a medicinal product at one time during follow-up, but unexposed at another time point. Since the population exposure during follow-up is known, incidence rates can be calculated. In many cohort studies involving exposure to medicinal product(s), comparison cohorts of interest are selected on the basis of medication use and followed over time. Cohort studies are useful when there is a need to know the incidence rates of adverse events in addition to the relative risks of adverse events. They are also useful for the evaluation of multiple adverse events within the same study. However, it may be difficult to recruit sufficient numbers of patients who are exposed to a product of interest (such as an orphan medicinal product) or to study very rare outcomes. The identification of patients for cohort studies may come from large automated databases or from data collected specifically for the study at hand. In addition, cohort studies may be used to examine safety concerns in special populations (older persons, children, patients with co-morbid conditions, pregnant women) through over-sampling of these patients or by stratifying the cohort if sufficient numbers of patients exist.

VIII.App1.1.2.3. Case-control Study

In a case-control study, cases of disease (or events) are identified and patients from the source population that gave rise to the cases but who do not have the disease or event of interest at the time of selection are then selected as controls. The odds of exposure are then compared between the two groups. Patients may be identified from an existing database or using a field study approach, in which data are collected specifically for the purpose of the case control study. If safety information is sought for special populations, the cases and controls may be stratified according to the population of interest (e.g. the older persons, children, pregnant women). Existing large population-based databases are a useful and efficient means of providing needed exposure and medical outcome data in a relatively short period of time. Case-control studies are particularly useful when the goal is to investigate whether there is an association between a medicinal product (or several products) and one specific rare adverse event, as well as to identify multiple risk factors for adverse events. Factors of interest may include conditions such as renal and hepatic dysfunction that might modify the relationship between the exposure to the medicinal product and the adverse event. If all cases of interest (or a well-defined fraction of cases) in the catchment area are captured and the fraction of controls from the source population is known, a case-control study may also provide the absolute incidence rate of the event.

When the source population for the case-control study is a well-defined cohort or catchment area, it is then possible to select a random sample from it to form the control series. In these situations, because the sampling fractions of cases and controls are known, a case-control study may also provide the absolute incidence rate of the event. The name "nested case-control study" has been coined to designate those studies in which the control sampling is density-based (e.g. the control series represents the person-time distribution of exposure in the source population). The case-cohort is also a variant in which the control sampling is performed on those persons who make up the source population regardless of the duration of time they may have contributed to it. A case-control approach could also be set up as a permanent scheme to identify and quantify risks (case-control surveillance). This strategy has been followed for rare diseases with a relevant aetiology fraction attributed to medicinal products, including blood dyscrasias or serious skin disorders.

VIII.App1.1.2.4. Case-only Designs

Case-only designs have been proposed to assess the association between intermittent exposures and short-term events, including the self-controlled case-series, the case-crossover and the case-time-control studies. In these designs, only cases are used and the control information is obtained from person-time experience of the cases themselves. One of the important strengths of these designs is that confounding variables that do not change over time within individuals are automatically matched. However, case-only designs cannot be used under all circumstances, for instance when the exact date of disease onset is difficult to establish or when evaluating chronic exposures.

VIII.App1.1.3. Clinical Trials

When important risks are identified from pre-approval clinical trials, further clinical trials might be called for to evaluate the mechanism of action for the adverse reaction. If the study is a clinical trial, provisions of Directive 2001/20/EC shall apply. In some instances, pharmacodynamic and pharmacokinetic studies might be conducted to determine whether a particular dosing regimen can put patients at an increased risk of adverse events. Genetic testing may also provide clues about which group of patients might be at an increased risk of adverse reactions. Furthermore, based on the pharmacological properties and the expected use of the medicinal product in clinical practice, conducting specific studies to investigate potential drug-drug interactions and food-drug interactions might be called for. These studies may include population pharmacokinetic studies and therapeutic drug monitoring in patients and normal volunteers.

Sometimes, potential risks or unforeseen benefits in special populations might be identified from pre-approval clinical trials, but cannot be fully quantified due to small sample sizes or the exclusion of subpopulations of patients from these clinical studies. These populations might include older persons, pregnant women, children or patients with renal or hepatic disorders. Children, older persons and persons with co-morbid conditions may metabolise medicinal products differently than patients typically enrolled in clinical trials. Further clinical trials may be used to determine and to quantify the magnitude of the risk (or benefit) in such populations.

VIII.App1.1.3.1. Large Simple Trials

A large simple trial is a specific form of clinical trial where large numbers of patients are randomised to treatment but data collection and monitoring are kept to the minimum, consistent with the aims of the study to be a relatively low burden. Likewise, standardised follow-up generally consistent with normal clinical practice for the patient population may be included. This design may be used in pharmacovigilance to elucidate the risk-benefit profile of a medicinal product outside of the formal/traditional clinical trial setting and/or to fully quantify the risk of a critical but relatively rare adverse event. The use of the term 'simple' refers to data structure and not data collection. It is used in relation to situations in which limited information is collected regarding exposure, outcome and potential confounders to help ensure feasibility of recruiting large patient numbers in an experimental design, and the term may not adequately reflect the complexity of the studies undertaken. These studies qualify as clinical trials. As used in this context, the definitions of a pragmatic trial and of a large simple trial are synonymous.

VIII.App1.1.4. Drug Utilisation Studies

Drug utilisation studies (DUS) describe how a medicinal product is prescribed and used in routine clinical practice in large populations, including older persons, children, pregnant women or patients with hepatic or renal dysfunction. These populations are often not eligible for inclusion in randomised clinical trials. Stratification by age, sex, concomitant medication and other characteristics allows a comprehensive characterisation of treated patients, including the distribution of those factors that may influence clinical, social, and economic outcomes. Denominator data may be derived from these studies to determining rates of adverse events. DUS have been used to describe the effect of regulatory actions and media attention on the use of medicinal products in everyday medical practice, to examine the relationship between recommended and actual clinical practice, to monitor medication errors and to determine whether a medicinal product has potential for abuse by examining whether patients are taking escalating dose regimens or whether there is evidence of inappropriate repeat prescribing. DUS are particularly useful as a first step in the design of post-authorisation safety studies, to obtain sufficient understanding of the characteristics of the user population of the medicinal product under study and the determination of the most appropriate comparator as well as important potential confounders to consider. They are also useful to provide a first indication of the level of public health impact anticipated if there is a true causal association between the exposure of interest and an adverse event, for example given the size of the population exposed, the extent of off-label use, and so on. For regulatory purposes, DUS for which the main aim is to add knowledge to the safety of medicinal products or the effectiveness of risk minimisation measures may be classified as PASS (see VIII.B.1.).

VIII.App1.2. Data Sources

Pharmacoepidemiological studies may be performed using a variety of data sources. Traditionally, field studies were required for retrieving the necessary data on exposure, outcomes, potential confounders and other variables, through interview of appropriate subjects (e.g. patients, relatives) or by consulting the paper-based medical records. However, the advent of automated healthcare databases has remarkably increased the efficiency of pharmacoepidemiological research. Generally, there are two main types of automated databases: those that contain comprehensive medical information, including prescriptions, diagnosis, referral letters and discharge reports, and those mainly created for administrative purposes, which require a record-linkage between pharmacy claims and medical claims databases. These datasets may include millions of patients and allow for large studies. A major limitation however often is the lack of long-term follow up and the consequent left- and right-censoring of data. In addition, these databases may not have the detailed and accurate information needed for some research, such as validated diagnostic information or laboratory data, and paper-based medical records should be consulted to ascertain and validate test results and medical diagnoses. Depending on the outcome of interest, the validation may require either a case-by-case approach or just the review of a random sample of cases. Other key aspects may require validation where appropriate. There are many databases in place for potential use in pharmacoepidemiological studies or in their validation phase.

Marketing authorisation holders should select the best data source according to validity (e.g. completeness of relevant information, possibility of outcome validation) and efficiency criteria (e.g. time span to provide results). External validity should also be taken into account. As far as feasible the data source chosen to perform the study should include the population in which the safety concern has been raised. In case another population is involved, the marketing authorisation holder should evaluate the differences that may exist in the relevant variables (e.g. age, sex, pattern of use of the medicinal product) and the potential impact on the results. In the statistical analyses, the potential effect of modification of such variables should be explored.

With any data source used, the privacy and confidentiality regulations that apply to personal data should be adhered to.

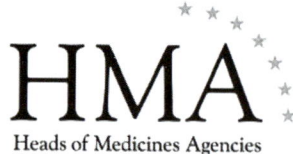
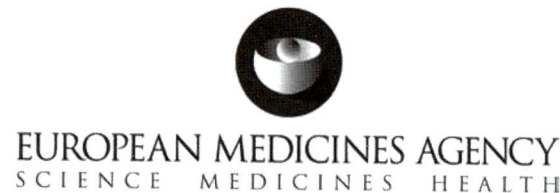

4 August 2016
EMA/395730/2012 Rev 2*

GUIDELINE ON GOOD PHARMACOVIGILANCE PRACTICES (GVP)

Module VIII Addendum I — Requirements and Recommendations for the Submission of Information on Non-Interventional Post-Authorisation Safety Studies (Rev 2)

Date for coming into effect of first version	2 July 2012
Date for coming into effect of Revision 1*	25 April 2013
Draft Revision 2 finalised by the Agency in collaboration with Member States	23 June 2015
Draft Revision 2 agreed by the European Risk Management Facilitation Group (ERMS FG)	16 July 2015
Draft Revision 2 adopted by Executive Director	3 August 2015
Release for public consultation	11 August 2015
End of consultation (deadline for comments)	9 October 2015
Revised draft Revision 2 finalised by the Agency in collaboration with Member States	14 April 2016
Revised draft Revision 2 agreed by ERMS FG	15 July 2016
Revised draft Revision 2 adopted by Executive Director as final	4 August 2016
Date for coming into effect of Revision 2*	9 August 2016

***Note:** Revision 2 contains the following:
- Change of the title;
- Deletion of Tables XIII Add I.1. and XIII Add I.2. and simplification of presentation of submission requirements and recommendations based on legislation related to non-interventional post-authorisation safety studies;
- Update of submission requirements for study protocols and progress reports according to Art 107m(5) based on updated information provided by Member States;
- Addition of information regarding study registration in the EU PAS Register.

VIII.ADD.I.1. INTRODUCTION

This Addendum provides additional information on legal requirements (identifiable by the modal verb "shall") and recommendations (identifiable by the modal verb "should") for the submission of study protocols, progress reports and final study reports of non-interventional post-authorisation safety studies (PASS) to national competent authorities and the Agency. It also provides additional information as regards the registration of non-interventional PASS in the EU PAS Register. It does not provide recommendations for the transmission of information to ethics committees, national review boards or other bodies in place according to national legislation.

VIII.ADD.I.2. STUDY REGISTRATION

According to IR Annex III.3 (Format of the final study report), the date of study registration in the electronic study register shall be included as a milestone in the final study report for non-interventional post-authorisation safety studies (PASS) imposed as an obligation. VIII.B.2. also states that marketing authorisation holders should register all non-interventional PASS conducted voluntarily in the EU or included in the risk management plan agreed in the EU. Non-interventional PASS should be registered before the study commences or at the earliest possible date, and the study protocol (and its updates), the progress reports and the study reports should be uploaded in the register.

The EU PAS Register is a register of post-authorisation studies publicly available through the EU PAS Register webpage[1] that serves as the electronic study register mentioned in IR Annex III. The information requested at the time of study registration in the EU PAS Register includes administrative details, targets of the study and methodological aspects. The study protocol, the study report and other documents can be uploaded. Administrative information includes whether the study has been requested by a regulatory authority, the RMP category if applicable, information about the percentage of funding from different sources and the country(-ies) where the study will be conducted. In case the record for a new registered study indicates that the study has been requested by a regulatory authority, is funded even partially by a pharmaceutical company and is conducted in at least one EU country, the Agency sends a notification message with the full study title, the name of the funder(s), the name of the country(-ies) where the study will be conducted and a link to the current study record to all national competent authorities of the EU Member States. This notification aims to systematically inform Member States of the public registration of a post-authorisation study requested by a regulatory authority, funded by a marketing authorisation holder and conducted on their territory.

Uploading of the study protocol, the progress report(s) and the final study report in the EU PAS Register is not a legal obligation. Therefore, registration of a non-interventional PASS in the EU PAS Register cannot be the only channel for the submission of these documents to national competent authorities and the Agency.

VIII.ADD.I.3. REQUIREMENTS AND RECOMMENDATIONS FOR NON-INTERVENTIONAL PASS CONDUCTED PURSUANT TO AN OBLIGATION IMPOSED BY AN EU COMPETENT AUTHORITY

These studies include non-interventional PASS of categories 1 and 2 of studies of GVP Module V.

The draft protocol, the updated study protocol following substantial amendment and the final study report shall be submitted according to the normal procedure to the Pharmacovigilance Risk Assessment Committee (PRAC) and the Agency, or to the national competent authority of the Member State that requested the study if the study is conducted in only one Member State [DIR Art 107n to 107p]. The final study report shall be submitted within 12 months after the end of data collection [DIR Art 107p(1)].

According to DIR Art 107m(5), the marketing authorisation holder may be required by the national competent authority to submit the progress reports to the competent authorities of the Member States in which the study is conducted. The national competent authority of all Member States in which

---

1. http://www.encepp.eu/encepp_studies/indexRegister.shtml

the study is conducted, except Denmark, stated they require submission of the progress reports. The progress reports should also be submitted to the Agency for centrally-authorised products.

VIII.ADD.I.4. REQUIREMENTS AND RECOMMENDATIONS FOR NON-INTERVENTIONAL PASS CONDUCTED VOLUNTARILY

These studies include non-interventional PASS of category 3 of the GVP Module V and other non-interventional PASS voluntary conducted by marketing authorisation holders.

According to DIR Art 107m(6), the final study report shall be submitted according to national procedures to the competent authorities of the Member States where the study was conducted within 12 months of the end of data collection.

According to DIR Art 107m(5), the marketing authorisation holder may be required by the national competent authority to submit the study protocol and the progress reports to the competent authorities of the Member States in which the study is conducted. The national competent authority of the following Member States in which the study is conducted stated they require submission of the study protocol and progress reports through national procedures:

Austria, Bulgaria, Croatia, Czech Republic, France, Germany, Italy, Lithuania, The Netherlands, Portugal, Romania, Slovakia, Slovenia, Spain.

For studies of category 3, progress reports should also be submitted to the Agency for centrally-authorised products.

For studies of category 3, the study protocol should also be submitted with the risk management plan according to the recommendations of GVP Module V.

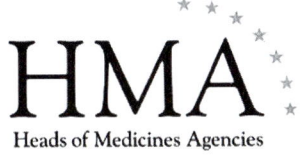 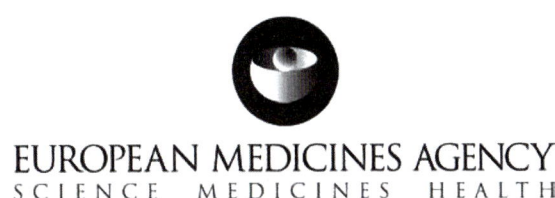

22 June 2012
EMA/827661/2011

GUIDELINE ON GOOD PHARMACOVIGILANCE PRACTICES (GVP)

Module IX – Signal Management

Draft finalised by the Agency in collaboration with Member States and submitted to ERMS FG	19 January 2012
Draft agreed by ERMS FG	24 January 2012
Draft adopted by Executive Director	20 February 2012
Released for consultation	21 February 2012
End of consultation (deadline for comments)	18 April 2012
Revised draft finalised by the Agency in collaboration with Member States	20 June 2012
Revised draft agreed by ERMS FG	21 June 2012
Revised draft adopted by Executive Director as final	22 June 2012
Date for coming into effect	2 July 2012

IX.A. INTRODUCTION

The Report of the Council for International Organisations of Medical Sciences Working group VIII Practical Aspects of Signal Detection in Pharmacovigilance (CIOMS, Geneva 2010) defines a signal as *information that arises from one or multiple sources (including observations and experiments), which suggests a new potentially causal association, or a new aspect of a known association, between an intervention and an event or set of related events, either adverse or beneficial, that is judged to be of sufficient likelihood to justify verificatory action.*

For the purpose of this Module, only new information related to adverse effects will be considered.

In order to suggest a new potentially causal association or a new aspect of a known association, any signal should be validated taking into account other relevant sources of information.

The signal management process can be defined as the set of activities performed to determine whether, based on an examination of individual case safety reports (ICSRs), aggregated data from active surveillance systems or studies, literature information or other data sources, there are new risks associated with an active substance or a medicinal product or whether known risks have changed. The signal management process shall include all steps from initial signal detection; through their validation and confirmation; analysis and prioritisation; and signal assessment to recommending action, as well as the tracking of the steps taken and of any recommendations made [IR Art 21(1)].

In the European Union, the signal management process concerns all stakeholders involved in the safety monitoring of medicinal products including patients, healthcare professionals, marketing authorisation holders, regulatory authorities, scientific committees and decision-making bodies (such as competent authorities in the Member States and the European Commission (EC)).

Whereas the EudraVigilance database will be a major source of pharmacovigilance information, the signal management process covers signals arising from outside the EudraVigilance database or not directly supported by the EudraVigilance database. For the purpose of monitoring data in EudraVigilance database, only signals related to an adverse reaction shall be considered [IR Art 19(1)].

Regulation (EU) No 1235/2010 amending Regulation (EC) No 726/2004, Directive 2010/84/EU amending Directive 2001/83/EC and Commission Implementing Regulation (EU) No 520/2012 on the Performance of Pharmacovigilance Activities Provided for in Regulation (EC) No 726/2004 and Directive 2001/83/EC include provisions for signal management in the European Union.

In this Module, all applicable legal requirements are referenced as explained in the GVP Introductory Cover Note and are usually identifiable by the modal verb "shall". Guidance for the implementation of legal requirements is provided using the modal verb "should".

The objectives of this Module are:
- To provide general guidance and requirements on structures and processes involved in signal management (section IX.B.);
- To describe how these structures and processes are applied in the setting of the EU pharmacovigilance and regulatory network (section IX.C.).

IX.B. STRUCTURES AND PROCESSES

IX.B.1. Sources of Data and Information

The sources for identifying new signals are diverse. They potentially include all scientific information concerning the use of medicinal products including quality, non-clinical, clinical, pharmacovigilance and pharmacoepidemiological data. Specific sources for signals include spontaneous adverse drug reaction (ADR) reporting systems, active surveillance systems, non-interventional studies, clinical trials, scientific literature and other sources of information.

Signals from spontaneous reports may be detected from monitoring of individual case safety reports (ICSRs), ADR databases, articles from the scientific literature or review of information provided by marketing authorisation holders in the context of regulatory procedures (e.g. variations, renewals, post-authorisation commitments, periodic safety update reports (PSURs), Risk Management Plan (RMP) updates or from other activities related to the on-going benefit-risk monitoring of medicinal products.

Spontaneous reports of ADRs may also be notified to poison centres, teratology information services, vaccine surveillance programmes, reporting systems established by marketing authorisation holders, and any other structured and organised data collection schemes allowing patients and healthcare professionals to report suspected adverse reactions related to medicinal products. Competent authorities should liaise with other institutions or organisations managing such reporting system so as to be informed of these suspected adverse reactions.

Due to the increase in volume of spontaneous reports of (ADRs), the introduction of electronic safety reporting by patients and healthcare professionals and the mandatory electronic transmission of case reports from marketing authorisation holders to competent authorities, signal detection is now increasingly based on periodic monitoring of large databases such as the EudraVigilance database.

Signals may arise from a wide range of different study types, including quality, non-clinical, interventional and non-interventional studies, systematic reviews and meta-analyses. Interventional trials and observational studies may, by design, recruit and follow-up a defined population of subjects who may experience ADRs. Review of aggregated data and statistical analyses may also point to an elevated risk of an adverse event to be further investigated as a signal.

Published results of relevant studies should be identified by marketing authorisation holders by screening the scientific literature. For general guidance on performing literature searches, refer to Module VI.

Marketing authorisation holders should regularly screen internet or digital media under their management or responsibility as specified in Module VI, for potential reports of suspected ADRs, which may characterise a new signal. Marketing authorisation holders and competent authorities should seek further information related to suspected ADRs they become aware of from any source. Suspected serious ADRs should be confirmed if possible through other data sources such as EudraVigilance.

IX.B.2. Methodology for Signal Detection

As a general principle, signal detection should follow a recognised methodology, which may vary depending on the type of medicinal product it is intended to cover. Vaccines may for example require other methodological strategies.

The detection of signals shall be based on a multidisciplinary approach. Signal detection within the EudraVigilance database shall be complemented by statistical analysis where appropriate [IR Art 19(2)].

In order to determine the evidentiary value (i.e. the supporting evidence) of a signal a recognised methodology shall be applied taking into account the clinical relevance, quantitative strength of the association, the consistency of the data, the exposure-response relationship, the biological plausibility, experimental findings, possible analogies and the nature and quality of the data [IR Art 20(1)].

Different factors may be taken into account for the prioritisation of signals, namely whether the association or the active substance/medicinal product is new, the strength of the association, the seriousness of the reaction involved and the documentation of the reports in the EudraVigilance database [IR Art 20(2)].

IX.B.3. The Signal Management Process

IX.B.3.1. Introduction

The signal management process covers all steps from detecting signals to recommending action(s) as follows:
- Signal detection;
- Signal validation;
- Signal analysis and prioritisation;
- Signal assessment;
- Recommendation for action;
- Exchange of information.

Although these steps generally follow a logical sequence, the wide range of sources of information available for signal detection may require some flexibility in the conduct of signal management e.g.:

- When signal detection is primarily based on a review of individual case safety reports (ICSRs), this activity may include validation and preliminary prioritisation of any detected signal;
- When a signal is detected from results of a study, it is generally not possible or practical to assess each individual case, and validation may require collection of additional data;
- Recommendation for action (followed by decision in accordance with the applicable legislation) and exchange of information are components to be considered at every step of the process.

For the purpose of this guidance, signals originating from the monitoring of data from spontaneous reporting systems are considered as the starting point of the signal management process. The same principles should apply for data originating from other sources.

IX.B.3.2. Signal Detection

Detailed guidance on methods of signal detection may be found in the Report of CIOMS Working group VIII Practical Aspects of Signal Detection in Pharmacovigilance (CIOMS, Geneva 2010) and in the Guideline on the Use of Statistical Signal Detection Methods in the EudraVigilance Data Analysis System (Doc. Ref. EMEA/106464/2006 rev. 1).

Whichever methods are employed for the detection of signals, the same principles should apply, namely:
- The method used should be appropriate for the data set; for example, the use of complex statistical tools may not be appropriate for smaller data sets;
- Data from all appropriate sources should be considered;
- Systems should be in place to ensure the quality of the signal detection activity;
- Any outputs from a review of cumulative data should be assessed by an appropriately qualified person in a timely manner;
- The process should be adequately documented, including the rationale for the method and periodicity of the signal detection activity.

Detection of signals may be performed based on a review of ICSRs, from statistical analyses in large databases, or from a combination of both.

IX.B.3.2.1. Review of Individual Case Safety Reports

As specified in Module VI, ICSRs may originate from a spontaneous reporting system, post-authorisation studies and monitoring of literature. Even a single report of a serious or severe adverse reaction (for example, one case of toxic epidermal necrolysis, aplastic anaemia or liver transplant) may be sufficient to raise a signal and to take further action. A review of ICSRs for this purpose should consider the number of cases (after exclusion of duplicates), the patient's demographics (including age and gender), the suspected medicinal product (including dose administered, formulation) and the suspected adverse reaction (including signs and symptoms), the temporal association, the clinical outcome in relation to drug continuation or discontinuation (i.e. de-challenge / re-challenge information). An assessment of causality of a suspected association should also consider, the presence of potential alternative causes including other concomitant medications, the underlying disease, the reporter's evaluation of causality and the plausibility of a biological and pharmacological relationship.

IX.B.3.2.2. Statistical Analyses

Signal detection is now increasingly based on a regular periodic monitoring of large databases of spontaneous reports of ADRs. Such databases allow generation of statistical reports presenting information on adverse reactions received over a defined time period for defined active substances or medicinal products. Various methods have been developed to identify statistics of disproportionate reporting, i.e. higher reporting than expected for an suspected adverse reaction for an active substance/medicinal product of interest compared to all other active substances/medicinal products in the database, (expressed e.g. as a lower bound of the proportionate reporting ratio >1). Given the limitations of these methods, statistics of disproportionate reporting alone do not necessarily indicate that there is a signal to be further investigated or that a causal association is present.

Use of statistical tools may not be appropriate in all situations. The size of the data set, the completeness of the available information and the severity of the adverse reaction(s) should be taken into account when considering the use of statistical methods and the selection of criteria for the detection of signals.

The periodicity at which statistical reports should be generated and reviewed may vary according to the active substance/medicinal product, its indication and any known potential or identified risks. Some active substances/medicinal products may also be subject to an increased frequency of data monitoring (see IX.C.2.). The duration for this increased frequency of monitoring may also vary and be flexible with the accumulation of knowledge of the risk profile associated with the use of the concerned active substance/medicinal product.

IX.B.3.2.3. Combination of Statistical Methods and Review of Individual Case Safety Reports

Statistical reports may be designed to provide tools for identifying suspected adverse reactions that meet pre-defined criteria of frequency, severity, clinical importance, novelty or statistical association. Such filtering tools may facilitate the selection of ICSRs to be reviewed as a first step. The thresholds used in this filtering process (for example, at least 3 cases reported) may vary according to the extent of usage of medicinal products and thus the potential public health impact.

Irrespective of the statistical method used, where statistical reports are used to automate the screening of a database, signal detection should always involve clinical judgement and the corresponding ICSRs should be individually reviewed, considering their clinical relevance (IX.B.3.2.1.).

The statistical method should therefore be a supporting tool in the whole process of signal detection and subsequent validation.

IX.B.3.3. Signal Validation

Signal validation is the process of evaluating the data supporting the detected signal in order to verify that the available documentation contains sufficient evidence demonstrating the existence of a new potentially causal association or a new aspect of a known association, and therefore justifies further analysis [IR Art 21(1)].

To validate a signal the following should be taken into account:
- Clinical relevance including, for example:
  - Strength of evidence for a causal effect (e.g. number of reports, exposure, temporal association, plausible mechanism, de/re-challenge, alternative explanation/confounders);
  - Seriousness and severity of the reaction and its outcome;
  - Novelty of the reaction (e.g. new and serious adverse reactions);
  - Drug-drug interactions;
  - Reactions occurring in special populations.
- Previous awareness:
  - The extent to which information is already included in the summary of product characteristics (SmPC) or patient leaflet;
  - Whether the association has already been assessed in a PSUR or RMP, or was discussed at the level of a scientific committee or has been subject to a regulatory procedure.

In principle only a new signal for which there is no previous awareness should be validated. However, an already known association may give rise to a new signal if its apparent frequency of reporting, its duration, its severity or a change in the previously reported outcome (such as new fatality) suggests new information as compared with the information included in the SmPC or previously assessed by the competent authority.

- Availability of other relevant sources of information providing a richer set of data on the same association:
  - Literature findings regarding similar cases;
  - Experimental findings or biological mechanisms;
  - Screening of databases with larger datasets (e.g. EudraVigilance when the signal was sourced initially by data from national or company-specific database).

The magnitude and clinical significance of a signal may also be examined by descriptive analyses in other available data sources or by analysis of the characteristics of exposed patients and their medicinal product utilisation patterns.

Signals for which the validity is not confirmed may deserve special attention in subsequent analyses i.e. it may be appropriate to continue to monitor the potential signal until there is enough evidence to confirm the signal. For example, there might be an inadequate case documentation or a supporting evidence of a causal association only in some of the ICSRs. In such scenarios, new cases of the same adverse reaction or follow-up reports of previously received cases should be reviewed at appropriate time intervals to ensure that all relevant cases are considered.

Marketing authorisation holders and competent authorities should establish tracking systems to capture the outcome of the validation of signals including the reasons why signals were not validated as well as information that would facilitate further retrieval of ICSRs and validation of signals.

IX.B.3.4. Signal Analysis and Prioritisation

A key element of the signal management process is to promptly identify validated signals with important public health impact or that may significantly affect the benefit-risk profile of the medicinal product in treated patients. These signals require urgent attention and need to be prioritised for further management without delay. This prioritisation process should consider:

- The impact on patients depending on the severity, reversibility, potential for prevention and clinical outcome of the association;
- The consequences of treatment discontinuation on the disease and the availability other therapeutic options;
- The strength and consistency of the evidence supporting an association, e.g., biological plausibility, a high number of cases reported in a short period of time, the measure of disproportionality of reporting and rapid increase of that measure over time and identification of the signal in different settings (e.g. general practice and hospital settings), data sources or countries;
- Clinical context (e.g. whether the association suggest a clinical syndrome that may include other reactions);
- The public health impact, including the extent of utilisation of the product in the general population and in special populations (e.g. pregnant women, children or the elderly) and the patterns of medicinal product utilisation (e.g. off-label use or misuse). The public health impact may include an estimation of the number of patients that may be affected by an adverse reaction and this number could be considered in relation to the size of the general population, the population with the target disease and the treated population;
- Increased frequency or severity of a known adverse reaction;
- Novelty of the suspected adverse reaction, e.g. when an unknown suspected adverse reaction occurs shortly after the marketing of a new medicinal product;
- If a marketing authorisation application for a new active substance is still under evaluation.

In some circumstances, priority can also be given to signals identified for medicinal products or events with potential high media and pharmacovigilance stakeholder interest in order to communicate the result to the public and healthcare professionals as early as possible.

The outcome of signal prioritisation should include a recommendation of the time frame for the management of the signal.

The outcome of the signal prioritisation process should be entered in the tracking system, with the justification for the priority attributed.

IX.B.3.5. Signal Assessment

The objective of signal assessment is to further evaluate a validated signal so as to identify the need for additional data collection or for any regulatory action. It consists of an assessment of the available pharmacological, non-clinical and clinical data and information from other sources. This review should be as complete as possible regarding the sources of information, including the application dossier, literature articles, spontaneous reports, expert consultation, and information held by marketing authorisation holders and competent authorities. When information is drawn from a range of sources, the strengths and limitations of each source should be considered in order to assess the contribution they can provide to the overall evaluation of the signal in terms of a recommendation for action. Summarising information from different data sources also requires the choice of an internationally agreed case definition (e.g. Brighton collaboration case definition for vaccines). If no such definition exists, an operational definition should be developed.

Signals may need to be assessed at a broader level e.g. at the therapeutic or system organ class level or at the level of a Standardised MedDRA[1] Query (i.e. SMQ). The search for information to assess the significance of a signal may also need to be extended to other products of the class and to other adverse reactions, such as to other terms linked to a complex disease (e.g. optic neuritis as a possible early sign of multiple sclerosis), to a prior stage of a reaction (e.g. QT prolongation and torsades de pointes) or to clinical complications of the adverse reaction of interest (e.g. dehydration and acute renal failure).

Gathering information from various sources may take time. For a new signal of a serious or severe adverse reaction, measures should be taken at any stage in the management of a signal including detection, if the information already available supports the conclusion that there is a potential risk that needs to be prevented or minimised in a timely manner.

IX.B.3.6. Recommendation for Action

Signal assessment results in a recommendation that either no further action is required at this point in time or a further action is needed. Although the recommendation for action normally takes place in a logical sequence after signal assessment based on the extent of the information, the need for action should be considered throughout the signal management process. For example, the first case of an adverse reaction indicating a manufacturing defect may require immediate recall of a product batch. The review of available information at the signal validation or signal prioritisation stages may similarly conclude that the evidence is sufficiently strong to introduce temporary measures. In such situations, it is still necessary to proceed with a formal assessment of the signal to confirm or not the safety issue in order to extend or lift the temporary measures.

The recommendation for action may include a request for:
- Immediate measures including the possibility of suspending the marketing authorisation of the medicinal product;
- Additional information to be provided by the marketing authorisation holder, e.g. in order to confirm if a conclusion is valid for all indications and patient groups;
- Periodic review of the signal, for example through PSURs (see Module VII);
- Additional investigations or risk minimisation activities;
- An update of the product information through a regulatory procedure;
- Conduct of a post-authorisation safety study (see Module VIII).

Whenever actions are requested of a marketing authorisation holder, the request should specify a timeframe by which they should be completed, including provision of progress reports and interim results, proportionate to the severity and public health impact of the signal.

IX.B.3.7. Exchange of Information

Information on validated signals, Emerging Safety Issues and the outcome of signal assessments should be exchanged between competent authorities and marketing authorisation holders.

Marketing authorisation holders should communicate signals that may have implications for public health and the benefit-risk profile of a product immediately to the competent authorities as an Emerging Safety Issue (see Module VI), and when appropriate this should include proposals for action.

The outcomes of signal assessment involving new or changed risks and risks that have an impact on the benefit-risk balance of the concerned active substance/medicinal products should be communicated to the public including health care professionals and patients (see IX.C.6.) as well as to the concerned marketing authorisation holders.

IX.B.4. Quality Requirements

IX.B.4.1. Tracking

All validation, prioritisation, assessment, timelines, decisions, actions, plans, reporting as well as all other key steps should be recorded and tracked systematically. Tracking systems should be used for documentation and should also include signals,

---

[1] MedDRA® the Medical Dictionary for Regulatory Activities terminology is the international medical terminology developed under the auspices of the International Conference on Harmonization of Technical Requirements for Registration of Pharmaceuticals for Human Use (ICH)

for which the validation process conducted was not suggestive of a new potentially causal association, or a new aspect of a known association. All records need to be archived [IR Art 24(1)] (see Module I).

IX.B.4.2. Quality Systems and Documentation

An essential feature of a signal management system is that it is clearly documented to ensure that the system functions properly and effectively, that the roles, responsibilities and required tasks are standardised, that these tasks are conducted by people with appropriate expertise and are clear to all parties involved and that there is provision for appropriate control and, when needed, improvement of the system. Therefore, a system of quality assurance and quality control consistent with the quality system standards should be in place and applied to all signal management processes (see Module I). Detailed procedures for this quality system should be developed, documented and implemented. The organisational roles and responsibilities for the activities and maintenance of documentation, quality control and review, and for ensuring corrective and preventive action need to be assigned and recorded. This should include the responsibilities for quality assurance auditing of the signal management system, including auditing of sub-contractors. Data and document confidentiality (per the applicable regulations), security and validity (including integrity when transferred) should be guaranteed.

Through their tracking system, all parties should keep an audit trail of their signal management activities and of the relevant queries and their outcomes, including how signals have been detected, validated, confirmed and assessed [IR Art 24(2)].

Documentation may be requested from the marketing authorisation holders demonstrating compliance with these provisions and reviewed before and after marketing authorisation.

Staff should be specifically trained in signal management activities in accordance with their roles and responsibilities. The training system and location of the training records should be documented, and curricula vitae and job descriptions should be archived.

IX.C. OPERATION OF THE EU NETWORK

IX.C.1. Roles and Responsibilities

Within the context of the operation of the EU regulatory network, the marketing authorisation holders, the Agency and national competent authorities should continuously monitor the data available in the EudraVigilance database to determine whether there are new risks or whether risks have changed and whether those risks have an impact on the benefit-risk balance. A recognised signal detection methodology should be applied and detected signals should be validated, as appropriate.

The Agency and national competent authorities shall cooperate in the monitoring of the data available in the EudraVigilance database [IR Art 18(1)].

Regarding medicinal products authorised in accordance with Regulation (EC) No 726/2004 (centrally authorised products (CAPs)) the Agency shall be assisted in the monitoring of data in EudraVigilance by the rapporteur appointed by the PRAC in accordance with Article 62(1) of that Regulation [IR Art 22(5)].

For medicinal products authorised in accordance with Directive 2001/83/EC in more than one Member State and for active substances contained in several medicinal products where at least one marketing authorisation has been granted in accordance with Directive 2001/83/EC, Member States may agree within the Coordination Group for Mutual Recognition and Decentralised Procedures - Human (CMDh), in collaboration with the PRAC, to appoint a lead Member State for the monitoring of data in the EudraVigilance database and for validation and confirmation of signals on behalf of the other Member States. The lead Member State may be supported by a co-leader, which shall assist the lead Member State in the fulfilment of its tasks. Any such appointment shall be reviewed at least every four years [IR Art 22(1)]. When appointing a lead Member State, and as appropriate a co-leader, the CMDh in collaboration with the PRAC, may take into account whether any Member State is acting as reference Member State, in accordance with Article 28(1) of Directive 2001/83/EC, or as a rapporteur for the assessment of periodic safety update reports in accordance with Article 107(e) of that Directive [IR Art 22(2)].

All Member States shall remain responsible for monitoring the data in the EudraVigilance database in accordance with Article 107h(1)(c) and Article 107h(3) of Directive 2001/83/EC [IR Art 22(4)].

The national competent authorities and the Agency shall validate and confirm any signal that has been detected by them in the course of their continuous monitoring of the data in EudraVigilance database [IR Art 21(4)].

For medicinal products or active substances where a rapporteur has been appointed by the PRAC, this rapporteur should confirm validated signals. For medicinal products or active substances where a lead Member State has been appointed, this lead Member State should confirm validated signals.

Confirmation by the PRAC rapporteur or the lead Member State means communication through the European Pharmacovigilance Issues Tracking Tool (EPITT) (see IX.C.5.) that the signal is valid. A justification should be provided when the signal is not confirmed. All confirmed signals shall be transmitted to the PRAC. For such medicinal products or active substances for which a lead Member State has been appointed, the lead Member State should validate and confirm as a single step the signals it has detected. For such medicinal products or active substances where a lead Member State has not been appointed, the national competent authority should validate and confirm as a single step the signals it has detected.

IX.C.1.1. Roles and Responsibilities of the Agency

The Agency:
- Shall make public on the European medicines web-portal a list of active substances/medicinal products and the authority (lead Member State, co-lead Member State or the Agency) responsible for their monitoring in EudraVigilance [IR Art 22(3)];
- Following consultation with the PRAC may publish a list of medical events that have to be taken into account for the detection of a signal [IR Art 19(2)];
- Shall support the monitoring of the data in the EudraVigilance database by providing national competent authorities with access to:
  - Data outputs and statistical reports allowing a review of all adverse reactions reported to EudraVigilance in relation with an active substance or a medicinal product;
  - Customised queries supporting the evaluation of individual case safety reports and case series;
  - Customised grouping and stratification of data enabling the identification of patient groups with a higher risk of occurrence of adverse reactions or with a risk of a more severe adverse reaction;
  - Statistical signal detection methods [IR Art 23];
- Shall ensure appropriate support for the monitoring of the data in EudraVigilance by marketing authorisation holders [IR Art 23];
- Should prepare a technical document establishing common requirements for signal detection and describing EudraVigilance data outputs and statistical reports;
- Shall administer the European Pharmacovigilance Issues Tracking Tool (EPITT) for validated signals that require further assessment [IR Art 21(5)];
- Shall take the lead for EudraVigilance data monitoring, signal detection and signal validation for CAPs and for active substances contained in several medicinal products, where at least one marketing authorisation has been granted in accordance with Regulation (EC) 726/2004;
- Shall enter validated signals it has detected into EPITT;
- Should validate (including, if appropriate, in the EudraVigilance database) and enter into EPITT any other signal communicated by a third party (e.g. regulatory authority from outside the EU), involving a CAP or an active substance for which the EudraVigilance data monitoring is performed by the Agency;
- Shall confirm in collaboration with the Member States as soon as possible and no later than 30 days from its receipt any validated signal communicated by marketing authorisation holders involving a CAP or an active substance for which the EudraVigilance data monitoring is performed by the Agency. In this context, where the validity of the signal is not confirmed, special attention shall be paid to any follow-up information which may allow for the signal's confirmation [IR Art 21(3)], see IX.B.3.3;

- Shall transmit confirmed signals to the PRAC for initial analysis and prioritisation in accordance with Article 28a(2) of Regulation (EC) No 726/2004 [IR Art 21(5)];
- Shall forthwith inform the concerned marketing authorisation holder(s) of the conclusions of the PRAC of the assessment of any confirmed signal [IR Art 21(6)];
- Shall keep an audit trail of its signal detection activities [IR Art 24(1)].

IX.C.1.2. Roles and Responsibilities of the Lead Member State

The lead Member State:
- Shall take the lead for EudraVigilance data monitoring, signal detection, signal validation and signal confirmation for active substances/medicinal products for which it has been appointed the lead;
- Shall confirm signals that have been detected and validated by a national competent authority for these substances/medicinal products;
- Shall enter into EPITT signals it has detected, validated and confirmed itself for these substances/medicinal products
- Should validate (including, if appropriate, in the EudraVigilance database) and enter into EPITT any other signal communicated by a third party (e.g. regulatory authority from outside the EU) for these substances/medicinal products;
- Shall confirm as soon as possible and no later than 30 days from its receipt any validated signal communicated by marketing authorisation holders for these substances/medicinal products. In this context, where the validity of the signal is not confirmed, special attention shall be paid to any follow-up information which may allow for the signal's confirmation [IR Art 21(3)], see IX.B.3.3.;
- Shall keep an audit trail of their signal detection activities [IR Art 24 (1)].

IX.C.1.3. Roles and Responsibilities of the National Competent Authorities

The national competent authorities shall specifically monitor data originated in their territory [IR Art 18(4)], including data arising from sources mentioned in IX.B.1.

If a lead Member State or the Agency has been appointed for the monitoring of an active substance/medicinal product, the national competent authorities:
- Should enter validated signals it has detected into EPITT for the lead Member State or the rapporteur appointed by the PRAC to confirm.

If no lead Member State or the Agency has been appointed for the monitoring of an active substance/medicinal product, the national competent authorities:
- Shall monitor the data of the EudraVigilance database for substances/medicinal products authorised in their territory;
- Shall validate and confirm any signal they have detected from EudraVigilance for substances/medicinal products authorised in their territory;
- Shall enter validated and confirmed signal they have detected into EPITT for substances/medicinal products authorised in their territory;
- Shall confirm as soon as possible and no later than 30 days from its receipt any validated signal communicated by a marketing authorisation holder for an active substance/medicinal product authorised in their territory. In this context, where the validity of the signal is not confirmed, special attention shall be paid to any follow-up information which may allow for the signal's confirmation [IR Art 21(3)], see IX.B.3.3.

The national competent authorities shall keep an audit trail of their signal detection activities [IR Art 24 (1)].

IX.C.1.4. Roles and Responsibilities of the Pharmacovigilance Risk Assessment Committee

The Pharmacovigilance Risk Assessment Committee (PRAC):
- Shall prioritise validated and confirmed signals for further assessment [REG Art 28a];
- Should nominate a rapporteur for the assessment of the validated and confirmed signals with a time frame for the assessment;
- Shall transmit to the CHMP or to the CMDh, as appropriate, any recommendations for action following the signal assessment;
- Shall perform a regular review of the signal management methodology to be used and publish recommendations as appropriate [IR Art 20 (3)];

- Should review at least every four years the lead and the co-lead Member States responsible for the monitoring of the data in EudraVigilance [IR Art 22(1)];
- Should review the list of medical events that have to be taken into account for the detection of a signal before their publication by the Agency [IR Art 19(2)].

IX.C.1.5. Roles and Responsibilities of Marketing Authorisation Holder

The marketing authorisation holder should continuously monitor the safety of its medicinal products and inform the authorities of any changes that might have an impact on the marketing authorisation.

The marketing authorisation holder:
- Shall monitor the data in EudraVigilance to the extent of their accessibility [IR Art 18(2)]. See also EudraVigilance access rights for stakeholder group III in the EudraVigilance Access Policy for Medicines for Human Use[2]. The frequency of the monitoring should be at least once monthly and shall be proportionate to the identified risk, the potential risk and the need for additional information [IM Art 18(3)];
- Shall validate any signal detected from EudraVigilance and shall forthwith inform the responsible competent authority for signal detection in line with the list as published by the Agency [IR Art 21(2)]. For the validation step, the elements of information presented in IX.B.3.3. should be taken into account;
- Should notify in writing as an Emerging Safety Issue to the competent authorities in Member States where the medicinal product is authorised and to the Agency via email (P-PV-emerging-safety-issue@ema.europa.eu) (see also Module VI), any safety issue arising from its signal detection activity which could have a significant impact on the benefit-risk balance for a medicinal product and/or have implications for public health;
- Should collaborate with the PRAC for the assessment of the signals by providing additional information upon request;
- Should keep an audit trail of its signal detection activities.

IX.C.2. Periodicity of Data Monitoring in EudraVigilance

National competent authorities and the Agency shall ensure the continuous monitoring of data in the EudraVigilance database with a frequency proportionate to the identified risk, the potential risk and the need for additional information [IR Art 18(3)]. The monitoring should be based on a periodic review of statistical outputs (e.g. reaction monitoring reports) to determine whether there are new or changed risks in the safety profile of an active substance/medicinal product. The statistical outputs should contain ADRs in a structured hierarchy (e.g. MedDRA hierarchy) by active substance(s)/medicinal product(s) and allow filters and thresholds to be applied on several fields as appropriate.

The baseline frequency for reviewing the statistical outputs from EudraVigilance should be once-monthly. An increase to the baseline frequency of data monitoring in EudraVigilance may be decided by the lead Member State, the national competent authority or the Agency if justified by the identified or potential risks of the product or by the need for additional information. The PRAC should be informed of the decision and the justification.

For products subject to additional monitoring (see Module X), the frequency for reviewing the statistical outputs should be every 2 weeks until the end of additional monitoring. A 2-week frequency for reviewing the statistical outputs may also be applied for any other product taking into account the following criteria:
- Any product considered to have an identified or potential risk that could impact significantly on the benefit-risk balance or have implications for public health. This may include risks associated with significant misuse, abuse or off-label use. The product may be moved back to baseline frequency of monitoring if risks are not confirmed;
- Any product for which the safety information is limited due to low patient exposure during

---

2. EudraVigilance access policy for medicines for human use published on 23 August 2011
http://www.ema.europa.eu/docs/en_GB/document_library/Other/2011/07/WC500108538.pdf

drug development, including products authorised under conditional approval or under exceptional circumstances, or for which there are vulnerable or poorly studied patient populations or important missing information (e.g. children, pregnant women, renal-impaired patients) while post-marketing exposure is likely to be significant;
- Any product that contains active substances already authorised in the EU but is indicated for use in a new patient population or with a new route of administration;
- Any product for which the existing marketing authorisation has been significantly varied (e.g. changes to indication, posology, pharmaceutical form or route of administration), thereby modifying the exposed patient population or the safety profile.

Confirmation of a signal arising from the EudraVigilance data monitoring activities does not necessarily imply that the product has to be more frequently monitored and a risk proportionate approach should be applied.

More frequent monitoring than every 2 weeks should be based on a proposal from the lead Member State, national competent authority or the Agency. It should be targeted to a safety concern of interest especially during public health emergencies (e.g. pandemics) and may be applied in the context of customised queries or near real-time alerts[3] conducted in the EudraVigilance Data Analysis System (EVDAS).

IX.C.3. Signal Analysis, Prioritisation and Assessment by the Pharmacovigilance Risk Assessment Committee (PRAC)

When the Agency or national competent authority validating or confirming a signal considers urgent action is required before the next PRAC meeting it should trigger the Rapid Alert procedure (see Module XII). All other signals that have been detected, validated and confirmed by the Agency or a national competent authority should be sent to the PRAC for consideration at its next meeting. In its consideration of a signal, the PRAC should agree on a prioritisation based on the individual patient and public health impact of the potential change to the benefit-risk balance. Depending on the prioritisation, an analysis of the need for further assessment or for any immediate recommendation for action should be made, taking into account the time frame proposed by the Agency or the national competent authority that detected the signal.

When PRAC considers a signal as a high priority at a given meeting, a recommendation on the action(s) required should be made during the same meeting and appropriate procedure(s) should be initiated by the Agency and/or national competent authorities in conjunction with the marketing authorisation holder.

When it considers that further signal assessment is needed, the PRAC should nominate a rapporteur and should define a timeframe for this assessment taking into account the prioritisation of the signal.

The rapporteur for the signal assessment should transmit to the PRAC an assessment stating whether there may be new risks, whether risks have changed or whether there is a change in the benefit risk balance in relation to the concerned active substance or medicinal product. The assessment should also include a proposed recommendation for action(s), if appropriate. The PRAC can also conclude that no action is required at EU level at this time point.

Following review of the rapporteur's assessment report, the PRAC should make a recommendation for action(s), stating the reasons on which it is based. The recommendation should include an implementation timetable for completion of any actions requested of the marketing authorisation holder commensurate with the extent and seriousness of the matter in accordance with Article 107h(2) of Directive 2001/83/EC and Article 28a(2) of Regulation (EC) 726/2004.

IX.C.4. Processes for EU Regulatory Follow-up

The recommendation for action of the PRAC should be sent to the CHMP in the case of an active substance that is centrally authorised and to the CMDh in the case of an active substance that is nationally authorised including authorisation through the mutual recognition or decentralised procedure.

---

3. EVDAS automated data processing and network transmission takes usually 1 day

The CHMP or CMDh may decide on any or a combination of the following actions:
- The marketing authorisation holder should conduct further evaluation of data and provide the results of that evaluation according to a defined timeline;
- The marketing authorisation holder should submit an *ad-hoc* PSUR;
- The marketing authorisation holder should sponsor a post-authorisation study according to an agreed protocol and submit the final results of that study;
- The marketing authorisation holder should be requested to submit a RMP or an updated RMP;
- The marketing authorisation holder should take any measures that are required for ensuring the safe and effective use of the medicinal product;
- The marketing authorisation should be varied, suspended, revoked or not renewed;
- The Member States or the Commission should initiate as appropriate, the procedure provided for in Article 31 or in Section 4, Urgent Union Procedure or in Article 31 where appropriate, of Directive 2001/83/EC;
- Urgent safety restrictions should be imposed in accordance with Article 22 of Regulation (EC) 1234/2008;
- An inspection should take place in order to verify that the marketing authorisation holder for the medicinal product satisfies the pharmacovigilance requirements laid down in Titles IX and XI of Directive 2001/83/EC;
- The medicinal product should be included in the list of medicinal products that are subject to additional monitoring within the scope defined in Article 23 of Regulation (EC) 726/2004.

Where recommended by the PRAC and agreed by the CHMP or the CMDh as appropriate, a procedure should be initiated with a timetable in which the marketing authorisation should be varied, suspended, revoked or not renewed where applicable.

IX.C.5. Record Management in the EU Regulatory Network

The Agency and the national competent authorities shall keep an audit trail of all their signal management activities relating to EudraVigilance and of the relevant queries and their outcomes.

Any signal that has been detected and validated by the Agency or a national competent authority in line with the processes described in Section IX.B. should be entered into the web-based European Pharmacovigilance Issues Tracking Tool (EPITT) administered by the Agency. All subsequent evaluations, timelines, decisions, actions, plans, reporting and all other key steps should be recorded and tracked systematically in EPITT by the Agency or the national competent authority in line with the guidance document Exchange of Information Relating to Signals through EPITT by the EU Regulatory Network (EMA/383041/2011).

IX.C.6. Transparency

Article 26(1) of Regulation (EC) 726/2004 states that the Agency shall, in collaboration with the Member States and the Commission, set up and maintain a European medicines web-portal for the dissemination of information on medicinal products authorised in the EU. This information will include the conclusions of the PRAC following the assessment of signals and any recommendations.

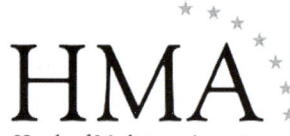
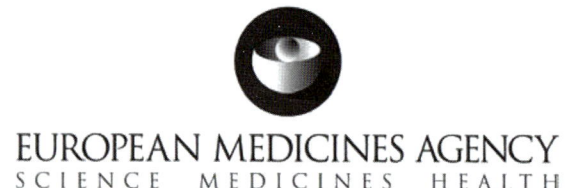

19 April 2013
EMA/169546/2012

GUIDELINE ON GOOD PHARMACOVIGILANCE PRACTICES (GVP)

Module X — Additional Monitoring

Draft finalised by the Agency in collaboration with Member States	25 May 2012
Draft agreed by ERMS FG	30 May 2012
Draft adopted by Executive Director	22 June 2012
Released for public consultation	27 June 2012
End of consultation (deadline for comments)	24 August 2012
Revised draft finalised by the Agency in collaboration with Member States	21 March 2013
Revised draft agreed by ERMS FG	27 March 2013
Revised draft adopted by Executive Director as final	19 April 2013
Date for coming into effect	25 April 2013

X.A. INTRODUCTION

Pharmacovigilance is a vital public health function with the aim of rapidly detecting and responding to potential safety hazards associated with the use of medicinal products.

A medicinal product is authorised on the basis that, its benefit-risk balance is considered to be positive at that time for a specified target population within its approved indication (s). However, not all risks can be identified at the time of initial authorisation and some of the risks associated with the use of a medicinal product emerge or are further characterised in the post-authorisation phase of the product's lifecycle. To strengthen the safety monitoring of medicinal products, the 2010 EU Pharmacovigilance legislation, further amended in 2012, has introduced a framework for enhanced risk proportionate post-authorisation data collection for medicinal products, including the concept of additional monitoring for certain medicinal products.

As defined in Article 23 of Regulation (EC) No 726/2004 (REG) and Article 11 of Directive 2001/83/EC (DIR), the Agency shall, in collaboration with the Member States, set up, maintain and make public a list of medicinal products that are subject to additional monitoring (hereafter referred to as "the list"). These medicinal products will be readily identifiable by an inverted equilateral black triangle ▼ as stipulated in the Implementing Regulation (EU) No 198/2013. That triangle will be followed by an explanatory statement in the summary of product characteristics (SmPC) as follows:

"This medicinal product is subject to additional monitoring. This will allow quick identification of new safety information. Healthcare professionals are asked to report any suspected adverse reactions. See section 4.8 for how to report adverse reactions."

A similar statement will also be included in the package leaflet. This explanatory statement should encourage healthcare professionals and patients to report all suspected adverse reactions.

The pharmacovigilance provisions of Regulation (EC) No 726/2004 and of Directive 2001/83/EC have been recently amended by Regulation (EU) No 1027/2012 and Directive 2012/26/EU respectively. These amendments have impacted on the content and the scope of Article 23 of the REG and will be applicable for centrally authorised products on 5 June 2013. This GVP takes into account the new provisions relating to the list of products which require additional monitoring.

Post-authorisation spontaneous Adverse Drug Reactions (ADR) reports remain a cornerstone of pharmacovigilance. Data from ADR reports is a key source of information for signal detection activities (see Module IX). Increasing the awareness of healthcare professionals and patients of the need to report suspected adverse drug reactions and encouraging their reporting is therefore an important means of monitoring the safety profile of a medicinal product.

The concept of additional monitoring originates primarily from the need to enhance the ADR reporting rates for newly authorised products for which the safety profile might not be fully characterised or for products with newly emerging safety concerns that also need to be better characterised. The main goals are to collect additional information as early as possible to further elucidate the risk profile of products when used in clinical practice and thereby informing the safe and effective use of medicinal products.

This Module is divided in two sections: X.B. provides general principles for assigning additional monitoring status to medicinal products and on communication and transparency aspects. X.C. describes the operation of the EU network regarding the supervision of additional monitoring status, the communication strategy and the impact on pharmacovigilance activities.

X.B. STRUCTURES AND PROCESSES

X.B.1. Principles for Assigning Additional Monitoring Status to a Medicinal Product

All medicines are authorised on the basis that the benefit of treatment is considered to outweigh the potential risks. To come to this conclusion for a marketing authorisation, data from clinical trials conducted during the development of a medicine are assessed. However, adverse reactions which occur rarely or after a long time may become apparent only once the product is used in a wider population and/or after long term use. In addition, the benefits and risks of a medicine may have been evaluated in conditions which may differ from those in everyday medical practice, e.g. clinical trials might exclude certain types of patients with multiple co-morbidities or concomitant medications. Therefore, after a medicine is placed on the market, its use in the wider population requires continuous monitoring. Marketing authorisation holders and competent authorities continuously monitor medicinal products for any information that becomes available and assess whether it impacts on the benefit-risk profile of the medicinal product. However, for certain medicinal products enhanced post-authorisation data collection is needed to ensure that any new safety hazards are identified as promptly as possible and that appropriate action can be initiated immediately. Therefore, in order to strengthen the monitoring of certain medicinal products and in particular to encourage the spontaneous reporting of ADRs, the concept of additional monitoring has been introduced.

Additional monitoring status can be assigned to a medicinal product at the time of granting a marketing authorisation or in some cases at later stages of the product life cycle for a medicinal product for which a new safety concern has been identified. The additional monitoring status is particularly important when granting marketing authorisation for medicinal products containing a new active substance and for all biological medicinal products, which are priorities for pharmacovigilance. Competent authorities may also require additional monitoring status for a medicinal product which is subject to specific obligations e.g. the conduct of a Post-Authorisation Safety Study (PASS) or restrictions with regards to the safe and effective use of the medicinal product.

X.B.2. Communication and Transparency

The additional monitoring status needs to be communicated to healthcare professionals and patients in such a way that it increases reporting of suspected adverse reactions without creating undue alarm. This can be achieved for example by highlighting the need to better characterise the safety profile of a new medicinal product by identifying additional risks but placing those potential risks in the context of the known benefits for this product. A publicly available list of medicinal products with additional monitoring status should be kept up to date by the Agency In addition, healthcare professionals and patients should be enabled to easily identify those products through their product labelling. The publication of the list together with appropriate communication should encourage healthcare professionals and patients to report all suspected adverse drug reactions for all medicinal products subject to additional monitoring.

X.C. OPERATION OF THE EU NETWORK

X.C.1. Criteria for Including a Medicinal Product in the Additional Monitoring List

X.C.1.1. Mandatory Scope

According to Article 23(1) of Regulation (EC) No 726/2004 (REG), it is mandatory to include the following categories of medicinal products in the list:
- Medicinal products authorised in the EU that contain a new active substance which, on 1 January 2011, was not contained in any medicinal product authorised in the EU;
- Any biological medicinal product not covered by the previous category and authorised after 1 January 2011;
- Products for which a PASS was requested at the time of marketing authorisation (point (cb) of Article 9(4) of Regulation (EC) No 726/2004 and point (b) of Article 21a of Directive 2001/83/EC);
- Products authorised with specific obligations on the recording or suspected adverse drug reactions exceeding those referred to in Chapter 3 of Directive 83/2001/EC (point (cb) of Article 9(4) of Regulation (EC) No 726/2004 and point (c) of Article 21a of Directive 2001/83/EC);
- Products for which a PASS was requested following the grant of marketing authorisation (Article 10a(1) of Regulation (EC) No 726/2004 and point (a) of Article 22a (1) of Directive 2001/83/EC);
- Products which were granted a conditional marketing authorisation (Article 14(7) of Regulation (EC) No 726/2004);
- Products authorised under exceptional circumstances (Article 14(8) of Regulation (EC) No 726/2004) and Article 22 of Directive 2001/83/EC).

X.C.1.2. Optional Scope

As set out in Article 23(2) of Regulation (EC) No 726/2004 there is the possibility to include in the list medicinal products subject to conditions, not falling under the mandatory scope. This can be done at the request of the European Commission or a national competent authority, as appropriate, following consultation with the Pharmacovigilance Risk Assessment Committee (PRAC).

As reflected in Article 23(2) of Regulation (EC) No 726/2004 the situations that could form the basis for a request for inclusion in the list are:
- When a marketing authorisation is granted subject to one or more of the following:
    - Conditions or restrictions with regard to the safe and effective use of the medicinal product [REG Art 9(4)(c), DIR Art 21a(d)];
    - Measures for ensuring the safe use of the medicinal product to be included in the risk management system [REG Art 9(4)(ca), DIR Art 21a(a)];
    - An obligation to conduct a post-authorisation efficacy study [REG Art 9(4)(cc)DIR Art 21a(f)];
    - The existence of an adequate pharmacovigilance system [DIR Art 21a(e)].

The scope of Article 23(2) of Regulation (EC) No 726/2004 does not only include medicinal products which are authorised or for which conditions are established after entry into force of the new pharmacovigilance legislation but also medicinal products which were authorised or made subject to conditions before such date, provided they fall within one or more of the above situations for the optional scope.

Pharmacovigilance rules in general and additional monitoring specifically take into account that the full safety profile of medicinal products can only be confirmed after products have been placed on the market. Due consideration should, therefore, be given to the merit of inclusion of a medicinal product in the list in terms of increasing awareness about the safe and effective use of a medicinal product and/or providing any additional information for the evaluation of the product. In this regard, the decision to include a medicinal product subject to conditions in the list should take account of the nature and scope of the conditions or obligations placed on the marketing authorisation including their potential public health impact. The decision should also consider the usefulness of the additional monitoring status in relation to other additional pharmacovigilance activities proposed in the risk management plan, for example in relation to the objectives of PASS.

X.C.2. Criteria for Defining the Initial Time Period of Maintenance in the Additional Monitoring List

X.C.2.1. Mandatory Scope

For medicinal products containing new active substances as well as for all biological medicinal products approved after 1 January 2011 the initial period of time for inclusion is five years after the Union Reference Date (URD) referred to in Article 107c(5) of Directive 2001/83/EC.

X.C.2.2. Optional Scope

The period of time for inclusion in the list of medicinal products authorised subject to conditions is decided by the European Commission or the national competent authority, as appropriate, is linked to the fulfilment of the conditions and obligations placed on the marketing authorisation.

If new conditions are imposed to the marketing authorisation during a product's lifecycle, it is envisaged that a medicinal product previously removed from the list can be added to the list again if for example the criteria stipulated in Article 23(2) of Regulation (EC) No 726/2004 are met again.

X.C.3. Roles and Responsibilities

X.C.3.1. The European Commission

The European Commission decides, based on a recommendation from the PRAC:
- If a particular centrally authorised medicinal product subject to conditions as set out in Article 23(2) of Regulation (EC) 726/2004 should be included in the list.

X.C.3.2. The Agency

The Agency:
- Is responsible for publishing the list of medicinal products that are subject to additional

- monitoring on the European web-portal with an electronic link(s) to a webpage where the product information and the summary of the RMP are publicly available;
- Will coordinate the gathering of information that should be sent by the competent authorities within the EU network in order to set up, maintain and publish the list;
- Is responsible for removing medicinal products from the list after a pre-determined time period;
- Will take into account the list of centralised medicinal products subject to additional monitoring in determining the frequency and processes of its signal detection activities;
- Will inform the relevant MAH when a centralised medicinal product has been included to the list of additional monitored products;
- Will support the process of consultation of the PRAC on the inclusion of medicinal products on the list.

X.C.3.3. National Competent Authorities

National competent authorities should:
- Inform the Agency which nationally authorised medicinal products are to be included in the list and provide the electronic links to the national webpage where the product information and the summary of the RMP are publicly available;
- Decide, based on a recommendation from the PRAC, if a particular nationally authorised medicinal product subject to conditions as set out in Article 23(2) of Regulation (EC) 726/2004 should be subject to additional monitoring and therefore included in the list;
- Make publicly available in their national web-portal the list of medicinal products authorised in their territory that are subject to additional monitoring. The list shall include an electronic link to a webpage where the product information and the summary of the RMP are publicly available;
- Inform the Agency of any update that needs to be made for nationally authorised medicinal products included in the list that is published by the Agency;
- Take into account the list of nationally authorised medicinal products subject to additional monitoring in determining the frequency and processes of their signal detection activities;
- Inform the relevant MAH when a nationally medicinal product has been included to the list of additional monitored products.

X.C.3.4. The Pharmacovigilance Risk Assessment Committee (PRAC)

The PRAC:
- Recommends, upon request of the European Commission or a national competent authority, as appropriate, if a medicinal product which is subject to conditions as set out in Article 23(2) of Regulation (EC) 726/2004 should be included in the list.

X.C.3.5. The Marketing Authorisation Holder

The marketing authorisation holder:
- Shall include in the SmPC and Package leaflet of their medicinal products subject to additional monitoring the black triangle symbol ▼ and the standardised explanatory statement on additional monitoring;
- Should include information on the status of additional monitoring in any material to be distributed to healthcare professionals and patients and should make all efforts to encourage reporting of adverse reactions, as agreed with national competent authorities;
- Should provide evidence to the competent authorities concerned on the status of any conditions imposed by the national competent authorities or the European Commission;
- Should submit the relevant variation to include/remove the black symbol, the statement, and the standardised explanatory sentence from the SmPC and PL, where applicable.

X.C.4. Creation and Maintenance of the List

As defined in Article 23 of Regulation (EC) 726/2004 the Agency shall, in collaboration with the Member States, set up, maintain and make public a list of medicinal products that are subject to additional monitoring. This list will include the names and active substances of all medicinal products approved in the EU subject to additional monitoring irrespective of the approval procedure (i.e. centrally or nationally authorised). In addition, as defined in Article 106 of Directive 2001/83/EC, each Member State shall make publicly available on their national web-portal the list of medicinal product authorised in their territory that are subject to additional monitoring, and take all appropriated measures to encourage patients and health care professional to report any suspected adverse drug reactions.

X.C.4.1. Process for the Creation of the List

The Agency in support of the European Commission will identify the centrally authorised products requiring additional monitoring. National competent authorities are responsible for identifying the nationally authorised products requiring additional monitoring.

Only medicinal products that fall under the mandatory scope according to Article 23(1) of Regulation (EC) 726/2004 will be automatically included in the list. For medicinal products that fall under the optional scope, consultation with the PRAC is required.

The Agency and the national competent authorities will maintain the information that is publicly available and ensure that it is up to date. While the Agency will have direct access to relevant data for centrally authorised products, for nationally authorised products, the Agency will rely on accurate and timely information provided by national competent authorities with regard to the inclusion or removal of medicinal products from the list and the provision of the electronic links to the national web-portals where the product information and the summary of the RMP are publicly available.

The Agency and the Members States will make the list available to the public.

X.C.4.2. Process for the Maintenance of the List

The list will be updated monthly following each PRAC meeting, as appropriate.

X.C.4.2.1. Inclusion of Medicinal Products in the List

Mandatory scope
According to Article 23(1) of Regulation (EC) 726/2004 medicinal product that fall under the mandatory scope will be automatically included in the list on an ongoing basis In case of medicinal products approved through the mutual recognition or decentralised procedures, the Reference Member State (RMS) should inform the Agency once authorisation for such products has been granted. In addition, each national competent authority included in such procedures should inform the Agency, within 15 days of granting the marketing authorisation nationally, and provide the electronic links to their national web-portal where the product information and the summary of the RMP are publicly available. The Agency will include medicinal products in the list within the next update following receipt of the European Commission decision, in case of centrally authorised products, or following receipt of the national competent authorities' notification.

Optional scope
According to Article 23(2) of Regulation (EC) No 726/2004 medicinal products that fall under the optional scope, consultation with the PRAC is required prior to inclusion in the list.

In case of mutual recognition or decentralised procedures, the RMS should be the lead and consult the PRAC as soon as relevant conditions are considered necessary and before the finalisation of the procedure.

In case of purely national procedures, the national competent authority should consult the PRAC as soon as relevant conditions are considered necessary and before the finalisation of the procedure.

The Agency will include centrally authorised products in the list within 15 days of receipt of the European Commission decision. For non-centrally authorised products, once a procedure is finalised each national competent authority should inform the Agency within 15 days on those particular medicinal products that are to be included in the list and provide the electronic links to their national web-portal where the product information and the summary of the RMP are publicly available.

X.C.5. Black Symbol and Explanatory Statements

For medicinal products included in the list, the SmPC shall include the statement:

"This medicinal product is subject to additional monitoring. This will allow quick identification of new safety information. Healthcare professionals are asked to report any suspected adverse reactions. See section 4.8 for how to report adverse reactions."

Preceded by an inverted equilateral black triangle (Implementing Regulation (EU) No 198/2013). A similar statement will also be included in the package leaflet. Once the medicinal product is included or removed from the list, the marketing authorisation holder shall update the SmPC and the package leaflet to include or remove, as appropriate, the black symbol, the statement, and the standardised explanatory statement.

If the decision to include or remove a medicinal product from the list is done during the assessment of a regulatory procedure (e.g. marketing authorisation application, extension of indication, renewal) the SmPC and the package leaflet should be updated before finalisation of the procedure in order to include or remove the black triangle symbol and explanatory statement from the product information.

If the decision to include or remove a medicinal product from the list is done outside a regulatory procedure, then the marketing authorisation holder is requested to subsequently submit a variation to update the product information of that product accordingly.

X.C.6. Transparency

Pursuant to Article 23 of Regulation 726/2004, the Agency will make publicly available the list of the names and active substances of all medicinal products approved in the EU subject to additional monitoring and the general criteria to include medicinal products in the list. The national competent authority shall also make publicly available the list of medicinal products authorised in their territory that are subject to additional monitoring.

The list will include an electronic link(s) to the relevant web-portal where the product information and the summary of the RMP are publicly available.

Annexure 8: Guideline on Good Pharmacovigilance Practices (GVP)

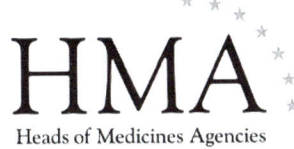

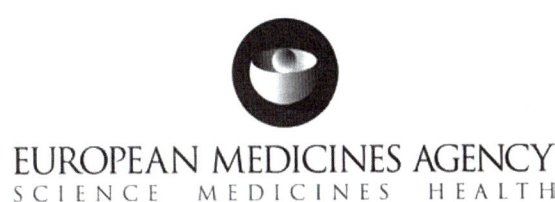

22 January 2013
EMA/118465/2012

GUIDELINE ON GOOD PHARMACOVIGILANCE PRACTICES (GVP)

Module XV – Safety Communication

Draft finalised by the Agency in collaboration with Member States and submitted to ERMS FG	12 July 2012
Draft agreed by ERMS FG	20 July 2012
Draft adopted by Executive Director	25 July 2012
Start of public consultation	26 July 2012
End of consultation (deadline for comments)	21 September 2012
Revised draft finalised by the Agency in collaboration with Member States	10 January 2013
Revised draft agreed by ERMS FG	16 January 2013
Revised draft adopted by Executive Director as final	22 January 2013
Date for coming into effect	24 January 2013

XV.A. INTRODUCTION

This Module provides guidance to marketing authorisation holders, competent authorities in Member States and the European Medicines Agency on how to communicate and coordinate safety information in the EU. Communicating safety information to patients and healthcare professionals is a public health responsibility and is essential for achieving the objectives of pharmacovigilance in terms of promoting the rational, safe and effective use of medicines, preventing harm from adverse reactions and contributing to the protection of patients' and public health (see Module I).

Safety communication is a broad term covering different types of information on medicines, including statutory information as contained in the product information (i.e. the summary of product characteristics (SmPC), package leaflet (PL) and the labelling of the packaging) and public assessment reports. Although some principles in this Module (i.e. Section XV.B.1 and B.2.) apply to all types of safety communication, the module itself focuses on the communication of 'new or emerging safety information', which means new information about a previously known or unknown risk of a medicine which has or may have an impact on a medicine's benefit-risk balance and its condition of use. Unless otherwise stated, the term 'safety communication' in this module should be read as referring to emerging safety information.

Experience so far has demonstrated the need to coordinate safety communication within the EU regulatory network. High levels of public interest are anticipated when new safety concerns arise and it is important that clear and consistent messages are provided across the EU in a timely manner. The new legislation on pharmacovigilance therefore includes a number of provisions to strengthen safety communication and its coordination[1].

Communication of important new safety information on medicinal products should take into account the views and expectations of concerned parties, including patients and healthcare professionals, with due consideration given to relevant legislation. This Module addresses some aspects of the interaction with concerned parties and supplements the specific guidance given in Module XI on public participation as well as the guidance on communication planning given in Module XII.

Communication is distinct from transparency, which aims to provide public access to information related to data assessment, decision-making and safety monitoring performed by competent authorities. The new EU legislation on pharmacovigilance envisages an unprecedented level of transparency. Transparency provisions applicable to each pharmacovigilance process are provided in the relevant GVP Modules.

Section XV.B. of this Module describes principles and means of safety communication. Section XV.C. provides guidance on the coordination and dissemination of safety communications within the EU network. Both sections give particular consideration to direct healthcare professional communications (DHPCs), and provide specific guidance for preparing them. This is because of the central importance of DHPCs in targeting healthcare professionals and because of the level of coordination required between marketing authorisation holders and competent authorities in their preparation.

Throughout this Module, legal obligations are referred to as stated in the GVP Introductory Cover Note and are usually identified by the modal verb 'shall' (e.g 'the marketing authorisation holder shall...'). When guidance is provided on how to implement legal provisions, the modal verb 'should' is used (e.g. 'the marketing authorisation holder should...'

XV.B. STRUCTURES AND PROCESSES

XV.B.1. Objectives of Safety Communication

Safety communication aims at:
- Providing timely, evidence-based information on the safe and effective use of medicines;

---

1. Directive 2010/84/EU amending Directive 2001/83/EC (the latter is referenced as DIR), Regulation (EU) No 1235/2010 amending Regulation (EC) No 726/2004 (the latter is referenced as REG) and in the Commission Implementing Regulation (EU) No 520/2012 on the Performance of Pharmacovigilance Activities Provided for in Regulation (EC) No 726/2004 and Directive 2001/83/EC (the Implementing Regulation is referenced as IR).

- Facilitating changes to healthcare practices (including self-medication practices) where necessary;
- Changing attitudes, decisions and behaviours in relation to the use of medicines;
- Supporting risk minimisation behaviour;
- Facilitating informed decisions on the rational use of medicines.

In addition to the above effective, high quality safety communication can support public confidence in the regulatory system.

XV.B.2. Principles of Safety Communication

The following principles of safety communication should be applied:
- The need for communicating safety information should be considered throughout the pharmacovigilance and risk management process, and should be part of risk assessment (see Module XII).
- There should be adequate coordination and cooperation between the different parties involved in issuing safety communications (e.g. competent authorities, other public bodies and marketing authorisation holders).
- Safety communication should deliver relevant, clear, accurate and consistent messages and reach the right audiences at the right time for them to take appropriate action.
- Safety communication should be tailored to the appropriate audiences (e.g. patients and healthcare professionals) by using appropriate language and taking account of the different levels of knowledge and information needs whilst maintaining the accuracy and consistency of the information conveyed.
- Information on risks should be presented in the context of the benefits of the medicine and include available and relevant information on the seriousness, severity, frequency, risk factors, time to onset, reversibility of potential adverse reactions and, if available, expected time to recovery.
- Safety communication should address the uncertainties related to a safety concern. This is of particular relevance for emerging information which is often communicated while competent authorities are conducting their evaluations; the usefulness of communication at this stage needs to be balanced against the potential for confusion if uncertainties are not properly represented.
- Information on competing risks such as the risk of non-treatment should be included where appropriate.
- The most appropriate quantitative measures should be used when describing and comparing risks, e.g. the use of absolute risks and not just relative risks; for risk comparisons, denominators should be the same in size. The use of other tools such as graphical presentation of the risk and/or the benefit-risk balance may also be used.
- Patients and healthcare professionals should, where possible, be consulted and messages pre-tested early in the preparation of safety communication, particularly on complex safety concerns (see Module XII).
- Where relevant safety communication should be complemented at a later stage with follow-up communication, e.g. on the resolution of a safety concern or updated recommendations.
- The effectiveness of safety communication should be evaluated where appropriate and possible (see XV.B.7.).
- Safety communications should comply with relevant requirements relating to individual data protection and confidentiality.

XV.B.3. Target Audiences

The primary target audiences for safety communication issued by regulatory authorities and marketing authorisation holders should be patients and healthcare professionals who use (i.e. prescribe, handle, dispense, administer or take) medicinal products.

As primary target audiences, healthcare professionals play an essential role. Effective safety communication enables them to give clear and useful information to their patients, thereby promoting patient safety and confidence in the regulatory system. Both healthcare professionals in clinical practice and those involved in clinical trials should be provided with appropriate information on any safety concern at the same time.

Patient, consumer and healthcare professional organisations can play a role as multipliers as they can disseminate important safety information to target audiences.

The media is also a target audience for safety communication. The capacity of the media to reach out to patients, healthcare professionals and the general public is a critical element for amplifying new and important information on medicines. The way safety information is communicated through the media will influence the public perception and it is therefore important that the media receives safety information directly from the competent authorities in addition to the information they receive from other sources, such as from the marketing authorisation holders.

XV.B.4. Content of Safety Communication

Taking into account the principles in XV.B.2., safety communication should contain:
- Important emerging information on any authorised medicinal product which has an impact on the medicine's benefit-risk balance under any conditions of use;
- The reason for initiating safety communication clearly explained to the target audience;
- Any recommendations to healthcare professionals and patients on how to deal with a safety concern;
- When applicable, a statement on the agreement between the marketing authorisation holder and the competent authority on the safety information provided;
- Information on any proposed change to the product information (e.g. the summary of product characteristics (SmPC) or package leaflet (PL));
- A list of literature references, when relevant or a reference to where more detailed information can be found;
- Where relevant, a reminder of the need to report suspected adverse reactions in accordance with national spontaneous reporting systems.

The information in the safety communication shall not be misleading and shall be presented objectively [DIR Art 106a(1)]. Safety information should not include any material or statement which might constitute advertising within the scope of Title VIII of Directive 2001/83/EC.

XV.B.5. Means of safety communication

Communication tools and channels[2] have become more numerous and varied over time, offering the public more information than was previously possible. The use of this increasing variety of means should be considered when issuing safety communication in order to reach the target audiences and meet their growing expectations. Different communication tools and channels are discussed below in sections XV.B.5.1.-XV-B.5.9.

XV.B.5.1. Direct Healthcare Professional Communication (DHPC)

A direct healthcare professional communication (DHPC) is defined in this document as a communication intervention by which important safety information is delivered directly to individual healthcare professionals by a marketing authorisation holder or a competent authority, to inform them of the need to take certain actions or adapt their practices in relation to a medicinal product. DHPCs are not replies to enquiries from healthcare professionals, nor are they meant as educational material for routine risk minimisation activities.

The preparation of DHPCs involves cooperation between the marketing authorisation holder and the competent authority. Agreement between these two parties should be reached before a DHPC is issued by the marketing authorisation holder. The agreement will cover both the content of the information (see XV.B.4.) and the communication plan, including the intended recipients and the timetable for disseminating the DHPC (see Module XII).

Where there are several marketing authorisation holders of the same active substance for which a DHPC is to be issued, a single consistent message should normally be delivered.

Whenever possible, it is advised that healthcare professionals' organisations or learned societies are involved as appropriate during the preparation of DHPCs to ensure that the information they deliver is useful and adapted to the target audience.

A DHPC may be complemented by other communication tools and channels and the

---

2. For the purpose of this section tools and channels are presented without distinction as they often overlap and there is no general agreement on their categorisation.

principle of providing consistent information should apply (XV.B.2.).

A DHPC may be an additional risk minimisation measure as part of a risk management plan (see Modules V and XV).

A DHPC should be disseminated in the following situations when there is a need to take immediate action or change current practice in relation to a medicinal product:
- Suspension, withdrawal or revocation of a marketing authorisation for safety reasons;
- An important change to the use of a medicine due to the restriction of an indication, a new contraindication, or a change in the recommended dose due to safety reasons;
- A restriction in availability or discontinuation of a medicine with potential detrimental effects on patient care.

Other situations where dissemination of a DHPC should be considered are:
- New major warnings or precautions for use in the product information;
- New data identifying a previously unknown risk or a change in the frequency or severity of a known risk;
- Substantiated knowledge that the medicinal product is not as effective as previously considered;
- New recommendations for preventing or treating adverse reactions or to avoid misuse or medication error with the medicinal product;
- Ongoing assessment of an important potential risk, for which data available at a particular point in time are insufficient to take regulatory action (in this case, the DHPC should encourage close monitoring of the safety concern in clinical practice and encourage reporting, and possibly provide information on how to minimise the potential risk).

A competent authority may disseminate or request the marketing authorisation holder to disseminate a DHPC in any situation where the competent authority considers it necessary for the continued safe and effective use of a medicinal product.

XV.B.5.2. Documents in Lay Language

Communication material in lay language (e.g. using a questions and answers format) helps patients and the general public to understand the scientific evidence and regulatory actions relating to a safety concern. Lay language documents should contain the competent authority's recommendations and advice for risk minimisation for patients and healthcare professionals in relation to the safety concern, and should be accompanied by relevant background information.

Lay language documents are generally useful to members of the public who have an interest in the subject but do not have a scientific or regulatory background. Reference should be made to other communication materials on the topic to direct readers to where they can find further information.

Competent authorities publish lay language documents on their national medicines web-portals and may additionally disseminate them to relevant parties such as patients and healthcare professionals' organisations.

Whenever possible, it is advised that patients and healthcare professionals are involved during the preparation of lay language documents to ensure that the information they deliver is useful and adapted to the target audience.

XV.B.5.3. Press Communication

Press communication includes press releases and press briefings which are primarily intended for journalists.

Competent authorities may send press releases directly to journalists in addition to publishing them on their websites. This ensures that journalists, in addition to obtaining information from other sources, receive information that is consistent with the authority's scientific assessment. Interaction with the media is an important way to reach out to a wider audience as well as to build trust in the regulatory system.

Press releases may also be prepared and published by marketing authorisation holders. Their press releases may reflect the position of the marketing authorisation holder on a safety topic but should also make reference to any regulatory action taken by the competent authority. Relevant ongoing reviews should be mentioned in any communication by the marketing authorisation holder.

Although aimed at journalists, press releases will be read by other audiences such as healthcare professionals, patients and the general public. Reference should therefore be made to related communication materials on the topic. In cases where a DHPC is also prepared, healthcare professionals should ideally receive it prior to or around the same time of the publication or distribution of a press release so that they are better prepared to respond to patients.

Press briefings with journalists should be considered by competent authorities for safety concerns or other matters relating to the safety of medicinal products that are of high media interest or when complex or public-health-sensitive messages need to be conveyed.

XV.B.5.4. Website

A website is a key tool for members of the public (including patients and healthcare professionals) actively searching the internet for specific information on medicinal products. Competent authorities as well as marketing authorisation holders should ensure that important safety information published on websites under their control is easily accessible and understandable by the public. Information on websites should be kept up-to-date, with any information that is out-of-date marked as such or removed.

The new legislation on pharmacovigilance foresees the creation of an EU medicines web portal which will contain information on all medicines authorised in the EU [Article 26 of Regulation (EU) No 1235/2010]. This web portal will become a key tool for communicating up-to-date safety information to EU citizens and will contain information in all EU official languages. Each Member State shall set up and maintain a national medicines web-portal which shall be linked to the EU medicines web-portal. [DIR Art 106a]. Until the web portal is fully established and into operation, the Agency's website will be acting as an interim platform to convey this important up-to-date safety information.

XV.B.5.5. Other web-based Communications

Online safety information may also be disseminated via other web tools. When using newer, more rapid communication channels, special attention should be paid to ensure that the accuracy of the information released is not compromised. Communication practices should take into account emerging communication tools used by the various target audiences.

XV.B.5.6. Bulletins and Newsletters

Bulletins and newsletters provide at regular intervals new information about medicines and their safety and effectiveness. Competent authorities can reach a large audience with these tools by using web-based and other available means.

XV.B.5.7. Inter-authority Communication

When one competent authority takes regulatory action on a particular safety concern, other competent authorities usually need to respond to enquiries or communicate on the same issue. The use of inter-authority communication material, such as lines-to-take should be considered. Lines-to-take are documents specifically prepared by a competent authority to assist its own staff and those of co-operating authorities in responding to external enquires or communicating on a specific safety issue.

XV.B.5.8. Responding to Enquiries from the Public

Competent authorities and marketing authorisation holders should have systems in place for responding to enquiries about medicines from individual members of the public. Responses should take into account the information which is in the public domain and should include the relevant recommendations to patients and healthcare professionals issued by competent authorities. Where questions relate to individual treatment advice, the patient should be advised to contact a healthcare professional.

In this respect, Article 86(2) and Article 98(1) of Directive 2001/83/EC apply to marketing authorisation holders.

XV.B.5.9. Other Means of Communication

In addition to those discussed above, there are other tools and channels such as publications in scientific journals and journals of professional bodies.

Some tools and channels may be used in the context of risk management; risk minimisation measures often include specific programmes for risk communication. Tools used in such programmes, such as patient alert cards or healthcare professional safety guidance, are outside the scope of this module and are described in more detail in Module XVI.

XV.B.6. Effectiveness of Safety Communication

Safety communication is considered effective when the message transmitted is received and understood by the target audience in the way it was intended, and appropriate action is taken by the target audience. Adequate mechanisms should be introduced in order to measure the effectiveness of the communication based on clear objectives. Measuring effectiveness allows lessons to be learned and helps in making decisions on prioritising and adapting tools and practices to meet the needs of the target audiences. A research-based approach will normally be appropriate in order to establish that safety communications have met the standard of XV.B.2. This approach may measure different outcomes, including behaviour, attitudes, and knowledge. When evaluating the effectiveness of safety communication, the scope of the evaluation may be broadened to include factors other than the performance of the individual tools used in the safety communication (see Module XVI).

In the case of DHPCs, the marketing authorisation holder should be responsible for evaluating the dissemination of the DHPCs they prepare and should inform the competent authorities of the outcome and of any difficulties identified (e.g. problems related to the list of recipients or the timing and mechanism of dissemination). Appropriate action should be taken as needed to correct the situation or prevent similar problems in the future.

XV.B.7. Quality System Requirements for Safety Communication

In accordance with the quality system requirements in Module I, procedures should be in place to ensure that safety communications comply with the principles in XV.B.2. as appropriate.

In particular, the communications should be subject to quality controls to ensure their accuracy and clarity. For this purpose review procedures with allocated responsibilities should be followed and documented.

XV.C. OPERATION OF THE EU REGULATORY NETWORK

XV.C.1. Coordination of Safety Announcements in the EU

In the EU, patients and healthcare professionals increasingly look at competent authorities as providers of important information on medicines. For safety communication to be effective, adequate coordination and cooperation is required within the EU regulatory network [3]. A good level of coordination of safety communication is of particular importance so that healthcare professionals and patients receive consistent information on regulatory decisions in the EU.

When issuing safety announcements, competent authorities may make use of the different tools and channels described in XV.B.5. Prior to the publication of a safety announcement, the Member States, the Agency or the European Commission shall inform each other not less than 24 hours in advance, unless urgent public announcements are required for the protection of public health [DIR Art 106a(2)].

For active substances contained in medicinal products authorised in more than one Member State, the Agency shall be responsible for the coordination between national competent authorities of safety announcements [DIR Art 106a(3)].

For practical reasons, considering the potential for overlap between transparency measures and active communications and in order to focus on those topics of major health relevance, not all safety information made public by a Member State or the Agency will be subject to systematic exchange and coordination. Only safety announcements that relate to the following and that pertain to active substances contained in medicinal products authorised in more than one Member State require coordination within the EU regulatory network:

---

3   i.e. the competent authorities in the Member States, the Agency and the European Commission.

- The suspension, withdrawal or revocation of a marketing authorisation due to changes to its benefit-risk balance;
- The start or finalisation of an EU referral procedure for safety reasons;
- Restriction of indication or treatment population or the addition of a new contraindication;
- Dissemination of a DHPC agreed by relevant competent authorities of a Member State or the Agency (see XV.C.2.1.);
- Other emerging safety concerns judged by a national competent authority or the Agency to be likely to give rise to public or media interest in more than one Member State (e.g. a publication of important safety findings in a (scientific) journal, safety-related regulatory action taken in a Member State or in a country outside the EU).

XV.C.1.1. Process for Exchange and Coordination of Safety Announcements

A competent authority of a Member State or the Agency shall inform the EU regulatory network prior to the publication of a safety announcement that pertains to active substances contained in medicinal products authorised in more than one Member State and that refer to any of the situations identified in XV.C.1. It shall include a timetable for the information being made public [DIR Art 106a(3)]. Whenever possible the safety announcement shall be sent to the network under embargo no less than 24 hours in advance of publication [DIR Art 106a (2)], in order to allow the members of the EU regulatory network to prepare or plan their own communication if necessary. Under the coordination of the Agency, the Member States shall make all reasonable efforts to agree on a common message [DIR Art 106a(3)].

The Agency should decide for each case, on the basis of the public health relevance and urgency of the safety concern, the population and number of Members States affected and the potential for media attention, whether further action in addition to the dissemination of the safety announcement is needed, such as:

- The preparation of lines-to-take (see XV.B.5.7.) which should be disseminated to the EU regulatory network. The lines-to-take document should help the EU regulatory network to respond to any request for information which may follow the publication of the safety announcement;
- The preparation of an Agency safety announcement in addition to that of the Member State, which should also be disseminated under embargo to the EU regulatory network together with a timetable for its publication.

The Agency should prepare lines-to-take documents and any Agency safety announcement together with the Member State(s) who originated the process and the PRAC Lead Member State or the PRAC Rapporteur, as appropriate. The PRAC, as well as the CHMP or CMDh, should also be consulted as necessary.

Coordination of safety announcements should be done in cooperation with the concerned marketing authorisation holder(s). Whenever possible, the Agency and the competent authorities in Member States should provide any safety announcement prior to its publication to the concerned marketing authorisation holder(s), together with the timetable for the information being made public. Any information of a personal or commercially confidential nature shall be deleted unless its public disclosure is necessary for the protection of public health [DIR Art 106a (4)].

The exchange and coordination of safety announcements within the EU regulatory network should make use of the EU Early Notification System (ENS). The ENS was developed for use by the Agency to provide advance notice to competent authorities in Member States and the European Commission of safety information on centrally authorised products. This system should also be used by competent authorities in Member States for the purpose of exchanging and coordinating safety announcements.

The ENS includes the Heads of Medicines Agencies (HMA), the members of the PRAC, CHMP, CMDh, the operational contact points for safety announcements at the competent authority in Member States, the European Commission and the Agency. Operational contact points should ensure that any information exchanged via the system reaches in a timely manner the relevant staff within each competent authority, including relevant staff working within the communications departments.

Safety announcements from the EU regulatory network should be shared with international partners in accordance with the guidance provided in Module XIV, subject to embargo and any specific confidentiality arrangements in place.

As a complement to the coordination of safety announcements within the EU regulatory network, competent authorities in Member States and the Agency should interact with concerned stakeholders in the EU (mainly patients' and healthcare professionals' organisations), who can play a key role in reviewing and disseminating information to the end users (patients and healthcare professionals). It is recommended that national competent authorities and the Agency keep up-to-date contact details of relevant patients, and healthcare professionals' organisations.

XV.C.1.2. Exchange of Safety Information Produced by Third Parties

There are situations where emerging safety information is to be published or has been published by a party other than a competent authority of a Member State or the Agency (e.g. scientific journals, learned societies). Competent authorities should bring to the attention of the EU regulatory network any such safety information that they become aware of, together with the timing of the publication if known. Where necessary and after evaluation of the information, the Agency should prepare and disseminate a lines-to-take document or an Agency safety announcement to address the information from the third party (see XV.C.1.1.).

In the context of collaboration with authorities outside the EU, the Agency or a competent authority of a Member State may become aware of safety announcements to be published by these authorities (see Module XIV). In these cases the Agency should, as necessary, prepare and disseminate lines-to-take or safety announcements within the EU regulatory network. In all cases, the terms of any relevant confidentiality agreements with non-EU regulatory authorities and the embargoes on the information received should be respected.

XV.C.1.3. Requirements for the Marketing Authorisation Holder in the EU

As soon as a marketing authorisation holder in the EU intends to make a public announcement relating to information on pharmacovigilance concerns in relation to the use of a medicinal product, and in any event at the same time or before the public announcement is made, the marketing authorisation holder shall be required to inform the competent authorities in Member States, the Agency and the European Commission [DIR Art 106a]. This should apply to announcements intended for the EU as well as outside the EU (when they concern products authorised in the EU or those for which an opinion under Article 58 of Regulation (EC) 726/2004 has been given). Informing the authorities at the same time as the public (i.e. without advance notice to the authorities) should only occur exceptionally and under justified grounds. Whenever possible, the information should be provided under embargo at least 24 hours prior to its publication.

The marketing authorisation holder shall ensure that information to the public is presented objectively and is not misleading [DIR Art 106a].

Whenever a marketing authorisation holder becomes aware that a third party (see XV.C.1.2.) intends to issue communication that could potentially impact the benefit-risk balance of a medicinal product authorised in the EU, the marketing authorisation holder should inform the relevant competent authorities in Member States and the Agency and make every effort to share the content of the communications with the relevant authorities.

XV.C.1.4. Consideration for Third Parties

Third parties (e.g. scientific journals, learned societies, patients' organisations) are encouraged to inform the Agency and the competent authorities in Member States of any relevant emerging information on the safety of medicines authorised in the EU and, if publication is planned, to share the information ahead of publication.

XV.C.1.5. Languages and Translations

Consistent messages should reach the public across the EU in a timely manner and in the official languages of the Member States as specified by the Member States where the medicinal product is placed on the market.

For the purpose of coordination, the Agency shall use English to inform the EU regulatory network of any safety announcement. When informing the Agency, the competent authorities in Member States are encouraged to provide English translations of their safety announcements for the purpose of initiating the coordination process. In the absence of a full text translation, an English summary should be provided.

XV.C.2. Direct Healthcare Professional Communications in the EU

In the EU, a direct healthcare professional communication (DHPC) (see XV.B.5.1.) is usually disseminated by one or a group of marketing authorisation holders for the respective medicinal product(s) or active substance(s), either at the request of a national competent authority or the Agency, or on the marketing authorisation holder's own initiative. The marketing authorisation holder should seek the agreement of the relevant national competent authorities or the Agency regarding the content of a DHPC (and communication plan) prior to dissemination.

XV.C.2.1. Processing of DHPCs

The situations when a DHPC is necessary or should be considered are provided in XV.B.5.1. When drafting a DHPC, the template (see Annex II) and the guidance provided in the annotations in the template should be followed as appropriate.

The roles and responsibilities of the competent authorities in a Member State, the Agency and marketing authorisation holders in the preparation and processing of DHPCs depend on the route of authorisation of the medicinal products concerned:
- For centrally authorised products and for products subject to an EU referral procedure for safety reasons, the relevant marketing authorisation holders should submit the draft DHPC and communication plan (including the intended recipients and the timetable for disseminating the DHPC) to the Agency, which should coordinate the review process by its scientific committees (i.e. PRAC and CHMP) and CMDh.
- For products authorised through the mutual recognition or decentralised procedure, the marketing authorisation holder should submit the draft DHPC and communication plan to the Reference Member State, which should co-ordinate the process with the marketing authorisation holder, while keeping the Concerned Member States informed of any proposed action.
- For nationally authorised products not authorised through the mutual recognition or decentralised procedure, the marketing authorisation holder should submit the draft DHPC and any communication plan to the competent authorities of the Member States where the products are authorised.

The marketing authorisation holder should allow a minimum of two working days for comments. However, whenever possible more time should be allowed. The timing may be adapted according to the urgency of the situation.

The Agency will coordinate the review of DHPCs within its scientific committees/groups as appropriate (i.e. involvement of PRAC, and finalisation by CHMP or CMDh) The PRAC should always be involved in the review of DHPCs related to a safety concern being discussed at the PRAC and the DHPC should form part of the PRAC assessment (see Module XII). The Agency may also request advice from the PRAC on issues related to other safety communications.

Once the content of a DHPC and communication plan from the MAH are agreed by national competent authorities or the Agency, the national competent authorities or the Agency should exchange the final DHPC and communication plan using the early notification system (see XV.C.1.1.), and the Agency should coordinate any subsequent safety announcement as appropriate using the process described in XV.C.1.1. The early notification system is only used if the DHPC concerns an active substance authorised in more than one Member State.

In cases where an authority outside the EU requests the dissemination of a DHPC in their territory for a product also authorised in the EU, the marketing authorisation holder should notify the relevant competent authorities in the EU. This is part of the legal requirement under which the marketing authorisation holder shall notify the competent authorities of any new information which may impact the benefit-risk balance of a medicinal product [REG Art 16(2) and DIR 23(2)]. The need for any subsequent communication, e.g. a DHPC, in the EU should be considered and agreed on a case-by-case basis.

A flow chart describing the processing of DHPCs is provided in Figure XV.I at the end of the Module.

Annexure 8: Guideline on Good Pharmacovigilance Practices (GVP)

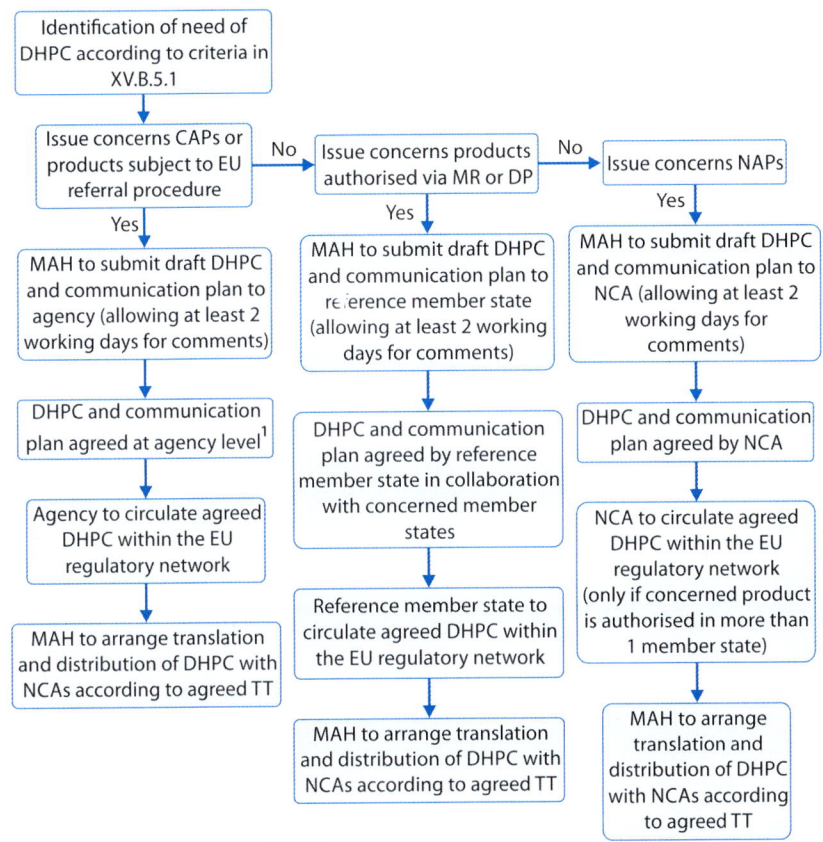

1. The Agency will coordinate the review of DHPC within its scientific committees (i.e. PRAC and CHMP) and CMDh.

FIG. XV.1: Processing of Direct Healthcare Professional Communications (DHPCs) in the EU.

XV.C.2.2. Translation of DHPCs

For centrally authorised products, products subject to an EU referral procedure for safety reasons and, in most cases, products authorised through the mutual recognition or decentralised procedure, the working language for preparing the DHPCs will normally be English.

Once the text of the DHPC is agreed, the marketing authorisation holder should prepare translations in the official languages of the Member States, as specified by the Member States where the DHPC is to be distributed. The draft translations should be submitted to the Member States for a language review within a reasonable timeframe (no more than two working days).

For centrally authorised products and products subject to an EU referral procedure for safety reasons, the relevant marketing authorisation holder should provide the Agency with a complete set of all final EU official language versions as well as any additional related communication documents.

XV.C.2.3. Publication of DHPCs

The competent authorities may publish the final DHPC. The timing for such publication should be aligned to that of the dissemination of DHPC in the Member States. The competent authorities may also issue an additional safety announcement, and disseminate the DHPC to relevant healthcare professionals' organisations as appropriate.

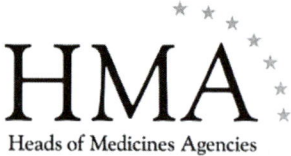
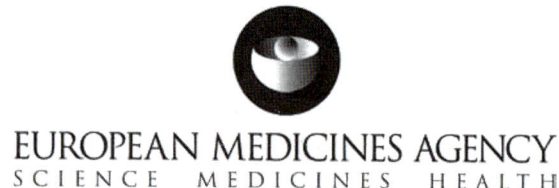

28 March 2017
EMA/204715/2012 Rev 2*

GUIDELINE ON GOOD PHARMACOVIGILANCE PRACTICES (GVP)

Module XVI — Risk Minimisation Measures: Selection of Tools and Effectiveness Indicators (Rev 2)

Date for coming into effect of first version	1 March 2014
Date for coming into effect of Revision 1	28 April 2014
Draft Revision 2* finalised by the Agency in collaboration with Member States	6 March 2017
Draft agreed by the EU Network Pharmacovigilance Oversight Group (EU-POG)	23 March 2017
Draft adopted by Executive Director as final	28 March 2017
Date for coming into effect of Revision 2*	31 March 2017

Note: Revision 2 includes the following:
- Changes to XVI.A. to delete the description of routine risk minimisation tools as they are detailed in GVP Module V and describe only additional risk minimisation tools in GVP Module XVI; therefore Modules V and XVI have to be read together for a full understanding of the selection of risk minimisation tools;
- Changes to XVI.C. to add a paragraph to emphasise the role of Member States in the implementation of risk minimisation measures;
- Changes to XVI.C.1. and XVI.C.2. to add text clarifying the responsibility of the marketing authorisation holder to implement all conditions or restrictions with regard to the safe use of the product in a particular territory;
- Changes to XVI.C.1.1.3. to clarify that patient alert cards included in the package are part of the product information; Editorial amendments throughout the Module to increase the clarity of the guidance and the consistency of its presentation with other GVP Modules.

This revision of the Module was not subject to public consultation because it concerns amendments with the specific objective to align its content with the changes in or adding text from GVP Module V Revision 2, which was subject to public consultation.

XVI.A. INTRODUCTION

Risk minimisation measures are interventions intended to prevent or reduce the occurrence of adverse reactions associated with the exposure to a medicine, or to reduce their severity or impact on the patient should adverse reactions occur. Planning and implementing risk minimisation measures and assessing their effectiveness are key elements of risk management.

The guidance provided in this Module should be considered in the context of the wider GVP guidance, in particular in conjunction with GVP Module V.

Risk minimisation measures may consist of routine risk minimisation or additional risk minimisation measures. Routine risk minimisation is applicable to all medicinal products, and involves the use of different tools, which are described in detail in GVP Module V. Additional risk minimisation measures are described in detail in this GVP Module XVI. Therefore both Modules have to be read together for a full understanding of the selection of risk minimisation tools.

Safety concerns of a medicinal product are normally adequately addressed by routine risk minimisation measures (see GVP Module V). In exceptional cases however, routine risk minimisation measures will not be sufficient for some risks and additional risk minimisation measures will be necessary to manage the risk and/or improve the risk-benefit balance of a medicinal product. This module provides particular guidance on the use of additional risk minimisation measures, including the selection of tools and the evaluation of their effectiveness. In specific circumstances, however, the effectiveness evaluation may also apply to routine risk minimisation measures associated with safety concern(s) which are described in the summary of product characteristics (SmPC) and package leaflet (PL) (e.g. the SmPC provides guidance for clinical actions beyond routine standards of clinical care for either the risk itself or management of the target population). In these circumstances, the guidance provided in this Module on effectiveness evaluation also applies to routine risk minimisation measures. On the basis of the safety concerns described in the safety specification (see GVP Module V), the appropriate risk minimisation measures should be determined. Each safety concern needs to be individually considered and the selection of the most suitable risk minimisation measure should take into account the seriousness of the potential adverse reaction(s) and its severity (impact on patient), its preventability or the clinical actions required to mitigate the risk, the indication, the route of administration, the target population and the healthcare setting for the use of the product. A safety concern may be addressed using more than one risk minimisation measure, and a risk minimisation measure may address more than one safety concern.

Directive 2001/83/EC indicates that the marketing authorisation holder shall "monitor the outcome of risk minimisation measures which are contained in the risk management plan or which are laid down as conditions of the marketing authorisation pursuant to Articles 21a, 22 or 22a" (DIR Art 104 (2) (d)). The Directive and Regulation (EC) No 726/2004 also include provisions for the Agency and the national competent authorities to monitor the outcome of risk minimisation measures which are contained in the risk management plans (RMPs) or measures that are laid down as conditions.

This Module provides guidance on the principles for:
- The development and implementation of additional risk minimisation measures, including examples of risk minimisation tools;
- The evaluation of the effectiveness of risk minimisation measures.

XVI.B. describes the development, implementation and co-ordination of risk minimisation measures and the general principles of the evaluation of their effectiveness. XVI.C. considers the application of those measures and principles in the setting of the EU regulatory network.

In this Module, all applicable legal requirements are referenced in the way explained in the GVP Introductory Cover Note and are usually identifiable by the modal verb "shall". Guidance for the implementation of legal requirements is provided using the modal verb "should".

XVI.B. STRUCTURES AND PROCESSES

XVI.B.1. General Principles

Risk minimisation measures aim to optimise the safe and effective use of a medicinal product throughout its life cycle. The risk-benefit balance of a medicinal product can be improved by reducing the burden of adverse reactions or by optimising benefit, through targeted patient selection and/or exclusion and through treatment management (e.g. specific dosing regimen, relevant testing, patient follow-up). Risk minimisation measures should therefore guide optimal use of a medicinal product in clinical practice with the goal of supporting the provision of the right medicine, at the right dose, at the right time, to the right patient and with the right information and monitoring.

The majority of safety concerns are addressed by routine risk minimisation measures (see GVP Module V). Exceptionally, for selected important risks, routine risk minimisation may be considered insufficient and additional risk minimisation measures may be deemed necessary. In determining if additional risk minimisation activities are needed, safety concerns should be prioritised in terms of frequency, seriousness, severity, impact on public health and preventability. Careful consideration should then be given to whether the goal can be reached with routine minimisation activities, and, if not considered sufficient, which additional minimisation measure(s) is (are) the most appropriate. Additional risk minimisation measures should focus on the most important, preventable risks and the burden of imposing additional risk minimisation should be balanced with the benefit for patients.

A variety of tools are currently available for additional risk minimisation. This field is continuously developing, and new tools are likely to be developed in the future. Technology advances, such as interactive web-based tools may gain prominence in addition to the paper-based educational materials.

Successful implementation of additional risk minimisation measures requires contributions from all stakeholders, including marketing authorisation applicants/holders, patients and healthcare professionals. The performance of these measures in healthcare systems requires assessment to ensure that their objectives are fulfilled and that the measures in place are proportionate taking account of the risk-benefit balance of the product and the efforts required of healthcare professionals and patients to implement the measures. It is therefore important to ensure that additional risk minimisation measures, including assessment of their effectiveness, do not introduce undue burden on the healthcare delivery system, the marketing authorisation holders, the regulators, and, most importantly, on the patients. To this aim, they should have a clearly defined objective relevant to the minimisation of specific risks and/or optimisation of the risk-benefit balance. Clear objectives and defined measures of success with milestones need to guide the development of additional risk minimisation measures, and close monitoring of both their implementation and ultimate effectiveness is necessary. The nature of the safety concern in the context of the risk-benefit balance of the product, the therapeutic need for the product, the target population and the required clinical actions for risk minimisation are factors to be considered when selecting risk minimisation tools and developing an implementation strategy to accomplish the desired public health outcome. The evaluation of effectiveness should facilitate early corrective actions if needed and may require modifications over time. It is recognised that this is an evolving area of medical sciences with no universally agreed standards and approaches. Therefore, it is important to take advantage of any relevant elements of methods from pharmacoepidemiology and other disciplines, such as social/behavioural sciences and qualitative research methods.

The introduction of additional risk minimisation should be considered as a "programme" where specific tools, together with an implementation scheme and evaluation strategy are developed. The description of risk minimisation measures, an integral part of the RMP (see GVP Module V), should therefore give appropriate consideration to the following points:

- Rationale: When additional risk minimisation measure(s) are introduced a rationale should be provided for those additional measures;
- Objectives: Each proposed additional risk minimisation measure(s) should include defined objective(s) and a clear description of how and which safety concern is addressed with the proposed additional risk minimisation measure(s);
- Description: This section of the RMP should describe the selected additional risk minimisation measures, including tools that will be used and key elements of content;

- Implementation: This section of the RMP should provide a detailed proposal for the implementation of additional risk minimisation measures (e.g. setting and timing or frequency of intervention, details of the target audience, plan for the distribution of educational tools; how the action will be coordinated where more than one marketing authorisation holder is involved);
- Evaluation: This section of the RMP should provide a detailed plan with milestones for evaluating the effectiveness of additional risk minimisation measures in process terms and in terms of overall health outcome measures (e.g. reduction of risk).

XVI.B.2. Risk Minimisation Measures

Risk minimisation measures aim to facilitate informed decision making to support risk minimisation when prescribing, dispensing and/or using a medicinal product. While routine measures are applied to every medicinal product (see GVP Module V), additional risk minimisation activities should only be introduced when they are deemed to be essential for the safe and effective use of the medicinal product (see also XVI.C.) and should be developed and provided by suitably qualified people.

Additional risk minimisation measures may differ widely in purpose, design, target audience and complexity. These measures might be used to guide appropriate patient selection with the exclusion of patients where use is contraindicated, to support on-treatment monitoring relevant to important risks and/or management of an adverse reaction. Additionally, specific measures may be developed to minimise the risk of medication error (see PRAC Good Practice Guide on Risk Minimisation and Prevention of Medication Errors[1]) and/or to ensure appropriate administration of the product where it is not feasible to achieve this through the product information and labelling alone. XVI.B.2. describes additional risk minimisation measures that may be considered in addition to the routine measures, including:

- Educational programmes;
- Controlled access programmes;
- Other risk minimisation measures.

XVI.B.2.1. Educational Programme

Educational programmes are based on targeted communication with the aim to supplement the information in the SmPC and PL. Any educational material should focus on actionable goals and should provide clear and concise messages describing actions to be taken in order to prevent and minimise selected risks.

The aim of an educational programme is to improve the use of a medicine by positively influencing the actions of healthcare professionals and patients towards minimising risk. Educational materials should therefore be built on the premise that there is an actionable recommendation for targeted education and that applying this measure is considered essential for minimising an important risk and/or for optimisation of the risk-benefit balance. In the context of an educational programme, the tools can have several different target audiences, can address more than one safety concern and can be delivered using a combination of tools and media (e.g. paper, audio, video, web, in-person training). Ideally, educational materials should be available in a range of formats so as to ensure that access is not limited by a disability or access to the internet. When feasible the appropriateness of the tool and media for the target audience (e.g. suitable language, pictures, diagrams, or other graphical support) should be user tested in advance, in order to optimise the success of the implementation phase.

The content of any educational material should be fully aligned with the currently approved product information for a medicinal product, such as the SmPC and PL, and should add rather than duplicate SmPC and PL information. Promotional elements, either direct or veiled (e.g. logos, product brand colours, suggestive images and pictures), should not be included and the focus of the educational material should be on the risk(s) related to the product and the management of those risk(s) requiring additional risk minimisation.

Any educational programme should be completely separated from promotional activities and contact information of physicians or patients gathered through educational programmes should not be used for promotional activities.

---

1. Pharmacovigilance Risk Assessment Committee. Good practice guide on risk minimisation and prevention of medication errors (EMA/606103/2014). London: EMA; 18 November 2015. Accessible at: www.ema.europa.eu.

The educational tools described below can be considered individually or in combinations while developing an educational programme for the purpose of additional risk minimisation.

XVI.B.2.1.1. Educational Tools

An educational tool should have a clearly defined scope and should include unambiguous statement(s) regarding the important risk(s) of concern to be addressed with the proposed tool, the nature of such risk(s) and the specific steps to be taken by healthcare professionals and/or patients in order to minimise those risks. This information should focus on clearly defined actions related to specific safety concerns described in the RMP and should not be diluted by including information that is not immediately relevant to the safety concern and that is already adequately presented in the SmPC or package leaflet. Educational tools should refer the reader to the SmPC and the package leaflet. In addition to an introductory statement that the educational material is essential to ensure the safe and effective use and appropriately manage important selected risks, elements for inclusion in an educational tool could provide:

- Guidance on prescribing, including patient selection, testing and monitoring;
- Guidance on the management of such risks (to healthcare professionals and patients or carers);
- Guidance on how and where to report adverse reaction of special interest.

Further guidance on the responsibilities of the applicant or marketing authorisation holder and the competent authorities are provided in XVI.C..

XVI.B.2.1.1.1. Educational tools targeting healthcare professionals

The aim of any educational tool targeting a healthcare professional should be to deliver specific recommendation(s) on the use (what to do) and/or contraindication(s) (what not to do) and/or warnings (e.g. how to manage an adverse reaction) associated with the medicine and the specific important risks needing additional risk minimisation measures, including:

- Selection of patients;
- Treatment management such as dosage, testing and monitoring;
- Special administration procedures, or the dispensing of a medicinal product;
- Details of information which needs to be given to patients.

The format of a particular tool should depend upon the message to be delivered. For example, where a number of actions are needed before writing a prescription for a patient, a checklist may be the most suitable format. A brochure may be more appropriate to enhance awareness of specific important risks with a focus on the early recognition and management of adverse reactions, while posters for display in certain clinical environments can include helpful treatment or dosage reference guides. Other formats may be preferable, depending on the objective of the tool.

XVI.B.2.1.1.2. Educational tools targeting patients and/or carers

The aim of tools targeting patients and/or carers should be to enhance their awareness of the early signs and symptoms of specific adverse reactions causing the need for additional risk minimisation measures and on the best course of action to be taken should any of those sign or symptoms occur. If appropriate, a patient' educational tool could be used to provide information on the correct administration of the product and to remind the patient about an important activity, for example a diary of dosing or a diagnostic procedures that need to be carried out and recorded by the patient and eventually discussed with healthcare professionals, to ensure that any steps required for the safe and effective use of the product are adhered to.

Patient alert card

The aim of this tool should be to ensure that special information regarding the patient's current therapy and its important risks (e.g. potential life-threatening interactions with other therapies) is held by the patient at all times and reaches the relevant healthcare professional when needed. The information should be kept to the minimum necessary to convey the key minimisation message(s) and the required action, in any circumstances, including emergency. Ability to carry the patient alert card with ease (e.g. it can be fitted in a wallet) should be a key design feature of this tool.

XVI.B.2.2. Controlled Access Programme

A controlled access programme consists of interventions seeking to control access to a medicinal product beyond the level of control ensured by routine risk minimisation measures, i.e. the legal status. Since a controlled access programme has large implications for all stakeholders, the use of such a programme should be limited and should be guided by a clear therapeutic need for the product based on its demonstrated benefit (e.g. it treats a serious disease without alternative therapies; it treats patients who have failed on existing therapies), the nature of the associated risk (e.g. risk is life-threatening), and the likelihood that this risk can be managed by such a programme. Therefore, controlled access should only be considered as a tool for minimising an important risk with significant public health or individual patient impact for a product with clearly demonstrated benefits but which would not otherwise be available without a programme where patient access is contingent on fulfilling one or more requirements prior to a product being prescribed or dispensed in order to assure its safe use.

Examples of requirements that need to be fulfilled before the product is prescribed and/or dispensed and/or used in a controlled access programme are listed below (they may be included individually or in combination):

- Specific testing and/or examination of the patient to ensure compliance with strictly defined clinical criteria;
- Prescriber, dispenser and/or patient documenting their receipt and understanding of information on the serious risk of the product;
- Explicit procedures for systematic patient follow-up through enrolment in a specific data collection system, e.g. patient registry;
- Medicines made available for dispensing only by pharmacies that are registered and approved to dispense the product.

On occasions, a requirement to test or to monitor a patient in a specific way can also be used as a controlled access tool. For example, monitoring of the patient's health status, laboratory values or other characteristic prior to and/or during treatment, e.g. electrocardiogram, liver function tests, regular blood tests, pregnancy tests (which can be part of a pregnancy prevention programme). Measures should be put in place to ensure that monitoring takes place according to the SmPC where this is critical to risk-benefit balance of the product.

XVI.B.2.3. Other Risk Minimisation Measures

XVI.B.2.3.1. Controlled Distribution System

A controlled distribution system refers to the set of measures implemented to ensure that the stages of the distribution chain of a medicinal product are tracked up to the prescription and/or pharmacy dispensing the product. Orders and shipments of product from a single or multiple identified distribution points facilitate traceability of the product. For instance, this sort of measures could be considered for those products controlled in each country under the respective national legislations to prevent misuse and abuse of medicines.

XVI.B.2.3.2 Pregnancy Prevention Programme

A pregnancy prevention programme (PPP) is a set of interventions aimed at minimising pregnancy exposure during treatment with a medicinal product with known or potential teratogenic effects. The scope of such a programme is to ensure that female patients are not pregnant when starting therapy and do not become pregnant during the course of and/or soon after stopping the therapy. It could also target male patients when use of a medicinal product by the biological father might have a negative effect on pregnancy outcome.

A PPP combines the use of educational tools with interventions to control appropriately access to the medicine. Therefore, the following elements should be considered individually and/or in combination in the development of a PPP:

- Educational tools targeting healthcare professionals and patients to inform about the teratogenic risk and required actions to minimise this risk (e.g. guidance on the need to use more than one method of contraception and guidance on different types of contraception, information included for the patient on how long to avoid pregnancy after treatment is stopped, information for when the male partner is treated);
- Controlled access at prescribing or dispensing level to ensure that a pregnancy test is carried out and negative results are verified by the healthcare professional before prescription or dispensing of the medicinal product;
- Prescription limited to a maximum of 30 days' supply;

- Counselling in the event of inadvertent pregnancy and evaluation of the outcome of any accidental pregnancy.

The design and implementation of a pregnancy registry (as a stand-alone activity or as part of a pregnancy prevention programme) should also be considered for universal enrolment of patients who become pregnant during treatment or within an appropriate time after the end of treatment (e.g. 3 months). Use of this systematic tool to collect pregnancy outcome information can be helpful in assessing the effectiveness of the pregnancy prevention programme and/or in facilitating further characterisation of the risk, particularly in the early period post-authorisation when human pregnancy data may be very limited and/or when the potential concern may be based on non-clinical data alone.

XVI.B.2.3.3. Direct Health Care Professional Communication (DHPC)

A direct healthcare professional communication (DHPC) is a communication intervention by which important information is delivered directly to individual healthcare professionals by a marketing authorisation holder or by a competent authority, to inform them of the need to take certain actions or adapt their practices in relation to a medicinal product (see GVP Annex I). For example, a DHPC may aim at adapting prescribing behaviour to minimise particular risks and/or to reduce the burden of adverse reactions with a medicinal product. Situations where dissemination of a DHPC should be considered are detailed in GVP Module XV.

XVI.B.3. Implementation of risk minimisation measures

Additional risk minimisation measures can consist of one or more interventions that should be implemented in a sustainable way in a defined target group. Careful consideration should be given to both the timing and frequency of any intervention and the procedures to reach the target population. For example, a one-off distribution of educational tools may be insufficient to ensure that all potential prescribers and/or users, including new prescribers and users, are reached. Additional periodic re-distribution of the tools might be necessary. Conversely, educational materials required at the time of launch of a new medicinal product may no longer be necessary or relevant once they have been available for a number of years (see GVP Module V). Because risk minimisation measures serve different specific objectives, some measures such as alert cards, controlled access programmes and pregnancy prevention programmes, will usually apply to all future applications for the same medicinal product, whilst others, such as DHPCs and training materials, may not necessarily be needed for all future applications. The appropriateness of each measure and whether these will be required for the future applications for the same medicinal products should be carefully considered at the time of authorisation of the product (and made clear in the RMP). Careful consideration should be given to the layout and content of the educational tools to ensure a clear distinction from any promotional material distributed. Submission of educational material for review by the competent authority should be separate from submission of promotional material and a cover letter should clearly state whether the materials are promotional or educational. Furthermore, educational tools should be distributed separately from promotional materials as a 'stand-alone' communication and it should be clearly stated that the tools are not promotional material, but rather have risk minimisation purposes. Quality assurance mechanisms should ensure that the distribution systems in place are fit for purpose and auditable.

XVI.B.4. Effectiveness of Risk Minimisation Measures

Evaluating the effectiveness of additional risk minimisation measures is necessary to establish whether an intervention has been effective or not, and if not why and which corrective actions are necessary. The evaluation should be performed for the additional risk minimisation tools individually and for the risk minimisation programme as a whole.

Effectiveness evaluation should be conducted at the most appropriate time, accounting for time required for launch of the risk minimisation measures, the estimated use of the product by the healthcare system and other relevant circumstances.

Periodic review of the effectiveness of one or more specific tools or the overall programme, as appropriate, should be planned. Time points of particular relevance are as follows:

- After initial implementation of a risk minimisation programme (e.g. within 12-18 months), in order to allow the possibility of amendments, should they be necessary;
- In time for the evaluation of the renewal of a marketing authorisation.

Whenever effectiveness is evaluated, careful consideration should be given on the need for continuing with the additional risk minimisation measure.

Effectiveness evaluation should address different aspects of the risk minimisation, i.e. the process itself (i.e. to what extent the programme has been implemented as planned), its impact on knowledge and behavioural changes in the target audience (i.e. the measure(s) in affecting behavioural change), and the outcome (i.e. to what extent the predefined objectives of risk minimisation were met, in the short- and long-term). In designing an evaluation strategy, due consideration needs to be made toward what aspects of process and outcomes can be realistically measured in order to avoid the generation of inaccurate or misleading data or placing an undue burden on the healthcare system or other stakeholders. The time point for assessing each aspect of the intervention as well as setting of realistic metrics on which the effectiveness of the tool is judged, should also be carefully considered and planned prior to initiation.

To evaluate the effectiveness of additional risk minimisation measures two categories of indicators should be considered:
- Process indicators;
- Outcome indicators.

Process indicators are necessary to gather evidence that the implementing steps of additional risk minimisation measures have been successful. These process indicators should provide insight into what extent the programme has been executed as planned and whether the intended impacts on behaviour have been observed. Implementation metrics should be identified in advance and tracked over time. Assessing the implementation process can also improve understanding of the process(es) and causal mechanism(s) whereby the additional risk minimisation measure(s) did or did not lead, to the desired control of specified important risks.

Outcome indicators provide an overall measure of the level of risk control that has been achieved with any risk minimisation measure in place. For example, where the objective of an intervention is to reduce the frequency and/or severity of an adverse reaction, the ultimate measure of success will be linked to this objective.

In rare circumstances when it is justified that the assessment of outcomes indicators is unfeasible (e.g. inadequate number of exposed patients, very rare adverse events), the effectiveness evaluation may be based exclusively on the carefull interpretation of data on process indicators.

The conclusion of the evaluation may be that risk minimisation should remain unchanged or modifications are to be made to existing activities. Alternatively, the assessment could indicate that risk minimisation is insufficient and should be strengthened (e.g. through amendment of warnings or recommendations in the SmPC or package leaflet, improving the clarity of the risk minimisation advice and/or by adding additional tools or improving existing tools). Another decision may be that the risk minimisation is disproportionate or lacking a clear focus and could be reduced or simplified (e.g. by decreasing the number of tools or frequency of intervention, or by eliminating interventions proved to be non-contributory to risk minimisation). In all circumstances, the burden on the patient and the healthcare system should be given careful consideration.

In addition to assessing the effectiveness of risk minimisation measures in managing safety concerns, it is also important to monitor if the risk minimisation intervention may have had unintended (negative) consequences relevant to the public health question under consideration, either in the short- and/or long-term. Examples of unintended consequences may include undue burden on the healthcare system, or discontinuation of a product in patients even if the risk-benefit balance was positive for them.

The legislation defines "Any study ....measuring the effectiveness of risk management measures" as a post-authorisation safety study [DIR Art 1 (15)]. Therefore, if a study is conducted to assess behavioural or safety outcome indicators the detailed guidance for conducting a post-authorisation safety study, which is provided in GVP Module VIII, should be followed. This guidance does not apply to the measurement

---

2. http://www.encepp.eu

of simple process markers (e.g. distribution of the tools reaching the target population). The ENCePP Guide on Methodological Standards in Pharmacoepidemiology[2] should be applied as appropriate.

XVI.B.4.1. Process Indicators

Process indicators are measures of the extent of implementation of the original plan, and/or variations in its delivery. Process indicators should complement but not replace the assessment of the attainment of the objectives of the risk minimisation measures (i.e. outcome indicators). Depending on the nature of the interventions various process indicators can be identified for the assessment of their performance.

XVI.B.4.1.1. Reaching the Target Population

When risk minimisation measures involve the provision of information and guidance to healthcare professionals and/or patients by means of educational tools, measures of distribution and receipt should be used to acquire basic information on implementation. These metrics should focus on assessing whether the materials were delivered to the target audience and whether they were actually received by the target population.

XVI.B.4.1.2. Assessing Clinical Knowledge

In order to assess the awareness of the target audience, their attitude and level of knowledge achieved by educational interventions or other information provision (e.g. via an educational programme with a goal of preventing drug exposure during pregnancy), scientifically rigorous survey methods should be applied. XVI.Appendix I summarises key methodological aspects to be considered for the design and implementation of a survey.

A survey generally includes a set of standard questions administered through telephone contact, in-person interview or self-administered through postal/electronic communication, which are repeated over time. Such an approach may be tailored to the monitoring of attitude and knowledge in a diverse sample that includes representatives from each audience segment of interest in the target populations of healthcare professionals and/or patients. Psychometric measures should be used as appropriate. Whenever feasible a randomised sample and an adequate sample size should be selected. In contrast, use of the advocacy groups or patient support groups to survey knowledge can be considered to be inherently biased through self-selection, and should be avoided.

Appropriate attention should be given to the research objectives, study design, sample size and representativeness, operational definition of dependent and independent variables, and statistical analysis. Thorough consideration should also be given to the choice of the most appropriate data collection instruments (e.g. questionnaires).

XVI.B.4.1.3. Assessing Clinical Actions

In order to evaluate the effectiveness of educational interventions and/or information provisions, not only clinical knowledge but also the resulting clinical actions (i.e. prescribing behaviour) should be measured. Drug utilisation studies by means of secondary use of electronic records or through medical chart abstraction are valuable options to quantify clinical actions if representativeness of the target population and adequate databases are provided. The analysis of prescription records, especially when linked to other patients records (e.g. clinical or demographic data), may allow the evaluation of prescribing behaviour, including co-prescribing of two interacting medicinal products, compliance with laboratory monitoring recommendations, as well as patient selection and monitoring. By applying appropriate statistical methods (e.g. time series analyses, survival analyses, logistic regression) to a cohort of medicines users, different aspects of prescribing or use may be analysed, which can provide insights beyond purely descriptive evidence. Careful consideration should be given to the conduct and interpretation of drug utilisation studies across countries, including the legal status of the medicine and how it is prescribed and dispensed, since prescription patterns may reflect not only the product information and any risk minimisation intervention, but also national guidelines, aspects related to healthcare services, local medical practice, and reimbursement constraints. Such a diversity of national healthcare delivery systems across the EU may justify the conduct of a study with the same objectives in multiple countries.

Studies of behaviour based on data collected through surveys should only be considered when no pre-existing data are available to evaluate clinical actions (i.e. conduct a drug utilisation study based on self-reported data collected in healthcare professionals and/or patients survey).

XVI.B.4.2. Outcome Indicators

The ultimate measures of success of a risk minimisation programme are the safety outcomes, i.e. the frequency and/or severity of adverse reactions in relation to patients' exposure to the medicine outside of an interventional study setting and these safety outcomes should be the outcome indicator(s). Such an evaluation should involve the comparison of epidemiologic measures of outcome frequency such as incidence rate or cumulative incidence of an adverse reaction, obtained, e.g. in the context of post-authorisation safety studies. The use of appropriate safety-related outcomes of interest should be considered (e.g. a surrogate endpoint such as an adequate biomarker as a substitute for a clinical endpoint) if such an approach facilitates the effectiveness evaluation. Under any approach, scientific rigour and recognised principles of epidemiologic research should always guide the assessment of the final outcome indicator of interest. Comparisons of frequency before and after the implementation of the risk minimisation measures (i.e. pre- post-designs) should be considered. When a pre-post design is unfeasible (e.g. when risk minimisation measures are put in place at the time of initial marketing authorisation), the comparison of an outcome frequency indicator obtained post-intervention against a predefined reference value obtained from literature review, historical data, expected frequency in general population, would be acceptable (i.e. observed versus expected analysis) and should take into account any stimulated reporting, changes in patient care and/or risk minimisation measures over time. The selection of any particular reference group should be justified.

Methods to measure the effectiveness of risk minimisation measure should be proportionate to the risks being minimised. As such use of spontaneous reporting rates (i.e. number of suspected adverse reaction reports over a fixed time period) may be acceptable in the context of routine risk minimisation. Spontaneous reporting should be considered with caution when estimating the frequency of adverse events in the treated population, while it may be useful in very specific circumstances, for instance when the adverse reaction with the product is rare, the background incidence of the adverse event in the general population negligible and a strong association between treatment and the adverse event. In those circumstances when a direct measure on the risk in the treated population is not feasible, spontaneous reporting could offer an approximation of the frequency of the adverse reaction in the treated population, provided that reasonably valid data can be obtained to evaluate the reporting rate in the context of product use. However, the well-known biases that affect reporting of suspected adverse reactions may provide misleading results. For instance, the introduction of a risk minimisation measure in response to a safety concern detected in the post-authorisation phase of a medicinal product may raise awareness regarding related adverse reactions which ultimately may result in an increased reporting rate. In these circumstances, an analysis of spontaneous reporting may lead to the erroneous conclusion that the intervention was ineffective. Decreasing reporting rates over time may also lead to the erroneous conclusion that the intervention was effective.

XVI.B.5. Coordination

If several products, including medicinal products authorised according to Articles 10(1) or 10(3) of Directive 2001/83/EC (herein referred to as "generics" or "hybrids", as appropriate), of the same active substance are available on a market, there should be a consistent approach in the use of additional risk minimisation measures coordinated and overseen by the competent authorities. When a coordinated action for a class of products is needed a harmonised approach should be agreed if appropriate. Under these circumstances advanced planning should ensure that the effectiveness of risk minimisation measures (see XVI.B.4.) can be considered for each individual product as well as for the products collectively.

XVI.B.6. Quality Systems of Risk Minimisation Measures

Although many experts may be involved in developing and implementing risk minimisation measures, the final responsibility for the quality, accuracy and scientific integrity of those measures and the plan describing them lies with the marketing authorisation holder and its qualified person responsible for pharmacovigilance (QPPV).

The marketing authorisation holder is responsible for updating the RMP when new information becomes available and should apply the quality principles detailed in GVP Module I. Tracked versions of the RMP should be submitted to facilitate regulatory assessment. These records, the RMP and the associated risk management systems, as well as any documents on risk minimisation measures may be subject to audit or inspection (see GVP Module III).

The marketing authorisation holder should ensure appropriate version control of the risk minimisation tools in order to ensure that all healthcare professionals and patients receive up-to-date risk minimisation tools in a timely manner and that the tools in circulation are consistent with the approved product information. For this purpose, the market authorisation holders are encouraged to keep track of the receipt of any risk minimisation tools by target audience. These records may be subject to audit and inspection.

The marketing authorisation holder should ensure that mechanisms for reporting the results of studies or analyses for evaluation of the effectiveness of risk minimisation measures are documented. These may be subject to audit or inspection.

XVI.C. OPERATION OF THE EU NETWORK

For centrally authorised products additional risk minimisation measures recommended by the Pharmacovigilance Risk Assessment Committee (PRAC) and agreed by the Committee for Medicinal Products for Human Use (CHMP) will become, once agreed by the European Commission through a Commission decision, conditions for the safe and effective use of a medicinal product.

Annex II of the CHMP opinion will outline the key elements of any additional risk minimisation measures imposed on the applicant or marketing authorisation holder as a condition for the safe and effective use of a medicinal product. Because of the specificities of the healthcare systems in Member States and of how particular risk(s) are managed within these systems, some risk minimisation measures may need to be implemented differently depending on national feasibility and require additional agreement with the Member States (e.g. pregnancy prevention programmes, controlled distribution). Therefore, for centrally authorised products, the legislation foresees that in addition to the Commission decision addressed to the marketing authorisation holder under Article 127a of Directive 2001/83/EC, there can be a Commission decision addressed to the Member States giving them the responsibility for ensuring that specific conditions and/or restrictions are implemented by the marketing authorisation holder in their territory.

Therefore, an annex in a Commission decision related to Article 127a of Directive 2001/83/EC may describe the responsibilities of national competent authorities in ensuring that the additional risk minimisation measures are implemented in the Member States in accordance with defined key elements. Further details or key elements on any additional risk minimisation measures should also be included in annex 6 of the RMP (see GVP Module V).

For products authorised under the mutual recognition and decentralised procedure, additional risk minimisation measures should be included in annex 6 of the RMP and may also be laid down as conditions of the marketing authorisation.

In all cases, implementation of additional risk minimisation measures takes place at national level and allows Member States to tailor the required conditions and restrictions to any national legal requirements and local healthcare systems.

XVI.C.1. Roles and Responsibilities within the EU Regulatory Network

This section outlines the responsibilities of different bodies in the process of developing, implementing and evaluating additional risk minimisation measures introduced for the safe and effective use of a medicinal product in the EU.

In order to respect the diversity of the different health care systems in Member States, key elements will be agreed at EU level, which need to be implemented in a coordinated manner across the Member States while providing for agreement of the detail of local implementation at national level. In circumstances where some key elements are specific for only some Member States (e.g. an activity is specifically linked to the healthcare system of one Member State) or where additional risk minimisation measures are not imposed as a condition for marketing authorisation these shall be included in the RMP.

XVI.C.1.1. The European Medicines Agency

The Agency shall, in collaboration with the Member States and facilitated through the PRAC, monitor the outcome of risk minimisation measures contained in RMPs and of conditions referred to in points (c), (ca), (cb) and (cc) of Article 9(4) or in points (a) and (b) of Article 10a(1), and in Article 14(7) and (8) of Regulation (EC) No 726/2004 [REG Art 28a(1)(a)].

In monitoring, the outcome of risk minimisation measures, the Agency should support the PRAC scientific assessment of the outcome of risk minimisation measures which comprise additional risk minimisation measures, through the integration of data provided by Member State resources and research activities. The PRAC will make recommendations to the CHMP or the Coordination Group – Human (CMDh), as appropriate, regarding any necessary regulatory action.

XVI.C.1.2. The Pharmacovigilance Risk Assessment Committee (PRAC)

The PRAC should evaluate the outcome of risk minimisation measures, including additional risk minimisation measures and make recommendations as appropriate regarding any necessary regulatory action.

In addition to advising on the studies and measures described in the RMP, the PRAC will assess both protocol and results of imposed post-authorisation safety studies which aim to evaluate the effectiveness of risk minimisation measures (see GVP Module VIII).

XVI.C.1.3. Competent Authorities in Member States

The national competent authorities are responsible for the oversight at national level of the implementation of additional risk minimisation measures imposed as a condition of the marketing authorisation for the safe and effective use of a medicinal product in the EU, irrespective of the route of marketing authorisation.

For those risk minimisation measures introduced after the initial marketing authorisation, the national competent authorities should ensure prompt consideration and agreement of the interventions with the marketing authorisation holder.

The national competent authorities assisted by the PRAC and CHMP or CMDh, as appropriate, may facilitate harmonisation of the implementation of risk minimisation tools for generic products of the same active substance. When additional risk minimisation measures are considered necessary for generic medicinal product(s) based on safety concerns related to the active substance, the risk minimisation measures applicable to the generic product(s) should be aligned with those for the reference medicinal product. Additional risk minimisation measures for hybrid products may be required in some circumstances beyond those of the reference medicinal product (e.g. different formulation or route of administration or incompatibility issues). To facilitate this, the PRAC may give advice on the key elements that should be implemented for all concerned nationally authorised products (as conditions of their marketing authorisation) and on agreement, may make these general requirements publicly available to facilitate harmonised implementation at national level.

In addition to the above, for centrally authorised products the responsibility of the national competent authorities in ensuring implementation of the risk minimisation measures may be addressed to them by means of Commission decision under Article 127a of Directive 2001/83/EC.

Additionally, the national competent authorities should agree the final content, format and media of the risk minimisation tools, including printed material, web-based platforms and other audio-video media, as well as the schedule planning of interventions with the applicant or marketing authorisation holder before a product is introduced to their market or at any time thereafter as needed (see GVP Module XVI Addendum I).

The national competent authority decides appropriate national educational materials and/or other risk minimisation tools as long as these are aligned with the key elements agreed at EU level and as outlined in the RMP (see GVP Module XVI Addendum I). Similarly, measurement of effectiveness of additional risk minimisation measures may be required in one Member State in reason of its specific health care delivery setting or when, due to national specificities, results of the effectiveness studies cannot be extrapolated from studies conducted in other Member States.

National competent authorities in collaboration with the Agency facilitated through the PRAC shall monitor at national level the outcome of risk minimisation measures contained in RMPs and of the conditions referred to in Articles 21a, 22 or 22a of Directive 2001/83/EC [DIR Art 107h(1)(a)]. Where patient alert cards (see XVI.B.2.1.1.2.) are included in the outer packaging, they are considered as part of the labelling, therefore the text and the format should be agreed by the authorising competent authority (full text included in annex III of the marketing authorisation).

For centrally authorised products, when specific national circumstances are required (e.g. multilingual documents), the patient alert card might not fit a wallet format. In such a case the card might not be included in the product package and should not be considered as part of the labelling. In this case, the national competent authorities should agree on the final content and format, as for other additional risk minimisation activities.

XVI.C.2. Roles and Responsibilities of the Marketing Authorisation Holder or Applicant in the EU

Marketing authorisation applicants/holders in the EU are responsible for ensuring compliance with the conditions of the marketing authorisation for their products wherever they are used within the EU. It is the responsibility of the marketing authorisation holder to implement all conditions or restrictions with regard to the safe use of the product in a particular territory.

The applicant or marketing authorisation holder should clearly define the objectives of any proposed additional risk minimisation measure and the indicators to assess their effectiveness.

The applicant or marketing authorisation holder is encouraged to discuss risk minimisation plans with the competent authorities in Member States as early as is feasible, e.g. when it seems likely that specific risk minimisation activities will need to be adapted to the different healthcare systems in place in the different Member States.

Any additional risk minimisation intervention should be developed in accordance with the general principles outlined in XVI.B.1. and XVI.B.2. and should be fully documented in the RMP (see GVP Module V).

The measures adopted in the RMP should be implemented by the marketing authorisation holder at national level after agreement with the national competent authorities.

The applicant or marketing authorisation holder should provide information regarding the status of implementation of additional risk minimisation measures as agreed with the national competent authorities and keep them informed of any changes, challenges or issues encountered in the implementation of the additional risk minimisation measures. Any relevant changes to the implementation of the tools should be agreed with the national competent authorities before implementation.

In the implementation of web-based tools the applicant or marketing authorisation holder should apply requirements specific for each Member State, with particular consideration of potential issues linked to accessibility, recognisability, responsibility, and privacy and data protection.

For generic products the applicant or marketing authorisation holder should develop risk minimisation in line with the scope, content, and format of the tools used for the reference medicinal product. Scheduling and planning of interventions should be carefully coordinated in order to minimise the burden on the healthcare systems.

The marketing authorisation holder shall monitor the outcome of risk minimisation measures which are contained in the RMP or which are laid down as conditions of the marketing authorisation pursuant to Articles 21a, 22 or 22a of DIR [DIR Art 104(3)(d)]. General principles for effectiveness evaluation are provided in XVI.B.3..

The applicant or marketing authorisation holder should report the evaluation of the impact of additional risk minimisation activities when updating the RMP (see V.B.11.4.).

The applicant or marketing authorisation holder should report in the periodic safety update report (PSUR) the results of the assessment of the effectiveness of risk minimisation measures which might have an impact on the safety or risk-benefit assessment (see VII.B.5.16.5. and VII.C.5.5).

For generic products, the effectiveness of risk minimisation measures should be assessed by the marketing authorisation holders in close cooperation with the competent authorities. Where formal studies are justified, joint studies for all medicinal products involved are strongly encouraged in order to minimise the burden on the healthcare systems. For instance, if a prospective cohort study is instituted, study entry should be independent from the prescription of a product with a specific invented name or marketing authorisation holder. Recording of specific product details would still be important to enable rapid identification of any new safety hazard with a particular product.

The applicant or marketing authorisation holder should ensure timely communication with the competent authorities for relevant regulatory evaluation and actions, as appropriate (see also XVI.C.2. and GVP Modules V and VII).

XVI.C.3. Healthcare Professionals and Patients

Healthcare professionals and patients hold no legal obligations with respect to the implementation of the pharmacovigilance legislation. Nonetheless the cooperation of healthcare professionals and patients is paramount to the success of educational programmes and/or controlled access programmes in order to optimise the risk-benefit balance. It is desirable that they give careful consideration to any additional risk minimisation measure which may be introduced for the safe and effective use of medicines.

XVI.C.4. Impact of Risk Minimisation Measures Effectiveness on RMP/PSUR in the EU

PSUR and RMP updates should include a summary evaluation of the outcome of specific risk minimisation measures implemented to mitigate important risks in the EU. In the RMP, the focus should be on how this informs risk minimisation and/or pharmacovigilance planning. In the PSUR, there should also be evaluation of how the implemented measures impact on the safety profile and/or risk-benefit balance of the product. In general, the focus should be on information which has emerged during the reporting period or since implementation of the most recent risk minimisation measure(s) in the EU. Where there is parallel submission of a PSUR and an RMP update to the competent authorities of the EU regulatory network, the use of a common content module should be considered (see GVP Modules V and VII). For the evaluation, the guidance in XVI.B.4. applies.

Results of the assessment(s) of the effectiveness of risk minimisation measures should always be included in the RMP. As part of this critical evaluation, the marketing authorisation holder should make observations on factors contributing to the success or weakness of risk minimisation measures. This critical analysis may include reference to experience outside the EU, where relevant.

The evaluation of the effectiveness of risk minimisation measures should focus on whether these have succeeded in minimising risk. This should be analysed using a combination of process and outcome indicators, as described in XVI.B.3.. It may be appropriate to distinguish between risk minimisation measures implemented at the time of initial marketing authorisation and those introduced later in the post-authorisation phase.

When presenting the outcome of an evaluation of the effectiveness of a risk minimisation measure, the following aspects should be considered:
1. The evaluation should provide context by a) briefly describing the implemented risk minimisation measure(s), b) defining their objective(s), and c) outlining the selected process and outcome indicators.
2. The evaluation should incorporate relevant analyses of the nature of the adverse reaction(s) including its severity and preventability. Where appropriate logistical factors which may impact on clinical delivery of the risk minimisation measure should also be included.
3. The evaluation should include an examination of the delivery of the risk minimisation measures in routine clinical practice, including any deviation from the original plan. Such an

evaluation may include the results of drug utilisation studies.
4. Outcome indicators should normally be the key endpoint when assessing the attainment of risk minimisation measures objectives.

Proposals for changes to enhance risk management should be presented in the regional appendix of the PSUR (see GVP Module VII). The RMP should be updated to take account of emerging information on the effectiveness of risk minimisation measures.

In general, generic products are exempt from routine PSUR reporting in the EU. The frequency of RMP updates should be proportionate to the risks of the product. In general, the focus of RMP updates should be on the risk minimisation measures and in providing updates on the implementation of those measures where applicable. If there is a consequential change to the summary RMP, this should also be highlighted in the cover letter. Changes to the product information should not be proposed via a standalone RMP update, but rather a variation application should be submitted. A PSUR can also result directly in an update to product information (if PSURs are being submitted by the marketing authorisation holder for a given generic product).

XVI.C.5. Transparency

Procedures should be in place to ensure full transparency of relevant information pertaining to the risk minimisation measures in place for the concerned medicinal products.

In accordance with Article 106 of Directive 2001/83/EC and Article 26 of Regulation (EC) No 726/2004, the Agency and national competent authorities shall make publicly available public assessment reports for medicinal products, as well as summaries of RMPs [IR Art 31], including risk minimisation measures therein described.

For centrally authorised products, the Agency shall make public:
- A summary of the risk management plan [REG Art 26(1)(c)], with specific focus on risk minimisation activities described therein [IR Art 31.1];
- The European public assessment report (EPAR) that includes any conditions of the marketing authorisation, such as additional risk minimisation measures [REG Art 26(1)(j)].

By means of the national medicines web-portals, the Member States shall make publicly available at least the following:
- Public assessment report; this shall include a summary written in a manner that is understandable to the public [DIR Art 21(4), Art 106(a)];
- Summary of product characteristics and package leaflets [DIR Art 21(3), Art 106(b)];
- Conditions of the marketing authorisation together with any deadlines for the fulfilment of those conditions [DIR Art 21(3)];
- Summaries of risk management plans [DIR Art 106(c)]; with specific focus on risk minimisation activities described therein [IR Art 31.1].

To promote public health, it is recommended that the Agency and the national competent authorities make the following information available via their websites:
- Details of additional risk minimisation measures required as a condition of the marketing authorisation (e.g. when risk communication tools consist of printed material, a copy is provided or whenever possible, provision of electronic access to the educational material, patient card, check lists or other risk minimisation tools is advised);
- Details of disease or substance registries requested as part of a restricted distribution system.

XVI. APPENDIX 1. KEY ELEMENTS OF SURVEY METHODOLOGY

Surveys are methods of systematically collecting primary data directly from a sample of participants of a larger population. These are conducted in order to characterise the larger population and may be cross-sectional (one-time only) or longitudinal (repeated over time).

In the context of the evaluation of the effectiveness of risk minimisation measures a survey can be conducted to evaluate understanding, knowledge and behaviour resulting from educational interventions in a specified target population with respect to the safety and risk management of a medicinal product.

A survey might not be the most appropriate approach for the evaluation of behaviour, since surveys often collect and analyse self-reported data from healthcare professionals and patients.

Furthermore, participation in a survey in itself may introduce behaviour changes or may not be representative of the target users given that participation is more likely amongst engaged healthcare professionals and/or more motivated or educated individuals.

As a minimum, the following elements should be considered in the design and implementation of a survey with a view to minimise potential biases and to optimise the generalisability of the results to the intended population:
1. Sampling procedures and recruitment strategy;
2. Design and administration of the data collection instrument(s);
3. Analytical approaches;
4. Ethics, privacy, and overall feasibility of a study.

XVI.App1.1. Sampling Procedures and Recruitment Strategy

In any survey, the sampling frame and recruitment of participants may be subject to selection bias leading to a study population that is not similar to, or representative of, the intended population in one or more aspects. Furthermore, it should be considered that a bias cannot be eliminated only by increasing the sample frame, sample size and response rate. Bias can be minimised by selecting the optimal sampling frame, taking into account age, sex, geographical distribution and additional characteristics of the study population. Bias can also be minimised by assuring the sample contains appropriate diversity to allow stratification of results by key population characteristics (e.g. by oversampling a small but important subgroup). Key elements to be considered in the sampling frame include age, gender, geographical distribution, and additional characteristics of the study population. For example, in a physician survey, the strategy for randomly selecting the study sample should consider whether a general random sample would be sufficient or if the sample should be stratified by key characteristics such as specialty, type of practice (e.g. primary care, specialist care, academic hospital). In a patient survey, income and education, medical condition(s), chronic vs acute use, should be considered.

In addition to the overall representativeness of the target population the recruitment strategy of a survey should give careful consideration of the potential recruitment sources. For the recruitment of healthcare professionals, sponsor lists, web panels, professional and learned societies may represent feasible approaches. However, their representativeness for the intended target population of physicians needs to be carefully reviewed for each study. For patient recruitment the relevant clinical setting, and existing web-panels should be considered. A recruitment strategy should be designed while accounting for the chances of achieving accurate and complete data collection. Efforts should be made to document the proportion of non-responders and their characteristics to evaluate potential influences on the representativeness of the sample.

XVI.App1.2. Design and Administration of the Data Collection Instrument(s)

Data collection approaches in a survey may vary from in-person interview, testing, and measurement or collection of biological samples as for routine clinical practice, to telephone interview, web-based or paper-based questionnaires. Audio computer-assisted self-interviewing (A-CASI), interactive voice response systems (IVRS), or mixed mode approaches may also be appropriate. The choice of the most suitable data collection approach will depend on the target population characteristics, the disease and the treatment characteristics and the type of data to be collected.

Each data collection approach will require the ad hoc design of one or more specific instruments. Nonetheless general design considerations that may apply to all instruments include the following:
- Burden to participant, e.g. length or duration, cognitive burden, sensitivity to participant;
- Clarity and sequence of questions, e.g. use of unambiguous language, minimising assumptions, starting with the most important questions and leaving sensitive questions until later;
- Completeness of responses, e.g. structure questions in order to lead to a single unambiguous answer, allow for choices such as "unknown" or "don't know";
- Layout of data collection instrument, e.g. clear flow, technology-assisted guides (avoid patterns, reminders for non-response and visual images);

- Testing and revision of instrument, e.g. formal testing using cognitive pre-testing such as one-to-one interviews, probing questions, interview guide or trained interviewer, and "think aloud" process;
- Incentives to improve response rate, e.g. fed back aggregated data to the survey participants.

XVI.App1.3. Analytical Approaches

The key analytical elements of a survey should include:
- Descriptive statistics, such as:
  - The percentage of participants responding correctly to knowledge questions;
  - Stratification by selected variable;
  - Data on no-response or incomplete response;
- Comparison of responders and non-responders characteristics (if data available);
- Comparison of responders and overall target population characteristics.
- When survey results are weighted, the following key points should be considered:
  - Differences in selection probabilities (e.g. if certain subgroups were over-sampled);
  - Differences in response rates;
  - Post-stratification weighting to the external population;
  - Clustering.

Examples of stratified analyses of physician's survey include the following:
- Specialty of physician;
- Geographic location;
- Receipt of any educational material;
- Volume of prescribing.

XVI.App1.4. Ethics, Privacy and Overall Study Feasibility

Ethical and data privacy requirements are not harmonised across Member States and have notable differences in national (or regional) processes. National (or regional) differences may exist regarding the appropriateness of providing incentives to survey participants. There may also be privacy considerations in allowing contact with physicians based on a prescriber list that is held by marketing authorisation holder.

The overall feasibility assessment of a study is a key step in the successful implementation of a survey. For clinical-based data collection, key elements of such an assessment include:
- Gathering information on site and characteristics of study population (patients or healthcare professionals);
- Estimating reasonable study sample size, the number of sites required to achieve the sample size, and approximate length of the data collection period (e.g. based on estimated patient volume, frequency of patient visits, and expected patient response rate);
- Evaluating site resources and interest in the study.

Key elements of a feasibility assessment may be different for other study designs (e.g. web-based recruitment and data collection) and for physician assessments.

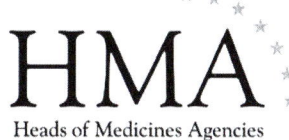 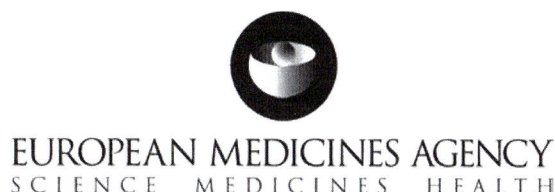

8 December 2015
EMA/61341/2015

GUIDELINE ON GOOD PHARMACOVIGILANCE PRACTICES (GVP)

Module XVI Addendum I — Educational Materials

Draft finalised by the Agency in collaboration with Member States for submission to ERMS FG	24 March 2015
Draft agreed by the European Risk Management Strategy Facilitation Group (ERMS FG)	30 March 2015
Draft adopted by the Executive Director	18 April 2015
Released for public consultation	27 April 2015
End of consultation (deadline for comments)	30 June 2015
Revised draft finalised by the Agency in collaboration with Member States	17 November 2015
Revised draft agreed by ERMS FG	24 November 2015
Revised draft adopted by Executive Director as final	8 December 2015
Date for coming into effect	16 December 2015

XVI. ADD I.1. INTRODUCTION

Educational programmes are additional risk minimisation measures (aRMM) (see GVP Module XVI) and usually include educational material(s) aimed to minimise an important risk and/or to maximise the risk-benefit balance of a medicinal product. The content of any educational material should be fully aligned with the currently authorised product information for the medicinal product, i.e. the summary product characteristics (SmPC), the package leaflet (PL) and the labelling, and should add rather than replicate SmPC and PL information.

When the development and distribution of educational material is recommended by the Pharmacovigilance Risk Assessment Committee (PRAC) and endorsed by the Committee for Medicinal Products for Human Use (CHMP) or the Coordination Group for Mutual Recognition and Decentralised Procedures-Human (CMDh), key elements of any educational material are agreed at EU level. Thereafter, drafts of the educational material(s) addressing the key elements should be submitted by the marketing authorisation holder to the competent authorities of Member States for assessment and then be implemented in Member States upon approval by the competent authorities.

Guidance on the requirements for including the key elements of the educational material(s) and/or the educational material(s) addressing the key elements as distributed in the Member States in an annex to the risk management plan (RMP) is provided in GVP Module V.

This Addendum to GVP Module XVI provides further guidance for marketing authorisation holders on the submission of draft educational material(s) to the competent authorities of Member States, as well as, guidance for these authorities to support the assessment of such materials, in particular with regard to format and content. Because of the specificities of the national healthcare systems and of how particular risk(s) are managed within these systems, individual Member States may have additional requirements. In this case, the guidance in this Addendum to GVP Module XVI should be followed together with national guidelines.

This Addendum is applicable to both centrally and nationally authorised products, including those authorised through the mutual recognition and decentralised procedures.

XVI. ADD I.2. PRINCIPLES FOR EDUCATIONAL MATERIALS

The following principles apply to educational materials:
- The need for educational materials may be agreed during a regulatory procedure, at the time of the initial marketing authorisation or in the post-authorisation phase, e.g. after introduction of a new RMP or an update of an existing RMP.
- Any educational material should be specifically designed to fulfil the risk minimisation objectives.
- It should focus on the specific safety concern(s) and provide clear statements and concise messages describing actions to be taken in order to prevent and minimise these risks.
- The national versions of the educational material should only be submitted, by the marketing authorisation holder, to the respective competent authorities of Member States, following the conclusion of the regulatory procedure in which the aRMM was agreed.
- Educational materials should be drafted in the official language(s) as required by the Member State.
- Educational materials should not include or be combined with promotional elements either direct or veiled (e.g. suggestive images and pictures).
- The methods for dissemination and the target audience in each Member State are determined at national level by the respective competent authority of the Member State.
- Based on the respective target audience, the marketing authorisation holder should provide to each national competent authority a proposal for the educational material(s). The target population determines which tool, content, format, language type and readability level is appropriate for the educational material. Specific efforts in adaption should be made when targeting patients (see GVP Module XV).
- The competent authorities of Member States where the medicinal product is/will be marketed should review the respective national version(s) of the educational material(s).
- The marketing authorisation holder should disseminate the educational material(s) in

a Member State only after approval by the competent authorities of that Member State.
- If the medicinal product is not placed on the market in a Member State dissemination of the material in that Member State is not required. In any case, the need for dissemination of any educational material should be discussed with the competent authority of each Member State.
- The marketing authorisation holder should exercise version control and ensure that only the latest agreed version of the educational material is disseminated. The date of approval by the competent authority the Member State should be included in the educational material, as reference for healthcare professionals and/or patients.
- Without prejudice to the originality of the format of the educational material, it is in the interest of public health that educational material used by different applicants/marketing authorisation holders for the same active substance should be kept as similar as possible, in order to deliver a consistent message and avoid confusion in the target audience. Therefore, marketing authorisation holders are strongly encouraged to share the content of their educational material(s) upon request from other marketing authorisation holders.

XVI. ADD I.3. SUBMISSION OF EDUCATIONAL MATERIALS

If no other national requirements apply, the draft educational material should be submitted to the competent authorities of Member States as follows:
- With a cover letter and/or request form including the following information:
  - The contact details of the marketing authorisation holder and, if applicable, another organisation to which it has subcontracted the submission (at least names and e-mail addresses);
  - The regulatory procedure which has led to the need of the educational material(s) with supportive documents (e.g. CHMP opinion, CMDh position and/or European Commission decision including conditions of the marketing authorisation and other annexes, national competent authority opinion, approved RMP, assessment report identifying the need for this aRMM);
  - A detailed implementation plan for the educational material with the following information:
    - Target population(s);
    - Dissemination method (e.g. paper, e-mail, via social media, learned societies and/or patient associations, publication on websites);
    - Time point when dissemination is anticipated to start and frequency of further disseminations;
    - Estimated date of launch or date of start of the marketing of the product (in the case of a new marketing authorisation);
- As documents in a common open text-processing electronic format of the proposed materials in language(s) required by the Member State(s);
- The intended layout and, where applicable, images and graphic presentations of the information (e.g. pictures, charts, diagrams, video).

When changes of the risk and/or the need for aRMM have been identified and changes in the key elements and/or in the content of the educational material(s) have been agreed at EU level and/or by the national competent authorities, the marketing authorisation holder should submit to the competent authorities of Member States revised proposals of the educational material for assessment and approval. In the revised educational material, the changes to the materials previously approved by the competent authority should be highlighted.

XVI. ADD I.4. FORMAT AND LAYOUT OF EDUCATIONAL MATERIALS

Educational materials should have an appropriate format and layout.

A title line identifying the type of educational material, e.g. administration guide, checklist for prescribing, alert card, educational leaflet for the patient, is recommended.

The format of educational material should include the following:
- The invented name of the medicinal product followed by the name of the active substance(s) and/or therapeutic class in brackets. However, if the educational material is applicable to several products from different marketing

authorisation holders in the Member State, the educational material should refer to the active substance only and a list of the invented names applicable in the Member State should be annexed;
- The black symbol next to the invented or active substance name, along with the explanatory standard statement for additional monitoring if the medicinal product is under additional monitoring (see GVP Module X).

The material should be formatted as follows:
- Bullet points should be used wherever appropriate to present the information clearly;
- Materials should be kept as brief as possible; however, if the educational material is long, an introductory text summarising the key messages should be added and an index may be included;
- If the marketing authorisation holder's and/or product's logo appear, it should appear only once in each educational material, preferably on the first or last page, respectively, and should not be larger than the document title;
- For version control, a unique document identifier should be used on each sheet of the educational material, and the date of last revision of the text (i.e. the approval date of the material by the applicable national competent authority) in the format of "<month> <year>" should be provided on the first and the last page, unless the type of educational material requires appropriate exceptions (e.g. a video should have the unique document identifier appearing at its beginning and ending).

XVI. ADD I.5. CONTENT OF EDUCATIONAL MATERIALS

The reference documents to be used in the preparation of educational materials are the agreed RMP (including its annexes), the product information and the conditions of the marketing authorisation.

The educational material should contain the messages of the key elements agreed, depending on the regulatory procedure, at EU level or with the competent authority of the Member State and laid down in the conditions of the marketing authorisation (as referred to in Article 9(4) of Regulation (EC) No 726/2004 and Article 21a(a) of Directive 2001/83/EC).

The educational material may also contain a reference to the website of the competent authority of the Member State, the Agency or the marketing authorisation holder's specific website (see XVI. Add I.7.), if the SmPC and/or PL are made publicly available on these websites.

References to other websites for "more information" will usually not be acceptable unless they refer to the SmPC/PL or unless specific circumstances apply, e.g. in order to refer to a specific antibody test or to refer to a video that instructs the patient how to take the medicine and/or to use a device, if agreed with the competent authority(ies) of Member State(s).

Images and graphic presentations of the information should only be used when text alone is insufficient to adequately convey the messages of the key element(s) and should not be promotional (e.g. use of a particular device to administer the medicinal product).

The scope of the information in the educational material should be limited to the agreed key elements. Additional information such as efficacy data, comparisons of safety with other medicinal products or statements which imply that the medicine is well tolerated or that adverse reactions occur with a low frequency should not be included. However, in certain circumstances the competent authorities of Member States might consider the inclusion of efficacy data provided that this is duly justified by the marketing authorisation holder. Referring to other medicinal products outside the scope of the educational material is not allowed.

A statement which encourages the reporting of any suspected adverse reaction and information on the modalities how to report in the Member State should be also included.

XVI. ADD I.6. ASSESSMENT AND PUBLICATION OF EDUCATIONAL MATERIALS BY THE COMPETENT AUTHORITIES OF MEMBER STATES

The timelines for the assessment of draft educational materials by the different competent authorities of Member States may vary, depending on e.g. the aRMM, the kind of requested educational materials, or the quality of the submitted drafts. Nevertheless, an average timeline of 60 days should be considered for assessment. This is without prejudice to any other timeline defined by competent authorities at national level.

In the interest of public health, the competent authorities of Member States, in accordance with national legislation, may publish the agreed educational material(s) in a dedicated section of their websites.

Marketing authorisation holders are solely responsible for the provision, to the competent authorities, of the latest agreed versions of the educational materials.

XVI. ADD I.7. PUBLICATION OF EDUCATIONAL MATERIALS ON THE MARKETING AUTHORISATION HOLDER'S SPECIFIC WEBSITE

The marketing authorisation holder may publish the educational material(s) on a specifically dedicated (or other suitable) website, provided that the marketing authorisation holder respects the following:

- The way in which dissemination via the website occurs should be agreed with the competent authority of the Member State, i.e. as primary or as an additional way for dissemination.
- The website address should be given to the competent authority of the Member State.
- A statement that the information of the website is consistent with the educational material approved by the competent authority should be submitted to the competent authority of the Member State.
- The specific website should not include any reference to documents or to other websites/pages or weblinks not agreed with the competent authority of the Member State.
- All elements and information on the specific website should be expressed in the official language(s) as required by the Member State or, in exceptional cases with the agreement of the competent authority of the Member State, in English.
- The specific website should not contain references to or information about medicinal products not marketed in that Member State.

Other relevant documents such as the SmPC, the PL and the summary of the RMP may be referred to.

ANNEXURE 9

ADR Report Form in English—China

Report can be returned by fax to 2319 6319
For Follow-up report (see Guidance),
Please provide previous case Ref. No.:_____

Department of Health
Adverse Drug Reactions (ADR) Report Form

Please read the following instructions:
1. Please read the Guidance for Healthcare Professionals (http://www.drugoffice.gov.hk/adr.html); and Guidance for Pharmaceutical Industry (http://www.drugoffice.gov.hk/adr_industry.html) before completing the ADR report form.
2. ADR can be briefly described as a noxious and unintended response to a pharmaceutical product (i.e. drug or vaccine).
3. If the ADR of a newborn/child may be related to the mother, please submit a separate report for the mother.
4. Please provide information to every section.
5. **Full name and any kind of personal identifier of the patient**, such as identity card number and hospital admission number, **should not be provided** on the report form.
6. Information of individual reporter will be treated in strict confidence. Please read the Statement of Purposes overleaf in respect of the collection of your personal data.
7. As limited space is provided, please use another page for additional information if necessary.
8. For further enquires, please contact the Pharmacovigilance Unit of Drug Office of the DH at 2319 2920.

Section (A): Patient Information
Patient initials or ref. no.: _____ **(Please read instruction 5 above)**
Sex: ❑ M ❑ F ❑ Unknown   For woman, is she pregnant? ❑ No ❑ Yes ❑ Unknown
Weight (if known): _____ kg   Date of birth: (dd/mm/yyyy) ____/____/____ or age (at last birthday):_____
Ethnic group: ❑ Chinese ❑ Asian (Not Chinese) ❑ African ❑ Caucasian ❑ Eurasian ❑ Unknown ❑ Others_____

Section (B): About the Adverse Drug Reaction

Date of onset of ADR: (dd/mm/yyyy) ____/____/____

Description of event: _____

ADR category (for vaccine related ADR only):
❑ Allergic reaction ❑ Local reaction ❑ Systemic reaction ❑ Neurological disorders
Severity (can tick more than 1 box if appropriate):
❑ Life threatening   ❑ Prolonged Hospitalization   ❑ Hospitalized on: (dd/mm/yyyy) ____/____/____
❑ Hospitalization NOT required
Laboratory result (if applicable):_____

All Drug Therapies/Vaccines Prior to ADR (Please use trade names and, for vaccine, indicate batch number. Please circle the suspected drug.)	Daily Dosage (dose number for vaccines e.g. 1st DTP)	Route	Date Begun	Date Stopped	Reason for Use

Section (C): Treatment & Outcome
Treatment for ADR: ❑ No ❑ Yes. Details (including dosage, frequency, route, duration) _____

Laboratory result (if applicable): _____

Outcome:❑ Recovered on: (dd/mm/yyyy) / /   ❑ Not yet recovered ❑ Unknown ❑ Died on: (dd/mm/yyyy) / /

Sequelae: ❑ No ❑ Yes: ❑ Persistent disability ❑ Birth defect ❑ Medically significant events   Details:_____

Allergies or other relevant history (including medical history, liver/kidney problems, smoking, alcohol use etc)
_____

Section (D): Reporter Details (Please read instruction 6 above)
Name of Reporter and Organization:_____   Sector of service: ❑ Private ❑ Public

Occupation: ❑ Doctor ❑ Chinese medicine practitioner ❑ Dentist ❑ Pharmacist ❑ Nurse ❑ Others_____

Correspondence Address:_____

Tel. no.: _____ Fax. no.: _____ Email: _____

Also report to: ❑Manufacturer ❑Distributor/Importer ❑Others_____   Date of this report:_____

DH 2580 (1/2015)

Annexure 9: ADR Report Form in English—China

Please fold inside along the dotted line and seal the edge

To: **Pharmacovigilance Unit**
Drug Office
Department of Health
Room 1856, Wu Chung House,
213 Queen's Road East, Wanchai,
Hong Kong

Please Affix Stamp

Statement of Purposes

Purpose of Collection

This personal data are provided by reporter for the purposes of reporting adverse drug reaction of the patient to the Department of Health (DH). The personal data provided will be used by DH for the following purposes:
(a) follow-up of the case report; and
(b) surveillance of drug-related events.

2. The provision of personal data is voluntary. If you do not provide sufficient information, we may not be able to assess the report properly.

Classes of Transferees

3. The personal data you provide are mainly for use within DH. Apart from this, the data may only be disclosed to parties where you have given consent to such disclosure or where such disclosure is allowed under the Personal Data (Privacy) Ordinance.

Access to Personal Data

4. You have a right of access and correction with respect to personal data as provided for in sections 18 and 22 and Principle 6 of Schedule 1 of the Personal Data (Privacy) Ordinance. Your right of access includes the right to obtain a copy of your personal data. A fee may be imposed for complying with a data access request.

Enquiries

5. Enquiries concerning the personal data provided, including the making access and corrections, should be addressed to:

Senior Pharmacist (PV&RM)1
Pharmacovigilance Unit
Pharmacovigilance and Risk Management Division
Drug Office
Department of Health
Room 1856, 18/F, Wu Chung House
213 Queen's Road East, Wan Chai, Hong Kong
Tel: 2319 2920

ANNEXURE 10

Blue-card-adverse-reaction-reporting-form

Australian Government
Department of Health
Therapeutic Goods Administration

TGA use only

Report of suspected adverse reaction to medicines or vaccines
See statement about the collection and use of personal information overleaf, and please attach any additional data to this form

Patient initials or medical record number:	Sex: M ☐ F ☐	Date of birth or age:
	Weight (kg):	

Suspected medicine(s)/vaccine(s)

Medicine/vaccine (please use trade names; include batch number and AUST R or AUST L number if known)	Dosage (Dose number for vaccines eg 1st DTP)	Date begun	Date stopped	Reason for use

Other medicine(s)/vaccine(s) taken at the time of the reaction

Medicine/vaccine	Dosage	Date begun	Date stopped	Reason for use

Reaction(s): Date of onset of reaction (for vaccines time after administration): / /

Describe: (please provide as much detail as possible and include any results of relevant laboratory data and other investigations)

Seriousness: Life threatening ☐   Hospitalised ☐   Required a visit to doctor ☐

Treatment of reaction:

Outcome: Recovered ☐ ▶ Date: / /   Not yet recovered ☐   Fatal ☐ ▶ Date: / /   Unknown ☐

Sequelae? No ☐   Yes ☐ ▶ Describe:

Reporting: Doctor ☐   Pharmacist ☐   Other ☐   Contact details (email or phone)

Name:

Address:

Postcode:

Signature:

Date: / /

Thank you for taking the time to complete this form   PTO

Annexure 10: Blue-card-adverse-reaction-reporting-form

Report of suspected reaction to medicines or vaccines ("Blue card")

Privacy statement

Personal information:
Personal information in this report about a patient is collected and used for the purpose of assessing the safety of medicines under the *Therapeutic Goods Act 1989* (the Act). All reports are assessed and entered into the TGA's Australian Adverse Drugs Reactions System (the ADRS). That information in this report is only disclosed: (i) under subsection 61(3) of the Act to State and Territory Health Departments (if the information relates to vaccine events); or (ii) where the disclosure is otherwise required by, or authorised under, a law. For example, the Secretary of the Department of Health can release information from this report under subsection 61(7) of the Act if it is necessary to do so to ensure the safe use of the medicine, including to the company responsible for its supply in Australia.
The reporter's details are recorded in the ADRS so that they can be contacted if further information is required about the reported adverse event. Personal information about a reporter is only disclosed: (i) under subsection 61(3) of the Act to State and Territory Health Departments (if the information relates to vaccine events); or (ii) where the disclosure is otherwise required by, or authorised under, a law.

Adverse event information:
Specified kinds of information about reported adverse events can be released to the public by the Secretary under subsection 61(5C) of the Act. The information includes such details as the medicine reported to have been involved in an adverse event, and statistics such as the number of cases of reported adverse events relating to a medicine for any particular period of time. This information does not include any "personal information" within the meaning of the *Privacy Act 1988* - that is, information from which an individual's identity might be apparent or reasonably ascertainable.
Further information about how the TGA uses adverse event information that is reported to it is available at <www.tga.gov.au/reporting-problems>.

Fold here first (Please do not use staples on this form)

Phone: 1800 044 114   www.tga.gov.au/reporting-problems   Email: adr.reports@tga.gov.au   Fax: 02 6232 8392

What to report
You do not need to be certain, just suspicious!
Any information related to the reporter and patient identifiers is kept strictly confidential.
Adverse drug reaction reports should be submitted for prescription medicines, vaccines, over-the-counter medicines (medicines purchased without a prescription), and complementary medicines (herbal medicines, naturopathic and/or homoeopathic medicines, and nutritional supplements such as vitamins and minerals). Please include timing of reactions relative to medicine administration where relevant.
The TGA particularly requests reports of:
- All suspected reactions to new medicines and vaccines
- All suspected drug interactions
- Unexpected reactions, that is not consistent with product information or labelling
- Serious reactions which are suspected of significantly affecting a patient's management, including reactions suspected of causing death, danger to life, admission to hospital, prolongation of hospitalisation, absence from productive activity, increased investigational or treatment costs, and birth defects.

Fold here second   D1073 October 2015

Delivery Address:
PO Box 100
WODEN ACT 2606

No stamp required
if posted in Australia

Medicines Safety Monitoring
Pharmacovigilance and Special Access Branch
Reply Paid 100
WODEN ACT 2606

ANNEXURE 11A

Mandatory Adverse Reaction Reporting Form for Industry Canada

 Health Canada / Santé Canada

Mandatory Adverse Reaction Reporting Form for Industry

Report of suspected adverse reaction to marketed health products* in Canada

CANADA VIGILANCE PROGRAM

How to Submit the Form

Completed forms should be

faxed to: 613-957-0335

or

mailed to: Canada Vigilance Program
Marketed Health Products Directorate
Health Canada
Postal Locator 0701E
Ottawa, Ontario K1A 0K9

Submission of a report does not constitute an admission that medical personnel or the health product caused or contributed to the adverse reaction.

For further information on adverse reaction reporting by Market Authorization Holders (MAHs) and source establishments, please refer to:

- **Drugs and Natural Health Products**:
  Guidance Document for Industry – Reporting Adverse Reactions to Marketed Health Products
  (http://www.hc-sc.gc.ca/dhp-mps/pubs/medeff/_guide/2011-guidance-directrice_reporting-notification/index-eng.php).

- **Cells, Tissues and Organs**:
  Guidance Document for Source Establishments – Reporting Adverse Reactions to Human Cells, Tissues and Organs
  (http://www.hc-sc.gc.ca/dhp-mps/pubs/medeff/_guide/2010-guid-dir_indust_cto/index-eng.php).

*   Use this form to report suspected adverse reactions to pharmaceuticals, biologics (including biotechnology products, fractionated blood products, and vaccines), natural health products, radiopharmaceuticals or human cells, tissues or organs.

A program of MedEffect™ Canada

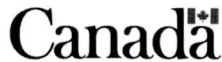

HC Pub.: 091086 (January 2011)

Annexure 11A: Mandatory Adverse Reaction Reporting Form for Industry Canada

INSTRUCTIONS ON COMPLETING THE MANDATORY ADVERSE REACTION REPORTING FORM FOR INDUSTRY

A. REPORTER INFORMATION

This section must be completed by the market authorization holder (MAH), or the source establishment (for cells, tissues and organs).

- **A1. Report Source:** Indicate the source of the report (from where the information originated). For literature sources, provide the full literature citation in box C6. Check "Not Available to MAH/Unknown" if the initial reporter did not specify the report source. Select "Other" to indicate that the report source is known, but does not fit into one of the categories provided.

- **A2. Reporter Qualification:** Indicate the type of reporter who initially reported the adverse reaction (AR) to the MAH or source establishment.

- **A3. Reporter Also Sent Report to the Canada Vigilance Program:** Indicate whether the initial reporter also reported the AR to the Canada Vigilance Program.

- **A4. MAH/Source Establishment Contact Office:** Enter the full name, civic address, and telephone and facsimile numbers of the MAH or source establishment. Include a contact name. For source establishments, include the establishment registration number.

- **A5. MAH/Source Establishment Report No.:** Indicate the MAH's or source establishment's identification number for the case. For follow-up reports, the report number should be the same as the number assigned to the initial report.

- **A6. Type of Report:**
  - Initial: Report has not previously been submitted by the MAH or source establishment.
  - Follow-up: Report is a follow-up to a previously submitted case.

- **A7. Date of Most Recent Information Received by MAH/Source Establishment:** Indicate the date when the MAH or source establishment received the information for this report.

- **A8. Date of this Report:** Indicate the date that this form was completed by the MAH or source establishment.

B. PATIENT INFORMATION

- **B1. Unique Identifier:** Provide a patient identifier in order to readily locate the case for follow-up purposes. Do not use the patient's name or initials.
- **B2. Age at Time of Reaction:** Provide the patient's age at the time of reaction.
- **B3. Sex:** Enter the patient's gender.
- **B4. Height:** Enter the patient's height, in centimetres (cm).
- **B5. Weight:** Enter the patient's weight, in kilograms (kg).

C. ADVERSE REACTION

- **C1. Country in which Reaction Occurred:** Indicate the country where the reaction took place.
- **C2. Date of Reaction:** Provide the date of onset of the adverse reaction.
- **C3. Serious Report:** Indicate if the report is serious.
- **C4. Criteria for Report Seriousness:** Check all boxes that apply to the definition of a serious adverse reaction per the *Food and Drug Regulations* (C.R.C., c.870), the *Natural Health Products Regulations* (SOR/2003-196), and the *Safety of Human Cells, Tissues and Organs for Transplantation Regulations* (SOR/2007-118).
  - For Drugs and Natural Health Products, a serious adverse reaction is a noxious and unintended response to a drug or natural health product that occurs at any dose and that requires in-patient hospitalization or prolongation of existing hospitalization, that causes congenital malformation, results in persistent or significant disability or incapacity, is life-threatening or results in death.
  - For Cells, Tissues and Organs, a serious adverse reaction means an undesirable response in the recipient to transplanted cells, tissues or organs, including the transmission of a disease or disease agent, that results in any of the following consequences in the recipient: their in-patient hospitalization or its prolongation; persistent or significant disability or incapacity; medical, dental or surgical intervention to preclude a persistent or significant disability or incapacity; a life-threatening condition; and death.

- **C5. Outcome:** Indicate the outcome of the adverse reaction.
- **C6. Describe the Reaction:** Provide a full description of the reaction(s) (e.g., body site and severity) and all relevant clinical information (medical status prior to the event, reported signs and/or symptoms, differential diagnosis for the event in question, clinical course, etc.).
- **C7. Relevant Tests/Laboratory Data:** Provide all appropriate information, including relevant negative tests and laboratory findings.
- **C8. Other Relevant History, Including Pre-existing Medical Conditions:** If available, provide information on the patient's history (e.g., race, allergies, pregnancy history, smoking and alcohol use, drug abuse) and other conditions known in the patient.

D. HEALTH PRODUCT(S)

Up to two suspected health products may be reported on one form. Attach additional forms if there were more than two suspected health products for the reported AR.

- **D1, D2 Suspected Health Product Name:** For each suspected product, provide the product name, check the box that applies to the type of health product, and provide the additional information below.
  - Drugs: Provide the Drug Identification Number (DIN) if available. Otherwise, list all active ingredients. Also provide the strength and dosage form.
  - Natural Health Products: Provide the label (preferably), or provide the Natural Product Number (NPN) or the Homeopathic Medicine Number (DIN-HM) if available. Otherwise, list all medicinal ingredients. Also provide the strength and dosage form.
  - Cells, Tissues and Organs: Also provide the donor identification code and the common name, followed by "cell", "tissue" or "organ" in parenthesis [e.g., Cornea (Tissue)].

- **D.i) Dose, Frequency & Route Used:** Describe how the product was used by the patient. For cells, tissues and organs, this box is only applicable to cells.

- **D.ii) Therapy Dates:**
  - Drugs and Natural Health Products: Provide the dates of therapy (start and stop dates of administration). If no dates are known, an estimated duration is acceptable.
  - Cells, Tissues and Organs: Provide the date of transplant.

- **D.iii) Indication for Use of Suspected Health Product:**
  - Drugs and Natural Health Products: Provide the indication for which the health product was prescribed or used in this particular patient.
  - Cells, Tissues and Organs: Provide the diagnostic reason or indication for the implantation, transplantation or infusion.

- **D.iv) Reaction Abated After Discontinuation or Dose Reduced:**
  - Drugs and Natural Health Products: Indicate if the adverse reaction abated after the suspected health product was discontinued, or the dose was reduced.
  - Cells, Tissues and Organs: Check "Does not apply".

- **D.v) Reaction Reappeared after Reintroduction:**
  - Drugs and Natural Health Products: Indicate if the adverse reaction reappeared after the suspected health product was reintroduced.
  - Cells, Tissues and Organs: Check "Does not apply".

- **D.vi) Lot #:** If known, indicate the lot number(s) of the suspected health product.
- **D.vii) Expiry Date:** If known, indicate the expiry date. For cells, tissues and organs, provide the date of expiration on the label, if any.

- **D3. Concomitant Health Products:** List and provide therapy dates for any other health products (drugs, biologics, including cells, tissues and organs, radiopharmaceuticals, natural health products, etc.) that the patient was using at the time of the event. Do not include health products used to treat the event.

- **D4. Treatment of the Adverse Reaction:** Describe the treatment of the adverse reaction, including other health products and/or therapies.

Mandatory Adverse Reaction Reporting Form for Industry
CANADA VIGILANCE PROGRAM
Mandatory fields are indicated by a *

PROTECTED B (when completed)
Page ___ of ___

A. REPORTER INFORMATION
(Must be completed by the Market Authorization Holder (MAH) or the Source Establishment)

1. Report Source*
○ Spontaneous ○ Study
○ Not available to MAH/Unknown ○ Other (specify): ____

2. Reporter Qualification
○ Physician ○ Lawyer
○ Pharmacist ○ Consumer
○ Other health professional ○ Other (specify): ____
(specialization): ____

3. Reporter Also Sent Report to the Canada Vigilance Program?*
○ Yes ○ No ○ Unknown

4. MAH/Source Establishment Contact Office*

5. MAH/Source Establishment Report No.

6. Type of Report*
○ Initial ○ Follow-up: ____

7. Date of Most Recent Information Received by MAH/Source Establishment*
(YYYY-MM-DD)

8. Date of this Report
(YYYY-MM-DD)

B. PATIENT INFORMATION

1. Unique Identifier

2. Age at Time of Reaction
____ ○ Years ○ Months ○ Other (specify:) ____

3. Sex
○ Male ○ Female ○ Unknown

4. Height ____ cm

5. Weight ____ kg

Privacy Notice Statement: For the purposes of the Canada Vigilance Adverse Reaction Monitoring Program, information related to the identity of the patient and/or reporter will be protected as personal information under the Privacy Act, including in cases of an access to information request. For details with regard to personal information collected under this program, visit the Personal Information Bank; Health Canada; Health Products and Food Branch; Branch Incident Reporting System; PIB# PPU 088 at: http://infosource.gc.ca/inst/shc/fed07_e.asp.

C. ADVERSE REACTION

1. Country in which Reaction Occurred:*

2. Date of Reaction (YYYY-MM-DD)

3. Serious Report:* ○ Yes ○ No

4. Criteria for Report Seriousness (check all that apply)
☐ Death ____ (YYYY-MM-DD) ☐ Life-threatening
☐ Caused/Prolonged hospitalization ☐ Disabling/Incapacitating
☐ Congenital anomaly/Birth defect
☐ Other medically important condition (specify): ____

5. Outcome:*
○ Recovered ○ Not Recovered ○ Recovering
○ Fatal ○ Recovered with Sequelae ○ Unknown

6. Describe the Reaction* (If more space is required, attach additional sheets.)

7. Relevant Tests/Laboratory Data (including dates) (YYYY-MM-DD)

8. Other Relevant History, Including Pre-existing Medical Conditions (e.g., allergies, pregnancy, smoking and alcohol use, hepatic/renal dysfunction)

** As per the Treasury Board of Canada Secretariat Government Security Policy
A program of MedEffect™ Canada
HC Pub.: 091086 (January 2011)

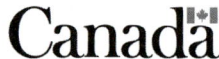

Annexure 11A: Mandatory Adverse Reaction Reporting Form for Industry Canada

Page ___ of ___

D. HEALTH PRODUCT(S)

If more than two health products are suspected, attach additional sheets.

1. Suspected Health Product Name*
Provide name, strength and dosage form, and check the circle that applies.
- ○ Drug – provide the DIN if available, otherwise list active ingredient(s)
- ○ Natural Health Product – provide the label, NPN or DIN-HM if available, otherwise list medicinal ingredients
- ○ Cells, Tissues and Organs – also provide the donor identification code and the common name followed by "cell", "tissue" or "organ" in parenthesis [e.g., Cornea (Tissue)]

2. Suspected Health Product Name
Provide name, strength and dosage form, and check the circle that applies.
- ○ Drug – provide the DIN if available, otherwise list active ingredient(s)
- ○ Natural Health Product – provide the label, NPN or DIN-HM if available, otherwise list medicinal ingredients
- ○ Cells, Tissues and Organs – also provide the donor identification code and the common name followed by "cell", "tissue" or "organ" in parenthesis [e.g., Cornea (Tissue)]

i) Dose, Frequency & Route Used

ii) Therapy Dates (if unknown, give duration) _____
From _____ to _____
    (YYYY-MM-DD)   (YYYY-MM-DD)

iii) Indication for Use of Suspected Health Product

iv) Reaction Abated After Discontinuation or Dose Reduced
○ Yes   ○ No   ○ Does not apply

v) Reaction Reappeared After Reintroduction
○ Yes   ○ No   ○ Does not apply

vi) Lot # (if known)

vii) Expiry Date (if known)

i) Dose, Frequency & Route Used

ii) Therapy Dates (if unknown, give duration) _____
From _____ to _____
    (YYYY-MM-DD)   (YYYY-MM-DD)

iii) Indication for Use of Suspected Health Product

iv) Reaction Abated After Discontinuation or Dose Reduced
○ Yes   ○ No   ○ Does not apply

v) Reaction Reappeared After Reintroduction
○ Yes   ○ No   ○ Does not apply

vi) Lot # (if known)

vii) Expiry Date (if known)

3. Concomitant Health Products (exclude treatment of reaction)

Name	Dose, Frequency & Route Used	Therapy Dates (yyyy-mm-dd)

4. Treatment of Adverse Reaction (health products and/or other therapy)

ANNEXURE 11B

ADR Form for Medical Device Problem Reporting Canada

 Health Canada / Santé Canada

Mandatory Medical Device Problem Reporting Form for Industry

Report of problems related to medical devices marketed in Canada

CANADA VIGILANCE - MEDICAL DEVICE PROBLEM REPORTING PROGRAM (CV-MD)

How to Submit the Report

Completed forms should be

emailed to: mdpr@hc-sc.gc.ca

or

faxed to: 613-954-0941

or

mailed to: Canada Vigilance - Medical Device Reporting Program
Marketed Health Products Directorate
Health Canada
Address Locator 0701E
200 Tunney's Pasture Driveway
Ottawa (Ontario) K1A 0K9

Submission of a report does not constitute an admission that medical personnel or the health product caused or contributed to the incident.

For further information on the Mandatory Medical Device Problem Reporting by Industry, please refer to: Guidance Document for Mandatory Problem Reporting for Medical Devices

http://www.hc-sc.qc.ca/dhp-mps/pubs/medeff/_guide/2011-devices-materiaux/index-eng.php

A program of MedEffect™ Canada

HC Pub.:110180 (October 2011)

Canada

Annexure 11B: ADR Form for Medical Device Problem Reporting Canada

INSTRUCTIONS ON COMPLETING THE MANDATORY MEDICAL DEVICE PROBLEM REPORTING FORM

A. REPORTER INFORMATION

This section contains information about the reporter, who is submitting the report to Canada Vigilance – Medical Devices Problem Reporting Program (CV-MD) to fulfil their obligations under sections 59, 60, 61 and 61.1 of the *Medical Devices Regulations*. It also includes details about the manufacturer and importer of the medical device that are responsible to submit the report to CV-MD.

- **A1. Reporter Type:**
  - **i.** Indicate if the reporter submitting this report to CV-MD is the manufacturer or the importer.
  - **ii.** Indicates if the importer submitting this report to CV-MD has also submitted reported this problem to the manufacturer of the device.
  - **iii.** Indicates if the importer is submitting on behalf of the manufacturer.
- **A2. Reporter Contact Information:** Includes the name of the individual, email, telephone and fax number of the reporter or his/her representative.
- **A3. Reporter File Number:** Indicates the manufacturer's or importer's file number for the case. For final reports, the report number should be the same as the preliminary report.
- **A4. Health Canada File Number:** A number provided in the acknowledgement letter for the preliminary report. It's a unique number assigned by Health Canada for the report.
- **A5. Type of Report:** Indicates if the report being submitted is a preliminary, update, final, or a preliminary and final. It also includes the anticipated date for the submission of the final report.
- **A6. Date Submitted:** Indicates the date at which the report is being submitted by the manufacturer/importer to CV-MD.
- **A7. Name and Address:** Indicates the name and address of the manufacturer and importer of the medical device.
- **A8. Health Canada assigned company identification number (if known):** The company identification number can be found either on the medical device licence or on the medical device establishment licence, as appropriate.
- **A9. Establishment Licence Number (if applicable):** Indicates the establishment licence (MDEL) number of the manufacturer and importer of the medical device in Canada.

B. INCIDENT INFORMATION

This section contains information about the incident that occurred with the medical device requiring a mandatory problem report to be submitted to CV-MD. It includes details about the incident and the patient consequences that occurred/could have occurred. In the context of mandatory problem reporting, information on the incident refers to the circumstances requiring reporting under section 59 of the *Medical Devices Regulations*.

- **B1. Classification of Incident:** Indicates
  - **i.** if the report is a 10 day or 30 day report, based on the seriousness of the incident associated with the medical device
  - **ii.** whether the incident occurred inside or outside Canada
  - **iii.** whether the incident occurred during investigational testing, or was caused by a medical device available only through the special access program or is a radiation emitting device (RED).
- **B2. Date of Incident:** Indicates the date at which the incident with the medical device occurred.
- **B3. Reporter's Awareness Date:** Indicates the date at which the manufacturer/importer of the medical device became aware of the potential problem associated with the device.
- **B4. Patient Consequences:** Includes information on the patient who was involved in the incident, and the consequences (or potential consequences) to the patient, user or other person(s) involved.
- **B5. Details of Incident:** Includes description of device(s), equipment, or drugs involved in the incident, and a detailed description of what happened in the incident.

C. MEDICAL DEVICE INFORMATION

This section contains details about the medical device involved in the incident, including its brand name and licence number.

- **C1. Trade/Brand Name:** Indicates the trade/brand name of the device and reported on the label.
- **C2. Control/Lot/Serial #:** Indicates the control number, lot number and/or serial number for the device.
- **C3. Expiration Date:** Indicates the expiration date issued to the medical device (if applicable).
- **C4. i. Device Classification:** Indicates the class of the device (I-IV).
  - **ii. Device Licence Number:** Indicates the medical device licence number issued by the Medical Devices Bureau on behalf of the Minister for Class II, III and IV medical devices sold in Canada.
  - **iii. Device Identification No:** Indicates the device identification number assigned by Health Canada in the license issued for the device.
  - **iv. Manufacturer's Medical Device Identifier:** Indicates the unique series of letters or numbers or any combination of these or a bar code that is assigned to a medical device by the manufacturer and that identifies it and distinguishes it from similar devices. Examples of an identifier for a device are a catalogue, model or part number.
- **C5. Software Version:** Indicates the version of the software contained within the device, if applicable for the device.
- **C6. Age of Device:** Indicates the number of years since the manufacturing date of the device.
- **C7. How long was the device in use?** Indicates how long the device was used.
- **C8. Was the device labelled as sterile?** Indicates if the device sold was manufactured and packaged in sterile conditions.
- **C9. Availability of Device:** Indicates if the device has been destroyed, or is available for the company/Health Canada for further evaluation to determine the root cause of the failure associated with the device.

D. COMPLAINANT INFORMATION

This section contains information about the complainant that contacted the reporter to inform them about the incident.

- **D1. Complainant is a:** Indicates if the complainant reporting to the manufacturer/importer was a consumer, a health professional etc.
- **D2. Name of Complainant:** Indicates the name of the person who informed the reporter about the incident.
- **D3. Name of Health Care Facility:** This section indicates the name of the health care facility where the problem occurred.
- **D4. Address:** Indicates the complete address of the complainant, including the postal code.
- **D5. Contact Information:** Indicates the telephone number and/or email address of the complainant.

E. INVESTIGATION INFORMATION

This section contains information about the investigation being carried out by the manufacturer/importer of the medical device to determine if there's any problem with the medical device, and if any corrective actions are necessary.

- **E1. Investigative Actions and Timeline:** Includes the rationale for the course of action taken to investigate the incident, the details of the action to be completed, and the timeline for its completion. If no investigation is to be done, a rational needs to be provided here.
- **E2. Root Cause of Problem:** To be completed once the investigation of the incident is complete, and the root cause of the incident identified. The root cause would ascertain the most likely reason why the problem occurred with the medical device. This section only applies for final reports.
- **E3. Corrective actions taken as a result of the investigation:** Includes information on actions taken to correct the problem, including any post-market surveillance, recalls, or corrective or preventive actions and the design and manufacture of the device. This should also include the rationale for performing the corrective action. This section only applies for final reports. If no corrective action is to be taken, a rationale needs to be provided here.

INSTRUCTIONS ON COMPLETING THE MANDATORY MEDICAL DEVICE PROBLEM REPORTING FORM

NOTE ON SUBMITTING REPORTS

Manufacturers and importers should ensure that all information requested in the form has been submitted to Health Canada through the use of preliminary, updates or final reports. Preliminary reports require that all sections (except E2 & E3) be filled. Sections of the form which must be filled when submitting a follow up to a preliminary report are indicated by an *. In addition to these sections, it's imperative that manufacturer/importers fill any other sections in the form that need to be updated to reflect any corrections to the information submitted previously to the Canada Vigilance - Medical Device Problem Reporting Program.

For example, if during the course of the investigation, additional steps were added as part of the course of action to investigate the incident, or there was additional information about patient outcomes, manufacturers and importers must submit this information in the relevant field.

Annexure 11B: ADR Form for Medical Device Problem Reporting Canada **607**

 Health Canada   Santé Canada

Mandatory Medical Device Problem Reporting Form for Industry
CANADA VIGILANCE - MEDICAL DEVICE PROBLEM REPORTING PROGRAM
If more space is required, please attach additional sheets
Fields required to be completed for updates/final reports are indicated by an *

Page ___ of ___

A. REPORTER INFORMATION

1. i. Reporter Type
   ○ Manufacturer   ○ Importer

   In the case where the reporter is the importer:
   ii. Did the importer report the incident to the manufacturer?
   ○ Yes   ○ No
   iii. Is the importer also submitting the report on behalf of the manufacturer?
   ○ Yes   ○ No

2. Reporter Contact Information *

3. Reporter File No. *

4. Health Canada File No. (if applicable) *

5. Type of Report *
   ○ Preliminary   ○ Update   ○ Final   ○ Preliminary & Final

   If "preliminary" only, anticipated date for the final report:
   (YYYY-MM-DD)
   If "update/final", date the previous report was submitted to Health Canada:
   (YYYY-MM-DD)

6. Date Submitted *
   (YYYY-MM-DD)

	Manufacturer	Importer
7. Name and Address		
8. Health Canada assigned company identification number (if known):		
9. Establishment License Number (if applicable):		

B. INCIDENT INFORMATION

1. Classification of Incident *
   i. ○ 10-Day   ○ 30-Day
   ii. ○ Canadian   ○ Foreign
   iii. ☐ Investigational testing   ☐ Special Access Program
       ☐ Radiation emitting device (if applicable)

2. Date of Incident
   (YYYY-MM-DD)

3. Reporter's Awareness Date
   (YYYY-MM-DD)

4. Patient Consequences

5. Details of Incident

A program of MedEffect™ Canada
HC Pub.: 110180 (October 2011)

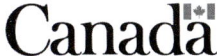

C. MEDICAL DEVICE INFORMATION

1. Trade/Brand Name *

2. Control/Lot/Serial No.

3. Expiration Date
   (YYYY-MM-DD)

4. i. Device Classification
   ○ I ○ II ○ III ○ IV

   ii. Device License No.

   iii. Device Identification No

   iv. Manufacturer's Medical Device Identifier (catalogue/model no.)

5. Software Version

6. Age of Device

7. How long was the device in use?

8. Was the device labelled as sterile?
   ○ Yes ○ No

9. Availability of device for evaluation
   ○ Destroyed ○ Returned to Manufacturer/Importer
   ○ Neither (with explanation)

D. COMPLAINANT INFORMATION

1. Complainant is a:
   ○ Consumer ○ Health professional ○ Other

2. Name of Complainant

3. Name of Health Care Facility (if applicable)

4. Address

5. Telephone No. and/or E-mail Address

Privacy Notice Statement: For the purposes of the Canada Vigilance - Medical Device Problem Reporting Program, information related to the identity of the complainant and/or reporter will be protected as personal information under the *Privacy Act*, and under the *Access to Information Act* in the case of an access to information request. For details with regard to personal information collected under this program, visit the Personal Information Bank; Health Canada; Health Products and Food Branch; Branch Incident Reporting System; HC PPU 088 at: http://infosource.gc.ca/inst/1476/1476-fedemp00-eng.asp

E. INVESTIGATION INFORMATION

1. Investigative Actions and Timeline

This section only applies for preliminary & final, and final reports

2. Root Cause of Problem

3. Corrective Actions taken as a result of the investigation

Page ___ of ___

ANNEXURE 11C

Side Effect Reporting Form Canada

SIDE EFFECT REPORTING FORM

Reporting suspected side effects (also known as adverse reactions) to marketed health products in Canada may contribute to the identification of previously unrecognized rare or serious side effects, which may lead to changes in the product's safety information.

Instructions on how to complete and submit this form and information about confidentiality can be found on Page 2. Complete all mandatory fields, marked by a *, and provide as much detail as possible for the remaining fields.

FAX completed form to 1-866-678-6789
For more information call 1-866-234-2345

PROTECTED "B" WHEN COMPLETED**

A) About the person who had the side effect

Reference # (if applicable)

1. Age*
   ___ Years
   ___ Months
2. Sex*
   ☐ Male
   ☐ Female
3. Height
   ___ cm
   ___ ft ___ in
4. Weight
   ___ kg
   ___ lbs ___ oz
5. Medical history and other related information (allergies, pregnancy, smoking/alcohol use, liver disease, etc.)

B) Reporter information

1. Name*
2. Telephone*
3. Province/Territory
4. Address
5. E-mail
6. Preferred language
   ☐ English
   ☐ French
7. Organization (if applicable)
8. Select one that best describes you
   ☐ Consumer or other non-health professional   ☐ Physician   ☐ Pharmacist
   ☐ Other health professional (specify) _____
9. Has this also been reported to the manufacturer?
   ☐ Yes   ☐ No

C) Side Effect

1. Seriousness of the side effect
   ☐ Death (yyyy-mm-dd) _____
   ☐ Life-threatening
   ☐ Admitted to hospital
   ☐ Lengthened hospital stay
   ☐ Disability
   ☐ Birth defect
   ☐ Needed medical attention
2. Recovered after the side effect*
   ☐ Yes   ☐ No   ☐ Unknown
   ☐ Recovering (explain)
3. Side effect start date* (yyyy-mm-dd)
4. Side effect end date (yyyy-mm-dd)
5. Describe the side effect (timeliness, treatment, etc.)*

D) Suspected health product

1. Product name*
2. Strength
3. Manufacturer
4. Lot #
5. DIN #/NPN #
6. Country of purchase
   ☐ Canada
   ☐ United States
   ☐ Other (specify): _____
7. Where it was purchased/obtained
   ☐ Pharmacy
   ☐ Grocery store
   ☐ Internet
   ☐ Other (specify): _____
8. Product start date (yyyy-mm-dd)*
9. Product end date (yyyy-mm-dd)

At the time of the side effect, specify:

10. Dosage* (strength and quantity)
11. Frequency (e.g. twice daily)
12. How the product was taken (e.g. by mouth)

13. What was the product prescribed/taken for?*

14. Did use of the product stop after the side effect appeared?
    ☐ Yes   ☐ No
15. If the product was stopped did the side effect stop?
    ☐ Yes   ☐ No   ☐ Does not apply
16. Was the product restarted after the side effect stopped?
    ☐ Yes   ☐ No   ☐ Does not apply
17. If the product was restarted, did the side effect return?
    ☐ Yes   ☐ No   ☐ Does not apply
18. Likelihood that the product caused the side effect
    ☐ Certain   ☐ Not available/Unable to assess
    ☐ Probably/Likely   ☐ Unlikely
    ☐ Possible   ☐ Unrelated
19. Other health products taken at the time of the side effect, excluding treatment (length of use, timelines, etc.)

20. Related test/laboratory results

** As per the Treasury Board of Canada Secretariat Government Security Policy.

Pub.: 150142 | Date: August 2016

 Health Canada / Santé Canada

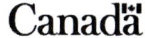 Canada

How to complete the Side Effect Reporting Form

- All sections of the form should be filled in as completely as possible. Use a separate form for each patient. Attach an additional form if there is more than one suspected health product. Additional pages may be attached if more space is required. Please provide the product label where possible.
- Follow-up information for a side effect that has already been reported can be submitted using a new form, indicating that it consists of follow-up information, including, if known, the date of the original report and the report number provided in the acknowledgement.

What is a side effect?

A side effect (also known as adverse reaction) is a harmful and unintended response to a health product. Health products include prescription and non-prescription medications; natural health products; biologics (includes biotechnology products, vaccines, fractionated blood products, human blood and blood components, as well as human cells, tissues and organs) radiopharmaceuticals; and disinfectants and sanitizers with disinfectant claims. This includes any undesirable patient effect suspected to be associated with health product use. An unintended effect, health product abuse, overdose, interaction (including drug-drug and drug-food interactions) and unusual lack of therapeutic efficacy are all considered to be reportable side effects.

What is considered a serious side effect?

A serious side effect is one that requires in-patient hospitalization or prolongation of existing hospitalization, causes congenital malformation, results in persistent or significant disability or incapacity, is life-threatening or results in death. Side effects that result in significant medical intervention to prevent one of these listed outcomes are also considered to be serious.

What types of side effects should be reported?

All suspected side effects should be reported, especially those that are:

- *unexpected*, regardless of their severity (i.e. not consistent with product information or labelling;
- *serious*, whether expected or not;
- reactions to *recently marketed* health products (on the market less than five years), regardless of their nature or severity.

How to submit your completed form	Other ways to report a side effect
Fax: 1-866-678-6789	**Online:** www.health.gc.ca/medeffect
Mail: Canada Vigilance Program Marketed Health Products Directorate Health Canada Address locator 0701E Ottawa ON K1A 0K9	**Telephone:** 1-866-234-2345 *Do not send reports by e-mail. Health Canada is not able to ensure secure transfer of information by e-mail.*

Other information

- Reporting a side effect does not constitute an admission that medical personnel or the product caused or contributed to it.
- Side effect reports are, for the most part, only suspected associations. A temporal or possible association is sufficient for a report to be made. Reporting of a side effect does not imply a definitive causal link.
- Health professionals and consumers may also report side effects to the market authorization holder. Indicate on your form sent to Health Canada if a case was also reported to the product's market authorization holder.

For more information about side effect reporting, call Health Canada at 1-866-234-2345 or contact a regional office directly:	
British Columbia CanadaVigilance_BC@hc-sc.gc.ca	**Ontario** CanadaVigilance_ON@hc-sc.gc.ca
Alberta, Northwest Territories and Yukon CanadaVigilance_AB@hc-sc.gc.ca	**Québec** CanadaVigilance_QC@hc-sc.gc.ca
Saskatchewan and Nunavut CanadaVigilance_SK@hc-sc.gc.ca	**New Brunswick, Nova Scotia, Prince Edward Island, and Newfoundland and Labrador** CanadaVigilance_ATL@hc-sc.gc.ca
Manitoba CanadaVigilance_MB@hc-sc.gc.ca	

Confidentiality

In the context of Health Canada's side effect reporting program (the Canada Vigilance Program), personal information is collected pursuant to section 4 of the *Department of Health Act*, for the purpose of monitoring licensed products, detecting potential emerging safety issues and trends, mitigating the risks and improving the safe use and efficacy of the health products. Information related to the identity of the patient and/or reporter will be protected as personal information under the *Privacy Act*, and in the case of an access to information request, under the *Access to Information Act*. Suspected health product side effect-related information that is voluntarily submitted to Health Canada is maintained in a secure computerized database. The program endeavours to use and disclose only de-identified information but may use and disclose personal information that is not de-identified as permitted under the *Privacy Act*. For further details regarding the personal information collected under this program, visit the Personal Information Bank; Health Canada; Health Products and Food Branch; Branch Incident Reporting System; PIB#PPU 088 at: www.hc-sc.gc.ca/ahc-asc/activit/atip-aiprp/infosource/index-eng.php#a2. Every Canadian individual has the right to access their own personal information and is entitled to request correction to ensure accuracy of their information. If you wish to exercise this right, contact the Treasury Board of Canada Secretariat (www.tbs-sct.gc.ca/tbsf-fsct/350-58-eng.ASP).

Index

Page numbers followed by *b* refer to box, *f* refer to figure, *fc* refer to flowchart, and *t* refer to table.

A

Absinth 158
Absinthe 158
Absinthium 158
Absorption interactions 58*t*
Active implantable medical device 231
Acute leukemia, treatment of 117
Adderall XR mixed amphetamine salts 23
Additional monitoring 556
    communication and transparency 558
    creation and maintenance of 560
    initial time period of maintenance in 559
    medicinal product in 558
    operation of EU network 558
    principles for assigning 557
    roles and responsibilities 559
    status 558
    structures and processes 557
Adenomatous Polyp Prevention on Vioxx 21
ADME interactions 57
ADR *See* Adverse drug reaction
Adult respiratory distress syndrome 161
Adverse drug interactions 56
    classification of 56
    indirect pharmacodynamic 57
    pharmaceutical 59
    pharmacodynamic 56
    pharmacokinetic 57
Adverse drug reaction 1, 19, 40-42, 49, 63, 81, 127, 141, 152, 153, 175, 176, 180, 206, 216, 269
    advisory committee 197
    assessment of 20
    classification of 40, 41*t*
    detection of 19, 183
    direct effects of 41
    disease related factors 42
    drug related factors 42
    economic burden of 219
    expected 3
    first book on 12*f*
    form for consumers in Hindi 273
    form for health care professionals 271
    form for medical device problem reporting Canada 604
    frequency of 48
    hospitalization due to 216
    idiosyncratic 55*t*
    incidence of 55
    indirect effects of 41
    interaction 40
    management of 219
    mechanism of 40, 49
    monitoring 100
    monitoring centres 86, 109
    patient related factors 42
    prevention of 20
    report form in English—China 596
    reporting form
        suspected 26
        types of different 205
    responsible factors for type A 50*t*
    social factors 42
    type A 49, 49*f*
        absorption 50
        distribution 51
        drug elimination 53
        drug excretion 53
        metabolism 51
        pharmaceutical causes 49
        pharmacodynamic causes 54
        pharmacokinetic causes 50
    type B 54
        pharmaceutical causes 54
        pharmacodynamic causes 55
        pharmacokinetic causes 54
Adverse event following immunization 34, 36
    common programme errors leading to 35*t*
    isolated and clusters of 34
    process of reporting serious 36
    types of 34, 34*t*
Adverse event notifications, types of database of 197
Adverse event of special interest 1
Adverse event relationship 259
Adverse event reporting 160
    system 203, 267
Adverse experience 40
Adverse health effect 111
    benefit 111
    benefit-risk analysis 112
Adverse incident tracking system 231
Adverse reaction
    numbers of 517*t*
    reporting form, mandatory 600
    suspected serious 47
    unexpected 47, 86
    type B 55
    unexpected 7
Adverse reactions to medicinal products
    collection of reports 408, 420
    data management 412
    electronic exchange of safety information in EU 428
    follow-up of reports 411
    management of 405
    operation of EU network 416
    post-authorisation studies in EU 416
    quality management 413
    reporting 405
        modalities 415, 426
        of individual case safety reports 415
        rules for clinical trials 416
        time frames 426
    scope 406
    special situations 413
    structures and processes 408
    terminology 406
    validation of reports 410
AEFI *See* Adverse event following immunization

AERS *See* Adverse Event Reporting System
Aflatoxin B1 55
Agcomposer 263
Age and gender specific terms 170
Agency's stakeholders 182
Agranulocytosis 117
agSignals 262
agXchange 262
AIMD *See* Active implantable medical device
AITS *See* Adverse incident tracking system
Albumin fraction 57
Alcohol 59
  consumption 5
Allergic phenomenon 48
Allium sativum 155
Allopathic medicine 7
Allopathy 1
Allopurinol 89
Alosetron hydrochloride 22
Alzheimer's disease 219
American Medical Association 12
Amlodipine 87
Amoxicillin 81, 82
Amphotericin-B 86
Ampicillin 59
Anaphylaxis 28, 34, 37
Anatomical therapeutic chemical codes 81
Anemia 154
Angiodema 153
Anorexia 154
Antiarrhythmics 175
Antipsychotics, atypical 88
Aplastic anemia 118
Applicable regulatory authority 80
Applicant's pharmacovigilance system 343
Approval system 228
Aprotinin 23
Argus 253
ARIS G 253
  for complaints 262
ARIS global total safety suite 261
Aristolochia debilis 161
Aristolochia fangchi 161
Aristolochic acid nephropathy 155
Artemisia absinthium L 158
Aspirin 58, 117
Atenolol 58, 87
Audit reporting in EU, requirements for 377

Auxiliary nurse midwife 36
Azathioprine 51, 59

B

Bacillus-Calmette-Guerin 38
  vaccine 87
Barbiturates 59
Baxtra 23
Bayesian confidence propagation neural network 2, 71, 143
BCG *See* Bacillus-Calmette-Guerin
Benefit-risk
  actual versus perceived 112
  analysis 2
Benefit-risk assessment 112*f*, 116
  in pharmacovigilance 111
  quantitative approach to 117
  semi-quantitative approach to 117
  stepwise approach to 115
Benefit-risk balance 114
  stepwise process of assessing 115*f*
Beta-blockers 175
Biological medicinal products, identification of 440
Biological products 2
Biotransformations 53
Bleeding disorder 176
Blood products 19
Blood supply, adequate 195
Blue-card-adverse-reaction-reporting-form 598
Bones 51
Brachial neuritis 36
Bromfenac sodium 22
Bronchial asthma 169
Bupivacaine 86
Burning 154
Business process map 456*f*, 459*f*, 465, 467*f*
  suspected adverse reaction reporting in EU
    final arrangements 454*f*
    interim arrangements. 449*f*
Business profile 263

C

Cabergoline 87
Canada Vigilance Programme 198
Canadian adverse drug reaction information system 197

Canadian risk-based classification system 246
Cancer 171
CAPA *See* Corrective and preventive actions
Carboxylic acids 155
Cardiac disease 154
  history of 90
Cardiac risk factors 90
Cardiovascular disease, development of 93
Case report in literature 67
Case report management, computer software for 145
Case-control study 212
  retrospective 31*f*
Causality assessment 2
Causality classification 45
  certain 45
  conditional 46, 47
  doubtful 47
  inaccessible 46
  likely 46
  possible 46, 47
  probable 46
  unclassifiable 46
  unclassified 46
  unlikely 46
Caveat document 2
CBER *See* Centre for biologics evaluation and research
CDER *See* Centre for drug evaluation and research
CDSCO *See* Central Drug Standard Control Organization
Cefixime 87
Celecoxib 178
Central Drug Standard Control Organization 15, 26, 86, 108, 231, 243, 244, 248
Central Drugs Authority 192
Centre for biologics evaluation and research 206
Centre for devices and radiological health 243
Centre for drug evaluation and research 206
Centres for Disease Control and Prevention 217
Cephalexin 58
Cerivastatin 22
Chemically reactive metabolite 54
Chest pain 153

China Adverse Drug Reaction Monitoring System 194
China Food and Drug Administration 194
Chinese Centres for Disease Control and Prevention 194
Chlorambucil 51
Chloramphenicol 12
Chlorinated hydrocarbon 55
Chloroform anesthesia 11
Chloroquine 45
Chlorpromazine 59
CHM *See* Commission of Human Medicines
Cholinergic drug 57
Chronic disease 221
Ciprofloxacine 58
Cirrhosis 53
Cisapride monohydrate 22
Clavulanic acid 82
Clinical data management
 systems 252
 tools for 252
Clinical safety data management 40
Clinical trial
 and studies in EU, types of 417*f*
 characteristics of 78*b*
 limitations of 18*b*
 management system 252
Cluster adverse event following immunization 35
Codes 188
Codex Alimentarius Commission 111
Cohort studies 2, 31, 32, 93, 213
 advantages 93
 disadvantages 93
Collaborative perinatal project 94
Coma 154
Combinations database 2, 73
Commission implementing regulation 184
Commission of Human Medicines 185, 206
Committee for medicinal products
 for human use 592
 for veterinary use 182
Committee on safety
 of drugs 84
 of medicines 185
Common adverse reactions 119
Communicable disease 221
Communication 20
Community health centre 36

Comorbid disease 218
Competent authorities in member states 456
Computer-based
 methods 254
 systems, role of 251
Concentration-effect relationships 209
Concomitant medications, effect of 259
Congenital limb abnormality 180
Corneal opacities after thioridazine 45
Coronary artery disease 87
Coronary stents 225
Coronary thrombosis 256
Corrective and preventive actions 231
Corticosteroids 59
Cost, types of 221
Coumarins 59
Council for International Organizations of Medical Sciences 14
Crisis
 characteristics of 127, 127*b*
 handling 133
 intrinsic 130
 perceived 130, 131
 planning team, establishing strategic 134
 prevention principles 139
 response 131
Crisis in pharmacovigilance 128
 threat sources for 129
Crisis management 128, 129
 communication division 137
 cycle 130, 132*f*
 division 137
 in pharmacovigilance 127
 issues related to 134
 model 131, 134*f*
 operational division 137
 Plan 138*t*
 planning for 133
 planning, stages of 135*f*
 team, establishing tactical 136
Cross-sectional studies 3, 91, 92*f*, 212
 advantages of 92
 disadvantages of 92
Cumulative exposure from marketing experience 516*t*
Cyclophosphamide 51

Cyclosporine 59
Cylert 23
Cytochrome p450 enzyme family 175

D

DAEN-medical devices 197
DAEN-medicines 197
Data analysis 258
Data collection instrument
 administration of 589
 design of 589
Data management and pharmacovigilance, methods of safety 255
Data monitoring in EudraVigilance, periodicity of 553
Data protection in EU 339
Data standards and interoperable systems 255
Data warehouses 268
Database
 large size of 258
 research and monitoring 95
 searches 442
Data-mining 3
DCGI *See* Drug Controller General of India
Death 154, 169
 accidental 169
 homicide 169
 natural 169
 suicide 169
Decision-making in benefit-risk assessment, Principle of three framework for 118*f*
Defective medicines report centre 185
Deleterious substances 195
Dermatitis 153
Dermatological conditions 154
Development safety update report 3
Device adverse reporting systems 232*t*
Dexatrim 22
Dexfenfluramine hydrochloride 22
Dextran 59
Diabetes, type 2 221
Diabetic ketoacidosis 169
Diarrhea 153

Diazepam 58
Diet 5
Dietary Supplement
   and Infant Formulas 84
   Health and Education ACT 151
Diethylene glycol 12
Diethylstilbestrol 79
Digoxin 14, 50
Diphtheria, pertussis tetanus 38
Direct cost 221
Directorate General of Health
   Services 26
Disability-adjusted life years 220
Disease Control and Prevention 217
Disease progression 171
Disease registry 29, 30
Disease related factors 44
Disease severity 28
Disease-modifying antirheumatic
   drugs 117
Disseminated Bacillus-Calmette-
   Guerin infections 37
Distribution interactions 58t
District immunization officer 36
Docetaxel 87
Domestic reporting in Japanese
   format 262
DPT *See* Diphtheria, pertussis
   tetanus
Draft regulatory policies for
   medical devices 240
Drug
   and drug addiction, European
      monitoring centre for 428
   dynamic process of increasing
      use of 113f
   event monitoring 29
   exposure 93
   for systemic absorption 49
   interactions 53, 171
      due to absorption of 57
      due to distribution of 57
      due to excretion of 59
      due to metabolism of 58
   labelling, pregnancy categories
      used in 79t
   lists, essential 20
   miracle 11
   molecules, large number of 100
   monitoring centres, initiation
      of 101
   name errors 257
   object 56
   primary pharmacological
      characteristics of 49f
   prime 56
   reaches 51
   regulatory agency 5
   substance, active 3
   transporters, role of 53
   use investigations 196
Drug Controller General of India
   26, 191, 206, 244
Drug development 251f
   process 77f
Drug related factors 43
   drug dose and frequency 43
   polypharmacy 43
Drug safety
   alerts 87t
   and evaluation branch 196
   technology vendors 261
Drug utilization
   research 3
   study 33
Drug-associated syndrome 66
Drug-drug interaction 49, 50,
   63, 66
   detection of 63
Drug-induced hypersensitivity
   syndrome 89
Drugs and Cosmetics Act 243
Duract 22
Dyskinesia, exacerbation of 170

E

Echocardiography 168
Educational materials 591
   assessment of 594
   content of 594
   format and layout of 593
   principles for 592
   publication of 593-595
Educational programmes 592
Efficient pharmacovigilance
   system 17
Electronic submission of copies
   of articles published in
   scientific literature 445
EMA *See* European Mdicines
   Agency
Emergency department 217
Emerging technologies 259
Encephalopathy 37
Encoding pharmacodynamic
   parameters 176
Environmental risk assessment
   working party 182
Enzymatic cellular defense
   mechanisms 55
Enzyme 21
   induction 53, 59
   inhibition 59
Epilepsy, treatment of 118
Erectile dysfunction 154
Etanercept 88
Ethics, privacy and overall study
   feasibility 590
Eudralex 182
Eudravigilance 3, 181
   system 343
European Commission, role of
   367
European economic area 3, 181
European Medicines Agency 3,
   181, 206
   role of 366
European Medicines Evaluation
   Agency 181
Excretion interactions 60t
Experimental study designs 213
Exposure (drug) registries 29
Eye 51

F

Face edema 153
Factors affecting benefit-risk
   assessment 114f
   balance 114
FAERS *See* FDA adverse event
   reporting system
Fatal disease, treatment of 117
Fats 51
FDA *See* Food and Drug
   Administration
Federal food drug 243
Fenfluramine hydrochloride 22
Ferrous sulfate 58
Fever 34, 37, 66, 153
Field safety
   corrective actions 231
   notice 231
First information report 299
First investigation report 300
Flu 117
Food and Drug Administration
   11, 278, 206, 231, 245
   adverse event reporting
      system 206
   Amendments Act 204
Food, Drug and Cosmetics Act 270

Framingham heart study 93
French agency for safety of health products 188
French Pharmaceutical Manufacturers Association 188
French pharmacovigilance system 188
Frequency classification 48
FSCA *See* Field safety corrective actions
FSN *See* Field safety notice
Furosemide 87

G

Garden heliotrope 158
Gastric mucosa, protection of 21
Gastrointestinal bleeding 117
Gastrointestinal disorders 81
Gene polymorphisms 176*t*
General medical devices 247*t*
Generate toxic intermediates 55*t*
Generation III cohort 94
Genetic factors 5
Genetic variability leading 175*fc*
Genotype 178*t*
Gentamicin 86
Germander hepatotoxicity 156
Giddiness 154
Ginkgo biloba 155, 156
  induced thrombocytopenia 155
Glibenclamide 58
Global harmonization task force 227, 243
Glomerular filtration rate 42
Good clinical practice 4
Good pharmacovigilance practice 4, 184, 196, 206, 247
  development of 319
  history of 317
  guideline on 316, 322, 341, 356, 370, 379, 405, 470, 520, 540, 543, 556, 563, 574, 591
  legal basis for 319
  principles for 324
  referencing of legal requirements in 320
  scope and process for 319
  structure of 320
Good postmarketing surveillance practice 196
Grapefruit juice 157

induced herb-drug interactions 157
Grepafloxacin hydrochloride 22
Gut motility, alteration of 58
GVP *See* Good pharmacovigilance practice
Gynura root 161

H

Hair 51
  loss 1
Halogenated hydrocarbons, number of 51
Harmful drugs 75
Hazard 4
HBLR *See* Hierarchical Bayesian Logistic Regression
HBsAG *See* Hepatitis B surface antigen
HCV *See* Hepatitis C virus
Headache 153
Health care
  professional communication 28
  system, crucial components of 225
Health products and food branch 197
Health professionals and patients 129
Health Professions Council of South Africa 249
Healthcare professional communications
  direct 572
  processing of direct 573*f*
Healthcare system's requirements 248
Heart valves 225
Heliotrope 158
Heliotropium europaeum 158
Hematologic disease, risk of 80
Hemorrhagic tendency of warfarin 56
Hemovigilance 186
Hemovigilance Program of India 87
Hepatic carcinoma 53
Hepatic disease 170
Hepatic dysfunction 90
Hepatic veno-occlusive disease 161
Hepatitis 53, 82, 153, 154
  B surface antigen 244
  C virus 244

Herbal 19
Herbal drugs 152, 153, 155
  adverse effects of 152
  safety monitoring of 153
  side effects 152
  toxicities of 152
Herbal materials 154
Herbal medicines 4, 150, 152, 156
  advisory committee 186
  and products 150
Herbal product 150, 153
  assessment of safety of 159
Herbal reports in WHO database 156*f*
Herbo-mineral formulations, metals present in 154*t*
Heterogeneous patients 258
Hierarchical Bayesian Logistic Regression 260, 267
High level group terms and system organ class, relationship between 168*f*
High level term and high level group terms, relationship of 167*f*
High quality safety data 256
High-dimension of data 258
High-grade fever 36
High-tech medical equipment 248
Hindering signal generation 64*t*
Hismanal 22
HIV *See* Human immunodeficiency virus
Homeopathy 4
Homogenous population sample 18
Human adverse reaction online monitoring system 254
Human and animal health, promotion of 181
Human beings 407
Human dishonesty 129
Human errors 129
Human genome 177
Human immunodeficiency virus 244
Human resource 102
HVPI *See* Hemovigilance Program of India
Hyderabad Chloroform Commission, second 11
Hydromorphan, extended release 23
Hypertension 45, 153
  accelerated 45
Hypothesis generation methods 25

Hypothesis testing methods 25
Hypotonic hyporesponsive
　　episode 36

I

ICSR *See* Individual case safety
　　reports
Idiosyncratic reactions 50f
Illness
　　diagnosis of 225
　　prevention of 225
　　treatment of 225
IMDTS *See* Implantable
　　medical device tracking
　　subcommittee
Implantable medical device
　　tracking subcommittee 231
Impotence 1
In vitro diagnostic device 187, 244
Indexing and hyperlinking 254
Indian Pharmacopoeia
　　Commission 15, 85, 192, 206
Indirect cost 221
Individual case safety reports 4,
　　86, 101, 192, 206
　　duplicate detection and
　　　management of 467
　　transmitted electronically, data
　　　quality monitoring of 465f
Indomethacin 50
Influence drug responses 175
Information, sharing of 366
Infrastructure 102
　　database 102
　　equipments 102
　　　computer system 102
　　　fax 102
　　　internet connection 102
　　　multi-connection
　　　　telephone 102
　　　photocopier 102
　　　printer 102
　　location 102
In-hospital settings 28
Injection reaction 34
Injection site abscess 36, 37
Intensive hospital-based drug
　　surveillance system 66
Intensive Medicines Monitoring
　　Programme 177
Interacting agent 56
International Conference on
　　Harmonization 14, 190

International Drug Information
　　System 69
International Drug Monitoring
　　Programme 157
Interval exposure from marketing
　　experience. 516t
Intravenous 244
　　injection 54
Intrinsic benefit-risk balance 120t
Intrinsic crisis 130
Investigation report, detailed 309
Investigational drug from
　　completed clinical trials,
　　cumulative subject
　　exposure to 515t
Investigator's brochure 3, 4
Ion channels 177
IPC *See* Indian Pharmacopoeia
　　Commission
Irinotecan 176
Isoniazid 176
　　acetylation of 52
Isotretinoin 89
Itch severity 28
Itraconazole 87
IV *See* Intravenous
IVD *See* In vitro diagnostic device

J

Japanese adverse drug event
　　report 196

K

Ketoconazole 58
Kidneys 51
Knowledge-detection 4

L

Lancet thalidomide infant 13
Lennox-Gastaut epilepsy 118
Levodopa 58
Life-threatening 47
　　diseases, treatment of 414
Limited concomitant drug use 80
Literature searches, record of 444
Lithium
　　carbonate 58, 87
　　NSAIDs 50
Liver 51
　　injury 154

Longer-lasting disease, case of 92
Lotronex 22
Lowest level term with preferred
　　term, relationship of 167f
Lumiracoxib 23
Lungs 51
Lyell's syndrome 73
Lymphadenitis 37
Lymphatic system disorders 81

M

Madderwort 158
Magenkraut and herba absinthii
　　158
Manufacturer and user facility
　　device experience 204
Marketed health products
　　directorate 197
Marketing authorisation
　　application 562
　　holders 4, 188, 376, 456, 586
　　and applicants, role of 368
Martindale 5
MDR *See* Medical device
　　reporting
Mechanism classification 48
　　drug interaction 49
　　hypersensitivity 48
　　idiosyncracy 48
　　intolerance 49
　　pharmacologic 49
MedDRA versioning 172
Medical device 19, 197, 225, 229
　　agency 184
　　classification 229
　　market 247
　　pre- and postmarket
　　　supervision of 228
　　regulation 187, 228, 228t, 243
　　　and need for harmonization
　　　　240
　　　and reporting pathway
　　　　245fc
　　regulatory authority of india 243
　　reporting 231
　　tracking 229
Medical dictionary for regulatory
　　activities 165, 203, 253, 257
　　applications of 165
　　criteria for term selection 168
　　objectives of 165
　　regulatory status 166
　　rules 168

Index 617

structure 166
Medical error 5
Medical terms coding, levels of 166f
Medication errors 171
Medication-related adverse events 216
Medications, concomitant 80
Medicinal drugs, listing of 3
Medicine
　alternative 161
　complementary 161
　control agency 184
　essential 3
Medicines and Healthcare Products Regulatory Agency 160, 184, 206, 226, 231
　classification 247t
Member states, role of 367
Mentha pulegium 156
Mercaptopurine 59
Meropenem 87
Meta-analyses 95
Metabolism interactions 59t
Metabolism of warfarin 52
Metabolizing enzymes 176
Methyserzide 45
Metoclopramide containing products 88
Metronidazole 86
Mexiletine 58
MGPS *See* Multi-item gamma poisson shrinker
MHRA *See* Medicines and Healthcare Products Regulatory Agency
MHRA-yellow-card-healthcare-professional-form-february-2017 277
MHRA-yellow-card-patient-form-to-report-side-effects 275
Mibefradil dihydrochloride 22
Mingwort 158
Ministry of Health and Family Welfare 108, 192, 243, 248
Ministry of Health, Labor and Welfare 195
Missing information 257
Modalities for reporting 449
　final arrangements 454
　interim arrangements 449
Montelukast 87
Mucosal pain severity 28
Mugwort 158

Multi-criteria decision analysis 119, 121f
Multi-item gamma poisson shrinker 260, 267
Multiple drugs 218
　together 260
Myocardial infarction 169

N

N-acetylation of isoniazid, ethnic variation in 52t
N-acetyltransferase 176
Natalizumab 23, 88
National AIDS Control Organization 109
National and International Pharmacovigilance Programmes 21
National Centre for Adverse Drug Reaction 193
　monitoring 194
National Centre for Drug Monitoring 148
National Centre for Pharmacovigilance 82
National Coordination Centre 15, 85, 109, 206
National Health Insurance Scheme 249
National Health Policies
　elements of effective 242
　strategies, and plans 242
National Health Programmes 109
National Heart, Lung, and Blood Institute 93
National Immunization Programmes 34
National Institute for Health and Clinical Excellence 187
National Patient Safety Agency 187
National Pharmacovigilance Centre 5, 67, 109
National Pharmacovigilance Programme 15, 108, 191
National Programme of Prevention and Control of hospital infections 190
National Regulatory Agency for Medical Devices, global distribution of 241f
National Sanitary Surveillance System 190

National Vector-borne Disease Control Programme 109
Natural history of disease 33
Natural products 153
Nausea 66, 153
NCC *See* National Coordination Centre
Neoplasms 171
Nervous system
　disorders 81
　drugs 81
Neural network 5
Neuroleptic agents 177
New adverse reaction signals 143
　analysis 143
　identification 143
New drug
　application 12, 260
　development 63
New pharmaceutical affairs law 247
Neyman bias 92
Nitrofurantion 86, 87
Non-representative patient selection 79
Non-sterile injection 35
Nonsteroidal anti-inflammatory drugs 21, 50
Norfloxacine 58
Nortryptyline 50
NSAIDs *See* Nonsteroidal anti-inflammatory drugs
Nucleic acids 51
Nucleotide polymorphisms 174
Nullification of cases 462
Numerical data errors 257
Nurse 26
　prescribers' extended formulary 186
Nutritional products, special 84

O

Observational study design 214
Obstructive jaundice 53
Offspring cohort 94
Olanzapine 87, 89
Omeprazole 86
Ophthalmopathy 45
OPV *See* Oral polio vaccine
Oracle adverse event reporting system 254, 267
Oracle pharmaceutical applications 267
Oral anticoagulant 175

Oral contraceptives 59
Oral hypoglycemics 59
Oral polio vaccine 38
Orange card 186
Organosulfur compounds induced CYP inhibition 157
Original cohort 93
Osteitis 37
Osteomyelitis 37
Ovarian cancer, malignant 171

P

PADE *See* Postmarketing adverse drug experience
Pain, abdominal 153
Palladone 23
PaniFlow 254
Paper-based method 254
Para amino benzoic acid 52
Paracetamol 55, 58
Paraplegia 154
Parkinson's disease 168, 219
Patient compliance 80
Patient group directions 186
Patient related factors 42
    age 42
    allergy 43
    body weight 43
    creatinine clearance 43
    fat distribution 43
    fetal development 42
    gender 42
    maternity status 42
Pelargonium reniforme 151
Pelargonium sidoides 151
Pemoline 23, 51
Penicillamine 58
Penicillin, conversion of 51
Penicilloic acid 51
People's republic of China 195
Pergolide 23
Periodic safety update report 196, 206, 263, 470
    assessment in EU network, processes for 501
    assessment procedure 503*f*, 505*f*
    format and contents of 475
    objectives of 472
    operation of EU network 494
    principles for evaluation of risk-benefit balance within 472
    principles for preparation of 473
    procedure 495*f*
    quality systems for 492, 511
    record management systems for 511
    reference information 474
    renewal of marketing authorisations 513
    sections/subsections, signals and risks 493*f*
    standard submission schedule of 494
    structures and processes 472
    submission, conditions for 497*f*
    training of staff members related to 493
    transition and interim arrangements 514
    transparency 513
Peritoneal fibrosis 45
Persistent inconsolable screaming 36, 37
P-glycoprotein 176
Pharmaceutical and Medical Device Agency 195, 196, 247
Pharmaceutical and Medical Safety Bureau 195
Pharmaceutical manufacturing 129
Pharmaceutical marketing strategies, changing 17, 18
Pharmaceutical preparations 54
Pharmacists 26
Pharmacoepidemiologic
    designs 212*t*
    studies, methodologies in 211
Pharmacoepidemiology 5, 209
    in drug development 214
Pharmacogenetics 5, 174
Pharmacogenomics 5
    practical challenges of 177
Pharmacological adverse reactions 49
Pharmacological characteristics of drug, secondary 49*f*
Pharmacological classification 44
Pharmacological properties 10
Pharmacology 5
Pharmacovigilance 1, 5, 14, 174, 209, 251, 270, 557
    activities, additional 393*t*
    and widening horizons 17
    basics of 14
    before 18th century 9
    computer-based tools for 259
    conduct of 4
    current methods of 25
    data management in 251
    data to competent authorities, reporting of 527
    discipline of 19
    equipment for 326
    evaluation 65
    facilities for 326
    global 147
    historical perspective 9
    in 18th century 9
    in 19th century 11
    in 20th century 11, 13
    in Europe 180
    informatics in 255
    inspection
        follow-up 364
        process 363
        scope 361
    need and objectives 17
    need for 17*b*
    numerical methods to 71
    objectives of 251, 318
    of plasma-derived medicinal products 189
    option analysis 122
    overall quality objectives for 324
    plan 390
    potential of 19
    practices, maintenance of good 319
    priority areas of 19
    purpose of 19
    qualification and training of inspectors 365
    record management and archiving 365
    regulations 180, 204*t*
    regulatory actions and sanctions 364
    responsible body 204
    risk assessment committee 541, 554, 592
    role of 25
    science of 19
    scope of 19
    signal detection in 63
        signal generation 64
        signal strengthening 64
        signal testing 65
    sites to be inspected 361
    softwares for 253

specific aims of 19
stakeholders in 129*b*
training of personnel for 325
working party 184
Pharmacovigilance audit 205, 370
   and objective 372
   policy framework and organizational structure 376
   risk-based approach to 373
Pharmacovigilance centre 100
   advisory committee 103
   associations 108
   communication 107
   continuity 103
   funding 108
   human resource 102
   in India 108
   infrastructure 102
   practicalities in organization of 102
   services provided 103
   setting up of 100
Pharmacovigilance in public health emergencies
   preparedness planning for 330
   preparedness planning in EU for 340
Pharmacovigilance inspection 205, 356
   planning 360
   process, quality management of 366
Pharmacovigilance method 25
   active surveillance 25, 28
   comparative observational studies 25, 30
   descriptive studies 25, 33
   passive surveillance 25, 26
   stimulated reporting 25, 28
   targeted clinical investigations 25, 32
Pharmacovigilance of herbal
   drugs 150
   medicines 157, 161
Pharmacovigilance Programme of India 85, 109, 192, 206
Pharmacovigilance system 181, 101, 323
   master file 205, 341
      accessibility of 354
      information to be contained in 346
      presentation 352
   monitoring of performance and effectiveness of 329

quality systems 322
   representation of 344
Phenylpropanolamine 22
Phenytoin 50, 57, 59, 87, 175
Phocomelia 5, 180
Physician and patient preferences, changing 17, 18
Physician's and nurse's health study 94
Physicochemical properties 22
Physiological function, modification of 216
Phytotherapy 5
PIR *See* Preliminary investigation report
Placebo 5
Plant derivatives 150
Plastic anemia 28
PMA *See* Postmarket approval
Poisonous
   regulation of 195
   solvent 12
Polymorphism in genes encoding pharmacokinetic parameters 175
Polymorphisms of cyp450 enzyme gene 175*t*
Polypharmacy 5, 260
Pondimin 22
Population epidemiology of disease 214
Posicor 22
Post-authorisation safety studies 520
   data protection 531
   impact on risk management system 531
   methods for 535
   operation of EU network 531
   principles 522
   procedure for imposing 531
   publication of study results 530
   quality systems, audits and inspections 531
   reporting of adverse
      events 527
      reactions 527
   structures and processes 522
   study designs 535
   study protocol 524
   study registration 523
   supervision of non-interventional 532
Post-crisis 131

Postmarket approval 245
   process 246
Postmarketing adverse drug experience 206
Postmarketing data, MGPS and HBLR for analysis of 260
Postmarketing phase vigilance, early 28
Postmarketing reporting of adverse drug experiences 199
Postmarketing surveillance 77, 78
   activities 229
   methodologies 80
   system 13
   tools for 254
Post-thalidomide era 13
Potential threat sources 129*b*
Practolol oculomucocutaneous syndrome 85
Prazosin 45
Preclinical safety data, unreliability of 17
Pre-crisis
   conditions 130
   planning 131
Predisposing factors 5
Pre-existing disease, effect of 259
Pre-existing medical conditions 170
Preferred term with high level term, relationship of 167*f*
Pregnancy and breastfeeding, exposure during 171
Preliminary investigation report 302
Prescription Drug User Fee Act 204
Prescription event monitoring 5
Prescription only medicine 5
Prescription-event monitoring 67
Prevention quality indicators 218
Prexige 23
Primary Health Centre 36
Procainamide 176
Programme error 34
Programme for International Drug Monitoring 100, 193
Propagest 22
Prophylaxis 6
Propulsid 22
Protein P-glycoprotein 53
Pruritus 153
PSUR *See* Periodic safety update report
Public consultation, practical advice for 321
Public health code 188
Pulegone toxicity 156

Pulmonary fibrosis 45
Purpura 82, 153
PvPI *See* Pharmacovigilance Programme of India

Q

QPP *See* Qualified personnel for pharmacovigilance
Qualified personnel for pharmacovigilance 206
Quality management of audit activities, competence of auditors and 375
Quality objectives 323
Quality requirements 323
Quality system 323
   and record management practices 375
   documentation of 327
   procedures and processes, specific 326
   within organisation, responsibilities for 324
Quantitative signal detection 71
Quinine containing preparations 23

R

RAE *See* Remedial action exemption
Randomized clinical trials 94
Randomized controlled trial 6
Rapacuronium 22
Rare adverse reactions 119
Rash 153
   erythematous 153
Rational drug use 6
Raxar 22
Reactions 34
   type A 44*t*
   type B 44*t*
   types of 48
Recall communication 231
Record 231
   linkage 6
   management 327
Redness at injection site 34
Redux 22

Regional pharmacovigilance centres 188
Registration and maintenance 343
Registry 29
Regulatory authorities 6, 129, 204
   of Japan 195
Regulatory pharmacovigilance 182
   process of 182
Regulatory submission studies 253
Remedial action exemption 231
Renal and hepatic dysfunction 31
Renal dysfunction 154
Renal failure 154, 169
Reportable adverse events 37*t*
Reporting time frame 230
Reporting, criteria for 229
Reports in VigiBase, processing of 70*f*
Restructuring capabilities 257
Revised National Tuberculosis Control Programme 109
Rezulin 22
Rheumatoid arthritis 117
   registry of 29
Risk classification 228
Risk management 6
   of medicines 185
   plan, content of 382
   principles of 381
   responsibilities for 382
   system 205, 379
Risk minimisation measures 577
   effectiveness indicators 574
   general principles 575
   healthcare professionals and patients 587
   impact of 587
   selection of tools 574
   structures and processes 575
   transparency 588
Rofecoxib 22, 178
Royal College of Physicians 10

S

Safe and rational use of medicines 68*f*
Safety announcements, coordination of 569
Safety communication 206, 563
   content of 566
   effectiveness of 569
   means of 566
   objectives of 564

   operation of EU regulatory network 569
   principles of 565
   quality system requirements for 569
   structures and processes 564
   target audiences 565
Safety data analysis, methods of 254
Safety database
   mining 269
   querying 269
Safetymart 262
Salvia miltiorrhiza 155
Sampling procedures and recruitment strategy 589
SAS *See* Statistical analysis system
Scientific literature 445
   database searches 442
   day zero 445
   duplicates 445
   guidance on monitoring of 442
   record keeping 444
   review and selection of articles 444
   start and stop searching in 442
Seizures 34, 38
Seldane 22
Sender's diagnosis 439
Sender's syndrome 439
Sepsis 38
Septicemia 169
Serious adverse blood reactions and events 187
Serious adverse effect 120*t*
Serious adverse event 6, 15, 187
   from clinical trials, cumulative tabulation of 516*t*
Serious adverse reaction 6, 187
Serious hazards of transfusion 187
Seriousness classification 47
   expected adverse drug reaction 48
   unexpected adverse drug reaction 47
Severe disease 210
Severe local reaction 36, 38
Severity classification 47
   mild 47
   moderate 47
   severe 47
Side effect 7
   reporting form Canada 609
Signal arising, confirmation of 554

Signal detection
   application of quantitative methods for 71
   automated quantitative 69
   data mining and 268
   methods of 65
   sources of 65
Signal management 543
   methodology for 545
   operation of EU network 550
   process 545
   quality requirements 549
   sources of data and information 544
   structures and processes 544
Skin 51
SLE *See* Systemic lupus erythematosus
Smoking 93
Social factors 43
   race and ethnicity 43
   smoking 43
Sodium valproate 86
Software-based systems, role of 251
Solvent diethylene glycol 12*f*
Sophisticated life-saving implants 225
Spontaneous disease 66
Spontaneous reporting 7
   methods for evaluation of 27*b*
   system 65, 80, 196
      strengths of 89*t*
      weaknesses of 89*t*
Stakeholders 128
Standard treatment guidelines 20
State Drug Administration 193
State Food and Drug administration 193
Statistical analysis system 268
Statistical classification 49
   non-specific 49
   specific 49
Steven-Johnson syndrome 28, 73, 82, 86, 87
Streptokinase 86
Study designs, classification of 211*fc*
Submission data tabulation model 260
Sugar pill 5
Suicide 169
Sulfamethoxazole 58
Sulfanilamide 12, 58, 176
Sulfonylureas 57
Surgical and medical procedures 171
Surveillance, active 29
Survey methodology, key elements of 588
Swiss Medicines Agency 146
Systemic lupus erythematosus 176

T

Tardive dyskinesia 177
Taste, loss of 1
Terfenadine 22
Tetracycline 58, 91
Teucrium chamaedrys 156
TGA *See* Therapeutic goods and administration
Thalidomide 7, 55
   disaster 13
   infant 13*f*
Theophylline 59
Therapeutic drugs 100
Therapeutic goods
   amendment regulation 197
   and administration 196, 197, 231
   Australian register of 197
Therapeutic Products Division of health Canada 246
Therapy of disease 216
Thiopurine methyltransferase 176
Thrombocytopenia 36, 153, 155
Thyroxine 58
Ticlopidine 117
Tigan 23
Tissue localization of drugs 51
Tolbutamide 57-59, 175
Toxic epidermal necrolysis 28
Toxic shock syndrome 38
Toxicities 54, 153
Toxins 33
Traditional and complementary medicines 19
Traditional Chinese medicine 161, 195
   regulations for 195
Traditional Herbal Medicines Registration Scheme 186
Traditional medicines 7
Training and consultancy support, providing 145
Tramadol 86
Transparent uniform risk benefit overview 119
Trasylol 23
Tremors 154
Tricyclic 59
   antidepressant 59, 175
Trimethobenzamide suppositories 23
Trimethoprim 58
Troglitazone 22
TSS *See* Toxic shock syndrome
Typical antisychotics 175
Tysabri 23, 88

U

UDP *See* Uridine diphosphate
UK Yellow card system 84
Ulcerative colitis 170, 171
UMC *See* Uppsala Monitoring Centre
Uppsala monitoring centre 1, 71, 82, 100, 183, 206, 269, 270
   signaling process 73, 74*f*
   signaling triage, algorithm used in 73*b*
Uridine diphosphate 176
   glucuronosyltransferase 176
Urothelial cancer, development of 155
Urticaria 153
Urticarial rash 154
US Food and Drug Administration 198, 225

V

Vaccine 19
   adverse event reporting system 36, 204
   reaction 34
   safety, methods for 33
   transportation 35
Valdecoxib 23, 96
Valeriana officinalis 158
Valvular heart disease 90
Vascular disorders 81
Vendor profile 261, 263
   eResearch technologies 265
   Galt Associates Inc. 263
   insightful 263
   Oracle Corp 264
   phase forward 264

Relsys Inc. 265
SAIC 266
SAS 266
Veterans affairs, department of 217
Vigi methods and tools 72
VigiBase 7, 69, 254
  cumulative increase 147f
VigiFlow 7, 72, 83, 254, 268, 270
VigiGrade 72
Vigilance exchange 231
  form 231
Vigilance of medicines 185
Vigilance systems 229t
  for medical devices 225
VigiLyze 72, 254
VigiMatch 72
VigiMed 7
VigiMine 73
VigiPoint 72
VigiRank 72
VigiSearch 7
Vioxx 21, 22
  saga 21
Volume of data for analysis 259
Vomiting 66, 153, 171

W

Warfarin 57, 58, 175
  S-enantiomer of 176
Warmot 158
Weakness 154
Weber effect 89
  in postmarketing 89
WedSDM 267
Wermuth 158
Wheezing 169
WHO *See* World Health Organization
WHO Programme for International Drug Monitoring, role of 143
World Health Assembly 240
  Resolution 240
World Health Organization 14, 25, 40, 100, 145, 190, 216, 225, 428
  adverse reactions terminology 253
  Collaborating Centre for International Drug Monitoring 459f
  herbal dictionary 145
  pharmaceutical newsletter 143
  Pharmacovigilance Programme for Global Drug Monitoring 141
  Programme for International Drug Monitoring 82
  UMC classification 45
Wormwood 158

Y

Yellow card
  reporting 185
  scheme 84, 185, 186

Z

Zelnorm 23